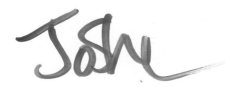

Introduction to Massage Therapy

Introduction to Massage Therapy

Mary Beth Braun, BA, MT, NCTMB
Stephanie J. Simonson, BS, MT

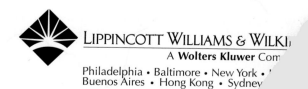

LIPPINCOTT WILLIAMS & WILKI

A **Wolters Kluwer** Com

Philadelphia · Baltimore · New York ·
Buenos Aires · Hong Kong · Sydne

Editor: Pete Darcy
Development Editors: David Payne, Tom Lochhaas
Marketing Manager: Christen DeMarco
Project Editor: Jennifer Ajello
Indexer: Lillian Rodberg
Designer: Doug Smock
Artwork: Dragonfly Media Group
Photography: Don Distel
Typesetter: Graphic World
Printer: RR Donnelly—Willard Division

Printed in the United States of America

Library of Congress Cataloging-in-Publication Data

Braun, Mary Beth.
    Introduction to massage therapy / Mary Beth Braun, Stephanie J. Simonson.
       p. ; cm.
    Includes index.
    ISBN 0-7817-8597-9
    1. Massage therapy. I. Simonson, Stephanie J. II. Title.
    [DNLM: 1. Massage. WB 537 B825i 2004]
    RM721.B785 2004
    615.8'22--dc22   2004046575

To purchase additional copies of this book, call our customer service department at **(800) 638-3030** or fax orders to **(301) 824-7390**. For other book services, including chapter reprints and large quantity sales, ask for the Special Sales department.

For all other calls originating outside of the United States, please call **(301)714-2324**.

Visit Lippincott Williams & Wilkins on the Internet: **http://www.lww.com**. Lippincott Williams & Wilkins customer service representatives are available from 8:30 am to 6:00 pm, EST, Monday through day, for telephone access.

06 07 08 09
1 2 3 4 5 6 7 8 9 10

For my Grandpa, Clarence John Pickard,
who taught me many things
including the power of knowledge gained through reading books

and

For my parents, Leo and Mary Jane,
who taught me that I could accomplish anything

—Mary Beth Braun

For those who want to learn massage

and

those who want to teach massage

—Stephanie J. Simonson

PREFACE

Introduction to Massage Therapy is primarily a textbook for entry-level massage therapy students who are seeking fundamental and practical knowledge for becoming professional massage therapists. It integrates functional anatomy and physiology information with massage therapy techniques and introduces students to the foundations of history, medical terminology, documentation and communication skills, and business and self-care practices for massage therapists.

This book also serves as a functional approach reference for practicing massage therapists. Practicing therapists need a functional understanding of anatomy and physiology as it pertains to the soft tissues, and they need to understand the various components of a massage therapy practice. This text is designed to provide practical information regarding the assessment and treatment of clients. Specifically, the special muscle section provides an excellent guide to treating clients for their particular areas of concern.

This book was born from our desire for a more functional and practical curriculum for beginning massage therapy students as well as our need for a text that provides guidance and support for massage therapy instructors. With extraordinary care and teamwork, we have created a massage therapy textbook that enables the reader to translate the fundamental knowledge base for massage into practical applications both inside and outside the classroom.

Unique Organization and Features

The 14 chapters in this book are in progressive order, with each building on the one before it. It is designed to lead the student through the process of accepting a new client, gathering intake information, assessing the client, treating the client, and developing a treatment plan and ultimately helps the reader learn how to build a massage therapy business while maintaining health and energy through self-care.

The approach of this book is extraordinarily visual, with a wealth of illustrations and photos to facilitate comprehension of basic information and hands-on practice. Additionally, the book contains many outstanding features, including the following:

- **Step-by-step procedure boxes** enable the reader to practice techniques both in and outside of the classroom.
- **Progressive case studies** walk the reader through the documentation process as sample clients are presented at different stages of a massage session.
- **Special muscle section** (at the end of Chapter 4) presents in an easy-to-reference format the specific movements and muscles involved in a client's soft tissue area of concern. This section is also linked to a group of extraordinary art plates from *Basic Clinical Massage Therapy: Integrating Anatomy and Treatment* by James H. Clay and David M. Pounds, Lippincott Williams & Wilkins.
- **Key points** emphasize information that is particularly important for practical application and client education.
- **Alert** boxes point out potential contraindications and precautions to take in situations that may arise during a massage therapist's practice.
- **Key terms** with definitions at the beginning of each chapter as well as in the glossary introduce students to basic terminology associated with massage therapy.
- **Chapter exercises** help students review and retain the information they have encountered in each chapter.
- **FREE 3D Anatomy CD-ROM** from Primal Pictures graphically depicts the layered structure of muscles and soft tissues to help reinforce student's knowledge of anatomy.

For Schools and Instructors

The book contains a solid core of basic information that is flexible enough to use in any massage therapy program. It can be supplemented with other textbooks to accommodate any given massage curriculum. For example, a program with a clinical focus can use more advanced anatomy and physiology books, and a program that focuses more on spa massage can supplement this text with hydrotherapy and aromatherapy books. The material is presented in a format so instructors can develop a curriculum and teach with ease. Additionally, there is a complete package of instructor resources available. The resources are available on a CD-ROM or on our companion website at http://connection.lww.com/go/braun and include the images from the book to be used in lectures and handouts, PowerPoint presentations for each chapter, additional case studies, web links to internet sites for more information, chapter objectives from the book,

and a Test Generator with more than 750 questions. Plus, students have access to our Student Resource Center at http://connection.lww.com/go/braun, which includes an interactive quiz bank with additional review questions.

Summary

The functional and practical approach of this text makes it appropriate for both entry-level massage therapy students and practicing massage therapists. The special muscle section enables practicing massage therapists to use the book as a resource for treating specific client conditions. The step-by-step procedures will help students to learn and practice basic massage techniques relatively easily.

We wish every reader success in learning about massage therapy, and we hope that this book will serve as a valuable resource to practitioners in all settings.

Mary Beth Braun
Stephanie Simonson

HOW TO USE THIS BOOK

Introduction to Massage Therapy provides the fundamentals you need to develop as a massage therapist. This exquisite text gives you a well-rounded and informed understanding that will help build your understanding of massage therapy including basic techniques, fundamentals of history, medical terminology, pharmacology, assessment, documentation, ethics, pathology, self-care, and more. This User's Guide shows you how to put the book's features to work for you.

Learning Objectives

Objectives listed at the start of each chapter clearly outline what you should be able to accomplish upon completion of the chapter.

Terminology

Key terms with definitions at the beginning of each chapter as well as in the glossary introduce you to basic massage therapy terminology.

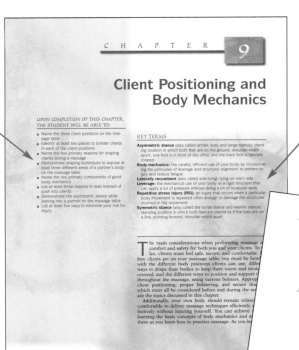

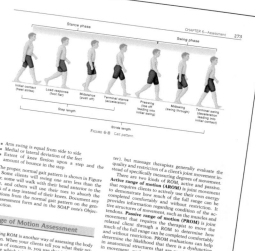

Key Points

Key points, highlighted in a different color, emphasize information that is particularly important for client education and practical application.

Special Boxes

Special boxes warn you about special circumstance, provide step-by-step procedures, and offer the latest information on massage therapy techniques

Procedure boxes offer step-by-step procedures for specific treatments or assessments for practice both in and outside the classroom.

Alert boxes, marked with ![], warn you about special circumstances in which caution is necessary.

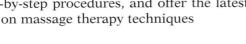

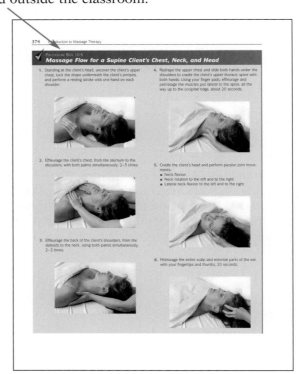

Clear Illustrations

Numerous high-quality illustrations and photographs throughout the book illustrate the most important information, make complex details easy to understand, and facilitate comprehension of basic information and hands-on practice.

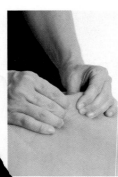

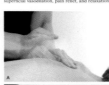

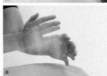

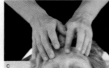

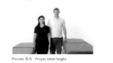

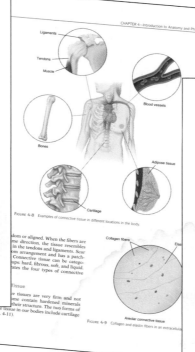

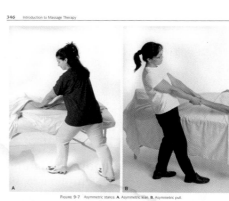

Case Studies

Progressive case studies present sample clients and walk you through the documentation process for different stages of a massage session.

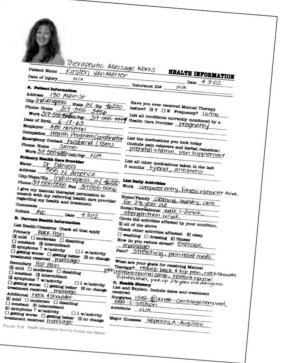

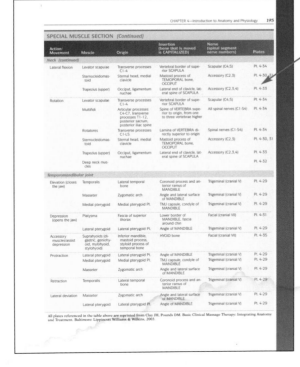

Muscle Table

Special muscle section, at the end of Chapter 4, *Introduction to Anatomy and Physiology,* presents, in an easy-to-reference format, the specific movements and muscles involved in the soft tissue area of concern with reference to color plates to identify the muscle.

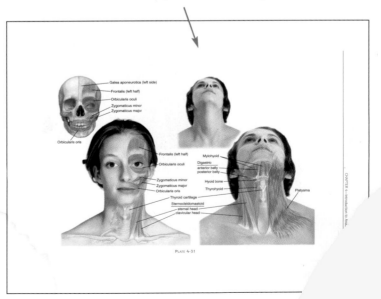

Review Materials

Challenging, thought-provoking exercises and case studies help you reinforce and apply the main topics and concepts.

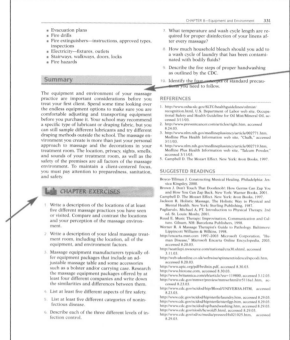

Chapter Summaries review key topics and concepts of the chapter that should be understood and retained.

Student exercises, at the end of each chapter, provide review questions for testing your knowledge of the material.

Free student resource CD-ROM

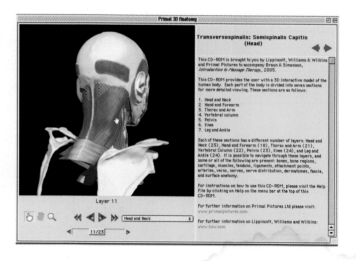

This free **3-D Anatomy CD-ROM** from Primal Pictures provides a wealth of anatomical 3-D information to help reinforce your knowledge of anatomy. Anatomical models of the human body can be rotated to give a full range of insightful perspectives. Layers of anatomy can be added or subtracted, allowing you to develop a unique familiarity with the human body.

ACKNOWLEDGMENTS

We extend our sincere appreciation to The Crew at Lippincott Williams & Wilkins for working tirelessly on this project since its inception. In particular, we want to thank

- Pete Darcy, Senior Acquisitions Editor
- Nancy Peterson, Development Manager
- David Payne, Development Editor
- Doug Smock, Designer
- Christen DeMarco, Senior Marketing Manager
- Kate Staples and Joseph Latta, Editorial Assistants
- Leigh Wells, Sales Manager (and all of her crew)
- Eric Branger, Managing Editor
- Karen Gulliver, Art Editor

We especially thank our developmental editor, Tom Lochhaas, for his time, guidance, and knowledge. His expertise has undoubtedly made this an extraordinary book. This book has been through an extensive review process by professionals in the massage therapy field (see the reviewer list), each of whom we thank for their time and input.

We also thank our artists, Rob Duckwall and Dragonfly Media Group, and our photographer, Don Distel, for their incredible contributions to our book.

Ruth Werner, friend, book diva, and author of *A Massage Therapist's Guide to Pathology*, connected us with Victoria Isaacs, Sales Associate for Lippincott Williams & Wilkins, to present our idea for this text. We extend many thanks to Ruth and Victoria for believing in and encouraging us to proceed with this project. We also thank Diana Thompson, notable author of *Hands Heal*, who helped us with the details of documentation.

We thank everyone who served as volunteer models throughout the book: Rob Blackwell, Jeff Braun, Kylie Clevenger, Karla Eggart, Anne Jordan, Larry Marietta, Andy Simonson, Bob Simonson, Claire Simonson, Dr. Robert T. Simonson, Annie VanderLinden, and Kirsten VanMarter-Clevenger.

Mary Beth Braun would particularly like to thank her family, friends, and clients for their encouragement and unwavering support throughout this incredible book project, including her parents, Leo and Mary Jane Braun; Jim Braun; Jeff Braun; Cathy and Scott Seibert; Rita and Bob Englum; Jim Pickard; John and Sandy Pickard; Kirsten VanMarter-Clevenger; Larry Marietta; Annie VanderLinden; Anne Jordan; Marcia Gilson; Tyler Ray; Rob Blackwell, Kathy Kane (a.k.a Super K); Kathy Latimer; Nancy McGuire; Margi Cangany-Lane; Christopher Sovereign; Cynthia Ribeiro; Carolyn Talley-Porter; Laurel and Howard Freeman; Charna Rosenholtz and Randa Cherry.

Stephanie J. Simonson thanks Andy, Kieran, and Keely for their willingness and ability to develop independence through the years spent on this project. The experience of living with someone who is writing a book is at times as challenging as writing one. Also, she is grateful to her parents, who taught her the value of hard work and showed her how to work hard. This book could not have been written without both. Marilyn and Horace Davis showed her that there are many ways to learn and even more ways to teach. They, along with her students, have inspired this book.

CONTENTS

CHAPTER 4   INTRODUCTION TO ANATOMY AND PHYSIOLOGY, *cont'd*

Welcome to the World of Massage Therapy!

UPON COMPLETION OF THIS CHAPTER, THE STUDENT WILL BE ABLE TO:

- Identify the four ancient river valley civilizations that used massage
- Describe the essence of the Hippocratic Oath and its relation to massage therapy
- Name at least three ancient Greek and Roman physicians who recommended massage
- Explain the difference between development of the arts, science, and massage in Europe and that in the Arab countries during the Middle Ages
- Describe how massage therapy was affected by the Renaissance period
- Identify the transition that occurred in American healthcare in the 19th century
- Describe the difference between massage and bodywork
- List the nine categories of bodywork modalities
- Name at least two indications that massage is evolving in the American healthcare system
- Identify at least two attributes of a massage therapist that are needed for successful employment in a spa
- Name at least three current trends in massage education

KEY TERMS

Anointing: ritualistic or religious activity of rubbing oil into the skin

Bodywork: treatment that involves manipulation of the client's body as a way to maintain or improve health

Gymnastics: activity at ancient gymnasiums that included exercise, massage, and baths

Massage: manual therapy involving pressure applied with the hands (term started by the French explorers in the 1700s)

Masseur: male person who administers massage

Masseuse: female person who administers massage

Mechanical effects: therapist applies pressure or manipulation to physically change the shape or condition of the client's tissues

Metabolic effects: combined result of mechanical and reflex effects on the whole body

Modality: a collection of manual therapies that tends to use similar applications of movement or massage strokes to reach a similar goal

Movement Cure: American version of Ling's movement system

Reflex effects: therapist stimulates the client's sensory neurons, which triggers the client's nervous system to change the shape or condition of the tissues in areas that were addressed as well as other, related areas

Swedish Gymnastics: a therapeutic movement system developed by Per Henrik Ling

Swedish Movements: Europe's version of Ling's movement system

Qi (CHEE): a dynamic, changing energy force that runs through the whole body, supplying and being supplied by body processes and activities

Welcome to the world of massage therapy! You are about to embark on a most rewarding journey, discovering what is involved in becoming a professional massage therapist. This chapter covers the history of massage and events that led to the current practice of massage. We define massage and distinguish it from bodywork because so many different bodywork techniques have been developed, and there is a lack of clarity regarding the difference. Whereas **bodywork** is a manipulative treatment of a client's body that is intended to maintain or improve health, **massage** requires manual pressure on the client's tissues, applied with the therapist's touch, to maintain or improve health. We identify nine categories and briefly summarize some of the massage modalities that have developed over time. The active development of so many kinds of specialized bodywork is partly due to the latest touch research. We introduce the concept of touch and illustrate the increased interest in scientific research on the topic. As the academic and scientific world proves the value of touch, massage becomes more a part of the American healthcare system. Continued involvement in the medical and healthcare communities is accompanied by some changes in massage education, also discussed in this chapter. A general understanding of these concepts can provide a solid foundation for you as you build your professional massage practice.

History of Massage

Throughout thousands of years and a myriad of cultures, people have used massage for communication, relieving pain or discomfort, healing, protecting, or improving one's overall health. Most people have experienced the instinctive or intuitive use of massage when stopping to rub or hold an injury, bruise, or area of discomfort on the body.

TABLE 1-1

"Massage" Roots and Terms from Around the World

ROOT/TERM	MEANING	CULTURE/PERSON
Amma	to calm by rubbing or press-rub	China
Anatripsis	to rub up	Greek/Hippocrates
Anma	to calm by rubbing or press-rub	China
Anmo	to calm by rubbing or press-rub	China
Kampo	"the Chinese way"	Japan
Makeh	to press softly	Sanskrit
Mass	to press softly	Arabic
Mass'h	to press softly	Arabic
Massa	to touch, handle, squeeze, knead	Latin
Massein	to touch, handle, squeeze, knead	Greek
Masser	to knead by hand	French
Masso	to touch, handle, squeeze, knead	Greek
Mordan	to rub	Indian
Samvahana	hand rubbing	Indian

Historical references to massage have been found in cultures around the world. To better comprehend that massage is found in many cultures, you can examine the different terms used to describe the same or similar activity (Table 1-1). Even cultures without written language have passed down the tradition of massage and techniques, shown by the notes of early explorers who "discovered" these native peoples.

In the most primitive civilizations, medicine was ritualistic and oftentimes combined with magical or mystical activities, as people believed that illness came from demons, spirits, or sins. Shamans and priests used massage, among other practices, to help rid people of these evil entities. The spiritual and medical traditions were passed on from generation to generation, perpetuating the practice of massage. Evidence of this is found everywhere from Australia to Africa, including ancient Egypt, to the Pacific Islands, Russia and the Ukraine, and North and South America.

Ancient civilizations used massage in conjunction with many variations of water therapy to cleanse and purify the body of disease-causing spirits: bathing, steam rooms, hot springs, and sweat lodges. These rituals that combined massage with water therapies persisted throughout history and still exist today.

ANCIENT RIVER VALLEY CIVILIZATIONS (7000–1000 BCE)

The oldest civilizations were created by groups of people who were able to feed and house large populations efficiently. Large-scale agricultural practices were developed, complex architectural structures were designed and built, political and religious organizations were established, the arts, sciences, and medicine were explored, and written records were kept. One of the most important requirements for civilization was a dependable source of water. Large rivers were able to sustain large populations and, as a result, there are four areas in the world where ancient river valley cultures were established: the Yellow River, the Indus River, the Tigris and Euphrates Rivers and the Nile River (Fig. 1-1).

The exact dates that these river valley civilizations were established are controversial because it is unclear from the remaining ancient records when they were actually written. Additionally, records have been translated and rewritten a number of times, occasionally making the original intent and message questionable. For the purpose of this book, civilizations in these four areas developed during the same time period, thousands of years before the common era (BCE).

Tracing massage history accurately is complicated because ancient references to massage do not use contemporary terminology or techniques. Early records

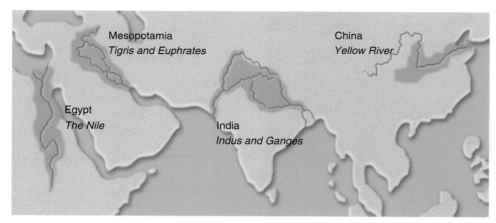

FIGURE 1-1 The four ancient river valley civilizations.

of massage being used in healthcare can be found in documents from all of the ancient cultures. Some of the earliest records of massage refer to **"anointing"** (ah-NOYN-ting), which is a process of rubbing oil into the skin, often used to banish evil influences that caused disease, again demonstrating the spiritual and religious basis for healthcare. This section of the chapter introduces massage as it evolved in different areas of the globe over time, eventually developing into the current massage therapy profession.

Ancient China

The Yellow River valley culture is also referred to as Shang China, or Ancient China. There is widespread and extensive massage information found in ancient Chinese records. One of the ancient Chinese documents of disputable age is the *Cong Fou*, which includes information on the use of medicinal plants, controlled breathing, and a system of exercises and positions for healthcare. It is questionable whether massage treatment was actually included, but many assume it was. Possibly started around 2700 BCE, it may have been completed over several generations.

The *Nei Ching* is the Yellow Emperor's classic of internal medicine and is one of the oldest medical references that still exist. Some claim that it was written around 2600 BCE because of its association with the Yellow Emperor of China, who died at about the same time. Others suggest that it was written from 475 BCE to 220 CE (common era, formerly called AD) as a series of entries by many different persons but linked to the famous and honorable emperor to establish its authority and bring it fame. The *Nei Ching* is more of a medical dialogue or discussion than a medical reference book and serves as the foundation for traditional Chinese medicine. Its main topics include the theory of five phases and the balance of yin and yang. These concepts are intro-

duced in Chapter 12, entitled "Special Techniques," which compares Eastern and Western approaches to healthcare.

In the Chinese language, words are represented by contextual pictograms. Translating, reading, and writing the words in English letters can be subjective and vague. A Chinese word written in English is an attempt to spell the pronunciation of the word. One of the oldest Chinese terms for a therapy involving massage-like activity is commonly written as moshuo (moh-SZH-woh). This term can be found in the *Nei Ching* in the context of massage and finger pressure used to energize someone or treat paralysis, chills, fever, and poor circulation of blood. As the Chinese language developed through time, massage techniques were called anmo (AHN-moh), to press and rub, and Tui-na (TOOY-nah), to push and hold.

From China, bodywork made its way into Japan and provided a source of employment for blind people. Since the Japanese culture tends to shun the disabled, few professions were available to the blind outside of acupuncture and massage therapy. With refined perceptions of touch, blind acupuncturists and massage therapists were very successful and were able to gain respect. While the Japanese developed many different forms of bodywork, Shiatsu is the best-known. Figure 1-2 is a photo taken prior to 1895 of a blind massage therapist performing Shiatsu on a client.

Ancient India

The Indus River is the site of the largest ancient river valley civilization discovered in the 20th century. This area of ancient India is near current day Pakistan. Unlike the others, the Indus Valley civilization did not leave a lot of written records to provide clues to their culture. There are four original scriptural texts,

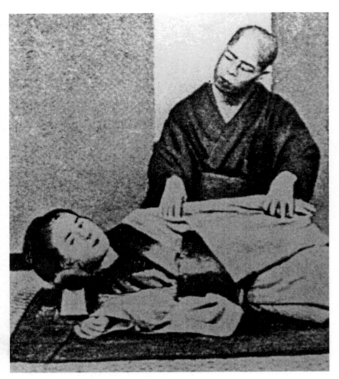

FIGURE 1-2   Blind Japanese masseur treating a patient. (Reprinted from Kellogg JH, Harvey JK. The Art of Massage. Battle Creek, MI: Modern Medicine, 1929.)

Ancient Mesopotamia

The area of ancient Mesopotamia lies between the Tigris and Euphrates Rivers, in the area that is now called the Middle East, near Iraq. The earliest people may have arrived in Mesopotamia somewhere around 7000 BCE, but civilization began around 3000 BCE.

Ancient Mesopotamians developed a written language called cuneiform. A series of wedge-shaped dents were made in wet clay, and when the clay dried, the clay tablets were portable, storable, and long lasting. Clay tablets and paintings on the walls of tombs have shown evidence of massage being used for healthcare. See Figure 1-3 for a photo of an ancient Babylonian clay tablet, circa 300 BCE, and its translation, which includes a reference to massage.

Physicians and priests both practiced medicine in Mesopotamia, another example of the relationship between illness and evil spirits. Even so, Mesopotamians had some understanding of anatomy and were able to diagnose and prescribe treatment for many specific medical conditions as well as perform surgeries. Babylonian King Hammurabi established a set of laws called the Code of Hammurabi, which includes the oldest code of medical ethics. It recommends an "eye for an eye" philosophy that is certainly questionable by today's standards.

the Vedas, which may have been written over 5000 years ago. It is believed that these lengthy, complex verbal messages from the gods were spoken directly to sages and only shared by word of mouth for generations. Eventually these messages were written down in poetic, lyrical form as the Rik Veda, Sama Veda, Yajur Veda, and Atharva Veda. Because the words were passed down only verbally for so many generations, the rhyming patterns may have been instrumental in the accuracy of the translation.

The Ayur Veda, a supplement to the Atharva Veda, discusses pharmacology and health. Its age is questionable, some claiming it was written around 3000 BCE, and others, 1000 BCE or later. The teachings of the Ayur Veda provided the basis for Ayurvedic healthcare, which is gaining popularity in the Western world. The holistic approach attempts to balance the body, mind, and spirit to maintain health and prevent illness. Some of the many therapies employed in this natural system of healing include herbs, diet, fasting, aromatherapy, massage, meditation, yoga, color, and metal therapy.

Ayurvedic references made to massage include samvahana (hand rubbing), mordan (to rub), and most importantly, shampooing. Shampooing was a medical treatment done with a brush and the hands for treating health problems. Massage was and continues to be used regularly in the Indian culture.

Ancient Egypt

Located on the Nile River, the fourth of the ancient river valley civilizations is now called Northern Africa. The history of ancient Egypt follows a timeline similar to that of China and Mesopotamia. Instead of using pictograms on walls and cuneiform on clay tablets to convey messages, the Egyptians developed a more complex writing system of hieroglyphics and invented papyrus (puh-PAHY-rus) paper.

The papyrus plant was a reedlike plant found along the banks of the Nile that was used to fabricate, among other things, a useful and durable paper with a secret recipe that no other culture could replicate. Produced in lengths of 35 feet or longer, the papyrus paper could be rolled up for storage and transport, unlike the Mesopotamian clay tablets. Unfortunately, the Egyptians used up the local supply of papyrus, their secret recipe was lost, and papyrus paper was not made again for thousands of years.

Many of the ancient papyrus records have been discovered, named, and translated. Topics covered all aspects of the culture, including literature, governmental tax records, religion, magic, and medicine. As in other early ancient civilizations, medicine was handled by priest-physicians who typically attributed health conditions to the work of gods and goddesses. Prayers, spells, amulets, herbal salves, and poultices

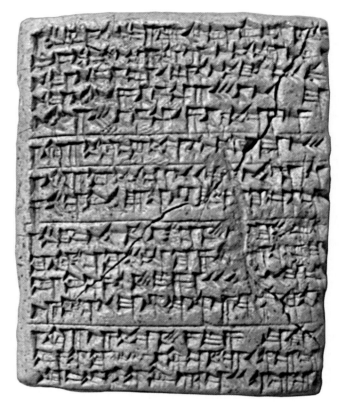

FIGURE 1-3 Clay tablet of medical text from Babylonia, 300 BCE. (Reprinted with Martin Schøyen's permission from the Schøyen Collection MS4575, Oslo and London.) Translation: "If a youth who has not known a woman suffers a prolapse of the rectum, you crush a . . . and a . . . and you have him drink it in beer, and/or massage him with it in oil . . . you anoint him with oil; you repeat this for 10 days. You repeat this for 20 days as with inflammation of the intestines, and he will recover." (Translated by one of the Leading Uruk scribes, Anu-Iksur of Iqisha.)

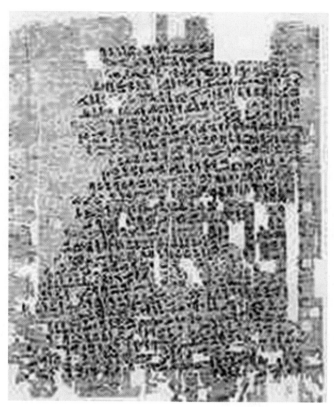

FIGURE 1-4 Kahun medical papyrus from 1825 BCE. Translation: "Examination of a woman aching in her legs and her calves after walking. You should say of it 'it is discharges of the womb.' You should treat it with a massage of her legs and calves with mud until she is well" (Translation by Stephen Quirke, available at http://www.petrie.ucl.ac.uk/digital_egypt/med/birthpapyrus.html, reprinted from Griffith FL. The Petrie Papyri: Hieratic Papyri from Kahun and Gurob. London: Bernard Quaritch, 1898. © Petrie Museum of Egyptian Archaeology, University College London UC 32057.)

were treatments often used in hopes of a cure. On the other hand, records of intricate surgeries and more advanced medical knowledge were also found. The Kahun Papyrus, written around 1800 BCE and found in fragments in 1889 CE, focuses on gynecological matters. One of the passages specifically indicates the use of massage for a woman whose legs ache (Fig. 1-4).

Medical conditions, prescriptions, diagnoses, and surgical treatments were documented in various papyri, as were details about the mummification process leading the deceased safely to the afterlife. The child king Tutankhamun's famous tomb and mummy demonstrate the extensive mummification process of the ancient Egyptians. The process required the removal of internal organs, leading the Egyptians to a thorough understanding of anatomy.

There is evidence of massage being used in ancient Egyptian healthcare from as early as 4000 BCE, when the mortal goddess Queen Isis included massage as treatment for health and healing. There is no evidence from the other ancient river valley cultures of any female healers, so it is probable that she was the first. She also trained her priestesses to perform the duties of a physician, massage being one of them.

The tomb of Ankhmahor, dated somewhere around 2350 BCE, has been called the Tomb of the Physician. His title as a physician has been disputed; one theory suggests that he was only a ka-priest who had farming duties and served the king. Regardless, Ankhmahor's tomb has images of foot manipulation and surgical operations such as circumcision. There are many who believe that the images depict foot reflexology, but it is also possible that foot surgery is being shown. The hieroglyphs accompanying the pictograph have been translated with the patient saying "Do not cause pain," and the therapist responding "I will act so you shall praise me" (Fig. 1-5).

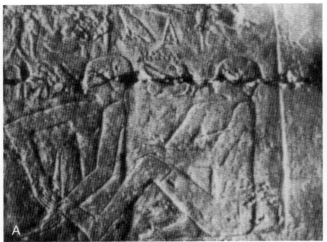
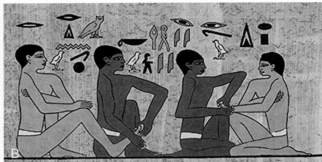

FIGURE 1-5 Ankhmahor's tomb illustrating bodywork. **A.** Photo of the tomb wall (by Trudy Baker, taken from www.foot-reflexologist.com/EGYPT). **B.** An artistic rendition of inscription, sometimes claimed to be a painting from the tomb.

ANCIENT GREECE (750 BCE–500 CE)

Although not one of the original river valley civilizations, there is evidence of human activity in Greece thousands of years before the common era. Written records can be found from about 2000 BCE, but what little has been deciphered does not reveal any advanced works of literature like those of the other civilizations of the time. Early evidence of the Greek alphabet dates from around 750 BCE, which provides most Greek history.

Massage in Ancient Greece

The Greek health regimen included exercise, massage, fresh air, rest, diet, and cleanliness. Exercise and competitive athletics were so much a part of the culture that the Olympic Games were held every four years as part of a religious festival. These games were very important to the Greeks, who even stopped wars to compete in them. Physical training was critical to good performance, giving rise to gymnasiums all over the country. Athletes and military of the day received their academic, art, and physical training at the gymnasiums. Baths, also an important aspect of the health regimen, were attached to or located near the gymnasiums. In time, the baths and gymnasiums served the general public as social, spiritual, mental, and physical gathering places.

Massage was one of the primary treatments provided at the Greek gymnasiums and baths throughout their existence. Athletes received special massage treatments to minimize exhaustion and tone the muscles. The aliptae were servants who provided this ritual before and after competition and became very knowledgeable about the muscles, the condition of muscles, and muscular activity during exercise. In a way, the aliptae were the predecessors to physical or athletic trainers. Although the ancient Greek records do not contain an abundance of specific information about massage, it was used so commonly in the gymnasiums that the term **"gymnastics"** referred to a combination of exercise, massage, and baths that were provided by the gymnasiums. There were, however, some detailed references to massage made by the famous Hippocrates, who made important scientific and medical advancements around 400 BCE.

Hippocrates of Cos

Hippocrates (hih-PAH-kruh-teez) was an ancient Greek physician who lived between 460 and 370 BCE. He is considered the "Father of Medicine" for a couple of reasons. He was the first influential physician to observe health and disease as a result of natural causes and establish medicine as a science, rejecting the theory of health and medicine as the work of magic and gods. Also, he was the first to introduce a medical code of ethics different from the "eye for an eye" philosophy outlined in the Laws of Hammurabi.

The Hippocratic Corpus is a series of 60 treatises discussing medicine and medical principles. Its several different styles of writing and many contradictory statements led to the belief that Hippocrates started the project but its completion occurred long after he was gone. Within the Corpus, the Hippocratic Oath is a statement in which physicians swear to respect, honor, and share knowledge with their teachers, promise to treat their patients to the best of

---

Box 1-1

A Translation of the Hippocratic Oath by Francis Adams

I swear by Apollo the physician, by Aesculapius, Hygeia and Panacea, and I take to witness all the gods, all the goddesses, to keep according to my ability and my judgment the following oath:

To consider dear to me as my parents him who taught me this art; to live in common with him and if necessary to share my goods with him; to look upon his children as my own brothers, to teach them this art if they so desire without fee or written promise; to impart to my sons and the sons of the master who taught me and the disciples who have enrolled themselves and who have agreed to the rules of the profession, but to these alone, the precepts and the instruction.

I will prescribe regimen for the good of my patients according to my ability and judgment and never do harm to anyone. To please no one will I prescribe a deadly drug, nor give advice which may cause his death. Nor will I give a woman a pessary to procure abortion.

But I will preserve the purity of my life and my art. I will not cut for stone, even for patients in whom the disease is manifest; I will leave this operation to be performed by practitioners (specialists in this art). In every house where I come I will enter only for the good of my patients, keeping myself far from all intentional ill-doing and all seduction, and especially from the pleasures of love with women or with men, be they free or slaves. All that may come to my knowledge in the exercise of my profession or outside of my profession or in daily commerce with men, which ought not to be spread abroad, I will keep secret and never reveal.

If I keep this oath faithfully, may I enjoy my life and practice my art, respected by all men and in all times; but if I swerve from it or violate it, may the reverse be my lot.

Box 1-2

Evidence of Massage in the Hippocratic Corpus, volume III, "On the Articulations" and "On the Surgery," translated by Francis Adams

"On the Articulations" is a discussion of a dislocated shoulder suggesting in Part 9

> the shoulder should be rubbed gently and softly. The physician ought to be acquainted with many things, and among others with friction; for from the same name the same results are not always obtained; for friction could brace a joint when unseasonably relaxed, and relax it when unseasonably hard; but we will define what we know respecting friction in another place. The shoulder, then, in such a state, should be rubbed with soft hands; and, moreover, in a gentle manner, and the joint should be moved about, but not roughly, so as to excite pain. Things get restored sometimes in a greater space of time, and sometimes in a smaller.

"On the Surgery" states in Part 17

> Friction can relax, brace, incarnate or attenuate: hard braces, soft relaxes, much attenuates, and moderate thickens.

---

their ability and only with good intentions, swear that they will not prescribe a deadly drug or treatment under any circumstance, and vow patient confidentiality in hopes of enjoying life and gaining respect from others. This is the philosophy with which Hippocrates practiced medicine, and it continues to be the foundation of the ethical codes for many healthcare professions including massage therapy. **The Hippocratic Oath to "Do no harm" provides the basis for professionalism**, which is discussed in the next chapter. See Box 1-1 for a translation of the Hippocratic Oath.

Hippocrates' original holistic methods included exercise, massage, fresh air, rest, diet, and cleanliness. **Hippocrates promoted the concept that the body is capable of curing itself.** As you move through your massage education, you will discover that massage techniques help the body to cure itself or to encourage self-healing. Human touch is an incredibly powerful part of this process.

Although there is only brief mention of massage in the Hippocratic Corpus, the information is detailed and specific. Anatripsis (to rub up) was developed by Hippocrates as a method of rubbing toward the heart, from the extremity to the core, to increase circulation. His technique for increasing circulation is still taught today and is one of the major benefits of massage. He recommended that all physicians be trained in anatripsis because it could promote healing, adjust the tension at a joint, and tighten, relax, or build muscle. See Box 1-2 for translation of the part of the Hippocratic Corpus that refers to massage.

ANCIENT ROME (750 BCE–500 CE)

Legends tell of illegitimate twin brothers, Remus and Romulus, who were left to die in the Tiber River but were rescued and raised by a wolf. One of the stories ends with Romulus murdering Remus and founding Rome in 753 BCE. Another story describes the two brothers founding the city of Rome together. With the beginning of Rome being based on myth, it is difficult to know what the ancient Roman lifestyle was truly like. Records dating to 500 BCE provide dependable history, but before that time, Roman lifestyle is somewhat of a mystery.

It is clear that the Greek culture influenced Roman religion, entertainment, sports, and medicine. The Greek physicians, who were considered superior to the Roman physicians, gained status and recognition within the Roman culture by serving Roman royalty. With Greek medicine came the Greek health regimen and its terminology, including gymnastics and baths. Exercise and massage were called "gymnastics" back in 400 BCE, and that term has maintained its association with massage throughout history.

Greek Physicians in Ancient Rome

Asclepiades of Bithynia (124–40 BCE) was a Greek physician who settled in Rome and promoted diet, exercise, bathing, and massage. His approach to medicine differed from Hippocrates' because his theory for health was based on a balance between tension, relaxation, and movement of very small, individual particles within the body, called atoms. He believed that free, fluid movement of the atoms promoted health, and irregular, inharmonious movement caused disease. To restore atomic harmony, he used movement therapies such as massage, swinging, and vibration. His methods were so popular that many other physicians adopted and practiced his theory.

Aulus Cornelius Celsus (25 BCE–57 CE) was another prominent figure in ancient Roman medicine and massage. A follower of Hippocrates, he wrote a series of eight texts called *De Medicina*, which covered many different facets of health and medicine. Its preamble reviews the philosophies of Celsus' contemporaries and follows with a summary of his own approach to the art of medicine. First, he describes how health providers should act, then he shares his observations of diseases, and finally he discusses treatments. There are numerous references to massage throughout the work, indicating its use in the treatment of the following[1]:

- Tone a weak body, relax a tense body, headaches, paralysis (Book II: Chapter 14)
- Fevers (Book III: Chapters 9, 11, 12, 14)
- Paralysis, headaches, head cold (IV:5); neck spasm (IV:6); asthma (IV:8); cough (IV:10); flatulence, ulcers (IV:12); stomach pain (IV:13); lung disorders (IV:14); liver disorders (IV:15); spleen disorders (IV:16); intestinal distress (IV:20–23); diarrhea (IV:26); menstrual cramps, urinary disorders (IV:27); joints (IV:29, 30); healing (IV:32)
- Eye disorders (VI:6); ear disorders (VI:7); nose disorders (VI:8); gum disorders (VI:13); fractures (VI:10)
- Dislocations (VIII:11)

At the time it was written, somewhere around 30 CE, *De Medicina* was just another piece of medical literature. However, in the late 1400s, the work was rediscovered in Italy, printed, published, and circulated and now is celebrated as one of the earliest remnants of Western medicine.

Claudius Galenus (130–201 CE), also known as Galen, is possibly the most famous of the Greek physicians in Rome. Another follower of Hippocrates, Galen revolutionized medicine not only by his many works on anatomy and medicine, but by developing the experimental method of scientific investigation. He encouraged physicians to practice dissection to discover anatomy and improve their surgical skills. One of his books, *Hygiene*, includes a discussion on morning and evening massage, a description of massage strokes and muscle fibers being rubbed in every direction, as well as an explanation of anointing with oil for health and well being.

The Fall of Rome

The culture of the Greeks continued to influence Rome around 150 CE, when the fall of Rome began. In a series of events, including loss of territory and control to other cultures and religions, the power and glory of the Roman Empire finally faded out around 500 CE.

THE MIDDLE AGES (400–1400)

As the last of the Roman emperors was ousted, world history was changing as Europe expanded northward with wars and battles for power and control. This period, which lasted from the year 400 until 1400, is called the Middle Ages. Understandably, European history took a unique path, different from that of the rest of the world. Europe was significantly affected by the expansion and resultant wars, and the Church took control of society and education. The Arab world, however, was not involved in the European conflicts and was not under the influence of the Church.

Middle Ages in Europe

The Middle Ages in Europe are sometimes called the Dark Ages because of the absence of art, science, and cultural development. Many written records were lost or destroyed amid the chaos of war, and with them went the luxurious lifestyle of the Romans. Despite the territorial battles, the Church maintained a strong presence throughout Europe. By salvaging and preserving some of the historical material, the Church became one of the primary sources of learning during the Middle Ages and became a powerful influence over society. Outside of the Church, art, literature, science, and medicine in Europe were absent.

The Christian influence over society affected European culture for a thousand years. Teachings of the Church were strongly enforced; heretics were severely punished; independent, creative, progressive thought was discouraged; and development of the arts and sciences came to a screeching halt. Public baths and gymnasiums were abolished by the Church because of the increase of sexual improprieties. Women who provided healthcare were often accused of being witches with supernatural or magical activities and burned at the stake, some theorize because they posed a threat to the male doctors. With the advent of the Christian era, massage became synonymous with witchcraft, and the practice declined in Rome and most of Europe.

Fortunately, there were women of the Dark Ages who managed to keep touch alive. The Church operated hospitals in which nuns were granted permission to provide basic care to victims of war. Eventually, women from all walks of life joined the nuns at the hospitals to care for patients. Massage and baths remained inexpensive treatments that women could provide. Incidentally, these oppressed women made great advances in women's rights toward the end of the Middle Ages, getting involved in politics, land ownership, science, literature, medicine, and education.

The Middle Ages in the Arab World

Women in the Arab world were also participating in healthcare during the Middle Ages, even if only serving as slaves who provided massage in the Turkish baths. While Europe suffered a thousand years with little progress, the Arab world continued to build upon the Greco-Roman knowledge base. The Arab countries were not constrained by the rules of the Church, which allowed them to use creativity, invention, and progressive thinking. They performed dissection on human cadavers, which was unacceptable in the Christian realm, and were able to advance anatomical knowledge. Al-Razi and Ibn Sina are Arabs who used massage and are famous for their contributions to medicine.

Al-Razi (854–935 CE), known in Latin as Rhazes, was an Islamic philosopher and physician. He wrote a medical encyclopedia that included knowledge from Arabic, Roman, and Greek physicians. He was especially interested in the interaction between psychology and physiology, gathering very detailed medical histories from his patients prior to diagnosing or prescribing. Because Al-Razi understood that health was affected by the state of mind, he considered preventive health maintenance very important. He perpetuated the use of massage as part of the health regimen as well as a treatment for disease.

Ibn Sina (980–1037 CE) is also known by his Latin name, Avicenna. He was a scholar, physician, and follower of the philosopher Aristotle. He wrote hundreds of books on a variety of subjects, but his greatest accomplishments were medical treatises. His *Canon of Medicine* is a systematic, useful, encyclopedic medical text that builds upon Galen's theories and observations. When revived after his death, it was quickly recognized as an excellent teaching text that was translated and used in medical schools across Europe for over 500 years. Ibn Sina recommended health maintenance that included the original Greek regimen of exercise, baths, and massage. He also included massage as a treatment for pain relief, for increasing blood flow, and for facilitating the healing process.

THE RENAISSANCE (1450–1600)

As Europeans tired of the cultural stagnation imposed by the Church, their curiosity and interest in the arts and sciences was revitalized. The Renaissance (French for rebirth) period started with this renewed burst of progressive thinking. During the Renaissance, medicine and art developed simultaneously, as renowned artists of the day studied and illustrated human anatomy and physiology.

Leonardo da Vinci's (1452–1519) illustrations of the human body and anatomy drawn during this period still exist today as some of the most admired medical illustrations. His studies of the human anatomy were often done in secret, since human dissection was not yet widely accepted in Europe. Figure 1-6 shows an example of Leonardo da Vinci's anatomical art.

Another anatomical artist from the Renaissance is Andreas Vesalius (1514–1564) of Belgium. As a child he felt compelled to learn anatomy, dissecting any unfortunate animals he could find. He found himself dissatisfied with his education at a medical school in Paris, partly because the teachers were fixed on Galen's philosophies and were still dissecting animals to understand anatomy. He returned to Belgium so passionate about learning human anatomy that he stole a cadaver to dissect the body. Vesalius paid special attention to the muscles and their attachments and actions, making his contribution to massage history especially notable. Figure 1-7 shows an example of the anatomical art of Andreas Vesalius.

In his distinguished book *De Humani Corporis Fabrica*, published in 1543, Vesalius states, "It was when the more fashionable doctors in Italy, in imitation of

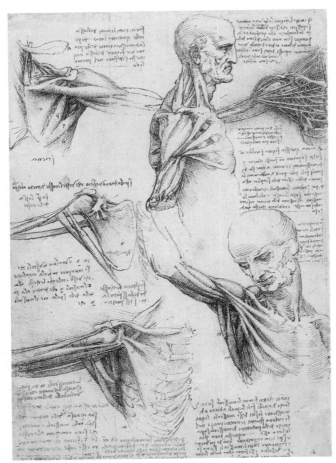

FIGURE 1-6 Leonardo da Vinci's anatomical illustrations. (Reprinted from Clayton M. *Leonardo da Vinci: A Singular Vision.* New York: Abbeville Press, 1996.)

the old Romans, despising the work of the hand, began to delegate to slaves the manual attentions they deemed necessary for their patients . . . that the art of medicine went to ruin."[2] This significant statement resonates with society today. Many people feel frustrated and disappointed with the medical community's personal disconnection and professional distancing, which fails to create a trusting relationship. Massage is a complementary therapy that can bridge the healthcare gap between clinical doctors who barely know their patients and the very personal and reassuring attention that human touch can provide.

The dualism theory of Rene Descartes (1596–1650), "I think, therefore I am," began the exploration into mind–body connection. In his book *Meditations VI,* he claims that the human body is like a machine: "so likewise if the body of man be considered as a kind of machine, so made up and composed of bones, nerves, muscles, veins, blood, and skin, that although there were in it no mind, it would still exhibit the same motions which it at present manifests involuntarily."[3] He

drew a distinction between the mechanical body and the emotional mind but also claimed that they were interconnected. He was the first to differentiate between the human body and a human being, which continues to be a philosophical argument of medical ethics even today.

THE 18TH CENTURY

The rediscovery of ancient cultures lasted until the next era, called the Age of Enlightenment, or the Age of Reason, occurred during the 1700s. The dogma and tradition of the Church were challenged, the sense of reason was explored and applied to different philosophies, humanitarianism blossomed, and education for everyone became a cultural norm. In America, reason, rationale, and education remained strong themes, but politics were the bigger part of history. The Declaration of Independence was signed, America became a free country, and the political system was established. The political and philosophical changes of the century bred inventions such as the bicycle, cotton gin, lightning rod, microscope, steam engine, telegraph, telescope, and thermometer.

Medical history was marked by the discovery of vaccination and inoculation. The ancient Chinese medical reference *The Cong Fou* was translated into French by Jesuit P. M. Cibot in 1779 CE. The text, which recommended controlled breathing and a system of exercises and positions for healthcare, was accompanied by illustrations in the French version. It is very likely that this text served as the inspiration for Per Henrik Ling's Swedish Gymnastics.

Per Henrik Ling

Per Henrik Ling of Sweden (1776–1839) started a bodywork revolution during the transition from the 18th to 19th century. Throughout his travels across Europe teaching, translating, and writing poetry and plays, Ling learned to fence. He noticed the repetitive motions and one-sided physical activity of fencing and their effects on his body. To balance the physical activity, he incorporated gymnastics into his health regimen and consequently relieved his chronic elbow pain. He never became a doctor, but he studied anatomy and physiology extensively and developed **Swedish Gymnastics,** a movement system with four categories:

- Aesthetic—giving expression to feelings, emotions, and thoughts
- Educational—developing the innate potential of the body with good posture and control
- Medical—correcting bodily defects with active, passive, and duplicated movements
- Military—strengthening and toughening the body

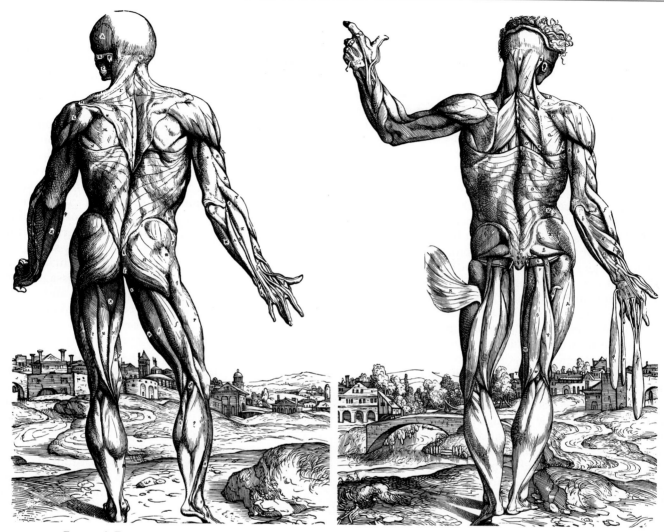

FIGURE 1-7   Anatomical illustrations by Andreas Vesalius showing muscular detail. (Reprinted from Saunders JB de CM, O'Malley CD. The Illustrations From the Works of Andreas Vesalius of Brussels. New York: Dover Publications, 1973.)

The system included classifications of active, passive, or duplicated movements. Active movements were defined as activities in which patients exercised or moved their own bodies. Passive movements required the patients to be relaxed and have their bodies moved by the attendant or to be relaxed and receive manipulation by the attendant. The terms "active" and "passive" are still used with the same definitions to describe movement today. Duplicated movements required physical work from both the patient and the attendant, in which the attendant physically resisted the patient's efforts to move his or her own body. Dr. Mathias Roth, an English physician, wrote one of the first books published in English about Swedish Gymnastics, *The Prevention and Cure of Many Chronic Diseases by Movements*, in 1851. His book included drawings of treatments and showed

the use of the low table, which was originally introduced by Ling. As the popularity and effectiveness of Ling's techniques spread across Europe and Russia, they were called the **Swedish Movements,** or the Swedish Movement Cure.

The use of the term "Swedish massage" likely stemmed from the Swedish movements, even though the inclusion of actual massage techniques as we know them today is questionable. Because of the popularity of the Swedish massage technique, Ling has been credited with leading the revival of the massage profession and is considered by some the "Father of Swedish Massage." The contribution of Ling's work is certainly better-known than that of other historical figures, but there are some people who are equally, if not more, important in massage history.

THE 19TH CENTURY

Bodywork made a significant step forward into the 19th century with the help of Ling. His ability to demonstrate the validity of Swedish Gymnastics as an independent therapy quickly spurred other forms of manual therapy. Specific massage and bodywork techniques were created, promoted, and published in Europe and America.

Massage in 19th Century Europe

Following the development of the Swedish Movements, there were people who specifically promoted the field of massage therapy. Dr. Johan Georg Mezger (1838–1909) of Holland coined some terms for massage techniques that are still used today: effleurage (EF-luhr-ahzh), petrissage (PEH-trih-sahzh), and tapotement (tuh-POHT-ment). It may seem odd that a Dutchman would choose French words for terminology, but the French words **"massage," "masseuse,"** and **"masseur"** were already gaining popularity. Table 1-2 lists massage terms with French roots.

Until Mezger's influence, gymnastics were primarily Ling's exercises and movements that sometimes included massage techniques. Dr. Mezger was the first to identify classic massage strokes and differentiate them from gymnastics and Swedish movements. He reinforced and popularized his terminology, which is still used as the standard worldwide.

In 1888, Swedish physician Dr. Emil Kleen studied the effects of effleurage, friction, pétrissage, and vibration on circulation and lymph flow. He documented his results in *Handbook of Massage*, in which he also emphasized the inclusion of massage and manual therapy in medical treatment. At the same time, he discouraged laypersons from practicing massage because of its medical applications. He identified medical gymnastics as a form of exercise or movement of the muscles and differentiated it from massage, which he defined as a manual therapy that is not exercise and is applied by another individual. He stressed the importance of anatomical and physiological education, palpation skills, hands-on techniques, and the use of mechanical instruments for assistance in some situations. He also included some guidelines for therapist self-care and acceptable lubricants and provided a general outline for a massage session.

In the late 1800s, some British doctors made some unfortunate discoveries in the field of massage. They were noticing false claims of education and abnormally high fees for massage treatment. As a result, the British Medical Association ordered an inquiry and revealed patterns of inconsistency in the massage profession. Schools with unqualified teachers and nonstandardized courses were recruiting girls from poor neighborhoods and preparing students inadequately. They were giving students false impressions regarding employment opportunities, and many graduates were finding themselves unemployed. Some schools opened massage school clinics and would forgive school debts to students who would work in their clinics. At best, these girls gave poor quality massages. At worst, these clinics were

TABLE 1-2

Massage Terms with French Roots

FRENCH WORD	FRENCH PRONUNCIATION	ENGLISH TRANSLATION	ENGLISH PRONUNCIATION (IF APPLICABLE)
Masser	MAH-say	to rub or knead with hands	
Masseur	mah-SUHR	male person who kneads with hands	muh-SOOR
Masseuse	mah-SUHZ	female person who kneads with hands	muh-SOOS
Massage	MAH-sahzh	a method of kneading with the hands	Muh-SAHZH
Effleurer	EF-luhr-ray	to touch lightly	
Effleurage	EF-luhr-rahzh	a method of light touching or stroking	EF-luhr-ahzh
Pétrir	pay-TREER	to knead	
Pétrissage	PAY-trih-sahzh	a method of kneading	PEH-trih-sahzh
Tapoter	TAH-poh-tay	to tap	
Tapotement	TAH-poht-mahn	a method of tapping or patting	tuh-POHT-ment

The word "massage" was first found formally in a French-German dictionary in 1812, but French colonists in India may have started using the term in the mid-1700s. When they found natives rubbing each other for therapy, they described the activity in their journals, using their own French language. The terms "massage," "masseuse," and "masseur" are still used in many cultures, but in the United States, as the profession has evolved, the term "massage therapist" or "massage practitioner" has become the norm.

considered houses of prostitution that deteriorated the reputation of massage practitioners. The rapid growth of the practice resulted in an excess of therapists who were unqualified and damaged the profession as a whole.

Legitimization of Massage

The negative repercussions of unregulated practice were accompanied by some clear advantages. Massage in hospitals and doctor's offices became more prevalent because the only massage therapists who were considered safe were directly associated with a doctor or hospital. Additionally, qualified massage therapists started organizing professional associations to protect the practice. The historical importance of this period relates to the steps that were taken to provide more legitimacy to the practice and to develop massage as a profession instead of an amateur trade.

Eight women founded the Society of Trained Masseuses in Britain in 1894 in an attempt to set a standard of high-quality massage therapists. They modeled their organization after the medical profession, where members had to meet specific academic requirements, pass an examination by a board of professionals including at least one physician, and receive training from a recognized school that received regular inspection and only hired qualified instructors. In 1900, it became the Incorporated Society of Trained Masseuses. When it expanded its membership to 12,000, it became the Chartered Society of Massage and Remedial Gymnastics. Massage practice was back on its way to being recognized as a legitimate profession.

Massage in 19th Century America

Healthcare made a transition in America during the 19th century, going from heroic, folk medicine and treatment to professional medical care. Massage first gained notice in the United States in the 1850s with Dr. George H. Taylor and his natural approach to medicine. He brought the Swedish movements to the American medical community, integrated them into his practice, and eventually founded the Remedial Hygienic Institute in New York. Patients were taught a holistic approach to their health and disease, including an education regarding the nature of their illness, good nutritional habits, and an explanation of the treatment regimen, including water and massage therapies. Dr. Taylor's **Movement Cure** was later combined with Mezger's massage terms and techniques, one of which had the client lie on a table for the entire session, creating a scene similar to the present-day massage session.

Dr. John Harvey Kellogg (1842–1953) was an American physician who pioneered the health food movement, encouraging people to eat dry cereals for breakfast as part of a healthy vegetarian diet. He became the superintendent of the Battle Creek Sanitarium, a medical and surgical center where patients were taught that a proper diet, exercise and massage, fresh air, good posture, and sufficient rest result in good health. The sanitarium specialized in water therapies and massage and became famous for being "the place where people learn to stay well."[4]

Dr. Kellogg made some very important contributions to the history of massage. He conducted extensive massage research at the sanitarium, defining and examining the **mechanical, reflex, and metabolic effects** of massage on the different systems of the body. Table 1-3 gives an explanation of the physiological effects of massage determined by Dr. Kellogg. He found significant effects on the nervous, muscular, skeletal, circulatory, respiratory, integumentary, and digestive systems as well as thermal regulation, cellular metabolism, and kidney and liver activity. In 1895, Kellogg wrote about these effects in his book *The Art of Massage*. The book is an excellent reference with detailed and accurate information regarding anatomical structures, physiological effects, massage techniques, therapeutic applications, joint movement, massage for specific body regions and diseases, rules for practice, and correct terminology. This text was published again in 1909, 1919, and 1923 because of its superior presentation of information.

THE 20TH CENTURY

Early in the 20th century, massage continued to establish a strong foundation for growth. Associations of massage professionals evolved to provide more legitimacy to the profession. The medical community respected the practice enough to allow it to continue in British hospitals and to be used to rehabilitate soldiers in World Wars I and II. In London, hospitals combined massage, physical exercise, physiotherapy, and orthopedic medicine departments. Massage services were particularly desired by private patients, so there was an increase in the number of nurses who took massage courses, studied for a Massage Certificate and became nurse masseurs. Other students studied for the examination of the Chartered Society of Massage and Remedial Gymnastics, which later became the Chartered Society of Physiotherapy.

Social conservatism, the advancement of physiotherapy, physical therapy, and the use of electronic devices restrained the use of massage to some degree. Despite the negative connotations and technological progress, massage remained a part of healthcare. The

TABLE 1-3

Dr. John Harvey Kellogg and His Determination of the Physiological Effects of Massage

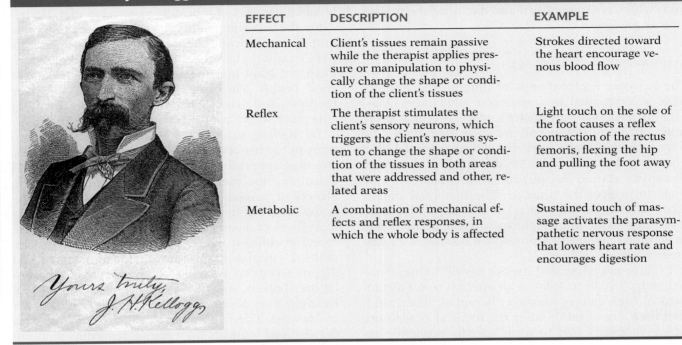

EFFECT	DESCRIPTION	EXAMPLE
Mechanical	Client's tissues remain passive while the therapist applies pressure or manipulation to physically change the shape or condition of the client's tissues	Strokes directed toward the heart encourage venous blood flow
Reflex	The therapist stimulates the client's sensory neurons, which triggers the client's nervous system to change the shape or condition of the tissues in both areas that were addressed and other, related areas	Light touch on the sole of the foot causes a reflex contraction of the rectus femoris, flexing the hip and pulling the foot away
Metabolic	A combination of mechanical effects and reflex responses, in which the whole body is affected	Sustained touch of massage activates the parasympathetic nervous response that lowers heart rate and encourages digestion

Photo courtesy of Robert Calvert, World of Massage Museum.

later part of the 20th century brought much change to the massage profession, especially as bodywork techniques were developed all over the world. There are so many forms of bodywork generated in the later part of the 20th century that we consider it a separate period in massage history (Fig 1-8).

CONTEMPORARY MASSAGE THERAPY

Bodywork has a long and rich history as a mode of physical, mental, and spiritual healing in various cultures and arenas that provides a solid foundation for the current massage therapy profession. For as much as bodywork has evolved over the previous thousands of years, massage has grown exponentially in the last 50 years. The rapid growth shows the popularity and validity of the practice, but it could also lead to the downfall of the massage profession. Although there is disagreement among current practitioners about standardization and governmental regulation, it encourages the safest and most dependable environment for massage clients.

Contemporary massage therapy in America began in the 1960s, when the younger generation rejected conservative habits and conformity in search of self-discovery. The Esalen Institute in Big Sur, California,

became one of the major places to explore the "human potential," or the world of unrealized human capacities. Founded in 1962, Esalen became famous for its beautiful landscape, its blend of Eastern and Western philosophies, its experiential workshops, and the steady influx of philosophers, psychologists, artists, and religious thinkers. Esalen is the one of the first modern places where massage was taught and considered bodywork as a pathway to well-being and transpersonal growth. The Esalen massage is a fluid and flowing combination of the structured Swedish movements with massage strokes delivered in a sensitive, personal way.

The very popular "human potential" movement resulted in numerous books written to accompany the explosion of new bodywork techniques. Since then, many people have contributed to the advancement of the massage profession by conducting research studies to prove its therapeutic legitimacy and writing books that include scientific proof. As a result, massage is regaining acceptance with the public and the medical community as a valid therapy. Contemporary massage is recapturing the historic roots of massage as a preventive and rehabilitative medical approach and is reviving the rich tradition of bathing and anointing in the progressive spa industry.

3000 BCE	Ancient Chinese medical texts, the *Cong Fou* and the *Nei Ching* are written Ancient forms of bodywork: anmo, anointing, mordan, samvahana, Tui-na
2500 BCE	Ancient Indian scriptures, the Vedas, are written
2350 BCE	Ankhmahor's tomb is inscribed with Egyptian drawings of bodywork
1825 BCE	Egypt's Kahun Medical Papyrus is written
1700 BCE	Babylonian laws called the Code of Hammurabi include "eye for an eye" medical ethics
1000 BCE	Ancient Greek health regimen included massage and baths
400 BCE	Hippocrates writes Hippocratic Corpus
30 CE	Aulus Cornelius Celsus writes *De Medicina*
175	Greek physician Claudius Galenus (Galen) of Rome develops early scientific research method
400–1400	The Middle Ages in Europe, influenced by the Church, is marked by cultural emptiness that results in a decline of massage in Europe The Middle Ages in the Arab world, less affected by the Church, generates the belief that health is affected by state of mind
1450–1600	The Renaissance brings anatomical art from Leonardo da Vinci and Andreas Vesalius René Descartes develops theory of mind–body connection, "I think, therefore I am"
1700s	Humanitarianism, reason, and education flood society, and many scientific inventions are created
1779	Jesuit P.M. Cibot translates the *Cong Fou* into French
1800's	Sweden's Per Henrik Ling creates Swedish Gymnastics Holland's Dr. Johan Mezger standardizes massage terminology and differentiates massage strokes from movement therapies Dr. George Taylor popularizes the Movement Cure in America Dr. John Kellogg pioneers the health food movement in America, researches the physiological effects of massage, and writes *The Art of Massage*, which is still a excellent reference British inquiry reveals unethical activity in the field of massage, which provides the stimulus for legitimization
1894	The first professional massage organization, the Society of Trained Masseuses, is founded in Britain
1913	Dr. William Fitzgerald develops Zone Therapy, a precursor to reflexology, based on reflex zones
1914-1918	Swedish massage rehabilitates injured soldiers in WWI
1920	The Society of Trained Masseuses grows, incorporates, and becomes the Chartered Society of Massage and Remedial Gymnastics Dr. Mikao Usui of Japan originates Reiki
1927	The first American massage association, New York State Society of Medical Massage Therapists, is founded
1930s	The first American massage association, New York State Society of Medical Massage Therapists, is founded Neuromuscular Therapy created in Europe by cousins, Boris Chaitow and Stanley Leif Dr. Emil Vodder and his wife, Estrid, a physical therapist, create Manual Lymph Drainage Eunice Ingham develops Reflexology
1939	The Florida State Massage Therapy Association, Inc. (FSMTA) organizes 85 charter members
1940	British osteopath James Cyriax creates deep transverse friction
1940s	Therese Pfrimmer creates cross-fiber muscle therapy, later called Pfrimmer Deep Muscle Therapy
1943	American Association of Masseurs and Masseuses (AAMM) formed in Chicago with dues of 50 cents The first Massage Act is passed by the Florida Legislature
1949	Massage Registration Act formulated by AAMM
1950s	Francis Tappan and Gertrude Beard write significant books and articles on massage techniques Dr. Randolph Stone develops Polarity Therapy
1952	Janet Travell researches trigger points
1958	AAMM becomes the American Massage and Therapy Association (AM&TA)
1960s	Esalen Institute establishes itself as a center to explore human potential
1960	Jin Shin Jyutsu, the Japanese art of circulation awakening, was brought to America by Mary Iino Burmeister
1964	Applied Kinesiology was founded by chiropractor George Goodheart
1970s	John F. Barnes, physical therapist, introduces his therapy called Myofascial Release to the public
1972	Moshe Feldenkrais develops his own method of movement therapy
1977	Paul St. John, LMT, develops the St. John Method of Neuromuscular Therapy
1978	Joseph Heller develops Hellerwork, a structural bodywork
1980	Dr. Milton Trager opens the Trager Institute and teaches the Trager Approach to movement therapy
1981	Dr. Lawrence H. Jones develops Strain Counterstrain neuromuscular techniques for relieving trigger points
1983	AM&TA becomes the current American Massage Therapy Association (AMTA)
1987	Associated Bodywork and Massage Professionals (ABMP)
1992	Dr. Tiffany Field opens the Touch Research Institute AMTA creates the National Certification Board for Therapeutic Massage and Bodywork (NCBTMB) National Institutes of Health establish the Office of Alternative Medicine

FIGURE 1-8   Timeline of bodywork and massage.

Massage and Bodywork Modalities

Historically, massage techniques were based upon the practices of anointing and bathing as well as variations of gymnastics and the Swedish Movements. Since then, numerous massage and bodywork modalities have emerged (Fig. 1-8). Keeping with the distinction that was made by Dr. Johan Mezger and Dr. Emil Kleen in the 1800s, we consider massage an activity that requires the therapist to apply manual pressure to the client's tissues. Bodywork can be characterized as treatment that involves manipulation of the client's body as a way to maintain or improve health. In other words, all forms of massage may be considered bodywork, but not all forms of bodywork may be called massage.

A **modality** is a collection of manual therapies that tends to use similar applications of movement or massage strokes to reach a similar goal. Currently, there is inconsistency with the categories that have been identified, but this text separates them into the following nine categories: Swedish, deep tissue, neuromuscular, circulation enhancement, energy, Oriental/Eastern approaches, structural/postural integration, movement bodywork, and special populations (Table 1-4). These categories are briefly introduced in this section, and most are covered in detail later in the text. The techniques not covered in detail likely require extensive study and training on their own. Table 1-5 provides a list of web sites with further information about bodywork modalities.

SWEDISH MODALITIES

Swedish massage is the most widely recognized and commonly used category of massage. While the public commonly identifies it as a gentle and superficial massage, the techniques vary from light to vigorous. Generally, Swedish includes a combination of long gliding (effleurage), kneading (petrissage), tapotement (percussion), and friction strokes applied to the superficial tissues of the body. They can be applied separately or mixed and matched to adapt to the needs of the client during the massage session. Oftentimes, these strokes are combined with active and passive movements to create a fluid, relaxing, circulatory-enhancing massage session.

Relaxation massage and health maintenance massage are considered Swedish modalities. Their **mechanical** and **reflexive benefits** are primarily intended to increase circulation of the blood and lymphatic fluid throughout the body as well as increase joint range of motion. These techniques and their effects are covered extensively in Chapter 7.

TABLE 1-4

Bodywork Modalities and Some Examples of Each

MODALITY	EXAMPLES
Swedish	Swedish massage Relaxation massage Health maintenance massage
Deep tissue	Connective tissue work Myofascial work Pfrimmer work Cross-fiber friction techniques Craniosacral work
Neuromuscular	St. John Method of Neuromuscular Therapy (NMT) Trigger point therapy Muscle energy techniques (MET) Proprioceptive neuromuscular facilitation (PNF) Reflexology
Circulation enhancement	Manual lymph drainage (MLD) Vodder technique Arterial enhancement Venous enhancement Abdominal massage
Energy	Polarity therapy Reiki
Oriental/Eastern approaches	Acupressure Shiatsu Jin Shin techniques Tui-na
Structural integration	Rolfing Hellerwork
Movement	Feldenkrais Alexander Technique Trager work
Special populations	Athletes Corporate massage Prenatal massage Infant massage Elderly massage Physically disabled Veterinary massage

DEEP TISSUE MODALITIES

The deep tissue modalities are intended to affect the tissues that are deep within the body and are often difficult to palpate. They are usually applied slowly and specifically and typically use long, sustained gliding strokes, prolonged direct pressure, and strokes that travel across the muscles, perpendicular to the muscle fibers. This category of massage modalities includes, but is not limited to, connective tissue, myofascial, Pfrimmer, cross-fiber friction, and craniosacral techniques.

TABLE 1-5

Bodywork Associations and Their Web Sites

MODALITY	ASSOCIATION	WEB SITE
Acupressure	Acupressure Institute	www.acupressure.com
Alexander Technique	Alexander Technique International	www.ati-net.com
Craniosacral	Upledger Institute	www.upledger.com
Esalen	Esalen Institute	www.esalen.org
Feldenkrais	Feldenkrais Guild of North America	www.feldenkrais.com
Hellerwork	Hellerwork International	www.hellerwork.com
Jin Shin techniques	American Association of Bodywork Therapies of Asia	www.aobta.org
Lymph drainage	Dr. Vodder School North America	www.vodderschool.com
Myofascial	John Barnes Myofascial Release	www.myofascialrelease.com
Neuromuscular therapy	St. John Method of Neuromuscular Therapy	www.stjohnseminars.com
Pfrimmer	Pfrimmer Deep Muscle Therapy	www.pfrimmer.com
Polarity	American Polarity Therapy Association	www.polaritytherapy.org
Reiki	The International Center for Reiki Training	www.reiki.org
Rolfing	The Rolf Institute of Structural Integration	www.rolf.org
Shiatsu	American Association of Bodywork Therapies of Asia	www.aobta.org
Trager	The United States Trager Association	www.trager-us.org
Tui-na	American Association of Bodywork Therapies of Asia	www.aobta.org

Connective tissue, myofascial, and Pfrimmer work are frequently used when there is some kind of restriction in the fascia or muscle. These restrictions, sometimes called adhesions, can form as a result of injury or chronic muscular tension patterns, may limit movement, create pain, and result in postural compensation patterns. These techniques may be uncomfortable for some clients, but by breaking up the restrictions and restoring space to the tissues, circulation and lymphatic flow are increased and health can be restored.

Dr. James Cyriax was an English physician who is considered the "Father of Orthopaedic Medicine." He developed the connective tissue technique of cross-fiber (deep transverse) friction that can be used to help heal muscular, tendinous, and ligamentous dysfunctions resulting from injury and overuse.

Deep tissue modalities often consist of applications of intense, localized pressure to access the deep tissue layers, but there are also some very subtle techniques that can accomplish the same thing. It may seem counterintuitive that a subtle technique could be a deep tissue modality, but there is a common misconception that "deep" means "hard." Consider the effect of vibrations. When you feel the rumbling of loud thunder or the booming bass of a car stereo or you strike a tuning fork and hold it against your skin, you may feel the vibrations resonate deep in your chest or throughout your whole body. Likewise, the deeper tissue layers can be affected with minimal energy and very little pressure by applying vibration or other subtle techniques such as craniosacral therapies or many of the energy modalities described later in this section.

Craniosacral therapy is a subtle technique that can affect very deep tissues and have very profound effects. This technique teaches practitioners to palpate and manipulate the rhythmic flow of cerebrospinal fluid that bathes the brain and spinal cord. Altering the rhythm of the flow can rearrange the fascia, restore space to the tissues, and increase lymph and blood flow to the area. The technique is applied very lightly, which is why it is sometimes considered an energy modality, but its purpose and effects classify it as a deep tissue modality.

NEUROMUSCULAR MODALITIES

Neuromuscular modalities engage the relationship between the nervous and muscular systems to create reflex responses. The organ systems of the body are separate but very interdependent processes. All of the activity of the muscular system depends on the nervous system, which is the main control system of the body. By using the physiological relationship between nerves and muscles, we can change muscle length and kinesthetic perception. Some of the neuromuscular modalities use massage, but this may be considered more of a bodywork modality. St. John Method of Neuromuscular Therapy (NMT), trigger point therapy, muscle energy techniques, proprioceptive neuromuscular facilitation, and reflexology can be categorized as neuromuscular modalities.

CIRCULATORY ENHANCEMENT MODALITIES

Circulatory enhancement modalities are massage techniques that use purely mechanical effects to manipulate the movement of blood, lymphatic fluid, and waste within the body. The flow of blood through the cardiovascular system can be enhanced through the arteries as well as the veins. Basic massage strokes are used in specific patterns to accomplish both arterial and venous enhancement.

Lymphatic fluid from the body tissues is collected and transported through the lymph vessels and is eventually emptied into the heart. The flow of lymph can also be encouraged with specific manual techniques such as manual lymph drainage (MLD) or the Vodder method.

Lastly, although not a circulatory system, the movement of waste through the large intestine can be encouraged with basic massage strokes applied over the abdomen in specific patterns.

ENERGY MODALITIES

Energy modalities are often associated with a sense of mystery and doubt, mostly because their validity may be unproven by scientific methods. There are several types of energy bodywork, most of which use very light touch or off-the-body application to manipulate the human body's energy fields. Polarity therapy and Reiki are two of the more common energy techniques.

The famous physicists Albert Einstein, Prince Louis de Broglie, and Max Planck suggested that matter is composed of an essence of energy, having electromagnetic fields and positive and negative poles. Polarity therapy, based on the concept that the human body creates an energy field, suggests that the human energy field is affected by internal and external inputs, including emotions, touch, sounds, and movement. While the central nervous system is the main component of our electrical or energetic existence, a whole host of biochemical reactions play a part as well. Basically, if biochemical reactions are hindered, the efficiency of nerve transmission and

other body systems is diminished. Theoretically, if the blockages are removed, function can be restored. Polarity therapy addresses the electrical field of the body, attempting to balance it out in an attempt to allow normal electrical activity to occur.

Briefly, Reiki is an energy modality that restores flow to the life force energy with spiritual guidance. The life force energy, or **Qi** (CHEE), is a dynamic, changing energy force that runs through the whole body, supplying and being supplied by body processes and activities. It can be vaguely compared to the flow of energy that you feel when you are enlightened, optimistic, or motivated. Unlike most bodywork modalities, Reiki is a technique that is transferred as a gift from one practitioner to another, requiring no intellectual or spiritual education. A very simplified explanation of Reiki portrays it as a spiritually guided manipulation of the life force energy.

ORIENTAL/EASTERN MODALITIES

In traditional Eastern philosophies, the Qi travels through a series of pathways called meridians. The philosophies teach that a balanced, unrestricted flow of Qi is required for the body to maintain good health, and disruptions or blockages to Qi cause disharmony in the body. Theoretically, removal of the disruptions and restoration of a balanced energy flow can restore health. The Oriental bodywork modalities manipulate the Qi mechanically to restore normal function and health to the body. These techniques use external, visible applications of pressure and manipulation, which classifies them as massage techniques. In addition to mechanical pressure, these techniques also use internal, energetic manipulations that are not visible. The internal work is the more profound of the two, which leads to the consideration of the Oriental techniques as forms of art as opposed to science. Acupressure, Shiatsu, Jin Shin techniques, and Tui-na are just some of the many Oriental modalities that use mechanical pressure from fingers, hands, thumbs, elbows, knees, and feet.

STRUCTURAL AND POSTURAL INTEGRATION MODALITIES

Structural and postural integration modalities, such as Rolfing and Hellerwork, may be considered massage techniques. They generally focus on realigning the skeletal system to relieve pain from postural compensations. Posture can significantly affect health, and although it often takes a lot of bodywork that may be accompanied by discomfort, structural realignment can be very beneficial. The assessment chapter of this text discusses the relationship between posture and health in further detail.

MOVEMENT MODALITIES

These bodywork modalities use movement to reorient the body for more optimal function. Feldenkrais (FEHL-den-krahys), Alexander Technique, and Trager (TRAY-ger) are examples of movement modalities.

Dr. Moshe Feldenkrais was a physicist, engineer, martial arts master, and teacher who developed his own bodywork method in the mid 1900s. Feldenkrais is a movement therapy that teaches body awareness, coordination, and flexibility through movement techniques. Habitual activities that may create dysfunctional movement patterns are studied and practiced in precise manners to reprogram the neuromuscular system. The neuromuscular component of this modality leads some to categorize it as a neuromuscular therapy, but its focus is on movement.

The Alexander Technique was developed by Frederick Matthias Alexander, a Shakespearean actor from the early 1900s. His technique studies the client's balance, coordination, flexibility, and support structure and encourages the client to be aware of reactive, habitual movements. The practitioner uses palpation skills and gentle movements to relieve muscular tension while the client demonstrates simple activities. By reprograming the body to make conscious movement choices instead of reactive, reflexive motions, the technique creates ease of movement and improves overall health.

Milton Trager, MD, developed a bodywork approach in the mid-1900s that uses active and passive components similar to ancient gymnastics. The client lies on a table for the passive component while the practitioner moves him in gentle, natural rocking and shaking patterns that are intended to feel unrestricted and effortless. The intent is to relieve chronic patterns of muscular tension. The active portion of the approach requires clients to shake and loosen their bodies to reinforce the practitioner's table work. Giving the clients exercises to use on their own allows them to take an active part in their healthcare and can have longer lasting or permanent results.

SPECIAL POPULATIONS

There are groups of clients who have special conditions or require special considerations to receive bodywork. This text refers to these groups as special populations, and the therapist must understand their specific needs to determine which techniques are appropriate and which should be avoided. Some special populations a therapist may encounter include athletes, corporate, geriatric, prenatal, infant, physically disabled, and veterinary clients. Essentially, the same massage strokes are used, but special considerations are given to session duration, pressure, areas to avoid, positions to avoid, precautions to take, and equipment to use. These special populations are covered in more detail later in the text.

Touch

Touch is one of the most basic of human needs and occurs in every culture and many animals. Touch can be used as a method of communication and learning, for comfort, and to provide self-esteem. Scientific research has indicated that it is required for healthy growth, development, and immune function. It has also been scientifically proven that deprivation of touch can cause significant developmental barriers in humans and animals. In essence, the sense of touch is required for our very survival.

From the time we are in the womb, we depend on touch to learn about the world. Infants commonly explore objects by putting them in their mouths, discovering the shapes, textures, and temperatures of objects in their world. When babies cry, they are comforted when they are picked up and held, stroked, or kissed. This comforting aspect of touch continues into adulthood. When we are upset, often we seek touch for comfort and validation. Handshakes, pats on the back, hand holding, hugs, and kisses are different forms of touch that provide comfort and validation, and they are also used as modes of communication. Adults use touch to communicate, evaluate, and navigate through the world. Again, touch is very powerful and, when used appropriately, can have incredibly positive outcomes on the human experience.

TOUCH PHYSIOLOGY

There is 18 square feet of skin on the average person, making the skin the largest sensory organ of the body. Unlike the other sensory organs, the skin remains in a constant state of readiness, sending pressure, temperature, and pain sensations to the central nervous system for the appropriate response. This function is especially critical when a person is blind or deaf or when other physiological changes affect sensory input. The skin is the major structure of the integumentary system and is covered in more detail in the chapter on anatomy and physiology.

TOUCH RESEARCH

Various forms of touch have long been a part of many cultures throughout history, but the formal, scientific study of touch is relatively new. As the massage profession continues to evolve, research is vital for validating the effects of massage. The hard scientific proof is helping the medical profession understand and accept the value of touch. Several medical schools such as Duke, Harvard, Johns Hopkins, and the University of Arizona offer integrated medicine electives and research opportunities to study the effects of touch and other bodywork modalities.

One very early example of touch research is the classic study conducted in 1958 by University of Wisconsin psychologist Harry Harlow. Infant monkeys were taken from their real mothers, isolated in metal cages, and offered different objects for sources of comfort and security. Harlow showed that the infants preferred cuddling with a soft cloth, artificial mother to a wire model with a head and face that held food. In fact, when the cloth model had the food as well, the infant monkeys didn't go to the wire model at all, suggesting that infants may instinctively prefer cuddling and tactile stimulation to food nourishment. There are so many people who believe in the power of touch that the government and private interest groups have funded research to prove its efficacy.

Government-Sponsored Research

The National Institutes of Health (NIH) established the Office of Alternative Medicine (OAM) in 1992 to study and recommend further research on unconventional medical treatments. In 1998, it expanded to become the National Center for Complementary and Alternative Medicine (NCCAM). "It is dedicated to exploring complementary and alternative healing practices in the context of rigorous science, training complementary and alternative medicine (CAM) researchers, and disseminating authoritative information to the public. To fulfill its mission, NCCAM supports a broad-based portfolio of research, research training, and educational grants and contracts, as well as various outreach mechanisms to disseminate information to the public."[5]

A growing number of Americans are using complementary approaches to healthcare and medical treatment and are seeking healthcare providers who treat the whole person instead of just an illness. As a result, then President Bill Clinton established the White House Commission on Complementary and Alternative Medicine Policy (WHCCAMP) by issuing Executive Order 13147 on March 7, 2000. The commission is composed of no more than 15 individuals who are knowledgeable in conventional, complementary, and alternative medicine. These representatives were appointed by the president and were asked to address the following issues:

- Research on CAM practices and products
- Delivery of and public access to CAM services
- Dissemination of reliable information on CAM to healthcare providers and the general public
- Appropriate licensing, education, and training of CAM healthcare practitioners

In March 2002, the WHCCAMP issued a final report covering all their charged issues. The following is the overview of the report, as written:

> Although heterogeneous, the major CAM systems have many common characteristics, including a focus on individualizing treatments, treating the whole person, promoting self-care and self-healing, and recognizing the spiritual nature of each individual. In addition, many CAM systems have characteristics commonly found in mainstream health care, such as a focus on good nutrition and preventive practices. Unlike mainstream medicine, CAM often lacks or has only limited experimental and clinical study; however, scientific investigation of CAM is beginning to address this knowledge gap. Thus, boundaries between CAM and mainstream medicine, as well as among different CAM systems, are often blurred and are constantly changing.[6]

Dr. Tiffany Field and the Touch Research Institute

Tiffany Field, PhD, is the pioneer of modern massage research and remains one of the foremost authorities on scientific proof of the benefits of massage (Fig. 1-9). Her interest in touch therapy began when her daughter was born prematurely. She conducted her first study as a psychology graduate student in 1982, determining that "infants given pacifiers during their tube feedings gained more weight, went off tube feedings earlier, did better on newborn behavior and neurological examinations, and were discharged earlier, at a much lower hospital cost, than infants not given pacifiers."[7]

Her remarkable work won her a start-up grant from Johnson & Johnson in 1992 to create the Touch Research Institute (TRI) at the University of Miami's School of Medicine. It was the first center in the world devoted to studying the scientific aspects and medical applications of touch, designing

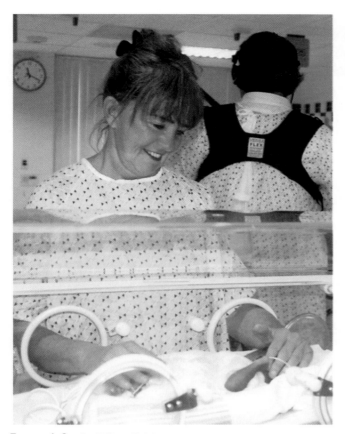

FIGURE 1-9 Dr. Tiffany Field.

research studies that can prove how touch promotes health and can be used to treat disease. The outcomes of these critical research studies will help validate the beneficial effects of massage. In fact, the TRI has already shown that massage is medically beneficial for premature infants and fibromyalgia, asthma, and diabetes patients. TRI research has shown that massage enhances the immune system by increasing production of natural killer cells and increases alertness and computational accuracy. See Research Box 1-1 for some specific research studies performed by the TRI.

AMTA Foundation

The American Massage Therapy Association (AMTA), covered in more detail in Chapter 2, created the AMTA Foundation in 1990. Its original goal was to generate and apply knowledge regarding the benefits of massage therapy and to disseminate the information to all aspects of society. The current mission also includes support of scientific research, community education, and community service. The AMTA Foundation relies on donations from individuals, schools,

massage therapy product vendors, and the AMTA to grant funds for research, community service, educational scholarship, and conferences. It also educates massage therapists about current research and provides direct consultation to the medical and research communities.

In 1998, the foundation established the AMTA Foundation Massage Therapy Research Database with hopes that it would become the primary source for massage-related articles with a focus on information from peer-reviewed research journals. It currently contains thousands of records, and the foundation hopes that future funding will allow foreign articles to be translated and all data to be summarized and analyzed. Some of the current sources of data are publications that are not included in standard medical indexes but are important for the field of massage.

INTERPRETATION OF TOUCH

While the physiological mechanisms for the touch response are basically the same in every human being, individual interpretation of touch can be vastly different. Influenced by emotion, gender, age, culture, spirituality, and religious customs, each person's unique intention and perception of touch make it one of the most powerful forms of communication.

There is a fine and often fuzzy line between all aspects of giving and receiving. In the world of massage therapy, the therapist gives his or her own form of touch to the client, but at the same time receives tactile input from the client. That input can be felt as basic muscular tension or reduced range of motion, but the input can also be a form of communication from the client. Any time a client is receiving bodywork, the therapist must be aware of the many ways a client's body can convey its reaction to the work. Clients may express discomfort by wincing, pulling away, getting quiet or talking excessively, holding the breath, or tensing the body. On the other hand, clients who are enjoying the bodywork might sigh or let out a big breath, their whole body might relax and go limp, breathing could slow down, or they could become quiet or go to sleep. All of these responses, which can be felt by the therapist's hands, are body language messages that might be telling the therapist to adjust the bodywork. Therapists must not let their own emotions, belief systems, or reactive responses influence sensory input from the client's body. This separation of the therapist's life experiences from the client's body is sometimes referred to as grounding, which is discussed later in the text.

General Information about TRI Research (Taken directly from the TRI web site: http://www.miami.edu/touch-research/index.html)

The Touch Research Institutes have conducted over 90 studies on the positive effects of massage therapy on many functions and medical conditions in varied age groups. Among the significant research findings are enhanced growth (e.g., in preterm infants), diminished pain (e.g., fibromyalgia), decreased autoimmune problems (e.g., increased pulmonary function in asthma and decreased glucose levels in diabetes), enhanced immune function (e.g., increased natural killer cells in HIV and cancer), and enhanced alertness and performance (e.g., EEG pattern of alertness and better performance on math computations). Many of these effects appear to be mediated by stress hormones. Several of these findings have been reviewed in the TRI newsletter ("Touchpoints") and in the volumes *Touch Therapy* (Harcourt Brace) and *Touch* (MIT Press).

References are cited below the subject/topic. Articles can be obtained by taking the reference to your local university library (not a public library) and asking the librarian to help you find a journal article. References listed as "in press," "in review," or "ongoing" are not yet available. To order a packet of articles from the Touch Research Institute, please go to the order form under "Touchpoints." You can select studies to receive for $20 per 4 articles.

Back Pain

Massage lessened lower back pain, depression, and anxiety and improved sleep. The massage therapy group also showed improved range of motion, and their serotonin and dopamine levels were higher.

Hernandez-Reif M, Field T, Krasnegor J, Theakston T. Low back pain is reduced and range of motion increased after massage therapy. Int J Neurosci 2001;106:131–145.

Breast Cancer

Massage therapy reduced anxiety and depression and improved immune function including increased natural killer cell number.

Hernandez-Reif M, Ironson G, Field T, et al. Breast cancer patients have improved immune functions following massage therapy. J Psychosom Res, in review.

Diabetes

Following 1 month of parents massaging their children with diabetes, the children's glucose levels decreased to the normal range and their dietary compliance increased. Also the parents' and children's anxiety and depression levels decreased.

Field T, Hernandez-Reif M, LaGreca A, et al. Massage therapy lowers blood glucose levels in children with diabetes mellitus. Diabetes Spectrum 1997;10:237–239.

Early Stimulation

Research is reviewed on the critical nature of rubbing the rat pup and the preterm newborn for their growth and development.

Schanberg S, Field T. Sensory deprivation stress and supplemental stimulation in the rat pup and preterm human neonate. Child Dev 1987;58:1431–1447.

Father–Infant Massage

Fathers gave their infants daily massages 15 minutes prior to bedtime for one month. The fathers in the massage group showed more optimal interaction behavior with their infants.

Cullen C, Field T, Escalona A, Hartshorn K. Father–infants interactions are enhanced by massage therapy. Early Child Dev Care 2000;164:41–47.

Fibromyalgia

Fibromyalgia patients slept better (showed lower activity levels, suggesting more deep sleep), and had lower substance P levels and less pain following a month of biweekly massages.

Field T, Diego M, Cullen C, et al. Fibromyalgia pain and substance P decrease and sleep improves after massage therapy. J Clin Rheumatol 2002;8:72–76.

Leukemia

Twenty children with leukemia were provided with daily massages by their parents and were compared with a standard treatment control group. Following a month of massage therapy, depressed mood decreased in the children's parents, and the children's white blood cell and neutrophil counts increased.

Field T, Cullen C, Diego M, et al. J Bodywork Movement Ther 2001;5:271–274.

Migraine Headaches

Massage therapy decreased the occurrence of headaches, sleep disturbances, and distress symptoms and increased serotonin levels.

Hernandez-Reif M, Field T, Dieter J, et al. Migraine headaches were reduced by massage therapy. Int J Neurosci 1998;96:1–11.

Massage as Part of the American Healthcare System

Contemporary massage therapy is evolving within and outside the American healthcare system. The practice of massage and bodywork is now considered a major component of complementary and integrated healthcare, as is evidenced by government sponsored research and development. Medical schools are incorporating complementary health education into their programs, and doctors are graduating with a general understanding of complementary healthcare. Hospitals are incorporating massage therapy into their services for both staff and patients, and massage is becoming more prevalent in medical clinics, pain clinics, and doctors' offices.

Even more exciting is the fact that insurance companies are beginning to recognize massage as a legitimate treatment instead of a luxury that has no medical benefit. Currently, American insurance companies are often looking to spend as little money as possible, they are notorious for delaying payment or denying claims, and they tend to raise premiums while reducing benefits. With the abundance of research to prove the benefits of massage, insurance companies are beginning to see that the low cost of massage may significantly reduce their overall costs. Massage may minimize or eliminate the need for pharmaceuticals, reduce the length of hospital stays, and reduce the number of physical therapy sessions a patient may need. Better yet, the side effects of massage do not require additional medical treatment, which often happens with prescription medications. Continued scientific research to validate the benefits of massage will help the public, healthcare community, and insurance companies validate the efficacy of touch.

Massage in the Spa Industry

In addition to the increased use in the healthcare system, the spa industry has greatly increased its interest in massage and bodywork over the last few years. The spa industry has a long history that includes massage and bodywork, and massage is offered in almost every spa in America now. In fact, it seems massage and water treatments have come full circle and are currently gaining extraordinary popularity as therapeutic treatments.

HISTORY OF THE SPA INDUSTRY

The ancient Romans discovered the therapeutic properties of hot mineral springs in the village of Spa, Belgium, and used them to heal wounded soldiers. The soldiers took their knowledge back to Rome, and the Roman baths were born. As the natural hot springs quickly became a standard part of health maintenance and improvement, the spa business was refined. Physicians recognized the therapeutic effects of spas and commonly set up practice in or near the spas to treat their patients. By 14 CE, there were over 150 spas in Rome being used by the general public for rest, relaxation, and stress reduction. Massage was one of the many rituals of the spa experience.

Native Americans were using hot springs for healthcare long before America was "discovered" by the Europeans. In 1790, Saratoga Hot Springs, in Saratoga, Wyoming, was the first commercial spa to be established in America. Spas have since become a standard community business. As stated above, massage and water treatments have come full circle and are currently gaining extraordinary popularity as therapeutic treatments.

The International Spa Association (ISPA) was founded in 1991 to provide a network for professional spa associates. ISPA's goals are to educate, set standards, provide resources, influence policy, and build coalitions for the spa industry worldwide. It has identified 10 elements of the spa experience, including a touch component for massage and bodywork (Fig. 1-10).

MEDICAL SPAS

For years, American spas focused on providing beauty and relaxation for their patrons, with little or no involvement of medical personnel. The 10 elements of a spa experience were incorporated into the services offered. The current industry trend, however, is showing a slow but steady increase in medical spas. With the philosophy that health and healing can be improved with a positive state of mind, medical spas offer a special approach toward healthcare by integrating client comfort and relaxation with conventional medical treatments.

Dentists, dermatologists, obstetricians, oncologists, and plastic surgeons are some of the medical professionals who can be found working at spas. The presence of these doctors and their services raises the profile of a beauty-related spa to a professional, health and medical treatment spa. The doctors offer medical and spa services to segments of the population who might not normally be able to take advantage of a spa. For example, an oncologist could determine which massage lubricants would not damage the skin or complicate the condition of a client undergoing chemotherapy. Likewise, an obste-

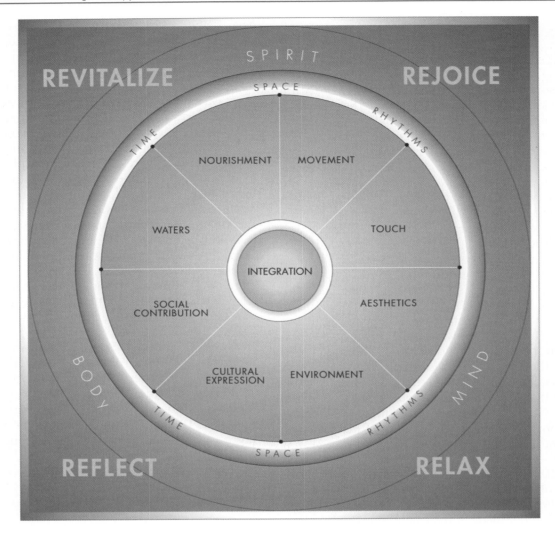

Waters: The internal and external use of water in its many forms.

Nourishment: What we feed ourselves: food, herbals, supplements, and medicines.

Movement: Vitality and energy through movement, exercise, stretching, and fitness.

Touch: Connectivity and communication embraced through touch, massage, and bodywork.

Integration: The personal and social relationship between mind, body, spirit, and environment.

Aesthetics: Our concept of beauty and how botanical agents relate to the biochemical components of the body.

Environment: Location, placement, weather patterns, water constitution, natural agents, and social responsibility.

Cultural Expression: The spiritual belief systems, the value of art and the scientific and political view of the time.

Social Contribution: Commerce, volunteer efforts, and intention as they relate to well-being.

Time, Space Rhythms: The perception of space and time and its relationship to natural cycles and rhythms.

Circle concept created by R. Zill for ISPA 2001

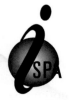

ISPA would like to thank the ISPA education committees past and present.

FIGURE 1-10   ISPA's ten elements. (Reprinted with permission from the International SPA Association. Circle concept created by R. Zill for ISPA 2001.)

trician would be able to recommend aromatherapy products that are safe during pregnancy, allowing the mother to enjoy a massage with therapeutic essential oils. The medical doctors on staff can ensure that all other spa services are safe for their patients and can monitor healing progress in addition to their patients' health.

SPA MASSAGE EDUCATION

Currently, spas are the largest employer of massage therapists. As American spas become more professional and medically oriented, massage training must be geared to support this direction. Self-employment tends to be the focus for most massage education, but many of those in the massage field work as employees for hospitals, clinics, fitness centers, and spas. Many of these jobs require group interaction, teamwork, and a willingness to take on other responsibilities.

Spas are now finding that they must spend time and resources training massage therapists to work as part of the team. Spa owners are looking for therapists who are team players. To fill this demand, esthetician schools, beauty schools, and cosmetology schools are starting to offer massage therapy training. They are graduating therapists who are more adept at working in a spa, but who have insufficient knowledge of anatomy, physiology, pathology, and pharmacology. The market will be better served by massage schools adding spa therapy training to their programs, preparing students for the hospitality environment and group interaction.

Group environments require cooperation, good communication skills, and an appreciation for the success of the business being a result of good teamwork. In addition to doing their own job very well, each person in the group must be aware of the other business activities and be willing to support and help the others accomplish those tasks. There are many occasions when therapists are asked to handle retail sales, housekeeping, front desk reception, body wraps, showers, and other spa services. When massage therapy is only one part of an assortment of business activities, it is important to work efficiently, keep appointments on schedule, cooperate, and support everyone else on the team.

Ego and superiority can be detrimental to a group. Many massage therapists are compassionate about the benefits of massage to the point where they may unknowingly project a superior attitude that alienates others in a group. Touch is so personal and individual that someone who receives the same simple stroke from two different therapists may find that the strokes feel completely different. Keep this in mind as you give and receive massage in class, comparing the feel of one person's touch to that of another and considering how different you feel after each massage. Outside school, you may find that your massage may not suit a particular client. To maintain a client-focused business, you can refer that client to a different therapist or to a different kind of treatment. Removing your ego from your massage will benefit you, your clients, and your coworkers.

Trends in Massage Education

When the "hippie" movement popularized massage in the 1960s, American massage education took an informal and nonscientific approach. People who felt gifted with touch often learned techniques from early texts, such as Dr. Kellogg's *The Art of Massage*. For the next 20 years, there was a sort of rebirth of the massage industry in America. Many people were learning techniques from individuals who specialized in massage, but the numbers of schools was steadily increasing.

Today, massage schools are opening up everywhere, with various levels of academic, technique, and business education. The more formal, extended study program is becoming increasingly common as the country moves toward regulation and standardization of the practice.

Insurance companies and their excessive trails of paperwork introduce an aspect to the practice that needs to be addressed. Medical coding, documentation, and billing procedures must be done correctly for insurance companies to even consider disbursing payment. Medical offices have higher incomes to offset the slow payment from insurance companies, but massage therapists often depend on fast payment to pay monthly bills. It may expedite payment from an insurance company if you are familiar with medical codes, paperwork, and billing procedures.

Another variable in massage education is the level of anatomy and physiology that is taught. Some schools include cadaver work to teach anatomy, which can be very helpful and is a unique educational experience; however, cadaver laboratories are very cost prohibitive. As an alternative, there are video tapes of cadaver dissections that offer students a visual approach to human anatomy. Remember that the academic education is only one part of the therapist's skills. Solid, substantial knowledge of science is necessary, but palpation and communication skills are just as important. Massage therapy is a hands-on activity that must be taught and learned with hands-on practice. One hopes that the future will bring regulations and standardization to all aspects of massage therapy, including education.

Chapter Summary

To better understand massage, it helps to understand the profession as it evolved through history. Basically, bodywork has existed as long as humans have walked the earth, used in both the spiritual and medical realms. The practice of massage has consistently been delivered by religious figures, laypersons, and folk healers, but the medical community exhibits a fluctuating pattern of acceptance and resistance of massage. Currently, the field of massage therapy is gaining acceptance in the medical community, and many people are suggesting that medical massage is a new modality. There is a push to separate medical massage treatment from spa massage, but this is really a moot point. The different applications of massage are based on the same physiological concept. In fact, some massage therapists work at both medical clinics and day spas, providing individualized treatment to all of their clients. Therapists who have sufficient academic education accompanied by adequate hands-on training can deliver the appropriate massage in any environment.

Throughout history, the associated use of massage and water therapies has also fluctuated in popularity. At this point, there is a renewed use of water and massage therapy as evidenced by hydrotherapy and spa treatments. These patterns of coexistence can be used as a guide to understand trends in the use of massage as a healthcare treatment.

Scientific research continues to prove the efficacy of massage as a medical treatment for a number of conditions and contributed to its growth in popularity. Science is showing the world the importance of touch in its many forms. Regardless of the science, there is a powerful human requirement for touch, and massage will continue to be used both intuitively as well as professionally.

History can guide us into a successful future for the world of massage therapy. Excessive growth in the field of massage in the 1800s flooded society with inadequately trained therapists. Lack of regulation and standards of practice damaged the reputation of massage, but the decline was stopped because steps were taken to legitimize the practice. Understanding historical lessons, you can better appreciate the importance of standardization and regulation to legitimization of massage therapy (Box 1-3).

CHAPTER EXERCISES

1. List at least three ancient Greek and Roman medical texts and their references to the use of massage treatment.

2. Identify at least three examples throughout history where massage was associated with the spiritual realm. Are there any scenarios in today's culture that illustrate a connection between massage and the spiritual realm?

3. Name at least four factors that influence a person's interpretation of touch. Write a paragraph describing a tactile experience with another person in which your interpretation of the event differed from theirs.

4. Draw lines to match the following individuals listed in the left column with their historical contributions listed in the right column:

Kellogg	wrote De Medicina
Vesalius	developed terminology for massage: "effleurage" "petrissage" "tapotement"
Hippocrates	popularized Movement Cure in America
Cibot	originated theory of mind-body connection "I think, therefore I am"
Per Henrik Ling	created Swedish Gymnastics
Mezger	identified physiological effects of massage in his book *The Art of Massage*
Celsus	promoted medical ethical code to "do no harm"
Taylor	translated the *Cong Fou* from Chinese to French
Field	promoted medical ethical code to treat "an eye for an eye"
Hammurabi	created anatomical illustrations focusing on musculature
Descartes	established the Touch Research Institute

Box 1-3

Suggested Web Sites for Further Information

- AMTA Foundation: www.amtafoundation.org
- *De Humani Corporis Fabrica* by Andreas Vesalius: http://www.stanford.edu/class/history13/Readings/vesalius.htm
- *De Medicina* by Aulus Cornelius Celsus: http://www.ku.edu/history/index/europe/ancient_rome/E/Roman/Texts/Celsus/1*.html
- National Library of Medicine's PubMed: www.nlm.nih.gov/nccam/camonpubmed.html
- NCCAM: www.nccam.nih.gov
- WHCCAMP's final report: www.whccamp.hhs.gov/
- World of Massage Museum: www.worldofmassagemuseum.com

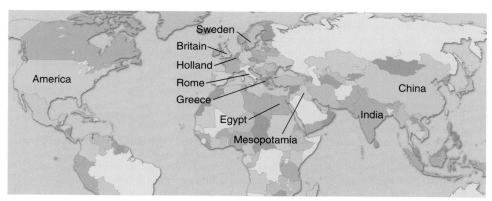

FIGURE 1-11   Global Map for Exercise 7.

5. Choose one of the following events from the history of massage. Write a paragraph about its effect on history and how history might have been different without it.

Hippocrates writes the Hippocratic Corpus
Dr. Mezger popularizes French massage terms
Dr. Kellogg studies the physiological effects of massage
The British Medical Association finds inconsistency and inadequacy in the field of massage therapy
Dr. Tiffany Field opens the Touch Research Institute

6. Organize the following historical events in chronological order and number the list:

Kahun Medical Papyrus is written in Egypt
Doctors find inconsistent and inadequate massage practices in Britain
Code of Hammurabi's medical ethics are written in Mesopotamia
Greek ritualistic health regimen included massage
Dr. Johan Mezger initiates massage terminology in Holland
Per Henrik Ling develops Swedish Gymnastics in Sweden
Ancient texts, the *Cong Fou* and the *Nei Ching*, written in China
The New York State Society of Medical Massage Therapists is the first professional American massage association
Ancient Indian scriptures, the Vedas, are written
Galen of Rome develops scientific method for research

7. Trace the history of massage across the world by using the map and events from Exercise 6. Identify the location of each event by writing its number on the map in Figure 1-11.

8. There is currently a lot of touch research being conducted in the public and private sectors. List at least three examples of massage research that you would want someone to do and explain why. (For example: I am interested in seeing how massage influences a person's physical coordination because of the neuromuscular effects on proprioceptors.)

9. Identify at least five doctors who were notable in the history of massage therapy and describe their contributions.

10. List the nine categories of bodywork, identify each one's classification as a bodywork or massage modality, and explain why it has been classified as such.

REFERENCES

1. Celsus AC. De Medicina. http://www.ku.edu/history/index/europe/ancient_rome/E/Roman/Texts/Celsus/1*.html
2. Vesalius A. De Humani Corporis Fabrica. http://www.stanford.edu/class/history13/Readings/vesalius.htm
3. Descartes R. Meditations. Veitch J (transl), 1901. http://philos.wright.edu/DesCartes/Meditation6.html
4. Kellogg JH. The Art of Massage. From the Historical Society of Battle Creek web site: http://www.geocities.com/Athens/Oracle/9840/kellogg.html
5. NCCAM web site: www.nccam.nih.gov
6. WHCCAMP web site: www.whccamp.hhs.gov/
7. Field T. Touch. Cambridge, MA: MIT Press, 2001.

SUGGESTED READINGS

Aten J. A Part of Something Great. Carthage, IL: Good Apple, 1980.
Crabtree C, Nash GB, Gagnon P, Waugh S, eds. Lessons from History, Essential Understandings and Historical Perspectives Students Should Acquire, A Project of the National Center for History in the Schools. A Cooperative UCLA/NEH Research Program. Los Angeles: National Center for History in the Schools, 1992.
DeBaz P. The Story of Medicine. New York: Philosophical Library, 1975.

Field T. Touch. Cambridge, MA: MIT Press, 2001.

Field TM, Ingatoff E, Stringer S, Brennan J, et al. Nonnutritive sucking during tube feedings: Effect on preterm neonates in an intensive care unit. Pediatrics 1982;70(3):381–384.

Finney S, Kindle P. China Then and Now, Dynasties to Dragon Boats, Pagodas to Pavilions. Carthage, IL: Good Apple, 1988.

Garrison FH. An Introduction to the History of Medicine, with Medical Chronology, Suggestions for Study and Bibliographic Data. 4th ed. Philadelphia, PA: WB Saunders, 1929.

Harlow H, Zimmerman RR. The development of affectional responses in infant monkeys. Proc Am Philos Soc 1958;102: 501–509.

Jackson R. Holistic Massage, the Holistic Way to Physical and Mental Health. New York: Sterling Publishing, 1987.

Kellogg JH. The Art of Massage. Battle Creek, MI: Modern Medicine Publishing, 1975.

Knasta M. Energy, Eastern style. Massage Ther J 1998; Fall.

Libby W. The History of Medicine in its Salient Features. Boston: Houghton Mifflin, 1922.

Partin RL. The Social Studies Teacher's Book of Lists. Englewood Cliffs, NJ: Prentice Hall, 1992.

Saunders JB de CM, O'Malley CD. The Illustrations from the Works of Andreas Vesalius of Brussels. New York: Dover Publications, 1973.

Tappan FM, Benjamin PJ. Tappan's Handbook of Healing Massage Techniques, Classic, Holistic, and Emerging Methods. Old Tappan, NJ: Appleton & Lange, 1998.

Taylor GH. A Sketch of the Movement Cure, with Illustrative Cases. New York: New York Institute for Movement Cure, 1860.

Van-Why RP. The Bodywork Knowledgebase: Lecture on the History of Massage in Four Parts. Richard P. Van-Why, 1991.

Waltz SK. Handbook of Instructional Devices for Intermediate Social Studies. Darien, CT: Teachers Publishing Corporation, 1968.

http://books.mirror.org/gb.hippocrates.html

http://emuseum.mnsu.edu/prehistory/egypt/dailylife/papyrus.html, accessed 5.3.03.

http://orientalmedicine.com/acu-faq.html, accessed 5.23.03.

http://philos.wright.edu/DesCartes/Meditation6.html, accessed 5.17.03.

http://ragz-international.com/sumeria.htm, accessed 5.2.03.

http://scriptorium.lib.duke.edu/papyrus/texts/world.html, accessed 5.4.03.

http://spas.about.com/library/weekly/aa063002ga.htm, 5.20.03.

http://www.aim25.ac.uk/cgi-bin/search2?coll_id=3919&inst_id=23, accessed 4.7.03

http://www.ama-assn.org/sci-pubs/amnews/pick_02/prca0128.htm, accessed 5.9.03.

http://www.aota.org/about.asp, accessed 5.14.03.

http://www.ayurvedicscience.com/clinic_intropage.htm#what, accessed 5.14.03.

http://www.bbc.co.uk/history/historic_figures/galen_claudius.shtml, accessed 5.9.03.

http://www.bmp.state.mn.us/Apfactsh.htm, accessed 5.14.03.

http://www.body-balancing.com/Massage_and_Spa_History.htm, 5.20.03.

http://www.careerinsports.com/sweden.html, accessed 5.20.03.

http://www.cmtbc.bc.ca/information.htm, accessed 5.14.03.

http://www.cmto.com/facts.htm, accessed 5.14.03.

http://www.compwellness.com/eGuide/deept.htm, accessed 4.7.03.

http://www.csp.org.uk/thecsp/about/history.cfm accessed 4.7.03.

http://digilander.libero.it/debibliotheca/Arte/Leonardoana_file/page_01.htm accessed 5.23.03.

http://www.experienceispa.com/conferences/articles/american_spa.html, 5.20.03.

http://www.experienceispa.com/conferences/articles/american_spa.html, 5.21.03.

http://www.experienceispa.com/learn/who_is_ispa.html, accessed 5.20.03.

http://www.famousamericans.net/georgehtaylor/ accessed 5.24.03.

http://www.fonetiks.org/sou2chx.php, accessed 5.14.03.

http://www.foot-reflexologist.com/EGYPT_1.htm, accessed 5.23.03.

http://www.geocities.com/Athens/Oracle/9840/kellogg.html, accessed 5.23.03.

http://www.geocities.com/unclesamsfarm/drtaylor.htm, accessed 5.24.03.

http://www.healthy.net/pan/pa/homeopathic/natcenhom/hnm21cen.htm, accessed 4.7.03.

http://www.healthy.net/pan/pa/homeopathic/natcenhom/WHtmed.htm, accessed 4.7.03.

http://www.kfki.hu/~arthp/html/l/leonardo/10anatom/index.html, accessed 5.23.03.

http://www.iskcon.org/main/twohk/philo/roots/script.htm, accessed 5.3.03.

http://www.itmonline.org/arts/japacu.htm, accessed 4.29.03.

http://www.ku.edu/history/index/europe/ancient_rome/E/Roman/Texts/Celsus/1*.html, accessed 5.5.03.

http://www.ku.edu/history/index/europe/ancient_rome/E/Roman/Texts/secondary/SMIGRA*/Aliptae.html, accessed 5.23.03.

http://www.ku.edu/history/index/europe/ancient_rome/E/Roman/Texts/Celsus/1*.html, accessed 5.23.03.

http://www.mendiseasestcm.com/translatione.htm, accessed 4.29.03.

http://www.meridianinstitute.com/eamt/files/articles/artfasse.htm, accessed 5.5.03.

http://www.miami.edu/touch-research, accessed 4.7.03.

http://www.miami.edu/touch-research/index.html, accessed 4.7.03.

http://www.naprapathy.edu, accessed 4.20.03.

http://www.naturalchoice.net/glossary.htm, accessed 4.20.03.

http://www.nb.no/baser/schoyen/5/5.5/#4575, accessed 5.23.03.

http://www.nb.no/baser/schoyen/5/5.5/index.html#4575, accessed 5.23.03.

http://www.ncbtmb.com/handbook/handbk1.htm#WhoIsEligible, accessed 4.7.03.

http://www.nccam.nih.gov, accessed 4.14.03.

http://www.nccam.nih.gov/nccam/an/general/index.html, accessed 4.14.03.

http://www.nefertiti.iwebland.com/timelines/topics/medicine.htm, accessed 5.3.03.

http://www.pbs.org/wgbh/aso/databank/entires/bhharl.htm, accessed 4.7.03.

http://www.petrie.ucl.ac.uk/digital_egypt/med/birthpapyrus.html, accessed 5.23.03.

http://www.petrie.ucl.ac.uk/digital_egypt/lahun/ucarchivelahun/uc32057page1-2small.gif, accessed 5.23.03.

http://www.qigonghealing.com/html/qigong.html, accessed 4.29.03.

http://www.spamassagealliance.com/researchlibrary/article.asp?id=7, accessed 5.20.03.

http://www.spas.about.com/library/weekly/aa030199.htm, accessed 5.20.03.

http://www.spa-therapy.com/about_history.asp, 5.21.03.

http://www.stanford.edu/class/history13/Readings/vesalius.htm, accessed 5.12.03.

http://www.thebodyworker.com/history.htm, accessed, 4.7.03

http://www.unani.com/avicennastory2.htm, accessed 5.23.03.

http://www.vitinc.com/pdoa/podiatry.html, accessed 5.20.03.

http://www.whccamp.hhs.gov/, accessed 4.15.03.

http://www.wischik.com/marcus/essay/med2.html, accessed 5.6.03.

https://www.apta.org/Consumer/whoareptsptas/profile, accessed 4.8.03.

Ethics and Professionalism

UPON COMPLETION OF THIS CHAPTER, THE STUDENT WILL BE ABLE TO:

- Identify the four characteristics of a profession
- Describe the general scope of practice for massage therapy
- Explain how a code of ethics affects the massage therapy profession
- Identify the two different levels of massage therapy scope of practice
- Identify seven steps for resolving an ethical dilemma
- List five aspects of a massage therapist's professional attire
- Identify at least two professional massage therapy associations
- List at least three business practices that demonstrate professionalism
- Define a dual relationship

KEY TERMS

Accountability: the quality of accepting the consequences of your actions and claiming responsibility for your decisions

Certification: the act of issuing someone a certificate of completion or validation of authenticity

Client-centered: when attitudes, decisions, and activities of a practice are in the best interest of the client's health and well being

Code of ethics: commonly accepted guidelines or principles of conduct that govern professional conduct

Confidentiality: the principle that client information revealed to a health professional during an appointment is to be kept private and has limits on how and when it can be disclosed to a third party

Ethics: conduct rules based on integrity and differentiating right from wrong

Informed consent: a client's agreement to participate in an activity after the purpose, methods, benefits, risks, and rights to withdraw at any time have been explained

Licensure: legal authority or permission to practice massage when the state laws or regulations require it

Professionalism: ethical conduct, goals, and qualities characterized by a profession

Registration: the act of enrolling in a system or database that keeps track of recorded information

Scope of practice: a practitioner's service limits and boundaries as determined by legal, educational, competency, and accountability factors

Standards of practice: specific rules and procedures for professional conduct and quality of care that are to be followed by all members of a profession

Ethics and professionalism are the cornerstones of a successful massage practice. The massage therapy profession follows a set of guiding principles based on right and wrong, commonly referred to as **ethics.** They provide guidelines for appropriate and safe decisions and behaviors. The fundamental ethical principle for massage therapy is **client-centered care,** which focuses all of the attitudes, decisions, and activities on whatever is best for the client's health and well being. Client-centered care is the key component that determines a therapist's **professionalism,** which is the combined qualities of integrity, competency, effective communication and interpersonal skills, respectful behavior, and good business practices. Ethics and professionalism are closely intertwined and sometimes inseparable as they reinforce and support each other. The relationships you develop as a professional can be complicated and rewarding, but ethics and professionalism can provide guidance. There are some specific concepts outlined in this chapter that can help to establish and maintain appropriate, professional relationships. Combining ethics and integrity with professionalism establishes a foundation for developing yourself as an effective, successful, professional massage therapist.

Characteristics of a Profession

A profession is an occupation that requires a specialized academic education and is characterized by specialized education, scope of practice, code of ethics, and standards of practice. The massage therapy profession requires a lot of academic knowledge and hands-on training, and each of these components is of equal importance. You can learn massage from a book without practicing on a person; however, without adequate anatomy and physiology knowledge, your massage may be harmful to your clients. A **scope of practice** outlines the limits of a massage therapist's service determined by legal, educational, and competency factors. The scope of practice for massage therapy has yet to be standardized, but the determining factors could lead to the development of two separate scopes within the profession: a wellness massage scope of practice and a therapeutic massage scope of practice. There is a **code of ethics,** or commonly accepted guidelines or principles of conduct, that governs professional conduct. **Standards of practice** are specific rules and procedures for professional conduct and quality of care that all members of a profession should follow. These standards involve the public image of a practitioner as well as the legal and ethical obligations that protect both clients and therapists. Unfortunately, the current massage therapy profession has not been standardized, and as a result, there is some confusion within and from outside the profession regarding education, scope of practice, code of ethics, and standards of practice. The professional characteristics outlined by some of the current professional massage associations are fairly similar and are used as a basis for the information in this chapter.

EDUCATION

Massage is a hands-on activity that requires hands-on training. Massage also requires scientific education because therapists need to understand what tissues are being touched and how the body responds to the touch. Both of these aspects of a high-quality massage education are equally important, but you may find one easier than the other. Some persons find that when they have their hands on a human being to practice techniques, everything makes sense and comes easily, but when they read the textbooks and do the homework, it is a struggle. Others sail through the academic work without trouble, but find that when they put their hands on a body, nothing makes sense. In both of these situations, there may be frustration and disappointment. Remember that this is a learning process that will take time and effort. Although it may not be easy, your massage education will help you understand more about yourself and will provide a solid foundation for building a successful practice.

Historical Perspective of Massage Education

Recognizing the historical events in massage therapy education can be used to guide future education in a better direction by preventing similar unfortunate outcomes. Very early on, many ancient medical practices were passed down from generation to generation or from masters to apprentices. Massage and other forms of natural treatment were taught as part of the medical treatments. Later, as massage became more popular with patients, the hospitals developed specific educational programs for massage, and British nurses started studying massage therapy. The reputation of massage was so quickly rising that it became a very popular occupation. Unfortunately, along with the many massage therapists with a good education, there were also a number of poorly trained therapists flooding the market. At the time, lack of regulation resulted in unqualified teachers, inferior schools, incompetent therapists, and unscrupulous practices. There was downfall in the reputation of massage therapy that led to a split between professional massage therapists and those with little or no formal training. The division allowed massage to continue its acceptance within the medical community, and the lack of regulation started a movement toward legitimizing the practice.

As illustrated in Chapter 1, massage therapy prevailed, and several techniques of massage and bodywork were created during the 19th century (see Fig. 1-8, Timeline of bodywork and massage). In the 1960s, massage experienced a revival in America. The long-time tradition of passing massage from person to person became more prevalent. One place

---

Box 2-1

AMTA Scope of Practice (this is NOT a legally binding scope of practice!)

AMTA defines the Scope of Practice of its members as follows:

Massage or massage therapy is any skilled manipulation of soft tissue, connective tissue, and/or body energy fields with the intention of maintaining or improving health by affecting change in relaxation, circulation, nerve responses, or patterns of energy flow.

Massage or massage therapy may be accomplished manually with or without the use of the following: movement, superficial heat or cold, electrical or mechanical devices, water, lubricants, or salts.

---

normal massage education resurfaced was at the Esalen Institute in Big Sur, California. History was repeated as massage education became a widely variable experience.

Current Perspective of Massage Education

As the popularity of massage continues, there are a myriad of avenues for massage education today. You can find courses that only take a couple of days to programs that last 2 years. You will see programs that offer absolutely no anatomy or physiology, and you will find programs that study human cadavers to learn human anatomy. Some therapists receive a certificate of completion and consider themselves "certified," and others are required to pass a national written exam to be considered "certified." Regulation of the profession exists in some states, but not all, and you will find that the level of education varies from state to state. Standardizing massage education will benefit therapists, clients, and the profession.

In states without massage regulation, massage continues to be taught through apprenticeship or by schools and instructors that may have different levels of experience and/or varied qualifications. That is not to say that unregulated states have unqualified or incompetent educators, but you cannot assume that the educators are qualified. In fact, there are some excellent massage training programs in unregulated states.

Currently, it is difficult to determine the information that is fundamental to the entry-level massage therapist. With enough motivation and support, massage education will continue to evolve toward a more specific knowledge base requirement for entry into the profession.

Education should not end once you have entered the profession. You can continue to develop professionally by taking continuing education classes. There

are hundreds, possibly thousands, of courses offered around the world that teach various specialties of massage and bodywork. By continuing the educational process you show your concern and dedication to the wealth of knowledge that exists in the field of massage. In turn, you may share that knowledge and expertise with your clients. **Knowledge is power!**

SCOPE OF PRACTICE

Boundaries exist in all aspects of life, and although they are be seen by some as constraints, they give everyone the same ground rules and provide everyone with an aspect of safety by giving us a better idea of what to expect. Massage therapists provide a service that is limited by legal, educational, and competency factors. Collectively, these boundaries are called the scope of practice. They paint a clear picture of which services are and are not acceptable for massage therapists to provide. The American Massage Therapy Association (AMTA) is one of the largest professional massage organizations in the country. Its scope of practice is a short description of the activities that are considered massage therapy by the AMTA. One must understand that this is a scope of practice as the professional organization defines it, and that it is NOT a legally binding document. See Box 2-1 for the AMTA scope of practice.

Some, but not all, states have created legislation to regulate the massage therapy profession. In those states, the scope of practice has been outlined for practice protection, which identifies specific activities that determine who is and who is not considered a part of that practice. The scopes of practice vary from state to state, so you can consult Box 2-2 for a

---

Box 2-2

Web Sites for Further Information

American Massage Therapy Association (AMTA) web site: www.amtamassage.org
Associated Bodywork and Massage Professionals (ABMP) web site: www.abmp.com
Constitutions, statutes, legislative information, Cornell Law School's Legal Information Institute web site: http://www.law.cornell.edu/statutes.html
National Certification for Therapeutic Massage and Bodywork (NCBTMB) web site: www.ncbtmb.com
Nationwide massage therapy laws:
  AMTA web site:
    http://www.amtamassage.org/about/lawstateguide.htm
  careeratyourfingertips.com web site:
    http://www.careeratyourfingertips.com/laws.htm
State and federal listings for laws regarding abuse and neglect: http://www.prevent-abuse-now.com/govhome.htm

web site that will refer you to nationwide massage therapy laws. Box 2-3 shows Ohio's brief but thorough legal description of massage.

Currently, the scope of practice for massage therapy is not standardized, but the factors used to determine it may lead to the development of two separate scopes within the profession. Wellness massage is provided for general relaxation and health maintenance. Its primary intent is to increase circulation for general physiological benefit. The therapist typically uses only basic massage strokes and does not address specific muscular conditions or client complaints.

Therapeutic massage requires a higher level of education and uses advanced massage techniques. These techniques are covered in the hands-on and therapeutic application chapters later in the text. With a thorough understanding of anatomy and physiology and with practical knowledge of specific techniques, the scope of practice for therapeutic massage is wider. It allows therapists to treat clients with specific muscular or soft tissue conditions and complaints of pain or dysfunction.

CODE OF ETHICS

In the same way that a scope of practice limits the services a massage therapist can perform, a code of ethics is a set of principles or guidelines for decisions and professional conduct that all massage therapists should follow. It serves as a basis for establishing and maintaining the reputation of massage therapists as honest, respectable professionals. Codes of ethics are often established by professional organizations as guidelines for their members to use in their practices. At the same time, a code of ethics helps the public understand the expected behavior of professional massage therapists.

Box 2-3

State Medical Board of Ohio's Scope of Practice for Massage

4731-1-05 Scope of practice: massage.

(A) Massage is limited to the treatment of disorders of the human body by the systematic external application of touch, stroking, friction, vibration, percussion, kneading, stretching, compression, and passive joint movements within the normal physiologic range of motion; and adjunctive thereto, the external application of water, heat, cold, topical preparations, and mechanical devices.

(B) A practitioner of massage shall not diagnose a patient's condition except as to whether the application of massage is advisable. In determining whether the application of massage is advisable, a practitioner of massage shall be limited to taking a written or verbal inquiry, visual inspection, touch, and the taking of a pulse, temperature and blood pressure.

(C) A practitioner of massage may treat temporomandibular joint dysfunction provided that the patient has been directly referred in writing for such treatment to the practitioner of massage by a physician currently licensed pursuant to Chapter 4731. of the Revised Code, by a chiropractor currently licensed pursuant to Chapter 4734. of the Revised Code, or a dentist currently licensed pursuant to Chapter 4715. of the Revised Code.

(D) Massage does not include:
 (1) The application of high velocity-low amplitude force;
 (2) The application of ultrasound, diathermy, and electrical neuromuscular stimulation or substantially similar modalities; and
 (3) Colonic irrigation.

(E) As used within this rule:
 (1) "External" does not prohibit a practitioner from performing massage inside the mouth or oral cavity; and
 (2) "Mechanical devices" means any tool or device which mimics or enhances the actions possible by the hands.

Box 2-4

American Massage Therapy Association Code of Ethics

This Code of Ethics is a summary statement of the standards by which massage therapists agree to conduct their practices and is a declaration of the general principles of acceptable, ethical, professional behavior.

Massage therapists shall:
1. Demonstrate commitment to provide the highest quality massage therapy/bodywork to those who seek their professional service.
2. Acknowledge the inherent worth and individuality of each person by not discriminating or behaving in any prejudicial manner with clients and/or colleagues.
3. Demonstrate professional excellence through regular self-assessment of strengths, limitations, and effectiveness by continued education and training.
4. Acknowledge the confidential nature of the professional relationship with clients and respect each client's right to privacy.
5. Conduct all business and professional activities within their scope of practice, the law of the land, and project a professional image.
6. Refrain from engaging in any sexual conduct or sexual activities involving their clients.
7. Accept responsibility to do no harm to the physical, mental and emotional well being of self, clients, and associates.

The AMTA's code of ethics includes seven guidelines for the profession that address high-quality service, respect for others, self-assessment, confidentiality, scope of practice, professionalism, the exclusion of sexual activity, and the promise to intend no harm. Box 2-4 lists the AMTA code of ethics.

The Associated Bodywork and Massage Professionals (ABMP) is a membership organization that includes a variety of bodywork therapists and esthetic professionals. Its professional code of ethics is separated into four sections: client relationships, professionalism, scope of practice and image/advertising claims. It covers client-centered care, quality service, confidentiality, self-assessment, exclusion of sexual

activity, specifies professional behaviors that are acceptable and not acceptable, specifies scope of practice limitations, specifies a physiological understanding to determine when to use and when not to use techniques and stresses professional public image, public education and honest advertising. Box 2-5 includes the ABMP professional code of ethics.

As you can see by the examples, these codes look very different on a quick glance, but their content is similar. It may seem like common sense to follow these codes, but ethical conduct is not always clear cut. There are many situations in which the ethical decision between one choice and another is unclear and difficult. Codes of ethics are not just the rules and

---

Box 2-5

ABMP Code of Ethics

Professional Code of Ethics

As a member of Associated Bodywork & Massage Professionals, I hereby pledge to abide by the ABMP Code of Ethics as outlined below.

Client Relationships

I shall endeavor to serve the best interests of my clients at all times and to provide the highest quality service possible.

I shall maintain clear and honest communications with my clients and shall keep client communications confidential.

I shall acknowledge the limitations of my skills and, when necessary, refer clients to the appropriate qualified health care professional.

I shall in no way instigate or tolerate any kind of sexual advance while acting in the capacity of a massage, bodywork, somatic therapy or esthetic practitioner.

Professionalism

I shall maintain the highest standards of professional conduct, providing services in an ethical and professional manner in relation to my clientele, business associates, health care professionals, and the general public.

I shall respect the rights of all ethical practitioners and will cooperate with all health care professionals in a friendly and professional manner.

I shall refrain from the use of any mind-altering drugs, alcohol, or intoxicants prior to or during professional sessions.

I shall always dress in a professional manner, proper dress being defined as attire suitable and consistent with accepted business and professional practice.

I shall not be affiliated with or employed by any business that utilizes any form of sexual suggestiveness or explicit sexuality in its advertising or promotion of services, or in the actual practice of its services.

Scope of Practice/Appropriate Techniques

I shall provide services within the scope of the ABMP definition of massage, bodywork, somatic therapies and skin care, and the limits of my training. I will not employ those

massage, bodywork or skin care techniques for which I have not had adequate training and shall represent my education, training, qualifications and abilities honestly.

I shall be conscious of the intent of the services that I am providing and shall be aware of and practice good judgment regarding the application of massage, bodywork or somatic techniques utilized.

I shall not perform manipulations or adjustments of the human skeletal structure, diagnose, prescribe or provide any other service, procedure or therapy which requires a license to practice chiropractic, osteopathy, physical therapy, podiatry, orthopedics, psychotherapy, acupuncture, dermatology, cosmetology, or any other profession or branch of medicine unless specifically licensed to do so.

I shall be thoroughly educated and understand the physiological effects of the specific massage, bodywork, somatic or skin care techniques utilized in order to determine whether such application is contraindicated and/or to determine the most beneficial techniques to apply to a given individual. I shall not apply massage, bodywork, somatic or skin care techniques in those cases where they may be contraindicated without a written referral from the client's primary care provider.

Image/Advertising Claims

I shall strive to project a professional image for myself, my business or place of employment, and the profession in general.

I shall actively participate in educating the public regarding the actual benefits of massage, bodywork, somatic therapies and skin care.

I shall practice honesty in advertising, promote my services ethically and in good taste, and practice and/or advertise only those techniques for which I have received adequate training and/or certification. I shall not make false claims regarding the potential benefits of the techniques rendered.

Box 2-6

AMTA Standards of Practice Document

Purpose Statement: These American Massage Therapy Association (AMTA) Standards of Practice were developed to assist the professional massage therapist to:
- provide safe, consistent care
- determine the quality of care provided
- provide a common base to develop a practice
- support/preserve the basic rights of the client and professional massage therapist
- assist the public to understand what to expect from a professional massage therapist

This document allows the professional massage therapist to evaluate and adapt performance in his/her massage/bodywork practice. The professional massage therapist can evaluate the quality of his/her practice by utilizing the Standards of Practice in conjunction with the Code of Ethics, the Bylaws and Policies of AMTA, and precedents set by the AMTA Grievance, Standards, and Bylaws Committees.

1. Conduct of the Professional Massage Therapist or Practitioner, hereinafter referred to as "Practitioner"
   - AMTA members must meet and maintain appropriate membership requirements.
   - Individual AMTA members who engage in the practice of professional massage/bodywork, shall adhere to standards of professional conduct, including the AMTA Code of Ethics.
   - The Practitioner follows consistent standards in all settings.
   - The Practitioner seeks professional supervision/consultation consistent with promoting and maintaining appropriate application of skills and knowledge.

2. Sanitation, Hygiene and Safety
   - Practitioner provides an environment consistent with accepted standards of sanitation, hygiene, safety and universal precautions.
   - Pathophysiology (Contraindications)
   - The Practitioner maintains current knowledge and skills of pathophysiology and the appropriate application of massage/bodywork.
   - The Practitioner monitors feedback from the client throughout a session.
   - The Practitioner makes appropriate referrals to other reputable healthcare providers.

3. Professional Relationships with Clients
   - The Practitioner relates to the client in a manner consistent with accepted standards and ethics.
   - The Practitioner maintains appropriate professional standards of confidentiality.
   - The Practitioner relates to the client in a manner which respects the integrity of the client and practitioner.
   - The Practitioner ensures that representations of his/her professional services, policies, and procedures are accurately communicated to the client prior to the initial application of massage/bodywork.
   - The Practitioner elicits participation and feedback from the client.

4. Professional Relationships with Other Professionals
   - The Practitioner relates to other reputable professionals with appropriate respect and within the parameters of accepted ethical standards.
   - The Practitioner's referrals to other professionals are only made in the interest of the client.
   - The Practitioner's communication with other professionals regarding clients is in compliance with accepted standards and ethics.
   - A Practitioner possessing knowledge that another practitioner:
     1. Committed a criminal act that reflects adversely on the Practitioner's competence in massage therapy, trustworthiness or fitness to practice massage therapy in other respects;
     2. Engaged in an act or practice that significantly undermines the massage therapy profession; or
     3. Engaged in conduct that creates a risk of serious harm for the physical or emotional well being of a recipient of massage therapy; shall report such knowledge to the appropriate AMTA committee if such information is not protected or restricted by a confidentiality law.

5. Records
   - Client Records: Practitioner establishes and maintains appropriate client records.
   - Financial Records: Practitioner establishes and maintains client financial accounts that follow accepted accounting practices.

6. Marketing
   - Marketing consists of, but is not limited to, advertising, public relations, promotion and publicity.
   - The Practitioner markets his/her practice in an accurate, truthful and ethical manner.

7. Legal Practice
   - American Massage Therapy Association members practice or collaborate with all others practicing professional massage/bodywork in a manner that is in compliance with national, state or local municipal law(s) pertaining to the practice of professional massage/bodywork.

8. Research
   - The Practitioner engaged in study and/or research is guided by the conventions and ethics of scholarly inquiry.
   - The Practitioner doing research avoids financial or political relationships that may limit objectivity or create conflict of interest.

regulations set forth by a profession to dictate what is right or wrong, they are living documents that continually evolve and serve to guide you in your words and actions.

STANDARDS OF PRACTICE

Standards of practice give the members of a profession a specific set of rules and procedures that help provide clients with a law-abiding, safe environment in a professional atmosphere. Basically, they include everything that contributes to high-quality care and client safety: professionalism, legal responsibilities, relationships, business practices, sanitation, hygiene, and safety. Professionalism, legal and ethical issues, and relationships are covered in this chapter, however business practice, hygiene, sanitation, and safety are detailed later in the text.

The ABMP does not have a separate document for its standards of practice because it has addressed the topics of professionalism and relationships in its code of ethics.

The AMTA has established its standards of practice to help its members provide safe and consistent care, determine quality of care, develop a practice, and protect and preserve client and therapist rights. It also gives the public a general understanding and expectation of professional massage therapy. Included are the topics of professional conduct, sanitation and safety, relationships with clients and other professionals, record keeping, marketing, legalities, and research. Box 2-6 includes the AMTA standards of practice.

Scope of Practice

The scope of practice for massage therapists is important to understand, especially as massage therapy evolves as a profession. The scope of practice identifies the limits and boundaries for a practitioner and is determined by several factors, including the law, education, and competency. The massage therapy scope of practice outlines

- Which activities are allowed
- When specific methods are used
- Where specific methods are applied
- How specific methods are applied
- Why specific methods are used

Generally, massage therapists are allowed to perform manipulation on the soft tissues or energetic fields of the body; however, they are prohibited from diagnosing medical conditions or prescribing specific treat-

ments, and they are prohibited from intentional joint manipulation and skeletal realignment.

LEGAL REGULATIONS

Government agencies and professional associations establish regulations for the practice of massage therapy. Since the United States has not standardized the scope of practice for massage, scopes vary from state to state. For example, some states include Reiki in the massage therapy scope of practice and require Reiki practitioners to conform to the same regulations as massage therapists. Other states exclude Reiki from the massage therapy scope, which gives the practitioners more freedom. Regulation is not intended to remove freedoms from practitioners, but many people equate regulation with restraint. Actually, its intention is to attempt to separate professional massage therapists from those who have unscrupulous practices. Some regulations even specify appropriate and inappropriate locations for practicing massage. Regulation intends to provide the public with a more dependable and qualified pool of massage therapists and motivate the profession to maintain high educational and ethical standards.

State, county, and local governments regulate the scope of massage therapy practice through the processes of licensure, certification, and registration. These terms are used interchangeably with vague and sometimes combined definitions, so it is especially important to learn about your own local laws and regulations before starting a practice. There are generally accepted definitions for licensure, certification, and registration that we have outlined below, but again, check your local regulations before assuming these definitions.

Licensure is the process of obtaining a license from the state government. Some states require that you have a license to practice massage therapy, making it illegal to practice massage without a license in those states. Licensure is intended to identify a level of proficiency that the state considers acceptable and safe. Typically, licensure requires a certain level of educational training or experience and the successful completion of some form of evaluation or testing. Licensure may also include title protection, which gives people who hold a license the exclusive use of particular titles such as "massage therapist," "massage practitioner," and "licensed massage therapist."

Certification is also a process of validation and authentication, but is usually voluntary. Certification programs are generally offered by nongovernmental agencies or organizations as a way to identify practitioners with advanced knowledge or skills. As with licensure, certification requires evaluation by the organizational body as well as sufficient education or experience. Certification is a form of title protection in which only persons who hold a certificate can identify themselves as "certified," but this can lead to some confusion. Unfortunately, there are persons who receive a certificate of completion for a 2-day course and consider themselves certified. True certification is typically granted by an organization that did not provide the education and can make an objective evaluation of the practitioner.

Registration is a process that allows an organization to keep track of therapists in a database. Some state government agencies, such as the Texas Department of Health, require massage therapists to hold a certificate of registration to practice massage therapy. To be eligible for registration, there are educational requirements, fees, and examinations, making the process very similar to licensure in other states. In essence, the registration policy in Texas is more of a licensure policy, differing mostly in terminology. Texas outlines the scope of practice for massage therapy that determines who is required to register as a massage therapist. Texas also includes an ineligibility statement that precludes a therapist from being registered if there is any kind of sexual misconduct conviction on public record. In addition to the other requirements, massage therapists in Texas have continuing education criteria. By keeping track of its registered massage therapists, the state has more control over who is practicing massage. Again, some may consider governmental regulation to be overbearing and controlling, but it is implemented with a client-centered philosophy.

Certification and licensure are the primary forms of regulation that promise consumer protection by requiring therapists to renew their credentials periodically with specific requirements for renewal and by creating an agency that can verify credentials, investigate and process grievances, and enforce discipline when necessary (Table 2-1).

EDUCATION

There is a basic level of knowledge required to practice massage that is used to determine the scope of practice. With the varied lengths and types of massage education and training programs, it has been difficult to establish consistent massage therapy regulations for scope of practice. Generally, massage programs teach some anatomy and physiology, massage techniques, hygiene and sanitation, ethics, and business practices, but the depth to which these topics are studied and the emphasis put on different topics is unique to each school. Regulation may define the number of hours required for training, but it does not guarantee the same knowledge base from gradu-

TABLE 2-1	
Licensure versus Certification	
LICENSURE	**CERTIFICATION**
Law that is **mandatory**	Law that is **voluntary**
Sets a scope of practice whose application **legally requires** practitioner to hold a license	Sets a scope of practice for **illustrative purposes** only
Usually lists some titles that legally require a license	**Always** specifies one or more titles that legally require certification
Restrictive levels of practice are established, such as wellness and therapeutic massage applications	Certification at higher levels of education could be built over a licensure program
It is mandatory, which implies that local laws are automatically preempted by state regulation	
It is mandatory, so practitioners who engage in related professions may need to be identified for exemption from licensure	It is voluntary, so it does not create exemption for other practices
It is mandatory, so any new licensing laws usually allow preexisting practitioners to be grandfathered into the new laws	It is voluntary, so there are no grandfathering provisions necessary for any new laws

ates of different schools. In states without regulation, the common knowledge base may be even more difficult to determine.

Massage schools or training programs may need to be accredited by a state education agency, meaning that the state has specific requirements for establishing any educational institution. Basically, the state tries to determine a school's legitimacy by investigating funding, intended location, property procurement, short- and long-term business plans, as well as the qualifications of the person interested in starting the school. Today, accredited massage training programs are offered by massage therapists turned educators, proprietary vocational schools, community colleges, and cosmetology schools.

Additionally, there are a myriad of continuing education options available after graduation. While regulations serve as a guide for initial training, adopting specialties through continuing education creates a unique scope of practice for each therapist. For example, a massage therapist who takes continuing education classes in neuromuscular therapy and craniosacral therapy may have a clientele and an approach to bodywork that differs from someone who takes classes in polarity and Reiki. These two therapists have different scopes of practice because of their education and competency.

COMPETENCY

In addition to education, scope of practice is influenced by the issue of competency. Competency raises two particularly poignant questions: What skills should an entry-level therapist have? What determines competency? At the time of publication, formal education hours and written and practical examinations are used to determine the laws and regulations for competency. The educational requirement for entry-level therapists in most regulated states generally begins at 500 hours and goes up from there. States that require licensure, certification, or registration may require continuing education courses and renewal examinations, both of which promote competency.

Academic knowledge is simple enough to test and evaluate, but as discussed in Chapter 1, touch is influenced by age, gender, experience, and emotions. Massage is especially difficult to measure objectively because of the perception of touch and the unique experience that each person experiences with touch. Practical examinations may determine general competence because the person who receives the massage can judge the therapist's knowledge, technique, and concern for safety. Some aspects of a practical examination are subjective, but it is difficult to fake competence when giving a massage.

While the determination of competency for entry into the massage profession is more established at this time, determining competency within specialized studies remains an issue. There are continuing education courses and workshops ranging in duration from a few hours to several years. The massage therapy profession is currently faced with the question of how to determine when a therapist is considered competent in a particular or specialty method. Polarity therapy, Reiki, craniosacral therapy, and shiatsu are some examples of bodywork modalities that are often introduced in massage school, but specialized, intense certification programs with hundreds of hours of education are available in each of these modalities. Some therapists consider the introductory education sufficient, but others recognize certification as a sign of competency.

National Certification Board for Therapeutic Massage and Bodywork

In 1992, the AMTA created the National Certification Board for Therapeutic Massage and Bodywork (NCBTMB). The NCBTMB offers an examination for National Certification in Therapeutic Massage and Bodywork (NCTMB) that has become the standard test for licensure in most of the states that currently regulate massage. The NCBTMB, which now operates independently from the AMTA, aims to establish and improve the basic competency parameters, provide a standard of proficiency, and promote professionalism for massage therapists in the United States.

Currently, national certification requires therapists to meet educational and eligibility criteria, pass a written examination, uphold the NCBTMB code of ethics and standards of practice, perform at least 200 hands-on hours or equivalent, complete a course on professional ethics, and continue their education in approved courses. It is a voluntary certification except when state licensure requires it. At the time of publication, 60,000 massage therapists have their NCTMB, and it is the closest thing we have to a national standard for massage therapy. Massage therapists who want to portray a professional image may want to consider becoming nationally certified.

In January, 2003, the NCBTMB established two new credentials that offer separate regulations for massage and bodywork: National Certification in Therapeutic Massage (NCTM) and the National Certification in Therapeutic Massage-Advanced (NCTM-A). These two new credentials require therapists to adhere to strict eligibility requirements, pass a rigorous examination, and observe NCBTMB's standards of practice and code of ethics. NCTM is an entry-level credential that certifies a practitioner's competence specifically in massage therapy and allows him or her to take higher-level courses and advanced techniques. Eventually, therapists with NCTM can take the NCTM-A examination, which is an advanced practice certification in massage therapy that represents advanced knowledge, skills, and abilities.

LIMITS OF PRACTICE

Although the specifics of massage therapy's scope of practice vary from state to state, there is enough consistency to understand the general limits of practice. Still, without specific limits, you have to make judgment calls regarding acceptable activity, which can lead to confusion. Limiting the practice can benefit clients by giving them an opportunity to seek treatment from several different people, all with different specialties and different scopes of practice. Often, it may be in the client's best interest to rely on a team of healthcare professionals instead of one person. There is no cure-all, and likewise, there is no individual who provides all facets of healthcare.

Given the factors that determine scope of practice, including legal, educational, and competency, the limits of practice can be applied within the field of massage therapy. As mentioned above, the NCBTMB offers three separate levels of certification to indicate the practitioner's level of skill. There is certification for therapeutic massage and bodywork, for entry-level massage, and for advanced massage.

Wellness Massage Scope of Practice

Wellness massage uses basic massage strokes to promote circulation, encourage relaxation, and reduce stress. The therapist's basic education will include general anatomy, physiology, and pathology as well as basic techniques for normalizing and treating soft tissue to promote homeostasis in the body. The NCTM certification is adequate for the wellness massage scope of practice, which does not require advanced knowledge or skill.

Therapeutic Massage Scope of Practice

Therapeutic massage intertwines the normalization of soft tissues with rehabilitative treatment. In addition to the basic knowledge for wellness massage, therapists will understand physical assessment, injury and tissue repair mechanisms, structural compensation patterns, and treatment techniques for soft tissue rehabilitation. This type of training allows therapists a wider scope of practice that includes treatment of specific soft tissue conditions and pain patterns and can be certified with NCTM-A.

Clients seeking therapeutic massage treatment may be under the care of another healthcare professional. If so, the therapist has an ethical responsibility to work cooperatively with the other caregivers to make sure that everyone is aware of all concurrent treatments, as they may compromise or enhance each other. **Overtreating is worse than not treating at all and may make the condition worse.** This concept is important for you to know when there are numerous treatments being used at the same time. The interactions can affect the client's well being, and sometimes not for the better. This goes for pharmaceutical medications as well as complementary therapies, which is evidenced by the computer crosschecking procedures that pharmacies install to avoid dangerous drug interactions that could go unnoticed.

In both wellness and therapeutic massage one must be able to evaluate a client's condition to determine whether a more thorough examination or medical diagnosis may be necessary and whether the client can safely receive massage. The client may need to be referred to another healthcare professional or refused massage treatment at the time. A massage therapist who is only qualified for wellness massage has an ethical responsibility to stay away from the therapeutic massage scope of practice by recognizing and respecting the limits of wellness massage. The scope of practice for therapeutic massage has more educational requirements and a higher competency level, allowing the therapist to provide more services to more clients. Also remember that if you are trained in therapeutic massage there are still limits, and as an ethical and professional therapist, you will not go beyond your scope of practice either.

Ethics

Everyone has a conscience. It is an internal feeling or regard for fairness or a sense of obligation to do the right thing. In essence, your conscience makes ethical decisions by helping you determine whether your behavior is acceptable or not. The decisions and behaviors regulated by your conscience are called ethics. You make ethical choices in your decisions and daily activities in your personal life, but you also use ethics in your professional life.

Ethics are one of the cornerstones of a successful massage practice, as they help you distinguish right from wrong and are established to keep you within your scope of practice and maintain client-centered care. An ethical practice is one that demonstrates the code of ethics in its attitudes, policies, procedures, and relationships. It not only serves the client and therapist's best interest, it supports and maintains the reputation of the profession as a whole. Remember, a code of ethics is only a guideline for behavior. The extent to which you follow the code depends on your conscience and your willingness to be responsible for your behavior.

ACCOUNTABILITY

Accountability is the quality of accepting the consequences of your actions and claiming responsibility for your decisions. Accountability requires that you look beyond the immediate moment or situation and consider all the consequences that may be your responsibility. Ethical behavior is influenced by our accountability when we choose to behave a certain way and are willing to accept the results of that behavior. Professional massage therapists understand the generally accepted scope of practice, they understand the repercussions of unacceptable behavior, and they make their own choices about what happens in the treatment room. In addition to holding yourself accountable for your behavior, you can also be held accountable by your clients, by a professional organization, by the profession as a whole, by your community, or by the law.

You have to be honest with yourself and others regarding the techniques and services you provide. Going outside your scope of practice is unethical behavior and, depending upon the situation, may be illegal. For example, telling a client to take ibuprofen for inflammation from an injury may be considered diagnosing, prescribing, or even practicing medicine without a license. These activities are out of the massage therapist's scope of practice, and it is against the law to perform them. On the other hand, recommending that the client apply ice to an area that has received specific massage treatment is most likely within the scope of practice for massage therapy.

Rules exist in all aspects of life, but it is an individual's choice to follow them. It is your responsibility to keep yourself within the limits set by regulation, certification, scope of practice, or membership in a professional organization. Your words and actions will affect the world around you and the massage therapy profession as a whole. Make thoughtful decisions based on accountability to maintain your integrity and stay within your scope of practice.

ETHICS FOR THE PROFESSION

Professional ethics are rules for acceptable behavior that are set forth for all members of a profession to follow to ensure a client-centered philosophy and maintain the integrity of the profession. You not only have a responsibility to use professional ethics in your own practice, but also have a responsibility to make sure your peers are practicing professional ethics. The reputation of the entire profession is at stake, and unethical behavior on the part of one massage therapist can quickly spread through a community and damage the reputation of massage for years.

At some point during your career, you may suspect a colleague of unethical or illegal behavior. This can be an awkward and difficult position. Sometimes we have been taught to mind our own business and that nobody likes a tattletale, and sometimes we feel compelled to rectify an inappropriate, unfair, or improper situation. If you suspect that a colleague has behaved unethically or illegally in some way, you have to decide whether you will attempt to investigate the situation further. It may be possible to resolve the situation without help, but it is probably better to let an outside source, such as a professional organization or the government, resolve the issue.

Reporting Unethical Activity

Professional organizations want to uphold their codes of ethics and are willing to spend time and resources to make sure that their members maintain a good reputation. The AMTA and the ABMP both have formal grievance procedures. The first step usually requires you to submit a description of the facts and nature of the suspected violation in writing. Once the grievance has been filed, the therapist in question will be informed of the suspected incident. From there, the rest of the resolution process is kept confidential, usually handled by the Board of Directors unless objective mediation or legal action is deemed necessary.

Resolving an ethical dilemma can be complicated if the therapist in question is not a member of a professional organization. You may need to look into the local or state laws that apply to massage therapy. In the states that do not regulate massage therapy with licensure, local regulations govern the practice of massage therapy. State licensure laws usually supersede the local regulation, meaning that the state laws carry more weight and are more consequential than the local laws. Each locale or state has its own process for filing and handling complaints and suspected illegal activity.

An example is Washington State's Department of Health Complaint and Disciplinary Process[1]. There are more than a dozen people designated by the Department of Health to be the decision makers. They review incoming complaints and determine whether public safety or a person's health may be affected by the situation in question. If health or safety is in danger, an investigation will be made. Disciplinary action can be applied in the form of a lawsuit, fines, limitations imposed on the practice, or suspension from practice. Washington's State Department of Health claims responsibility to public protection by imposing the disciplinary action, but they also attempt to rehabilitate the healthcare professional with counseling and retraining.

To locate other information regarding the governmental regulation of massage therapy, you can search the internet with state name + regulation + massage. If you prefer to have a hard copy version of this information, you can contact your local department of health to see if they can direct you to the appropriate regulatory body. Additionally, your massage school or training program will most likely be aware of the appropriate regulatory agencies you will need to contact upon graduation.

Resolving Ethical Dilemmas

There will most likely come a time when you, as a professional massage therapist, will be faced with making an ethical decision regarding your practice. Codes of ethics serve as guidelines for these decisions, but they do not guarantee that the decisions will be easy to make. When faced with an ethical dilemma, it is helpful to make a decision that is based on the highest good for all. The decision-making process outlined below, which is only one of many equally helpful methods, involves a series of steps for resolving ethical dilemmas:

1. Identify the problem or situation and gather any relevant information.
2. Identify the nature of the conflict: legal, moral, ethical, or a combination.
3. Identify the person, condition, or results that will be affected by the decision.
4. Brainstorm different decisions and the potential outcomes of each.
5. Consider different perspectives: your intuition, community, peers, legal.
6. Determine whether rules, codes of ethics, or laws invalidate any of the decisions.
7. Determine the best course of action. Will the client or you be harmed? Is it the most helpful thing to do?

Box 2-7 shows an example of using the 7-step guideline to ethical resolution.

Professionalism

Professionalism is defined as the conduct, goals, and qualities that generally characterize a profession. There is often a sense of maturity, patience, and awareness that accompanies professionalism. Typically, professionalism refers to conduct, business practices, legal and ethical responsibilities, and membership in professional associations that create your public image. **You never get a second chance to make a first impression** so the image you portray when people first come in contact with you on a professional level should be a good one.

CONDUCT

A respectable and reputable professional image is influenced by appropriate conduct. There are codes of ethics to provide guidelines for professionalism, which are discussed above, but there are other fac-

---

Box 2-7

An Example of Ethical Resolution Using the 7-Step Guideline

Dilemma
A client insists that you use a skeletal adjustment technique that you have not learned. How should you handle this situation?

1. **Identify the problem or situation and gather any relevant information**
   You have to decide whether to try an unfamiliar technique or disappoint your client

2. **Identify the nature of the conflict: legal, moral, ethical, or a combination**
   The technique is outside your scope of practice, which makes it a possible legal conflict, and you are unfamiliar with a technique, making it ethically wrong to try it because it may harm the client.
   However, your client is insisting that you use the technique, and your client-centered philosophy encourages you to serve the client's needs.

3. **Identify the person, condition, or results that will be affected by the decision**
   Your client could get hurt, your professional membership could be revoked, or your practice could be suspended by law if you attempt the technique.
   However, the client might not return because you will not address his or her needs, thus affecting your practice.

4. **Brainstorm different decisions and potential outcomes of each**
   a. You could explain your professional and ethical commitments to scope of practice and hope the client understands.

   b. You could attempt the technique and hope that it works and that the client does not get hurt.
   c. You could pretend to perform the technique and hope the client does not continue to push you.
   d. You could adamantly state that you will not attempt the technique because it is not a massage technique and tell the client that if he or she is not happy with your massage services, he or she can go elsewhere.

5. **Consider different perspectives: your intuition, community, peers, legal**
   Intuition tells you to explain things to the client and hope for understanding, which is probably the same thing your peers and community will suggest.
   The law does not have a preference how you handle it, as long as you do not attempt the technique.

6. **Determine whether rules, codes of ethics, or laws invalidate any of the decisions**
   By law, skeletal adjustments are outside the scope of practice for massage therapy, so you may not attempt the technique.
   Pretending to perform the technique and lying to the client about the technique not working is unethical.

7. **Determine the best course of action: Will the client or you be harmed? Is it the most helpful thing to do?**
   The best course of action is probably to gently explain scope of practice and hope for understanding. It protects the client from being hurt, it protects your practice from being sued or suspended, and it allows you to practice your ethics.

tors that contribute to your public image. Any input people receive with their eyes, ears, and nose will be used to develop an image of you as a professional, so your conduct includes the visual, auditory, and olfactory cues you project.

Visual Cues

Clients will see facial expressions, eye contact, posture, cleanliness, what you wear, and how you dress. Your facial expressions can convey emotion, exhaustion, stress, distraction, interest, or disinterest. Eye contact can express interest or disinterest, confidence, patience, and self-esteem. Posture can indicate your level of exhaustion, self-esteem, depression, shyness, or self-consciousness. Cleanliness of the practice, treatment room, equipment, your body, and your clothing may illustrate the level of pride in your practice or how careful you are.

Clothes are always used to evaluate people, both what they wear and how they wear it, so keep that in mind as you consider your professional image. The following are some guidelines for appropriate clothing and appearance for a professional massage therapist:

- Short sleeves
- Breathable fabrics
- Loose, comfortable clothes
- Long hair tied back
- Minimal or no jewelry
- Clean, intact clothes and shoes

Why short sleeves? Long sleeves interfere with massage strokes and pushing sleeves up throughout the massage is disruptive. Why breathable fabric? Massage is physical work that creates body heat, and cotton, linen, or cotton blends are cooler and more comfortable. Why loose clothing? Tight, form-fitting clothes restrict movement and can distract the client from the professional atmosphere. Why tie back long hair? Pushing hair out of your face throughout a massage is distracting, and you do not want your hair to accidentally touch the client during the treatment, for sanitation and hygiene reasons. Why limit jewelry? Excessive jewelry is a visual distraction that can also interfere with massage strokes and scratch skin. Why clean and intact clothes? Holes, tears, and stains are visually distracting. Visual input is the primary ingredient for a professional image. Figure 2-1 shows examples of professional attire.

There are some visual aspects of the practice that will also contribute to your professional image. Business cards and brochures are intended for public use, and they significantly influence your image. The quality of these marketing tools is measured by the paper, the colors, the layout, and the included information.

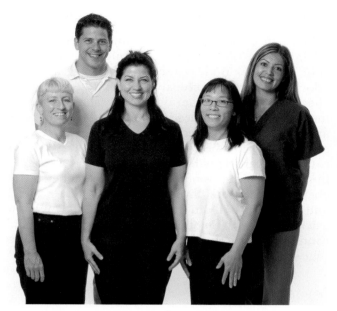

FIGURE 2-1 Examples of professional attire.

Business marketing tools are covered in more detail in the business chapter.

Auditory Cues

The words you speak, the tone you use, the volume, pace, and clarity of your speech, and the emotions you convey with your speech all contribute to a client's perception of your professional image. From the moment you exchange the first spoken words, whether over the phone or in a face-to-face meeting, you are creating a professional image that your client will associate with you. The fact that communication skills are critical may seem like common sense, so we address this topic very broadly. Discuss your policies and procedures with your clients and make sure there is no confusion. Use your answering machine, voice mail box, or e-mail as a communication tool. Let your clients know that you will return their messages within 24 to 48 hours, or let them know if you are unavailable for an extended period of time. Tone and attitude can be interpreted through your voice, so be careful to speak clearly and audibly, with a friendly and professional tone.

The sounds of your practice's environment add to your professional image. Traffic noise, nearby conversation, clocks, alarms, televisions, radios, bathroom noises, and pets may be distracting and detract from a professional image. Gentle music with a slow tempo and the natural sounds of water, birds, and wind can provide a more tranquil atmosphere that will encourage clients to relax and let go of their stress.

Olfactory Cues

Odors can evoke strong, emotional responses. Try to stay aware of any odors that might be present in your practice. Body odor, breath odor, and foot odor are especially offensive to a lot of persons, so check throughout the day and take preventive measures to avoid these problems. Many persons are sensitive to scented products, so perfumes and colognes should be used sparingly, if at all. Environmental smells will also affect your professional image. Garbage, food, pets, air fresheners, and chemical cleansers have odors that will be noticed, and not necessarily in a good way. You may want to ask a friend with an objective nose to check the surroundings of your practice and identify any odors that should be eliminated.

BUSINESS PRACTICES

Standards of practice for massage therapy include everyday business practices such as record keeping, sanitation, hygiene, safety, and marketing. These topics are detailed in a separate chapter, but they are outlined below.

The following are some aspects of your practice that require record keeping:

- Appointments
- Client information
- Client health history
- Massage session notes
- Meetings
- Work-related travel
- Business-related purchases (e.g., equipment, lubricants, business cards)
- Business-related expenses (e.g., laundry, professional memberships, utilities)
- Income

Sanitation, hygiene, and safety are concepts that support massage therapy's client-centered philosophy. Sanitation is the act of keeping your practice clean enough to prevent disease transmission. Professional standards of practice dictate a sanitary environment for the benefit of you, your clients, and the general public. A similar concept is hygiene, which is the act of keeping things clean to promote health. Safety is the condition that prevents physical harm to a person and applies to everything your clients will use: parking area, walkway, steps, bathroom, treatment room, equipment, floors, and furniture. Fire safety is specifically addressed by law, covering fire extinguisher placement, fire escape route, maximum capacity of people in a building, the use of open flames and smoke detectors. You can learn about sanitation and safety regulations from your local regulatory agency and fire department.

Marketing your business can be as low or high budget as you want. Word-of-mouth advertising is possibly the least expensive, and although it can be very effective, it is limited by the people who recommend your services. Business cards are an inexpensive but almost necessary marketing tool. Self-promotion involves you, sharing and educating people about the benefits of your services through demonstrations and public speaking. Promotional brochures and pamphlets are useful and attractive, but they can be expensive. Local media can provide some other avenues for marketing your services, including newspaper articles, television interviews or demonstrations, and radio shows or commercials. Whatever method(s) of marketing you choose should be professional and ethical.

LEGAL REQUIREMENTS AND ETHICAL RESPONSIBILITIES

There are legal requirements and ethical responsibilities associated with standards of practice that influence the foundation of the therapeutic relationship. We have covered legalities in terms of local or state regulations, including licensure, certification, and registration, scope of practice, and fire safety. Additionally, there are the two important principles of informed consent and confidentiality.

Informed Consent

Informed consent, sometimes called patient rights, is a client's agreement to participate in an activity after the benefits and risks of the activity have been explained and the client understands that he or she has the right to withdraw at any time. Basically, clients who are *informed* about a treatment give their *consent* to try it. Informed consent is a process that attempts to prepare all parties involved and avoid any unpleasant surprises. This concept started in the medical profession as a way to empower patients. Educating persons about their healthcare and allowing them to make an educated decision about whether they want to participate or not gives them a sense of comfort and control instead of feelings of vulnerability and powerlessness. Engaging clients in the massage treatment creates a teamwork approach to healthcare and maintains a client-centered practice. Informed consent benefits and protects clients because it

- Provides the client the opportunity to ask questions
- Allows the client to completely understand the rules and policies of the massage therapy session
- Clarifies what the massage session will and will not include

- Identifies the benefits and possible contraindications of massage or a particular technique
- Provides the opportunity to participate willingly in their healthcare by choosing to receive massage or specific techniques
- Allows the client to refuse treatment or stop treatment at any time
- Provides the opportunity to validate and verify the therapist's credentials

For the therapist, informed consent provides a signed statement that represents the therapist's good intentions and the client's education and awareness about massage. See Figure 2-2 for different examples of informed consent.

Clients are given the right of refusal and the control for session termination. While the therapist is ultimately responsible for maintaining boundaries and respecting limits, the client also has the capability and responsibility to do the same. Clients and therapists must adhere to the policies and procedures of the office, and both maintain the right to terminate or refuse treatment if there is reasonable cause. Specific conditions that would prompt session termination are often stipulated in the therapist's policies and procedures, which the client should have read and accepted during the initial intake. Generally, these situations include anything that violates or could interfere with safe and ethical treatment. Any activity that sexualizes the massage treatment is grounds for termination: sexual or lewd comments, gestures with a sexual connotation, intentional genital exposure, or intentional sexual contact of any kind. Clients who are repeatedly late or who repeatedly cancel appointments demonstrate a lack of respect for the therapist's practice and can be refused treatment if the therapist feels it is justified. The client must feel comfortable and agree to participate with a particular therapist, but it is equally important for the therapist to feel comfortable and agree to work with a particular client.

Confidentiality

Confidentiality is the principle that information revealed to a massage therapist during an appointment is to be kept private except under limited circumstances when that information is to be disclosed to a third party. Keeping client information confidential, or private, helps establish trust and respect between the client and the therapist. If clients want to tell people what is said or experienced in the therapeutic setting, it is up to them to do so. It is ethically, and may be legally, wrong for you to share that information without the client's permission, because you have promised to keep the information private. It is professionally wrong because you have agreed to uphold the professional standards of practice, which include confidentiality. Generally, as long as there is no direct or implied association to any specific person's identity, the shared information is probably allowed. There are many situations in which confidentiality may need to be broken, and each such circumstance will require that you make an ethical decision.

For example, you may want to discuss a client's condition or treatment plan with another healthcare professional and would need to share specific and thorough details about the client's condition. The best course of action would be to have a conversation with your client, explain your intention, and obtain the client's permission to disclose the information. The client should identify the details that can be shared, including names, dates, locations, conditions, treatments or outcomes, as well as any limitations on where, when, or how you plan to use the information. To allow professionals to exchange information, you can ask the client to sign a standard release form. See Figure 2-3 for examples of release forms.

You must break confidentiality in any situations that indicate a clear and imminent danger to someone's life, such as intended suicide, murder, personal endangerment, or abuse or neglect of a child, elderly person, or mentally challenged individual. It is your ethical responsibility to report these situations, but many states have established laws that require certain professionals to report suspected abuse.

Courts of law can subpoena any of your client files. Names, contact numbers, health histories, treatment notes, and account balances are all subject to being surrendered by subpoena. This situation does not occur frequently, but it does happen. Records should always be accurate, organized, and thorough, and extraneous and irrelevant notes, such as client's emotional state or comments on behavior, should never be kept in client files.

There are confidentiality issues to manage outside the treatment room as well. Unless clients approach you in public first, try to refrain from greeting them. They may not want people to know that they are receiving massage treatment, or they may not want their relationship with you to be public. Take your cues from the clients. If they openly acknowledge their professional relationship with you, respond with a professional demeanor. If you make eye contact with clients who do not openly recognize or acknowledge a relationship with you, let them go. It is possible that they do not remember you, but it is also possible that they are not interested in a public relationship.

Confidentiality is a standard of care that is imperative to the professional therapeutic relationship by guaranteeing the clients that whatever happens in the therapeutic setting is private and protected. There are

I understand that the massage therapy given here is for the purpose of stress reduction, relief from muscular tension, spasm or soft tissue injury, or for increasing circulation and energy flow. I understand that massage therapists **do not** diagnose illness or disease, nor do they prescribe any medical treatments or perform spinal manipulations. I acknowledge that massage **is not** a substitute for medical examination or diagnosis, and, it is recommended I see a healthcare professional for that service. I have stated all medical conditions and will update the massage therapist with any changes in my health status. I understand that sexual advances and/or comments will result in immediate termination of the massage session with full payment due. I understand that massage sessions are available by appointment only, and, if I am unable to keep my appointment, I will inform the massage therapist within 3 hours of the appointment or I will be charged a cancellation fee.

Signature: _____ Date: _____

I understand that massage therapy is intended to maintain and improve my general health by increasing circulation, reducing stress and promoting relaxation. In order to minimize any health risks, I have provided all my known medical information, and will inform the therapist of any new medical information I acquire as long as I am under the therapist's massage treatment. I acknowledge that manual therapy is not a substitute for medical treatment and that the massage therapist cannot diagnose or prescribe any medical conditions.

Signature:_____ Date: _____

I promise to participate fully in my healthcare as part of a team of professionals. I will make choices about my treatment based on the information provided regarding the benefits, risks and procedures involved. I agree to help choose and participate in any self-care activities that may be recommended in order to promote health and healing. I promise to inform my therapist(s) if I feel uncomfortable or that my health is being compromised during any treatment. In turn, I expect my therapist(s) to provide safe and effective, knowledgeable care that is in the best interest of my health and well being. I promise to keep my therapist(s) informed of any health or medical concerns, conditions or treatments while I am receiving massage therapy in order to minimize any risks.

Signature: _____ Date: _____

FIGURE 2-2 Examples of informed consent.

PATIENT'S RELEASE OF HEALTH CARE INFORMATION

Patient's Name __Darnel G. Washington__

Social Security Number __123-45-6789__   Date of Birth __4-22-37__

Health Care Provider/Facility __John Olson, LMP, GCFP__

is hereby authorized to release health care information, including intake forms, chart notes, reports, correspondence, billing statements, and other written information to my attorneys, employees, and designated agents of my attorneys, to wit:

Attorney's Name __B. Charma Storro, JD__   Phone __(612) 555-2337__

Address __5 Hive Lane__

City __Minnehaha__   State __MN__ Zip __55987__

This request and authorization applies to:

__✓__ Health care information relating to the following treatment, condition, or dates of treatment: __MVA 1-6-01__

____ All health care information:

____ Other: _____

Revocation of Prior Authorization: All medical authorizations by the patient or patient's authorized representatives given before the date of this release for any reason whatsoever are hereby revoked.

Information is not to be disclosed to any other person, including insurance agents or adjusters or other attorneys or their employees or agents, without my attorney's prior permission.

Effect of photocopy of this release shall have the same force and effect as a signed original.

Authorization expires 90 days from date of signature. Thereafter, no authorization exists unless an updated release is provided by: __B. Charma-Storro, JD__

__Darnel G. Washington__   __2-15-01__

Signature of Patient or Patient's Authorized Representative   Date

FIGURE 2-3 Examples of release forms. (Reprinted from Thompson D. Hands Heal: Communication, Documentation, and Insurance Billing for Manual Therapists. 2nd ed. Baltimore: Lippincott Williams & Wilkins, 2002:58, 286.)

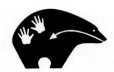

Helena LaLuna, CR
123 Sun Moon and Stars Drive
Capital Hill, WA   98119
TEL   206 555 4446

HEALTH INFORMATION

Patient Name _Zamora Hostetter_   Date _4-4-01_

Date of Injury _3-31-01_   Insurance ID# _C98-7654321_

A. Patient Information

Address _63 18th Ave. W_

City _Capitol Hill_   State _WA_ Zip _98119_

Phone: Home _(206) 555-1221_

   Work _555-2112_ Cell/Pgr _555-1122_

Date of Birth _5-22-80_

Employer _Howling Moon Cafe_

Occupation _Chef_

Emergency Contact _Mary Lou Hostetter_

Phone: Home _(206) 555-0909_

   Work _555-9090_ Cell/Pgr _555-9900_

Primary Health Care Provider

Name _Manda Rae Yuricich, DC_

Address _4041 Bell Town Wy, Ste. 200_

City/State/Zip _Capitol Hill WA 98119_

Phone: _555-3535_   Fax _555-4646_

I give my manual therapist permission to
consult with my referring health care provider
regarding my health and treatment. _& P.T._

Comments _re: work injury only_

Initials _ZH_   Date _4-4-01_

B. Current Health Information

List Health/Concerns Check all that apply

Primary _shoulder pain_

☐ mild ☐ moderate ☒ disabling
☒ constant ☐ intermittant
☒ symptoms ↑ w/activity   ☐ ↓ w/activity
☐ getting worse ☐ getting better ☒ no change
treatment received _ER-x-rays, sling_

Secondary _back pain_

☐ mild ☒ moderate ☐ disabling
☒ constant ☐ intermittant
☒ symptoms ↑ w/activity   ☐ ↓ w/activity
☐ getting worse ☒ getting better ☐ no change
treatment received _ER, DC-adjust._

Additional _neck pain & headaches_

☒ mild ☐ moderate ☐ disabling
☐ constant ☒ intermittant
☒ symptoms ↑ w/activity   ☐ ↓ w/activity
☐ getting worse ☒ getting better ☐ no change
treatment received _ER, DC_

Have you ever received Manual Therapy
before? ☐ Y ☒ N Frequency? _____

List all conditions currently monitored by a
Health Care Provider _none_

List the medications you took today
(include pain relievers and herbal remedies)
arnica, calcium, vitamins

List all other medications taken in the last 3
months _none_

List Daily Activities

Work _standing, lifting, cooking, chopping_

Home/Family _cooking, cleaning, yardwork_

Social/Recreational _biking, roller hockey, dancing_

Circle the activities affected by your condition,
☒ all of the above

Check other activities affected: ☒ sleep
☐ washing ☐ dressing ☒ fitness

How do you reduce stress? _sports, being outdoors_

Pain? _arnica, ice packs, visualization_

What are your goals for receiving Manual
Therapy? _get back to work & sports_

C. Health History

List and Explain. Include dates and treatment
received.

Surgeries _none_

Accidents _Broken arm ®, fell out of tree house in 1987, cast for 8 wks_

Major Illnesses _none_

FIGURE 2-3   *(continued)* Examples of release forms. (Reprinted from Thompson D. Hands Heal: Communication, Documentation, and Insurance Billing for Manual Therapists. 2nd ed. Baltimore: Lippincott Williams & Wilkins, 2002:58, 286.)

ethical and legal responsibilities that massage therapists should be aware of and understand.

PROFESSIONAL ASSOCIATIONS

A professional image is often supported by membership in professional organizations. The original massage associations were established to protect the massage profession, and they have since evolved to provide a number of benefits to their members. Different levels of insurance coverage, marketing and promotional media, networking groups, and continuing education are just some of the options available to members of professional massage associations.

Professional Associations in Britain

Chapter 1 covered the British Medical Association's discovery of unethical massage practices. The massage profession prevailed, despite its tarnished reputation. At that time, if a massage therapist was associated with a physician or hospital, the massage was still considered legitimate. A group of four women in Britain decided to protect the massage profession by forming the Society of Trained Masseuses in 1894. Lucy Marianne Robinson, Rosalind Paget, Elizabeth Anne Manley, and Margaret Dora Palmer founded the society, using the standards for the medical profession as their model. They established academic prerequisites for training, outlined criteria for qualified instructors, and inspected schools on a regular basis. Massage instructors and graduates were required to take written and practical examinations before a board, which included a physician. They maintained high standards and set membership regulations, requiring the massage professionals to only accept physicians' referrals and to avoid advertising through the media.

Many members abided by the many rules and regulations of the society, but there were still a number of massage therapists who continued to practice unethically. By 1900, the group became the Incorporated Society of Trained Masseuses. In 1920, a Royal Charter was granted, the group joined forces with the Institute of Massage and Remedial Gymnastics, and the Chartered Society of Massage and Remedial Gymnastics was established. With several branches throughout Britain, the widely respected society reached a membership of 12,000. In 1944, the society changed its name to the Chartered Society of Physiotherapy (CSP), which remains its name today.

Professional Associations in America

Soon after the British started the movement toward professional massage therapy, a flurry of professional activity began in the United States as well:

- 1927—The New York State Society of Medical Massage Therapists was America's first professional massage association to be established
- 1939—The Florida State Massage Therapy Association (FSMTA) was organized with 85 charter members
- 1943—The first Massage Act was passed by the Florida legislature
- 1943—The American Association of Masseurs and Masseuses (AAMM) was formed in Chicago
- 1949—AAMM established the Massage Registration Act, a state law requiring massage therapists to register with the state
- 1958—AAMM became the American Massage and Therapy Association (AM&TA)
- 1983—AM&TA became the current American Massage Therapy Association (AMTA)
- 1987—Associated Bodywork and Massage Professionals (ABMP) was founded in Colorado

The AMTA still exists today, providing massage therapists with professional liability and other insurance, membership standards for education and continuing education, a code of ethics, and standards of practice. The AMTA promotes research studies, supports involvement in regulatory efforts, and prints promotional information among other benefits. The AMTA's state chapters offer opportunities for community education, continuing education, and volunteer involvement in the organization. Therapists can volunteer in any capacity, from handling registration at a chapter meeting to being a national committee chairperson or director on the board.

In 1987, two massage therapists formed the Associated Bodywork and Massage Professionals (ABMP) organization in Evergreen, Colorado. The ABMP philosophy centers on the credo of "expect more" and helps massage, bodywork, somatic, and esthetic (skin care) practitioners build and sustain successful practices. The primary selling point for the ABMP is its claim to support the needs of its members by providing the necessary products or services. Currently, there is a companion magazine publication, an insurance program, and a business handbook for members in addition to its massage school relations program and support for regulation.

Relationships

Relationships can be complicated in any situation, but massage therapy can make them even more complex. Every relationship, whether personal or professional, is characterized by physical and conceptual boundaries. Physical boundaries describe the physical area that defines a person's comfort zone, and conceptual boundaries are the attitudes and behaviors that affect a person's level of comfort. The comfort provided by physical and conceptual boundaries can create a safe space for clients that allows a healthy professional relationship to grow. Professional relationships are made with clients, with other healthcare professionals, and in any situation in which you are representing yourself as a massage therapist. The physical and conceptual boundaries will play a part in each one of these relationships, so you must be aware of boundaries and respect them to maintain professionalism.

PHYSICAL BOUNDARIES

There is physical space around a person that is a boundary for outsiders. Anthropologist Edward T. Hall pioneered the field of proxemics, or the human behavioral use of space, in the 1960s. He defined the immediate space around a person as having four different zones:

- Intimate—for whispering and embracing, within 18 inches of your body
- Personal—for conversing with close friends, 18 inches to 4 feet away from your body
- Social—for conversing with acquaintances, 4 to 10 feet away from your body
- Public—for interacting with strangers, 10 to 25 feet away from your body

Personal space is like a protective bubble that insulates us from persons and things around us. You should respect others' personal space and stay out of it unless invited. When a person comes within a zone that is inappropriate for the relationship, Hall suggests that it makes the person being invaded feel uncomfortable and vulnerable and triggers an avoidance response. Americans typically require a space about six feet in diameter, or a little further than an arm's distance away, for social or comfortable public situations. This space is commonly called personal space, and the size of it varies with cultural, emotional, physical, and sexual experiences.

As mentioned above, personal space may vary individually depending upon perceived comfort and safety. During a massage session, you will be moving into different zones of your clients' space and need to be aware of their comfort level to make sure that you do not trigger avoidance or resistance. Understanding and maintaining physical boundaries is essential for preserving the therapeutic process before, during, and after the massage. Accountability is a quality that can help you maintain a safe personal space for your clients. It can be challenging to know for sure whether you are too far into a client's personal space,

so do not hesitate to ask periodically during the massage and suggest that the client respond. You can adjust the pressure and techniques according to the client's responses. In fact, you can inform clients prior to the treatment that during the massage you may ask about their comfort and can make the appropriate adjustments to the massage. In addition to the physical space that we use for protection and comfort, there are conceptual boundaries that do the same.

CONCEPTUAL BOUNDARIES

Conceptual boundaries, sometimes called comfort zones, provide us with a sense of safety or comfort. The intimate nature of massage can easily create a feeling of vulnerability, discomfort, nervousness, or hesitancy. Clients who feel safe, comfortable and trusting will ultimately receive more benefit from a massage than clients who feel unsure and uncomfortable. Comfort levels with the issues of emotions, intellect, energy, and sexuality are all forms of conceptual boundaries.

Emotions

Emotional boundaries determine the extent to which we expose emotions and feelings, based upon perceived levels of trust, safety, and comfort. The term "openness" expresses a person's willingness to share his or her emotions openly. Massage therapists must respect emotional boundaries as much as physical space boundaries. If you push clients to expose more emotion than they want to share or if you share too many of your own emotions with your clients, you may be met with resistance and avoidance. Clients' emotions and the issues that surround them may be interesting and can certainly affect the healing process, but managing them is not within the scope of massage therapy. Emotional factors in the healing process are addressed later in the text.

Intellect

Intellectual boundaries protect a person's thoughts, opinions, and belief systems. Culture, religion, spirituality, politics, nutritional habits, age, and gender can influence belief systems, so all of those topics should be respected and handled carefully without judgment. In a basic example, it may be challenging for a massage therapist who is a strict vegetarian to restrain from judging a junk food eater's nutritional habits. Even if the vegetarian therapist strongly believes that it is wrong to eat animal products, it is inappropriate for that therapist to think less of a client who disagrees. Another example of an intellectual boundary is a person sharing religious beliefs with his or her therapist. Therapists must respect the client's ideas, even if they seem absurd to them. Consider how a client in that situation would feel if the therapist responded with disbelief and surprise, saying "You actually believe that God does not exist!?"

Energy

Within human beings are endless chemical reactions and energetic transfers that create various energy fields in and around the body. Massage therapy affects physiological activities and consequently changes the energetic fields. Emotions can also affect physiological activity and energetic fields. Energy flows and patterns can influence each other, which is easily demonstrated by a magnet's ability to attract or repel, depending on the energy patterns of different objects. With increased awareness, you can prevent energetic influence from occurring between you and your clients.

In the beginning of your career as a massage therapist, you may become aware of increased physical stress on your body as a result of working with a client. For example, a client may come in with neck pain, and after the session, you feel discomfort in your neck. While this may seem strange, many therapists experience this phenomenon. It can also occur in reverse, with a transfer from the therapist to the client. Either way, it can affect the therapist's and the client's health and well being. Some grounding and centering techniques that can minimize the effect of these seemingly energetic influences are covered later in the text. Everyone who works with human bodies and receives work on his or her body is affected by the energy of another, so do what you can to protect yourself and your clients from negative effects.

Sexuality

Massage is an intimate and personal activity, and it is ultimately the therapist's responsibility to maintain a professional boundary. This is both a physical and conceptual boundary, but the conceptual limits are more sensitive and subtle than the physical limits. The therapist should be very clear in the informed consent process that sexualizing the treatment session is unacceptable and will result in immediate termination of the session. The treatment can be sexualized with a simple inappropriate comment, and there are also cases in which clients have asked for genital massage and for a sexual encounter. It should be very clear that there are absolutely NO exceptions to this boundary.

The intention of touch can significantly influence how a person perceives the touch, which is why you must make your professional policies absolutely clear prior to the session. In the somewhat puritanical American culture, any form of touch can be perceived as sexual. A client who is trying to sexualize the session can change a safe, ethical, and therapeutic touch into something that could be interpreted as sexual touch. Sexualizing a treatment session is the ultimate violation of professional boundaries, and it is undeniably unethical and probably illegal. If reported, you will most likely lose your right to practice and may face legal recourse.

With that in mind, you should know that sexual arousal may occur during a treatment session. Massage provides a lot of sensory stimulation in many different ways. Sometimes the slow massage strokes paired with a safe and caring touch can create feelings of intimacy and sexuality. Even if the feelings are unintentional, they can result from this excessive tactile experience and sometimes cause sexual arousal. The process of sexual arousal is a complex physiological and emotional response to many stimuli. We will cover this response very basically so you can be aware of what may occur during a treatment session and have an idea how to handle it if it does occur.

Sexual arousal may result from one or a combination of increased sensory stimulation, increased activity of the parasympathetic nervous system, and stimulation of the limbic system, which is the part of the brain that controls emotions. The primary intention of massage is to promote relaxation, which can be caused by the parasympathetic nervous system's response to some basic massage strokes. Many physiological changes occur during the parasympathetic response that allow the body to fall into a "rest and digest" mode, such as reduced heart rate, reduced blood pressure, dilation of the pupils, and increased blood flow to the digestive system and reproductive organs. The female's clitoris and the male's penis both become erect as a result of the parasympathetic response, but we all know that male erections are more apparent. The point here is that an erection does not necessarily mean that your client has sexual intent.

There are several thoughts and methods on how to handle this situation if it occurs, but in the end, you want to act with a client-centered frame of mind.

1. The first way to handle this situation takes place **BEFORE** any sexual arousal occurs. Your informed consent process can be used to educate clients about the parasympathetic system and its potential effect of sexual arousal.
2. You can speed up the tempo of the massage and switch to brisk, percussive strokes to induce the opposite physiological response, which will make the erection subside.

3. You can ignore an erection if you believe your client is either unaware of it or if you believe your client has no sexual intent.
4. If the client mentions or asks about his erection, and you believe that he has no sexual intent, you can explain the physiology briefly and assure him that it is a natural response and that his body is relaxing.
5. If a male client's erection is accompanied by inappropriate sexual gestures or comments, you must address the situation directly. You could temporarily stop the session, remind your client about your professional policies and intolerance of sexual behavior, and continue with the massage. You could also terminate the session, explain your professional intolerance for sexual behavior, excuse yourself from the room, ask the client to get dressed, and escort him to the door.

You may be embarrassed, upset, and afraid or confused when a client has an erection during a massage session. The way you handle the situation is a personal, professional, and ethical decision depending on the subtleties of the situation. Trust your intuition, respect the sexual boundaries of your clients and yourself, and keep professionalism in mind.

Safe Space

Safe space refers to the physical and emotional atmosphere of your practice. It provides an environment that is welcoming, comforting, noninvasive, safe, and secure, so clients can relax and get the most beneficial massage session. Security and safety in your practice can be conveyed by

- A safe location in the city
- A clean and well-maintained building
- An easily accessible treatment room
- Privacy in the treatment room
- Freedom from disruptive noises or odors
- Adequate lighting
- Appropriate music
- Proper draping techniques
- Professional image
- Professional knowledge, competence, compassion, and communication

CLIENT RELATIONSHIPS

The therapeutic relationship between the massage therapist and client is an important standard of practice to examine closely. The therapeutic relationship begins with your initial contact with the client and continues for as long as you and the client agree to work together. When the therapeutic relationship begins, there is usually an immediate power differential when the client assumes that the healthcare professional is an expert. Clients who seek massage treatment assume you have the training and knowledge to handle their condition appropriately. To emphasize the differential, massage clients take off some or all of their clothes and, while they are covered with appropriated draping, are in a more vulnerable position than the therapist. It may be easy to forget this power differential exists, so keep in mind that you are a person who represents authority and may seem more powerful in the client's eyes.

Dual Relationships

Dual relationships, which occur when personal and professional roles overlap, can enhance or detract from the therapeutic relationship depending upon how they are handled. **It is always the responsibility of the therapist to determine and communicate the risks, boundaries, and impact of dual or multiple relationships.**

When two people who are personal friends have a professional relationship of some kind, they have what is called a dual relationship. The overlap between professional and social interaction can jeopardize the personal and the professional relationships. Another issue that can complicate client relationships is transference. Basically, it is the experience in which expectations and behaviors from one relationship are placed upon another relationship, and it has a significant impact on your professional relationships.

This may be especially important when working with family and friends who become your massage clients. Family and friends do not intentionally take advantage of you as a professional, but they are more comfortable about canceling appointments at the last minute, not paying promptly, asking for massage outside the office and in social situations, and assuming that you will treat them anytime, anywhere. Some therapists describe these kinds of situations and let their friends and family know that if any of those situations occur, the professional relationship will be terminated. You may have to set definitive professional boundaries with them, and although it is not easy to do, it will make the professional relationship easier in the long run.

When assessing the risks of dual relationships, examine the impact it would have on the professional relationship. Since you are ultimately accountable for the therapeutic relationship, you must assess whether there is mutual benefit for establishing the secondary relationship and whether there could be any negative impact on your business and professional image. If you and the client decide that the risks are minimal, it is important to establish clear boundaries regarding the additional roles.

Transference

The concept of transference is found mostly in therapeutic relationships involving psychotherapy and healthcare relationships, and it is frequently present in massage therapy. You should be aware of the concept and understand the mechanism enough to recognize when it surfaces.

Transference is the process in which clients transfer expectations and behaviors of another relationship onto their therapeutic relationship with you. They may transfer or project unresolved feelings, needs, and issues onto you without good reason. Some examples of transference in the massage setting:

- The client brings you gifts in addition to your normal fees at every appointment
- The client repeatedly asks for personal psychological advice
- The client seems to linger in your office, unwilling to leave
- The client frequently tells you how much you look like another person
- The client repeatedly calls you at home despite your request that you only be called on your business phone
- The client always pushes for a longer session for the same price, despite your insistence that the session is finished

PROFESSIONAL RELATIONSHIPS

Similarly, there are social and professional relationships that may develop from the therapeutic relationship. You might cross paths with clients in social circles, business settings, or even in the dating scene. Dating and sexual activity with clients is unacceptable and unethical, but establishing a friendship is less definitive. It is especially important to stay within your scope of practice as a massage therapist, even if your clients ask you for help in the areas of psychological evaluation or nutritional advice. If you suspect the client needs additional expertise in an area in which you are not qualified, it is your ethical and professional responsibility to refer your client to the appropriate professional.

Countertransference

Countertransference is almost the same situation as transference, except it occurs when you, as the massage therapist, transfer or project feelings or needs from another relationship onto your client. Some

signs that you may be displaying countertransference include

- Disappointment when your client does not praise you
- Thinking that you are the best therapist for a particular client and that all other therapists only do more damage than good
- Feeling frustrated with a particular client for a vague reason
- Feeling strong emotions toward a particular client
- Thinking that a client is ungrateful because he or she mentioned that there was little improvement after the last session
- Frequently reaching out to clients for social interaction outside the practice

In a massage practice, the therapist is ultimately responsible for maintaining the therapeutic relationship. If you recognize transference or countertransference in your practice, it is your responsibility to examine the situation and decide what to do. You may need to terminate the professional relationship or discontinue the social relationship. You could discuss your awareness of the situation with your client and explain that the therapeutic relationship is being compromised. If you are uncomfortable with handling the situation directly, you may want assistance from a professionally trained counselor, a social worker, or a psychotherapist who has expertise in this arena.

Chapter Summary

The principles of ethics and professionalism are used as a guide in the massage therapy profession and promote and maintain the reputation of massage therapy. Understanding the professional standards of practice for a client-centered practice and having the accountability to follow the currently accepted codes of ethics will influence your thoughts and actions in creating and sustaining a successful massage therapy practice.

Legal regulations and scope of practice determine practice and technique parameters as well as the amount of education required to be considered a competent and professional massage therapist. Currently, the use of terminology is inconsistent and confusing, which makes it especially important to understand the specific requirement of your local and state laws.

The relationships you establish will present physical and conceptual boundaries that are different for every person, but if you are sensitive to and respect the limits, you can develop ethical and professional relationships. Massage therapy presents some complications to dual relationships and having a basic understanding about transference and countertransference can help you sort through those difficulties. Ultimately, being accountable for your behavior and actions and consistently behaving with a client-centered philosophy serve the best interest of everyone.

CHAPTER EXERCISES

1. Define the following terms and explain their importance in massage therapy:
   a. Ethics
   b. Code of ethics
   c. Standards of practice
   d. Informed consent
   e. Scope of practice

2. Explain what a client-centered philosophy is and why it is important to the massage profession.

3. Describe the following terms as they apply to the relationships of a massage therapist: dual relationships, transference, and countertransference.

4. What is scope of practice for
   a. Wellness massage
   b. Therapeutic massage

5. Explain the significance of the NCBTMB's levels of certification for determining scope of practice.

6. Define accountability and describe an experience from your own life in which your accountability influenced a decision you had to make.

7. Give at least five examples of boundaries that influence relationships.

8. What is the ultimate boundary violation and why?

9. How can you portray yourself as a professional massage therapist?

10. Use the 7-step process learned in this chapter to resolve the ethical dilemmas in each of the following scenarios:
    a. You accept free concert tickets from a client, but at the next appointment, your client expects a free session. What do you do?
    b. A new client makes sexual jokes during the massage session. What do you do?
    c. A long-time client who has recently been separated from his spouse begins scheduling more frequent appointments and repeatedly refers to his search for companionship throughout his massage sessions. What do you do?

REFERENCES

1. https://wws2.wa.gov/doh/hpqa-licensing/disciplinary/complaint.htm (Washington State's Health Department Complaint and Disciplinary Process, accessed 6.16.03)

SUGGESTED READINGS

Alpert A. Defining boundaries. Assoc Bodywork Massage Professionals Massage Bodywork Magazine (Evergreen, CO: Associated Bodywork and Massage Professionals) 1999;June/July: 76–78.

Benjamin B, Jordan D, Polseno D. Issues on sexuality. Am Massage Ther Massage Ther J (Evanston, IL: AMTA) 2000:Summer: 52–93.

McIntosh N. The Educated Heart. Memphis, TN: Decatur Bainbridge Press, 1999.

Polseno D. Informed consent. Am Massage Ther Massage Ther J (Evanston, IL: AMTA) 2001:Spring:136–141.

Rattray F, Ludwig L. Clinical Massage Therapy: Understanding, Assessing and Treating over 70 Conditions. Toronto, Ontario: Talus Incorporated, 2000.

Sohnen-Moe C, Benjamin B. The Ethics of Touch. Tucson, AZ: Sohnen-Moe Associates, 2003.

Torrenzano S. Ethics: The heart of the matter: Part 2. Assoc Bodywork Massage Professionals Massage Bodywork Magazine (Evergreen, CO: Associated Bodywork and Massage Professionals) 1999;June/July:62–70.

Torrenzano S. The heart of ethics. Lecture presented at the American Massage Therapy Association national convention, Quebec, Canada, 2001.

http://www.abmp.com, accessed 9.2.02.

http://www.amtamassage.org, accessed 9.12.02.

http://www.asinc.ca/en/services/licensure.html, accessed 6.16.03.

http://www.buzzle.com/editorials/text9-1-1999-11282.asp, accessed 6.19.03.

http://www.careeratyourfingertips.com/laws.htm, accessed 6.10.03.

http://www.findarticles.com/cf dls/go2601/0072601000774/article.jhtml, accessed 9.1.02.

http://www.law.cornell.edu/statutes.html, accessed 6.13.03.

http://www.m-w.com/cgi-bin/dictionary, accessed 6.14.03.

http://www.mdmassage.org/certnreg.htm, accessed 6.10.03.

http://www.ncbtmb.com, accessed 9.12.02.

http://www.prevent-abuse-now.com/govhome.htm, accessed 6.13.03.

http://www.stedmans.com accessed 6.14.03.

Medical Terminology

UPON COMPLETION OF THIS CHAPTER, THE STUDENT WILL BE ABLE TO:

- Identify the three word elements
- Translate at least five medical terms by using the five step guideline
- Describe the 10 directional terms
- Identify at least 20 surface anatomy body regions on self or a partner
- Name the two subdivisions of the posterior body cavity
- Name the three subdivisions of the anterior body cavity
- Describe the relationship between anatomy and physiology
- Describe the difference between an indication and a contraindication
- List at least three classes of pharmaceuticals

KEY TERMS

Anatomical position: describes a person standing up, feet shoulder-width apart, arms at the sides, and palms facing forward

Anatomy: the study of the structures of plants and animals

Anterior (ventral): refers to something on or toward someone's front side, or on the navel side

Contraindication: a condition or symptom for which massage should be avoided because it presents a risk for the client's health

Deep: refers to something farther from the surface of the skin, or more toward the inside of the body

Distal: refers to something that is farther away from the torso, toward the fingers or toes

Endangerment sites: particular areas of the body that contain superficial or unprotected organs, nerves, and blood vessels and require caution to prevent injury

Indication: a condition or symptom that points to massage as a potentially beneficial treatment

Inferior (caudad): refers to something being more toward the feet, or below

Pathology: the study of disease processes or of any deviation from a normal, healthy condition

Pharmacology: the science of the preparation, usage, and effects of medications

Physiology: the study of the normal functions of the organism or any part of the organism

Posterior (dorsal): refers to something on or toward someone's back

Prone: lying on the stomach, or face down

Proximal: describes something toward the attachment point of the limb to the body

Sidelying (laterally recumbent): refers to a person lying on his or her side

Superficial: refers to something closer to the surface of the skin

Superior (cephalad): refers to something being more toward the head, or above

Supine: refers to a person lying on his or her back or spine

This chapter introduces key medical terminology used in the field of massage therapy. This language will be completely foreign to some students but familiar for others. Learning a new language may be a difficult task, but the first step in the right direction is a personal commitment to learn, coupled with the willingness to practice, practice, practice. It is worth the time and effort to learn this language because a working knowledge of medical terminology has many benefits for the massage therapist. It will save time in communication with clients and other health care professionals and in record keeping, and it can minimize confusion, help maintain a professional image, and increase your knowledge base. **Knowledge is power!**

Begin by learning the basic rules of the medical language, and then learn some individual words. Over time and with practice, you will develop the confidence to use the words comfortably when speaking about healthcare. Most of the medical terms can be broken down into separate word elements that help simplify the meanings, and numerous medical dictionaries are available to help with spelling, pronunciation, and definitions. Having the appropriate references available and knowing how to use them is a more powerful tool than trying to memorize all the words.

The terms anatomy, physiology, and pathology are introduced in this chapter, but there is a separate chapter that covers them in detail. **Anatomy** (uh-NAT-uh-mee) explores the body's structures, **physiology** (fiz-ee-AH-loh-jee) studies the functions of those structures, and **pathology** looks at things that can go wrong with those functions. By understanding the basics of anatomy, physiology, and pathology and using additional reference books when they are needed for complex information, massage therapists can make better judgments about whether massage is appropriate for particular clients or could do more damage than good. This chapter provides the foundation for communicating with clients and other healthcare professionals. With practice and commitment, your mastery of this language will help you earn your professionalism and due respect.

Learning Medical Terminology

Communication is one of the keys to a successful business. For massage therapists, communication requires a working knowledge of medical terminology because we converse with many healthcare professionals. To be respected and considered professional, we need to understand what other health professionals are saying when they refer to a treatment or a body part, and we need to be able to respond to them using the same terms. In short, we must learn to speak a common language. Since modern medical terminology has its origins in Greek and Latin words, the language is consistent across the world, which makes it one of the most practical languages to learn. Medical language continues to evolve, and terms are added that are not based on either Greek or Latin. Some of these terms are named for people who discover a body part (Broca's area of the brain) or disease (Alzheimer's disease) or who develop a procedure (Heimlich maneuver), test (Tinel's test), or device (Foley catheter).

Using these unfamiliar terms in class and practicing them at home can raise your comfort level with your new language. You can increase your learning by reinforcing it with different combinations of processes. For instance, you can practice the language by writing terms on paper and spelling them aloud, by reading silently and saying the terms aloud, by reading the definitions, closing your eyes, and reciting the definitions, and by making up sentences that use the terms. The more ways you practice, using your eyes, ears, mouth, and hands, the more effective the learning. Eventually, you will be able to communicate with clients, keep professional records, and communicate with other healthcare professionals comfortably and easily.

Your learning process does not end when you can use the language on a functional level. As long as you practice massage, you will need to communicate with clients and other healthcare professionals, and you will not know every medical term that exists. One of the most useful tools for learning language is a dictionary that provides English translations and definitions. Medical dictionaries, which provide definitions and pronunciations for scientific and medical terminology, are widely available and are excellent tools to have in the office. When clients and other healthcare professionals refer to conditions, diseases, anatomical parts, or directional terms that you may not recognize or remember, you can use your medical dictionary to figure them out.

In addition to being a tool for your own knowledge, a medical dictionary can be an educational tool for clients. All therapists should understand medical language and be able to use it on a functional level, but the words and terms massage therapists use with their clients is an individual choice. Some clients expect their therapists to use medical terminology, but others are intimidated by it. You have to gauge your clients' comfort levels and use language that keeps your client at ease but still promotes professionalism. There are times when clients do not understand medical terms that their primary care physicians have mentioned but they are uncomfortable asking their doctors what those terms mean. Clients occasionally ask their massage therapists for explanations or definitions of medical words. By pulling out the medical dictionary and researching the term with your client, you have an opportunity to learn and teach at the same time, and you portray a professional image by showing interest in the client's concerns. More importantly, it is an admission that you do not know everything but are willing to learn, which generates trust and respect from your client.

Word Elements

The challenging process of learning your new language can be simplified by breaking medical terms down into smaller parts. Compound words are created by combining two or more words, and the definition of the compound word generally is a combination of the meanings of the two independent words. For example, the word "headache" is a compound word made up of the words "head" and "ache," and the definition is a simple combination of those two words. Likewise, most medical terms are created by combining two or three of the following word elements: the root, the prefix, and the suffix.

ROOTS

The root is the core building block that provides the basic meaning for the word. Typically it refers to an organ, an anatomical structure, body region, or disease. For example:

Organs
- hepat(o) refers to the liver
- cardi(o) refers to the heart

Anatomical structures
- brachi(o) refers to the arm
- cost(o) refers to the ribs
- my(o) refers to the muscle

Body regions
- abdomin(o) refers to the abdomen
- thorac(o) refers to the chest or thorax

Diseases
- carcin(o) refers to cancer
- toxic(o) and tox(o) refer to poison

The determination of some of these roots is not always so scientific. For instance, the word "muscle" comes from the Latin word meaning mouse, because the movement of a muscle under the skin resembles the scampering movement of a mouse. The coccyx is named after the cuckoo bird, because the shape of the bone resembles the cuckoo's bill.

Just as there are exceptions to every rule, there are oddball situations in which context and medical dictionaries are especially helpful. For instance, some roots have two different meanings, as illustrated below:

myel(o) refers to both
- spinal cord
- bone marrow

scler(o) refers to both
- hardening
- the white of the eye

cyst(i) and cyst(o) refer to both
- filled sac
- urinary bladder

There are also some instances in which two different roots refer to the same term. Since Greek and Latin serve as the basis for medical terms, sometimes each language provides a root for the same term. For example, the Greek root "nephr(o)" and the Latin root "ren" both refer to the kidney. Table 3-1 lists commonly used roots, their meanings, and examples of their usage.

PREFIXES

Prefixes are the word elements that come before the root, and they are indicated by a dash after them. They change, further specify, or alter the meaning of the root by referring to numbers, amounts, directions, positions, changes, and comparisons. For example:

Numbers or amounts
- bi- means two
- hyper- means excessive or too much
- hypo- means not enough or under
- poly- means many or much
- semi- means half or partial
- tri- means three

Directions and positions
- ab- means away from
- ad- means toward
- ante- means before
- endo- means inside
- post- means after or behind
- pre- means before or in front of
- syn- means together
- trans- means across or through

Changes
- a- means not or without
- anti- means against
- contra- means against
- dis- means separation or absence

Comparisons
- infra- means below
- iso- means the same or equal to

TABLE 3-1

Commonly Used Roots

ROOT	MEANING	EXAMPLE	DEFINITION
abdomin(o)	abdomen	rectus abdominus	abdominal muscle along midline of body
adrenal(o), adren(o)	adrenal	adrenaline	chemical produced by the adrenal gland
angi(o)	vessel	angioplasty	reconstructive surgery on blood vessels
arteri(o), arter(o)	artery	arterial	pertaining to the arteries
arthr(o)	joint	arthritis	inflammation of a joint
brachi(o)	arm	brachialis	muscle of the arm
bronch(i), bronch(o)	bronchus	bronchitis	inflammation of the bronchii in the lungs
cardi(o)	heart	cardiology	study of the heart
cephal(o)	head	cephalad	toward the head
cerebr(o)	cerebrum	cerebrospinal fluid	fluid that bathes the brain and spinal cord
cervic(o)	neck	cervical vertebrae	spinal segments of the neck
chondr(o)	cartilage	chondritis	inflammation of cartilage
cost(o)	rib	intercostals	muscles between ribs
crani(o)	skull	cranial nerves	major nerves in the skull
cyt(o)	cell	cytoplasm	fluid within the cell
dent(i), dent(o)	teeth	dentist	tooth and gum specialist
dermat(o), derm(o)	skin	dermatitis	inflammation of the skin
fibr(o)	fiber, fibrous	fibrositis	inflammation of fibrous connective tissue, muscles
gastr(o)	stomach	gastritis	inflammation of the stomach
gynec(o), gyn(o)	woman	gynecology	study of the female reproductive organs
hem(o), hemat(o)	blood	hematoma	localized collection or clot of blood
hepat(o)	liver	hepatology	study of the liver
hist(o)	tissue	histology	study of cells and tissues
hydr(o)	water	hydrotherapy	treatment using water internally and/or externally
ili(o)	ilium	Iliacus	muscle that attaches to the ilium
laryng(o)	larynx	laryngitis	inflammation of the larynx
my(o)	muscle	myositis	inflammation of the muscle
myel(o)	spinal cord, bone marrow	myelin	protective covering of nerves
nephr(o)	kidney	nephrology	study of the kidney
neur(i), neur(o)	nerve	neurology	study of the nervous system
ocul(o)	eye	oculomotor nerve	nerve that controls eye movement
oss, oste(o)	bone	osteoporosis	condition where bones become porous and fragile
ot(o)	ear	otitis	inflammation in the ear
ped(i), ped(o)	child	pediatrics	branch of medicine specializing in children
pneumat(o), pneum(o)	breathing, respiration	pneumonia	inflammation in the lungs
pod(o)	foot	podiatrist	foot specialist
psych(o)	mind	psychology	study of the mind
pulm(o), pulmon(o)	lung	pulmonologist	lung specialist
rhin(o)	nose	rhinoplasty	reconstructive surgery of the nose
stern(o)	chest	sternum	flat bone between ribs in center of chest
therm(o)	heat	thermometer	device for measuring heat
thorac(o)	chest, thorax	thoracic vertebrae	vertebral segments of the thorax
thyr(o)	thyroid	hypothyroidism	condition in which thyroid produces insufficient hormones
toxic(o), tox(o)	poison, toxin	toxicology	study of toxins, poisons
trache(o)	trachea	tracheostomy	surgical opening in trachea
troph(o)	growth	hypertrophy	excessive growth
ur(o), urin(o)	urinary tract, urination	urologist	urinary system specialist
ven(o)	vein	venule	a little vein
vertebr(o)	vertebra, spine	intervertebral disk	special tissue disks between vertebrae

- micro- means small
- ortho- means straight or correct
- pseudo- means false
- re- means again or back

Observe how prefixes modify roots in the following examples:

- hyper- + active = hyperactive, which is excessive activity
- hypo- + active = hypoactive, which means insufficient activity
- ad- + duct = adduct, which means movement toward something
- ab- + duct = abduct, which means movement away from something
- bi- + cycle = bicycle, or a cycle with two wheels
- tri- + cycle = tricycle, or a cycle with three wheels

Table 3-2 lists commonly used prefixes, their definitions, and examples.

SUFFIXES

Suffixes are word elements that are tacked on to the end of a root, and they are usually indicated with a dash in front of them. They can identify the medical term as a noun or an adjective and describe how the root is used, so they tend to be the starting point for interpretation of medical words. Briefly, suffixes can indicate a specific condition or a descriptive condition that refers to the root.

Noun indications
- –algia means characterized by pain in
- –esthesia means a sensation of
- –iatry means a medical specialty of
- –ism means a condition of
- –ist means a specialist of
- –itis means an inflammation of
- –logy means the study of

Descriptive indications
- –ac means pertaining to
- –al means pertaining to
- –form means like or resembling
- –oid means resembling
- –ous means pertaining to
- –es is the plural for –is
- –nges is the plural for –nx

COMBINING VOWELS

Pronunciation can get somewhat complicated when two word elements are combined that do not flow together well. When one element ends with a consonant and the word element after it begins with a con-sonant, a combining vowel is placed between the two to make the word easier to pronounce. You have probably noticed from many of the previous examples that most of the roots are followed with an (o), which is the most common combining vowel. For example, the root "electr" means electricity, the root "cardi" means heart, and "gram" means record. Combining the three elements into the word "electrocardiogram" uses a combining vowel between the parts for easier pronunciation. Try pronouncing the word without the combining vowel to see the difference.

Translating Terms

The three word elements—prefixes, roots, and suffixes—are the building blocks for medical terminology. Once you understand how each word element works, it becomes easy to figure out what a word means. Not all medical terms have a prefix, root, and suffix. Some only have two of the elements, and others have two roots and a suffix.

Terms can be translated in five methodical steps. The first step in translating medical terms is breaking up the term into its word elements. Because suffixes indicate how the term is used, the second step is defining the suffix. Next, go to the beginning of the term and define the elements in order. String all the definitions together and check the translation against a medical dictionary. We will demonstrate translation of the word "fibromyalgia":

1. Break it down into elements
   Fibromyalgia = "fibro" "my" "algia"
2. Start with the definition of the suffix
   "-algia" = painful condition of
3. Go to the beginning of the word and define each element
   "fibro" = fibrous
   "my" = muscle
4. String the definitions together
   painful condition of + fibrous + muscle
5. Check your definition with a medical dictionary or other source
   "painful condition of muscles, tendons, and joints"

For another example, we will translate "hypertonic."

1. "hyper" "ton" "ic"
2. "ic" = pertaining to
3. "hyper" = excessive
   "ton" = tone
4. pertaining to + excessive + tone
5. excessive tone in the muscles or excessive salt concentration in solution

TABLE 3-2

Commonly Used Prefixes

PREFIX	MEANING	EXAMPLE	DEFINITION
a-, an-	without, not, absent	anaerobic	without oxygen
ab-	away from	abduct	move away from
ad-	to, toward	adduct	move toward
ante-	before	anterior	on the front side or in front of
anti-	against	antibody	protein that fights against antigens and foreign substances
auto-	self	autoimmune	immune system attacks own body tissues
bi-	two	biceps brachii	arm muscle with two origins
bio-	life	biology	study of living objects
circum-	around	circumduct	to lead around, through full range of motion
contra-	against	contraindication	situation in which treatment should be avoided
de-	down, remove, loss	degenerative	condition of breakdown
dia-	across, through	diaphragm	muscle whose origin crosses entire thorax
dis-	apart, away from	disease	condition away from health
dys-	difficult, painful	dysfunction	function that is abnormal or painful
epi-	over, upon	epidermis	top layer of skin
ex-	out of	exhale	release air out of lungs
extra-	in addition, beyond	extracellular	area beyond or outside the cell
flex-	bent	flexion	movement that reduces angle at a joint
hemi	half	hemisphere	half of a sphere
hetero	the other	heterogeneous	characteristic of having dissimilar constituents
homeo	same	homeostasis	state of keeping everything the same or balanced
hyper	above, extreme, excessive	hypertonic	excessive tone or concentration
hypo-	under, below	hypotonic	insufficient tone or concentration
infra-	below	infraspinatus	below the spine
inter-	between	intercostals	muscles between the ribs
intra-	within, inside	intracellular	area between the cells
leuk-	white	leukocyte	white blood cell
macro-	large	macrophage	large cell that destroys foreign substances
mal-	abnormal, bad	malfunction	abnormal or bad function
medi-	middle	medial	beginning or occurring in the middle
micr(o)-	small	microscope	device that allows you to see small things
mono-	one, single	monoarticular	involving one joint
poly-	many	polyarticular	involving many joints
post-	after	posterior	the back or behind
pre-, pro-	before, in front of	precursor	forerunner, or event that happened before
quad-	four	quadriceps femoris	leg muscle with four origins
re-	again, back	recur	occur again
retro-	backward	retroactive	applying to events that occurred in the past
semi-	part	semipermeable	only allowing some things to permeate or move through
sub-	under, below	subcutaneous	below the skin
super-	above, in addition	superficial	on the surface or more toward the surface
supra-	above, over	suprahyoids	muscles that are above the hyoid bone
syn-	together	synergistic	working together
trans-	across	transverse process	projection of vertebrae that points outward, across the body
tri-	three	triceps brachii	arm muscle with three origins
uni-	one, single	unilateral	on one side

For one more example of translation, we will use "osteoarthritis."

1. "osteo" "arthr" "itis"
2. "itis" = inflammation of
3. "osteo" = bone
   "arthr" = joint
4. inflammation of + bone + joint
5. inflammation of the joints, especially the weight-bearing joints, characterized by degenerative condition of the articular cartilage

This process is straightforward, but you may need practice to become proficient at it. Table 3-3 is a list of commonly used suffixes, their definitions, and examples of terms that include them.

Some of the word elements that are used more commonly in massage therapy include

- Prefixes – dys- , hyper- , hypo- , pre-, and post-
- Roots – my(o), vertebr(o), cervic(o), fibr(o)
- Suffixes – -al , -algia , -itis

See Table 3-4 for some translations of terms used in the field of massage therapy.

Medical dictionaries contain thousands of terms and by learning the meanings of some of the more commonly used prefixes, roots, and suffixes, you will not need to look up as many medical terms for their definitions.

SPELLING AND PRONUNCIATION

Proper translation and communication requires proper spelling and pronunciation. Because of the Greek and Latin derivation of so many medical terms, their spelling and pronunciation may seem strange and unfamiliar. To make matters worse, regional accents can make familiar words sound unfamiliar. Slight differences in spelling usually mean very different terms. For example, the word "ilium" is a bone of the pelvis, and the word "ileum" is a part of the digestive tract. These completely different anatomical structures have the same pronunciation, so context is an important consideration when the terms are spoken. Correct spelling must also be used in documentation to keep accurate and useful records. Again, a

TABLE 3-3

Commonly Used Suffixes

SUFFIX	MEANING	EXAMPLE	DEFINITION
-al	pertaining to area	skeletal	Pertaining to the skeleton
-algia	pain, painful condition of	neuralgia	painful condition of the nerves
-ar	pertaining to area	muscular	Pertaining to the muscles
-ase	enzyme	lactase	breaks down lactose
-cyte	cell	leukocyte	white blood cell
-ectomy	removal of, excision	hysterectomy	surgical removal of uterus
-emia	blood condition	anemia	low numbers of red blood cells
-genic	causing, producing	allergenic	Causing allergic reaction
-gram	record	electrocardiogram	recording of the electrical activity of the heart
-ic	pertaining to	optic	pertaining to the eye
-itis	inflammation of	arthritis	inflammation of the joint
-logy	study of	biology	study of living things
-oid	resembling	fibroid	resembling fibers
-oma	tumor	lipoma	fatty tumor
-osis	condition of	lordosis	condition of increased lordotic curve
-pathy	disease or suffering	sympathy	suffering together
-phobia	irrational fear of	hydrophobia	fear of water
-plasty	surgical repair of	arthroplasty	surgical repair of a joint
-plegia	paralysis	paraplegia	paralysis of two limbs
-rrhage	excessive flow	hemorrhage	excessive loss of blood
-scope	instrument for viewing	microscope	tool for viewing very small things
-stomy	opening	tracheostomy	surgical opening in trachea
-tomy	incision	laparotomy	incision of the abdomen
-y	characterized by	bony	characterized by bones

TABLE 3-4

Translations of Terms Used in Massage Therapy

WORD	PREFIX	ROOT	SUFFIX	DEFINITION (specific reference to massage)
antagonist	ant- (against)	agon (struggle)	-ist (concerned with)	one that works against (a muscle with an opposing action)
atrophy	a- (without, not)	troph (growth)	-y (condition of)	condition of without growth (condition of muscular deterioration or no growth)
biceps brachii	bi- (two)	ceps (head) brachi (arm)	-i (plural)	two heads (specific arm muscle with two origins)
circumduction	circum- (around)	duct (to lead)	-tion (action of)	lead all the way around (circular movement of a body part through its range of motion)
contraindication	contra- (against)	indicate (to point)	-tion (action of)	indicating the other way (a situation in which treatment is inappropriate)
extension	ex- (away from)	ten (tendon)	-sion (action of)	action of away from the tendon (movement that opens the angle at a joint and stretches the tendon)
fibromyalgia		fibro (fiber) my (muscle)	-algia (painful condition of)	pain in fibers and muscles (condition with pain in muscles, tendons and joints)
hypertonic	hyper- (excessive)	ton (tone)	-ic (pertaining to)	condition of excessive tone (muscle that is too tense)
infraspinatus	infra- (below)	spin (spine)	-atus (refers to)	refers to below the spine (specific muscle that originates below the spine of the scapula)
isometric	iso- (equal)	metr (measure)	-ic (pertaining to)	pertaining to equal measure (muscle activity in which antagonists work equally and no movement occurs)
neuralgia		neur (nerve)	-algia (painful condition of)	nerve pain (condition of pain along the nerves)
osteoarthritis		oste (bone) arthr (joint)	-itis (inflammation of)	inflammation of bone and joint (condition of inflamed and degenerative joints)
proprioception		proprius (your own) cep (take)	-tion (action of)	action of taking your own (ability to sense stimuli from your own body's position in space)
tendinitis		tendin (tendon)	-itis (inflammation of)	inflammation of tendons

TABLE 3-5

Tips on Pronunciation

LETTERS	COMMONLY PRONOUNCED	EXAMPLE
c (before e, i, y)	S	quadriceps (KWAH-drih-seps)
c (before all other letters)	K	contraction (kon-TRAK-shun)
ch	K	cholesterol (koh-LESS-ter-ahl)
es (at the end of a word)	EEZ	meninges (meh-NIN-jeez)
eu	OO	aponeurosis (AP-oh-noo-ROH-sis)
	YOO	Eustachian tube (yoo-STAY-shun toob)
g (before e, i, y)	J	gemellus (juh-MELL-us)
g (before all other letters)	G (hard sound)	gluteus (GLOO-tee-us)
gm	M	diaphragm (DAHY-uh-fram)
gn	N	benign (bee-NAHYN)
i (at the end of a word)	AHY	nuclei (NOOK-lee-ahy)
pn	N	pneumonia (noo-MOHN-yuh)
ps	S	psoas (SOH-az)
pt	T	pterygoid (TAIR-ih-goyd)
x	Z	xyphoid (ZAHY-foyd)

medical dictionary is an indispensable tool for every massage therapist. Table 3-5 provides some general tips for pronouncing medical terms.

Terms for Positions, Planes, and Directions

As a massage therapist you will make observations while looking at a client's body. Some commonly used positions in massage therapy are the supine, prone, and sidelying positions. **Supine** refers to lying on the back, or spine (Fig. 3-1A). The supine position, unlike the other positions, gives you access to the client's anterior surface, including the face and abdomen, and lets you move the client's hips through a full range of motion. Clients who are uncomfortable about receiving massage can be more comfortable starting in the supine position because they can see the environment and feel less vulnerable. The **prone** position refers to lying on the stomach, or face down (Fig. 3-1B). The prone position gives the massage therapist full access to the client's back, neck, and gluteal muscles. **Sidelying,** sometimes referred to as laterally recumbent, describes lying on the side. It is not used as commonly as the supine and prone positions because it is a little more difficult to keep the client modestly draped. On the other hand, this position is superior for addressing the anterior, lateral, and posterior aspects of the neck. The sidelying position is a good alternative for pregnant women and persons who cannot lie on their stomach (Fig. 3-1C).

The **anatomical position** of the body describes a person standing up on both feet, with the feet shoulder-width apart, arms at the sides, and palms facing forward (Fig. 3-1D). The anatomical position is used as a reference when describing the locations of structures on the body. When being evaluated for posture, clients stand in the anatomical position because it provides a standard reference point for present and future observations. It is also used to determine the body's three planes of division: the sagittal, frontal, and transverse planes. These imaginary planes are like thin walls that divide the body or a specific organ into two parts, and they are used by anatomists as a reference tool (Fig. 3-2A). Any kind of physical observation is made in reference to these planes.

A **sagittal plane** (SA-jih-tuhl) plane runs vertically down the body, lengthwise, dividing the body into left and right parts (Fig. 3-2A). A sagittal plane can occur anywhere along the body, but if it runs exactly down the midline of the body, creating equal left and right halves, this plane is called the midsagittal or medial plane. Using the medial plane as a reference, two directional terms are generated: medial and lateral. Medial refers to something closer to the midline, and

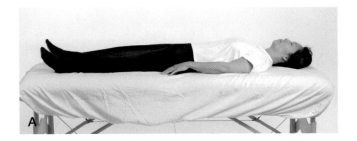

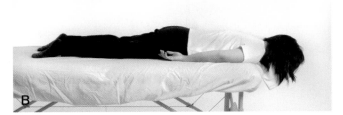

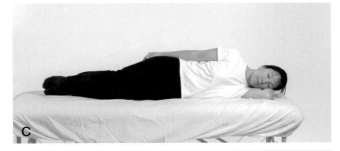

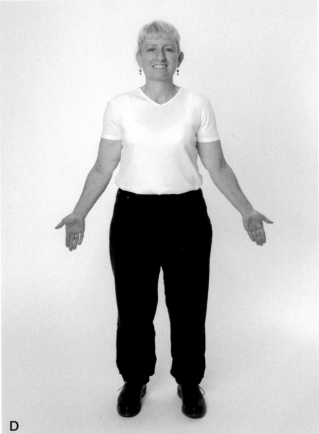

FIGURE 3-1   Terms for positions: **(A)** supine, **(B)** prone, **(C)** side lying (laterally recumbent), **(D)** anatomical position.

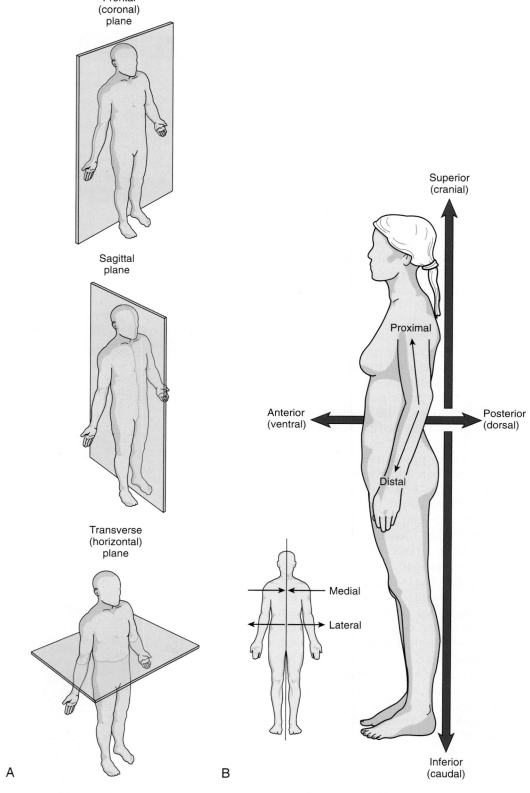

FIGURE 3-2   Planes of division **(A)** and directional terms **(B).** (Reprinted from Cohen BJ, Wood DL. Memmler's Structure and Function of the Human Body. 7th ed. Baltimore: Lippincott Williams & Wilkins, 2000:6, 7.)

lateral refers to something farther away from it. For instance, the ear is lateral to the eye because it is farther away from the midline.

A **frontal plane** (also called a coronal plane) also runs vertically, but divides the body into front and back parts (see Fig. 3-2A). It is used as a reference for the terms anterior and posterior. Although these terms are preferred in massage therapy, the terms ventral and dorsal are sometimes used. **Anterior** (ventral) indicates something on the front side of the body or more toward the front. **Posterior** (dorsal) indicates something on the back side of the body or more toward the back. For example, the nose is anterior to the ear because it is more toward the front side of the body.

A **transverse plane** runs horizontally through the body, dividing it into top and bottom parts (Fig. 3-2A). The transverse plane generates the terms superior and inferior. **Superior** (sometimes called cephalad) refers to something closer to a person's head, or above. **Inferior** (also called caudad) refers to something more toward the feet, or below. The knee is superior to the ankle because it is closer to the head.

There are other directional terms that refer to the anatomical position as well. To describe something on the extremities or limbs, proximal and distal are effective terms. **Proximal** describes something closer to the limb's attachment point on the body, and **distal** refers to something that is farther away from the torso, toward the fingers or toes. The elbow is proximal to the wrist, and the wrist is distal to the elbow

(Fig. 3-2B). Two more descriptive terms are often used, superficial and deep. **Superficial** refers to something closer to the surface of the skin, and **deep** refers to something farther from the surface of the skin, or deeper inside the body. Superficial and deep are commonly used in massage because they are used to describe the relative position of specific muscles in the body or to describe the depth to which the strokes are being applied. For example, the rhomboids are deep to the trapezius, and compression can access tissues that are too deep to reach with effleurage. Table 3-6 lists all the directional terms, definitions of each, and examples of their usage.

EXAMPLES USING DIRECTIONAL TERMS

It is much easier to use the terms that refer to positions, planes, and direction than to try to communicate without them. The following examples illustrate how helpful these terms can be.

Sometimes clients have preferences for positioning during the massage. When clients prefer starting supine, the massage therapist can include that information in the massage session notes. Rather than write, "The client likes to start the massage lying on her back," the therapist could note, "Client prefers to start supine." Similarly, some persons do not like the prone position at all. Instead of writing, "The client does not like to lie on his stomach," the therapist could note, "Avoid prone position." Client positioning is not the only time the medical terms come in handy.

TABLE 3-6		
Terms of Direction		
TERM	**DEFINITION**	**EXAMPLE**
anterior (ventral)	pertaining to the front side or toward the front of the body	the nose is anterior to the ears
deep	more internal, deeper into the body	the lungs are deep to the ribs
distal	farther from the point of attachment or farther from the torso	the fingers are distal to the elbow
inferior (caudad)	located lower or toward the feet	the knee is inferior to the hip
lateral[a]	farther away from the midline or toward the sides	the ear is lateral to the eye
medial[a]	closer to the midline or toward the middle of the body	the eye is medial to the ear
posterior (dorsal)	pertaining to the back side or toward the back of the body	the spine is posterior to the sternum
proximal	closer to the point of attachment or closer to the torso	the knee is proximal to the ankle
superficial	closer to the surface of the skin	the epidermis is superficial to the muscles
superior (cephalad)	located higher or toward the head	the nose is superior to the navel

[a]Remember that the body must be in anatomical position (palms forward).

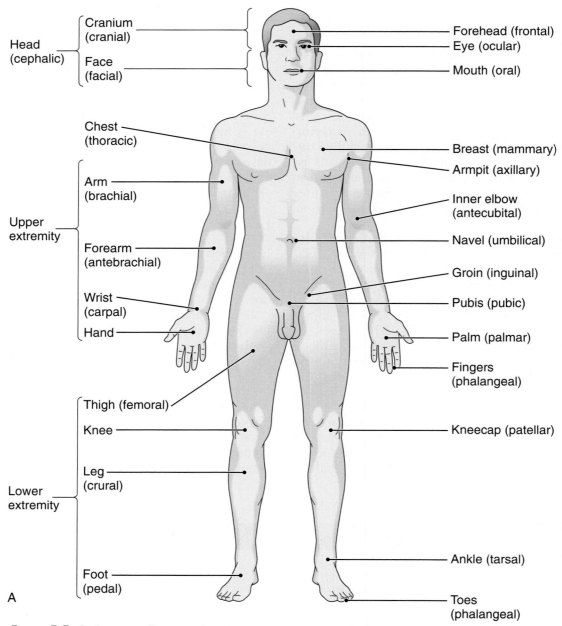

Figure 3-3   Body regions. (Reprinted from Cohen BJ. Medical Terminology: An Illustrated Guide. 4th ed. Baltimore: Lippincott Williams & Wilkins, 2004:69, 70.)

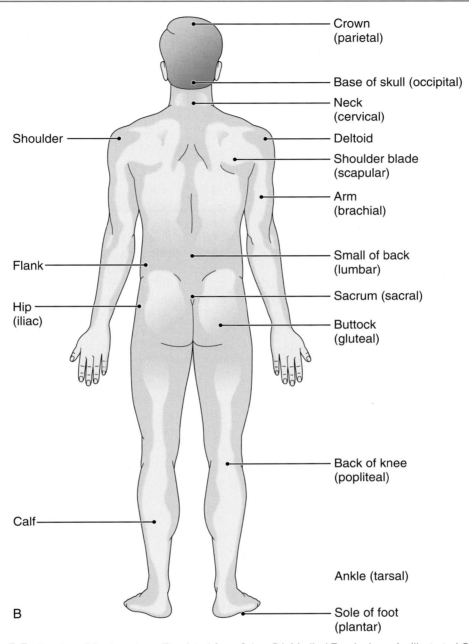

Crown
(parietal)

Base of skull (occipital)

Neck
(cervical)

Shoulder

Deltoid

Shoulder blade
(scapular)

Arm
(brachial)

Flank

Small of back
(lumbar)

Sacrum (sacral)

Hip
(iliac)

Buttock
(gluteal)

Back of knee
(popliteal)

Calf

Ankle (tarsal)

B

Sole of foot
(plantar)

Figure 3-3 *(continued)* Body regions. (Reprinted from Cohen BJ. Medical Terminology: An Illustrated Guide. 4th ed. Baltimore: Lippincott Williams & Wilkins, 2004:69, 70.)

If a client came to your office complaining of pain on the inside of her right wrist, it could mean any number of things. The "inside" of the wrist could refer to the anterior side of the wrist or the medial side of the wrist, and the pain could be on the proximal or distal side of the carpals. If you were to note the client's complaint of pain in your massage session notes, you could use one of the following descriptions:

- Client complained of pain on the medial side of the right wrist, proximal to the carpals.
- Client complained of pain on the medial side of the right wrist, distal to the carpals.
- Client complained of pain on the anterior side of the right wrist, proximal to the carpals.
- Client complained of pain on the anterior side of the right wrist, distal to the carpals.

The next time the client came in for a massage, the therapist could ask about the wrist and know what area to avoid, if the pain contraindicated massage.

Some clients who know medical terminology use it to describe things to their massage therapists. If a client came in and said that he had a hypertonic muscle in his back, just medial to the inferior angle of his right scapula, you would know to look for a muscle holding excessive tension, between the bottom of the right scapula and the spine.

Terms for Body Regions

The surface of the body is generally divided into different regions for orientation purposes. They are helpful terms when you want to refer to a general area of the body. We have identified 25 regions in Figure 3-3. The anterior landmarks include

- Cranial (KRAY-nee-uhl)
- Facial (FAY-shuhl)
- Thoracic (thoh-RASS-ik)
- Axillary (AK-sih-lair-ee)
- Brachial (BRAY-kee-uhl)
- Antecubital (an-tee-KYOO-bih-tuhl)
- Carpal (CAR-puhl)
- Phalangeal (fuh-LAN-jee-uhl)
- Abdominal (ab-DOM-ih-nuhl)
- Inguinal (IN-gwih-nuhl)
- Pubic (PYOO-bik)
- Femoral (FEM-or-uhl)
- Patellar (pah-TELL-er)
- Tarsal (TAR-suhl)

The posterior landmarks include

- Occipital (ok-SIP-ih-tuhl)
- Cervical (SER-vik-uhl)

- Deltoid (DELL-toyd)
- Scapular (SKAP-yoo-lahr)
- Thoracic (thoh-RASS-ik) – this region is identifiable on the anterior and posterior sides
- Lumbar (LUM-bahr)
- Sacral (SAY-kruhl)
- Gluteal (GLOO-tee-uhl)
- Popliteal (pop-lih-TEE-uhl)
- Plantar (PLAN-tahr)

Terms for Body Cavities

In addition to the surface anatomy references, there are special terms for identifying cavities and the organs inside the body. Figure 3-4 shows the two main cavities of the body, classified as the posterior and anterior cavities.

The posterior (dorsal) cavity has two subdivisions that are continuous with each other. The cranial cavity is enclosed by the bony cranium, and it holds and protects the brain. The spinal cavity is a continuation

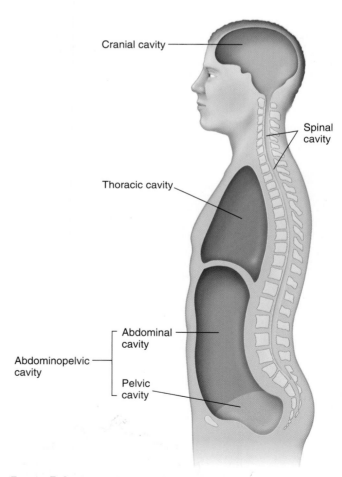

FIGURE 3-4 Interior body cavities.

of the cranial cavity that starts at the base of the skull and runs the length of the vertebral column. Surrounded by the vertebrae, the spinal cavity houses and protects the spinal cord.

The anterior (ventral) cavity, which includes all of the organs in the chest and abdomen, has three subdivisions: the thoracic, abdominal, and pelvic cavities. The thoracic cavity is more superior and contains the heart and lungs. The diaphragm is a large, umbrella-shaped muscle that separates the thoracic cavity from the abdominal cavity below it. Within the abdominal cavity are the stomach, intestines, liver, spleen, gall bladder, pancreas, and kidneys. There is no distinct separation between the abdominal and pelvic cavities, but an imaginary partition is created by a line that goes from the top of the pubic bone to the top of the sacrum. The pelvic cavity, which is located below that partition, is the most inferior of the anterior cavities and includes the reproductive organs, urinary bladder, and rectum. The abdominal cavity is more vulnerable to physical trauma than the thoracic and pelvic cavities, because there are no bones to surround and protect it.

Terms for Structure and Function

Anatomy is the study of the structures of plants and animals. Massage therapists need to know the correct terms for different structures of the body for the work they do, record keeping, and communication. In addition to learning the name of a structure, such as a specific organ, muscle, or bone, you need to learn its function or functions. Physiology is the study of the normal functions of an organism or of a particular part of an organism. Anatomy and physiology generally focus on normal conditions. The study of disease processes or of any deviation from a normal, healthy condition is called pathology. Pathological conditions are often treated with prescription medications to minimize their symptoms or treat their cause. **Pharmacology** (fahr-muh-KAH-loh-jee) is the science of the preparation, usage, and effects of these medications.

ANATOMY

The word anatomy is derived from the Greek roots "ana," meaning up or again, and "tomy," meaning cutting or dissection. The term refers to the first anatomists who had to cut open cadavers to discover anatomical structures. Science and technology has brought us a long way since then, and we now have amazing capabilities when it comes to looking at the

human body. Magnetic resonance imaging (MRI) and computerized tomography (CT) scans let us look at the hard and soft tissues inside the body with excellent clarity. In addition to the visible anatomical structures, there are invisible components that we cannot see with any current technology.

The structures of all living organisms are made up of individual components that can be organized from the simple to complex. The smallest element of structure is the invisible atom. Bonded together in specific arrangements, these atoms make up molecules. Various molecules combine to create cells. The cell is the basic building block for all living things. Groups of specialized cells are organized into tissues, each with a specific function. Different tissues coordinate their individual functions and form organs. Organs that all have a similar purpose are grouped together as organ systems, also called body systems. Finally, the most complex level of organization is the organism, which depends on all the organ systems working together (Fig. 3-5).

In total, there are eleven body systems. For functional purposes this text divides the systems as follows: skeletal, muscular, nervous, circulatory (cardiovascular and lymph), integumentary, and supportive systems (respiratory, digestive, urinary, endocrine, and reproductive). These body systems are discussed in detail in the anatomy and physiology chapter.

PHYSIOLOGY

Learning the individual structures of the body naturally leads to the discovery of the processes or responsibilities of those parts, called physiology. Massage therapists have to know at least the major anatomical structures and their physiological functions to provide safe and beneficial treatment. You need to know the physiological effects of massage to administer the appropriate treatments. You need to know the normal structures and functions to recognize abnormal ones that may need to be avoided. Massage therapists specialize in the muscular system, so they need to know a lot about muscles.

- Structural components of muscle
- Names of the major skeletal muscles
- Attachment points of different muscles
- Actions of different muscles
- Cooperative movement of muscle groups
- Neuromuscular control of muscle contraction
- Fascial involvement
- Interaction between the muscular system and other body systems

The physiology of each body system is covered in Chapter 4, Anatomy and Physiology.

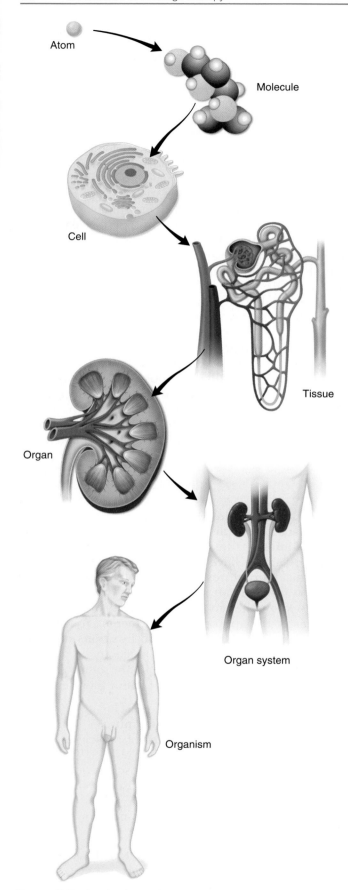

Atom

Molecule

Cell

Tissue

Organ

Organ system

Organism

FIGURE 3-5   Levels of organization.

Therapeutic Terms

There many therapeutic terms and concepts you will need to become familiar with, including pathology, indication, contraindication, and endangerment sites. Pathology is the study of disease. For massage therapy in particular, it is the study of disease or dysfunction to determine whether massage is appropriate. An **indication** for massage therapy is a condition or symptom that points to massage as a potentially beneficial treatment. A **contraindication** for massage therapy is a condition or symptom for which massage should be avoided because it presents a risk for the client's health. A local contraindication is one that can be avoided during a massage and will not be negatively affected by the massage. A systemic contraindication is one for which massage should be avoided altogether because the increase in circulation caused by massage could make the condition worse. This text presents a basic introduction to massage pathology. More comprehensive resources are available on this topic. A good rule when trying to determine whether massage is contraindicated is **"WHEN IN DOUBT, DON'T"**.

Endangerment sites are specific areas on the body where the organs, nerves, and blood vessels are more superficial or unprotected. You need to be aware of these endangerment sites when applying bodywork to prevent damage to the anatomy (Fig. 3-6).

Drug Terms

Pharmacology studies the sources, mechanisms, and applications for medications. Thousands of drugs are prescribed for various symptoms and pathological conditions. Many of them can be categorized into major groupings or classifications of medications by their purpose and the mechanism that makes them work. Because medications are so commonly used, you should be aware of basic drug classifications and how such drugs may interact with massage. Intentionally or not, massage can amplify the effect of a medication, reduce the effect of a medication, and it can relieve side effects of some medications. The *Physician's Desk Reference* (PDR) is a yearly publication that compiles the drug manufacturers and drug products as well as indications and contraindications. Although it is not necessary for you to get a new one each year, you should have access to at least one recently published PDR so you can look up specific drug names and identify possible contraindications for massage. Following are some

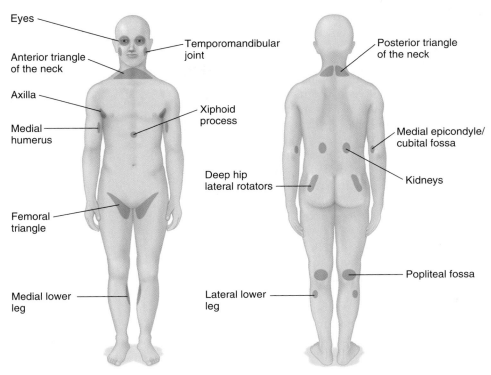

Eyes

Anterior triangle
of the neck

Axilla

Medial
humerus

Femoral
triangle

Medial lower
leg

Temporomandibular
joint

Xiphoid
process

Deep hip
lateral rotators

Lateral lower
leg

Posterior triangle
of the neck

Medial epicondyle/
cubital fossa

Kidneys

Popliteal fossa

FIGURE 3-6 Endangerment sites.

common drug classifications, their indications, how they work, and implications for massage.

Antibiotics: Used to treat bacterial infections, antibiotics disrupt the chemical processes within the offending microorganisms. Antibiotics sometimes have gastrointestinal side effects, and massage can reduce those symptoms. While the client's body is fighting a bacterial infection, with or without the aid of antibiotics, the immune system is compromised. During that time, it is important to avoid overstressing the body. Keeping the client's best interest in mind, use gentler massage techniques to minimize the mechanical and reflexive effects of massage.

Antidepressants: Many kinds of antidepressants are prescribed to eliminate or minimize depression, and sometimes these medications are prescribed also to relieve pain or to help someone stop smoking. Usually, antidepressants change the chemistry of the nervous system by increasing the production of certain chemicals or blocking specific chemical pathways. These medications sometimes cause constipation, a side effect that massage can help relieve. Because massage increases the levels of some of the critical brain chemicals involved in depression, be aware that the client may have an increased or decreased reaction to medication, and use massage in cooperation with the prescribing doctor.

Antihistamines: Chemicals called histamines are released when the body goes through an allergic response. Histamines cause capillaries to leak extra fluids, resulting in swelling and itching. In some cases, they can even cause contractions of involuntary muscles such as the bronchi, restricting or preventing the essential process of breathing. Antihistamines block the effects of histamines (the prefix, anti-, means against), reducing the itching and swelling associated with allergies. Common side effects of antihistamines are drowsiness, anxiety, as well as distorted or masked reactions to the massage. You must be aware of these effects and educate your clients so you and your clients do not worry if they occur.

Antiinflammatory drugs: Inflammation is the body's response to different kinds of irritants, including bacteria, exposure to extreme temperatures, chemicals, or an injury. Characterized by heat, redness, swelling, itching, and pain, inflammation can be reduced with various antiinflammatory medications. When clients are taking antiinflammatory medication, you want to be careful with techniques that require that the client monitor pain levels, such as positional release, because the medication sometimes reduces the client's perception of pain and pressure. Obviously, any massage techniques that create therapeutic inflammation, such as deep transverse friction, should be avoided. Creating inflammation may seem counterintuitive, but it can aid in the healing and normalization of tissue and is covered in detail in the technique section of this text.

Muscle Relaxants: Prescribed to reduce muscular tension, muscle relaxants reduce the chemical activity responsible for communication between the nervous system and the muscular system. As a result, the muscles receive fewer signals to contract. While taking muscle relaxants, clients may feel weak and tired, often with reduced sensitivity to pain. Massage techniques that require clients to monitor pain levels, such as positional release, should be used with caution.

Any time clients have reduced pain sensitivity, massage therapists must be especially cautious about moving clients' joints through their ranges of motion. There are different kinds of barriers that limit joint movement, and some of them involve hypertonic muscle or restricted fascia. Pushing the tissues past their barriers can injure anatomical structures. With experience, you can learn to feel the barriers to avoid hurting clients, but as a beginner, you may need input from your clients. Generally, clients feel discomfort when the limits of joint movement are being approached, but with reduced pain sensitivity, they may not.

Clients can feel weak or tired following a massage, and even more so when they are on medication. You must be aware of your clients' coordination and make sure that they are alert and awake enough to get home safely.

Chapter Summary

The language of massage therapy contains many medical and scientific terms. To learn this language you need commitment and lots of practice. Use your eyes, ear, mouth, and body in the process to reinforce and facilitate learning, but make sure you are learning correctly. In all modes of communication, whether oral or written, with the client or another healthcare professional, you must use correct spelling, pronunciation, and context. Knowing how to break down a word to determine its meaning will help you understand the universal language of healthcare and may make it easier to learn the basics of anatomy, physiology, pathology, and pharmacology.

Using medical terms for the body's positions, planes, and directions as well as structure and function will increase your knowledge and contribute to your professional image. It will save you time and prevent confusion in all modes of communication. The basics of medical language, coupled with the ability to use appropriate reference tools, will contribute to a safe and therapeutic environment for every client.

 CHAPTER EXERCISES

1. Name the three word elements and explain how they are used in a medical term.

2. Define each of the following prefixes:
   - ab-
   - ad-
   - bi-
   - circum-
   - contra-
   - dys-
   - hyper-
   - hypo-
   - infra-
   - inter-
   - poly-
   - post-
   - pre-
   - supra-

3. Define the following roots:
   - arthr(o)-
   - brachi(o)-
   - cervic(o)-
   - cost(o)-
   - crani(o)-
   - dermat(o)-
   - fibr(o)-
   - my(o)-
   - neur(o)-
   - oste(o)-
   - stern(o)-
   - thorac(o)-
   - vertebr(o)-

4. Define the following suffixes:
   - –algia
   - –asis
   - –iasis
   - –ism
   - –itis
   - –oma
   - –osis
   - –pathy
   - –stasis
   - –al
   - –ar

5. Break down the following words into separate elements and define:
   - osteoarthritis
   - fibromyalgia
   - neuropathy
   - tendinitis
   - intervertebral
   - unilateral

- hypertonic
- contralateral
- atrophy

6. Match the following:
   a. prone
   b. supine
   c. laterally recumbent
   d. anterior (ventral)
   e. posterior (dorsal)
   f. proximal
   g. distal
   h. lateral
   i. medial
   j. superior
   k. inferior
   l. superficial
   m. deep

   ____ toward the front of the body
   ____ closer to the midline of the body
   ____ lying face up
   ____ toward the feet, or below
   ____ on a limb, closer to the attachment point of the limb to the body
   ____ toward the side of the body, farther away from the midline
   ____ toward the surface of the skin
   ____ lying face down
   ____ toward the head or above
   ____ on a limb, farther away from the torso
   ____ farther into the body, below the skin
   ____ toward the back of the body
   ____ lying on your side

7. Use the *Physician's Desk Reference* to find the drugs listed below, determine what they are used for, identify at least one common side effect and generic name (if there is one):
   - Ceclor
   - Zithromax
   - Vioxx
   - Celebrex
   - Motrin
   - Flexeril
   - Seraphim
   - Wellbutrin
   - Tylenol
   - Heparin
   - Coumadin
   - Benadryl
   - Claritin

8. Fill in the blank:
   - The head is _____ to the feet.
   - Lying face down is called the _____ position.
   - The hand is _____ to the elbow.
   - The knee is _____ to the hip.
   - The navel is on the _____ side of the body.
   - The spine is on the _____ side of the body.
   - The wrist is _____ to the fingers.
   - The ear is _____ to the eye.
   - The lungs are _____ to the ribs.
   - The sidelying position is also called _____ _____.

9. Define the following:
   - Anatomy
   - Contraindication
   - Frontal plane
   - Indication
   - Pathology
   - Pharmacology
   - Physiology
   - Sagittal plane
   - Transverse plane

10. List at least 10 body regions that are used for surface anatomy orientation.

SUGGESTED READINGS

Austrin MG, Austrin HR. Learning Medical Terminology: A Worktext. 7th ed. St. Louis, MO: Mosby Year Book, 1991.

Chabner DE. Medical Terminology: A Short Course. Philadelphia: WB Saunders, 1999.

Cohen BJ. Medical Terminology: An Illustrated Guide. 3rd ed. Philadelphia: Lippincott-Raven, 1998.

Cohen BJ, Wood DL. The Human Body in Health and Disease. 8th ed. Baltimore: Lippincott Williams & Wilkins, 1996.

Fisher JP. Basic Medical Terminology. 5th ed. Westerville, OH: Glencoe-McGraw Hill, 1999.

Marieb EN. Essentials of Human Anatomy and Physiology. 5th ed. Menlo Park, CA: Benjamin Cummins, 1997.

McCann JAS. Medical Terminology Made Incredibly Easy. Springhouse, PA: Springhouse Corporation, 2001.

Moisio MA, Moisio EW. Medical Terminology A Student-Centered Approach. Albany, NY: Delmar Thomson Learning, 2002.

Random House Webster's College Dictionary. New York: Random House, 1997.

Sheaffer BP (project coord). Mary's Story: A Curriculum for Teaching Medical Terminology, Institute for the Study of Adult Literacy. University Park, PA: Penn State University, 1991–1992.

Stedman's Concise Medical Dictionary for the Health Professions. 4th ed. Baltimore: Lippincott Williams & Wilkins, 2001.

Willis MC. Medical Terminology The Language of Healthcare. Baltimore: Lippincott Williams & Wilkins, 1996.

Introduction to Anatomy and Physiology

UPON COMPLETION OF THIS CHAPTER, THE STUDENT WILL BE ABLE TO:

- Define homeostasis
- Name the 11 body systems
- Name the major structures of each body system
- Name the major functions of each body system
- Identify the bones in the axial and appendicular skeletons
- Name the three main types of joints
- Name the four common characteristics of all muscle tissue
- Describe the two attachment points of a skeletal muscle
- Demonstrate at least five pairs of antagonistic body movements on self or partner
- Demonstrate the difference between concentric and eccentric muscle contractions
- Describe the function of proprioceptors
- Identify at least five effects of the sympathetic and parasympathetic nervous systems
- Describe the difference between a local and a systemic contraindication

KEY TERMS

Acute: refers to a condition that has existed for only up to 3 days or has developed very quickly and severely

Antagonist: muscle whose contraction moves the body in the opposite direction from that of the prime mover

Artery: a tube that carries blood away from the heart

Atrophy (AT-roh-fee): a condition that results when a muscle is not used either by choice or by lack of nerve stimulation (e.g., with nerve damage)

Bony landmark: site for muscle attachment or safe passageway for nerves and blood vessels

Chronic: refers to a condition that develops slowly, recurs, or persists longer than 3 weeks

Concentric contraction: muscle shortens and the attachment sites of the muscle move closer together

Contraindication: a situation or condition in which massage is inappropriate

Eccentric contraction: muscle contraction in which the distance between the muscle attachments increases and the muscle effectively gets longer

Fascia (FASH-uh): a fibrous band or sheetlike tissue membrane that provides support and protection for the body organs

Fixator: special synergist (also called stabilizer) that holds a part of the body steady while the prime mover contracts to move that part

Homeostasis: the body's constant monitoring and adjustment of metabolic processes in an effort to maintain an internally balanced state of equilibrium

Insertion of a muscle: the point of attachment that moves most during contraction, often at the distal end

Local contraindication: a condition in which massage is appropriate except in the affected area

Metabolism: the overall cellular activity that breaks down nutrients to generate energy to build essential molecules

Motor neuron: neuron that carries messages away from the central nervous system (CNS) to the muscle or organs that must react (also called an efferent neuron)

Motor unit: one motor neuron and all of the muscle cells it stimulates

Muscle: a specially organized and packaged group of muscle cells, connective tissue wrappings, and blood vessels

Nerve: a specially organized and packaged bundle of neurons (individual nerve cells), connective tissue wrappings, and blood vessels

Nerve plexuses: large networks of intertwined nerves

Neuron: the basic unit of the nervous system, also called a nerve cell

Origin of a muscle: the attachment on the bone or connective tissue structure that is more stationary during muscle contraction

Parasympathetic response: autonomic nervous system response that stimulates organs to work in a "rest and digest" mode

Prime mover: muscle that performs most of the intended movement, also known as an agonist

Proprioceptor (PROH-pree-oh-SEP-tor)**:** sensory neuron responsible for detecting body position, muscle tone, and equilibrium

Sensory neuron: neuron that receives sensory input and transmits that information to the CNS, also called an afferent neuron

Stretch reflex: a protective muscle contraction that occurs when the tissues are stretched too far and/or too fast

Subacute: the period from about 3 days to 3 weeks after a health condition started

Synergist: assists the prime mover by contracting at the same time to facilitate more effective movement, also called an accessory muscle

Systemic contraindication: a condition or situation in which massage should be avoided altogether

Tendon reflex: a reflex that relaxes a muscle when a muscle and its tendon are subjected to slow and gentle tension.

Tissue: a group of cells with similar structure and function

Vein: a tube that transports blood from the capillaries of the body back to the heart

Anatomy is the science of body structures. Physiology is the science of the functions of the body and its individual parts. This chapter covers the basic anatomical structures and functions of the body, body conditions massage therapists commonly see in practice, and some common drugs used for different health conditions. The 11 body systems are presented in the following sections: Cells and Tissues, Integumentary System, Skeletal System, Muscular System, Nervous System, Circulatory Systems (cardiovascular and lymphatic), Respiratory System, Digestive System, Urinary System, Endocrine System, and Reproductive System.

The focus is not on rote learning of anatomy and physiology but on a more functional understanding of how the structures and systems relate to massage. This chapter serves only as an introduction to anatomy and physiology and is intended to give you a basic idea about the human body, what it is made of, and how it works.

Cells and Tissues

All living matter is made up of a variety of parts that range in size and complexity. The cell, which comes in many specialized forms, is the basic building block for structures of living things. **Tissues** are organized groups or layers of specialized cells that have similar structure and function. Organs are groups of tissue that perform specialized body functions. Tissues and organs that work closely together, cooperating to perform a particular function, are collectively called a body system, or organ system. Each body system works specifically to sustain a certain function in the body. Together, they work to sustain the life of the human body.

A basic cell has several different structural components, each with its own specific function. However, all of the components work together toward a common goal of maintaining the life of the cell. This section introduces the functions of the cells, the functions of the individual components of cells, and it identifies the different kinds of tissues that are created by cells.

Cellular Functions

A living cell is a powerhouse of chemical and molecular activity. There are three general functions of the cell: growth, maintenance, and reproduction. The physical and chemical processes of **metabolism** (meh-TAB-oh-liz-m) allow cells to grow. Maintenance and control of the metabolic processes is accomplished with **homeostasis** (HOH-mee-oh-STAY-sis). Cells reproduce by a series of steps called cell division, which consists of two major activities called mitosis (mahy-TOH-sis) and cytokinesis (SAHY-toh-kih-NEE-sis). The general functions of a cell are made possible by cooperative work of the cell's independent components.

METABOLISM

Metabolism is the overall cellular activity that breaks down nutrients to generate energy to build essential molecules. Catabolism (kah-TAB-oh-liz-m) is the destructive metabolic process that breaks down complex substances and releases energy for cellular activity, often in the form of adenosine triphosphate (ATP). Anabolism (an-AB-oh-liz-m) is the constructive metabolic process that requires energy to build larger, more complex molecules from simpler ones. When all of the metabolic processes are working properly and efficiently, the cell functions normally.

HOMEOSTASIS

The body is constantly monitoring and adjusting metabolic processes in an effort to maintain an internally balanced state of equilibrium called **homeostasis.** Through the dynamic process of responding to changes in the external environment, the body keeps fluid and chemical levels within very narrow limits, body temperature within a narrow range of safety, and oxygen demands of the tissues satisfied. Homeostasis is primarily controlled by negative feedback mechanisms that trigger the body to shut off or reduce certain metabolic activities when abnormal levels of chemicals, body temperatures, or pressures are detected in the body. Blood pressure, body temperature, oxygen level in the blood, carbon dioxide content, and heart rate are all controlled by negative feedback mechanisms. For example, the body is constantly monitoring its internal core temperature, which it typically maintains between 96.8 and 98.6°F. When the core temperature is too low, the body constricts the blood vessels in the skin to conserve heat and initiates shivering to generate heat when the environment is especially cold. As soon as the core temperature is detected within the normal range, the body stops shivering and relaxes the blood vessels in the skin.

CELL DIVISION

Cells can replicate themselves through the process of cell division, which occurs in a series of steps that replicate the genetic material of the cell and divide the components of the cell. Mitosis (mahy-TOH-sis) is the part of cellular division that divides the nucleus. The nucleus, which is an organelle inside the cell that holds the genetic material, is discussed below in this section. Cytokinesis divides the original cell and its contents into two separate cells. Cell divi-

sion is preceded by interphase, which is the part of the cell cycle in which there is no division taking place. Interphase prepares the cell for mitosis by replicating the genetic material called deoxyribonucleic acid (DNA). Following interphase, cell division occurs in the following four stages (Fig. 4-1):

1. Prophase—The chromosomes, which carry the now-duplicated DNA, thicken and resemble limp Xs that are identical pairs of chromatids. The nuclear membrane, which encloses the DNA inside the nucleus, breaks down and disappears.
2. Metaphase—The paired chromatids group together and arrange themselves along the midline of the cell.
3. Anaphase—The chromatids separate, sending each of the identical halves to opposite sides of the cell. Once the chromatids reach the opposite ends of the cell, they are again called chromosomes.
4. Telophase—The chromosomes lengthen and become thinner. Nuclear membranes form around each set of chromosomes to create two separate nuclei. At the same time, cytokinesis divides the rest of the cell into two separate cells, each with its own nucleus.

The entire process of cell division can last anywhere from several minutes to several hours, depending on the type of tissue. At the end of telophase, the original cell has become two cells that are slightly smaller than the original, but are genetically identical to it. The metabolic processes help the cell grow, and homeostatic processes maintain cell growth and life by adjusting metabolic activity.

The cellular function of homeostasis keeps cells safe, healthy, and alive, which keeps the tissues, organs, organ systems, and the whole body safe, healthy, and alive. A cellular imbalance will affect cell

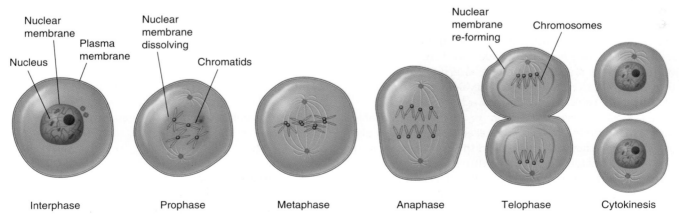

FIGURE 4-1 Stages of cell division.

growth, maintenance, and cell division, and can even result in cell death. This concept can be applied to massage when dealing with a hypertonic (excessively tight) muscle. Hypertonic muscles constrict blood flow, limiting the cell's ability to receive nutrition and eliminate waste. Insufficient oxygen or energy creates an imbalance in the cell and decreases the efficiency of cellular activity. Excessive buildup of waste does the same. Massage techniques can improve the circulation of the blood, which can restore cellular activity to a normal level and, consequently, restore the health of the organism.

Components of the Cell

The metabolic and homeostatic functions of cells are carried out by a number of different structures. A cell is a powerhouse of activity that serves as the basis for all anatomy and physiology. The basic components of a cell are the cell membrane, the cytoplasm, and the organelles. The cell membrane is the outer barrier of the cell and holds the contents of the cell. The cytoplasm is a fluid that suspends the many organelles, which are like separate little machines, each with specific functions to help keep the cell alive and functioning.

CELL MEMBRANE

The cell membrane, sometimes called the plasma membrane, is the outer layer of the cell that protects the contents and activities of the cell. The membrane is primarily composed of phospholipids, which are phosphorus molecules trapped within a double layer of lipid, or fat, molecules. The structure is also referred to as a lipid bilayer. Scattered throughout the membrane are proteins and receptor sites that are discussed below in this section (Fig. 4-2). The membrane provides a selective transport barrier that helps maintain a stable internal environment within the cell. The cell membrane allows nutrients to enter the cell, allows waste material to exit, and maintains appropriate chemical and fluid levels. When those levels are out of balance, cellular activity is affected, and extra energy is required to maintain homeostasis.

The most important function of the semipermeable plasma membrane is to be the "gatekeeper" of nutrient and waste exchange between the cell and the world outside it. If cells do not adequately receive nutrition or eliminate waste, cell growth is hindered, and cell death is possible. The semipermeable quality allows some, but not all, things to pass through the membrane, depending on shape, size, and chemical properties. The exchange

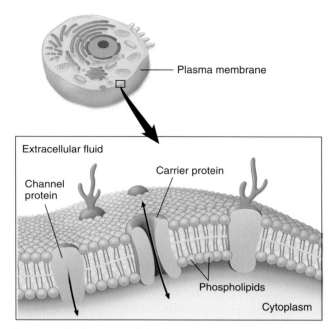

FIGURE 4-2   Structure of the plasma membrane.

can occur passively, without energy, or actively, requiring energy. Diffusion (dif-YOO-zhun), osmosis (oz-MOH-sis), and filtration are passive transport processes that occur without energy expenditure. Active transport processes, such as exocytosis (EK-soh-sahy-toh-sis) and endocytosis (EN-doh-sahy-toh-sis), require some cellular energy to take place.

Passive Transport Mechanism of Diffusion

Diffusion is a process in which molecules move from an area of higher concentration to an area of lower concentration until the molecules are evenly spread out throughout a solution or area. For example, over time and even without being stirred, a spoonful of sugar will dissolve and become evenly distributed throughout a glass of water, through the process of diffusion. The lipid bilayer structure of the membrane gives it some of its abilities to repel molecules that are fat insoluble (cannot dissolve in fat). It also allows fat-soluble molecules, small molecules, and ions to diffuse through. Fats and fat-soluble vitamins can be absorbed into cells via diffusion through the plasma membrane, oxygen and carbon dioxide molecules can diffuse across the respiratory membranes, and sodium ions can easily cross a membrane (Fig. 4-3A).

Passive Transport Mechanism of Osmosis

There are occasions when molecules that cannot pass through the semipermeable membrane are concentrated differently on either side of the membrane. To maintain homeostasis and keep everything balanced,

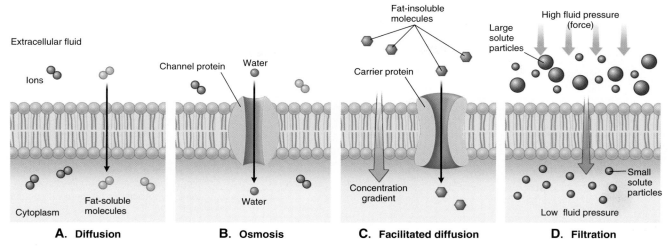

FIGURE 4-3 Mechanisms of passive transport.

the body moves water from the side that has a lower concentration of these molecules to the side with the higher concentration. The addition of water effectively lowers the concentration of these molecules. Most people recognize that oil and water do not mix. Because of its molecular structure, water is not soluble in oil or fat. Although water is not a fat-soluble molecule and it would typically be repelled by the lipid bilayer, water moves through the semipermeable cell membrane. Osmosis is the specific passive transport mechanism by which water crosses the membrane through channel proteins to balance concentrations on either side of the membrane. The best way to remember which direction water moves through the membrane is the phrase "Water follows concentration" (Fig. 4-3B). If there is a higher concentration of solutes outside the cell, water will move out of the cell in an attempt to balance the solutions on either side of the membrane. Conversely, if there is a higher concentration of solutes inside the cell, water will flow into the cell to achieve a balance.

Solutions possess osmotic pressure, which is the pressure exerted by dissolved particles in the solution. A solution whose osmotic pressure is the same as that within our cells is called an isotonic (AHY-soh-TAHN-ik) solution. When an isotonic solution surrounds our cells, the cells do not have to change their water levels to accommodate the new fluid. Intravenous fluids such as Ringer's lactate and 0.9% saline solution are isotonic solutions that have the same concentrations as our cells, so when they are injected into the bloodstream, the cells do not absorb or eliminate water.

When solutions that do not have the same concentration of dissolved substances as our cells are introduced into our bodies, the water content within the cell is adjusted to maintain a balance on either side of

the cell membrane. This homeostatic mechanism is used therapeutically when medical professionals give patients intravenous fluids. Hypotonic (HAHY-poh-TAHN-ik) solutions have a lower osmotic pressure (are less concentrated) than the fluid inside our cells and result in water moving into the cell by osmosis. Conditions of dehydration are sometimes treated with hypotonic solutions, which force water to move into and rehydrate the cells. Hypertonic (HAHY-per-TAHN-ik) solutions are used to treat edema, which is swelling due to an excess of fluid between the cells. The hypertonic solution, often 3–5% sodium chloride solution, causes water to move toward the higher concentration, outside the cells, and into the bloodstream. The excess fluid is then processed by the kidneys and excreted as urine (Fig. 4-4).

Passive Transport Mechanism of Facilitated Diffusion

Facilitated diffusion is a special form of passive membrane transport. Molecules that are too large or that would be repelled by the lipid bilayer use carrier proteins scattered along the membrane as trap doors that allow them to pass through easily. A carrier protein molecule attaches to the oversized molecule, slightly alters its shape or envelopes it, and pulls it through the membrane (see Fig. 4-3C). A good example of facilitated diffusion is the passage of glucose through a cell membrane. Glucose is a large molecule used for cellular metabolism that is not fat soluble, but can use a carrier protein to get through the membrane.

Passive Transport Mechanism of Filtration

Filtration is another mode of passive transport whereby water and dissolved substances (solutes) are

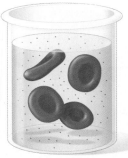 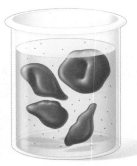 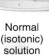 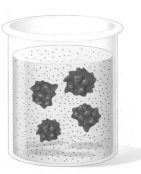

Normal
(isotonic)
solution

Hypotonic
solution

Hypertonic
solution

FIGURE 4-4 Effects of osmosis on red blood cells in different concentrations: isotonic, hypotonic, and hypertonic solutions.

pushed through a membrane by fluid pressure. This process moves the solution from an area of higher pressure to an area of lower pressure, again in an effort to keep a balance on either side of the membrane (see Fig. 4-3D). An example of filtration is urine formation in the kidneys, where the fluid pressure in the blood capillaries is higher than that in the kidney tubules. The difference in pressures forces the solution out of the blood capillaries and into the kidney tubules for elimination.

Active Transport Mechanisms

Active transport processes require ATP as a source of energy to move molecules through a membrane. There are several different situations in which molecules cannot be transported passively and energy must be used to move them:

- Molecules that are too large to pass through the membrane and cannot take advantage of carrier proteins
- Molecules that have to move against the concentration gradient, or from an area where they are lower in concentration to an area of higher concentration
- Molecules that are not fat soluble and cannot take advantage of carrier proteins

Solute pumping is the active transport process that uses energy from the breakdown of ATP to help protein carriers pull amino acids, some sugars, and many ions through the membrane.

Bulk transport is an active transport process that uses energy to package molecules and carry them across the membrane. Exocytosis is the bulk transport mechanism that takes cellular products from the inside of the cell to the outside of the cell. The products in the cytoplasm are packaged in a sac, the sac is incorporated into the membrane, and the contents of the sac are released into the extracellular fluid (the

fluid that surrounds the cell). Mucus is released outside the cell via exocytosis (Fig. 4-5B illustrates exocytosis). Active transport can work in the opposite direction via endocytosis, in which substances outside the cell are engulfed, transported inside the cell, and usually digested by enzymes (Fig. 4-5A). Bacteria and dead body cells are managed by the specific form of endocytosis called phagocytosis (FAY-goh-sahy-TOH-sis). When liquids that contain dissolved proteins or fats cannot diffuse through a cell membrane, pinocytosis (PEE-noh-sahy-toh-sis) is the special form of endocytosis that moves them into the cell. The prefix "exo-" means to "move out" and "endo-" means to "move in."

The cell membrane is a very active component of the cell that is involved in homeostasis, but there are a number of other structures that are equally important.

CYTOPLASM

The cytoplasm is the liquid substance inside the plasma membrane that houses most of the cellular activity. It is composed of a gellike substance called cytosol that contains nutrients, minerals, enzymes, and cytoplasmic organelles suspended in it. The cytoplasm makes up 50% of the cell's volume and contains everything necessary for protein synthesis as well as the enzymes for building and breaking down molecules. Imagine a pot of vegetable soup. The cellular membrane is similar to the pot that holds the soup, and the cytoplasm is like the soup inside the pot. The cytosol is like the liquid part of the soup, and the nutrients, minerals, enzymes, and organelles are like the vegetables in the soup. One difference is that the cellular membrane, unlike the cooking pot, allows passage of nutrients and other molecules into the cell and wastes out of the cell (Fig. 4-6).

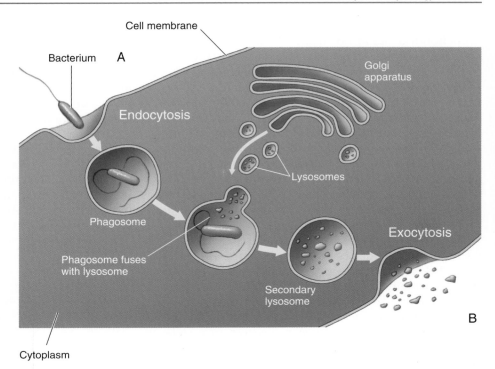

FIGURE 4-5 Bulk transport mechanisms. **A.** Endocytosis. **B.** Exocytosis. (Reprinted from Premkumar K. The Massage Connection: Anatomy & Physiology. 2nd ed. Baltimore: Lippincott Williams & Wilkins, 2004.)

CYTOPLASMIC ORGANELLES

The cytoplasmic organelles are the metabolic machinery of the cell that keeps the cell alive and dynamic. Organelles, including the nucleus, nucleolus, ribosomes, endoplasmic reticulum, mitochondria, Golgi apparatus, lysosomes, centrioles, cilia, and flagella, are all suspended in the cytosol. They have different shapes and functions, and any disruption of their activity will affect the homeostasis of the cell.

The largest organelle is the nucleus (NOOK-lee-us), located somewhere near the center of the cell. The nucleus is the control center for the cell. It is enveloped in a double-layered membrane that is perforated with pores that allow some molecules to pass between the nucleus and the cell. Within the nucleus is a small, spherical structure called a nucleolus (nook-lee-OH-lus), which builds the molecules required for protein synthesis. Occasionally, cells have two nucleoli, if there is a heavy demand for proteins. Among other molecules, the nucleus contains DNA, which is necessary for building protein fibers and reproducing cells and is the blueprint for building an entire organism.

Outside the nucleus are many organelles suspended in the cytoplasm that carry out other cellular operations. There are many ribosomes (RAHY-boh-zohmz) that serve as the framework for putting proteins together. Some are suspended in the cytosol, and some are attached to the rough endoplasmic reticulum. There are one or more endoplasmic retic-

ula within the cytoplasm, which are networks of tubes that carry newly made proteins from one area of the cell to another. The endoplasmic reticula also manufacture membrane lipids, synthesize and break down cholesterol, and metabolize fat.

Also within the cytosol are several elongated oval organelles called mitochondria (MAHY-toh-KON-

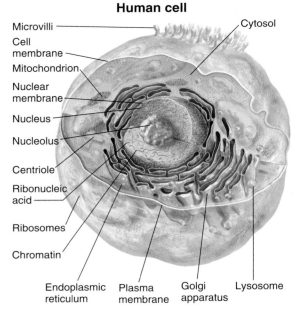

Human cell

Microvilli
Cell membrane
Mitochondrion
Nuclear membrane
Nucleus
Nucleolus
Centriole
Ribonucleic acid
Ribosomes
Chromatin
Cytosol
Endoplasmic reticulum
Plasma membrane
Golgi apparatus
Lysosome

FIGURE 4-6 Components of a cell. (Asset provided by Anatomical Chart Co.)

dree-uh). As the powerhouses of cellular function, mitochondria break down nutrients and release energy. Some of the energy is released as heat, but most of the energy is converted to ATP molecules through the process of cellular respiration, which is the primary source of energy for cellular metabolism. Because oxygen is required for cellular respiration, the process is sometimes referred to as aerobic respiration. Without oxygen, cells will suffer and eventually die. Generally, the more active the cell, the more oxygen and energy it requires and the more mitochondria it will have. Muscle cells that get regular exercise increase their numbers of mitochondria to generate more energy for the muscle cell.

The Golgi apparatus is an organelle that resembles a stack of flattened sacs that are suspended in the cytosol. Serving as a sort of packaging plant, the sacs receive proteins by way of the endoplasmic reticulum. The proteins are modified, sorted, and gathered in sacs until the sacs swell to the point that they pinch themselves off and become secretory vesicles. The final destination of the vesicles depends on their contents. Vesicles that contain mucus or digestive enzymes fuse with the plasma membrane and expel their contents outside the cell, illustrated above as the active transport mechanism of exocytosis (see Fig. 4-5). Some vesicles contain proteins and phospholipids that are taken to the plasma membrane and become part of its structure. Some vesicles containing digestive enzymes remain inside the cell, suspended in the cytosol.

Some of the smaller cytoplasmic organelles include lysosomes (LAHY-soh-zohmz), centrioles (SEN-tree-ohlz), and cilia (SIL-ee-uh). Varied in size, lysosomes are the vesicles from the Golgi apparatus that contain digestive enzymes. Inside the cell, lysosomes engulf and digest cellular waste, bacteria, and unwanted foreign substances. Centrioles are rod-shaped organelles located close to the nucleus that aid in chromosome separation during cell division. Some cells have cilia, which are small, hairlike projections on the outside of the cell that help sweep objects past the cell. They are located in respiratory and reproductive tracts to push mucus or an egg in a specific direction. An extra long form of cilium called a flagellum (fluh-JEL-uhm) is a whiplike extension that propels the cell itself. The human sperm cell has a single flagellum that moves the sperm from one place to another.

The many structures of a cell, with their many activities, work cooperatively to maintain the life cycle of the entire cell. As part of the whole picture, cells are the tiny building blocks that make up tissues, organs, organ systems, and the organism.

Tissues

A **tissue** is a group of cells that have a similar structure and work together to accomplish a similar function. There are four basic tissue types, each with a unique structure, specific function, and its own rate of healing. Structure and function are closely related, following the rule of "form follows function." Much of healing depends on nutrient delivery and waste removal, so the healing rate tends to be related to the tissue's blood supply. Epithelial (EH-pih-THEE-lee-uhl) tissue, connective tissue, muscle tissue, and nervous tissue are woven together within the body to provide coverings, support, movement, and control, respectively (Table 4-1).

EPITHELIAL TISSUE

Epithelial tissue, or epithelium (EH-pih-THEE-lee-uhm), covers the outside of our bodies, it lines cavities and tubes inside our bodies, and it forms some

TABLE 4-1

Types of Tissue

TISSUE TYPE	FUNCTION	LOCATION
Epithelium	Lines Covers Produces secretions	Skin, organs, glands
Connective tissue	Connects Protects Supports	Blood, bone, cartilage, fascia, fat, ligament, lymph, tendon

Muscle tissue
  Cardiac
  Skeletal
  Smooth
	
	Contracts the heart
	Moves and stabilizes
	Produces peristalsis
		
		Heart
		Attached to skeleton
		Organs

Nervous tissue	Communication and control	Brain, spinal cord, nerves

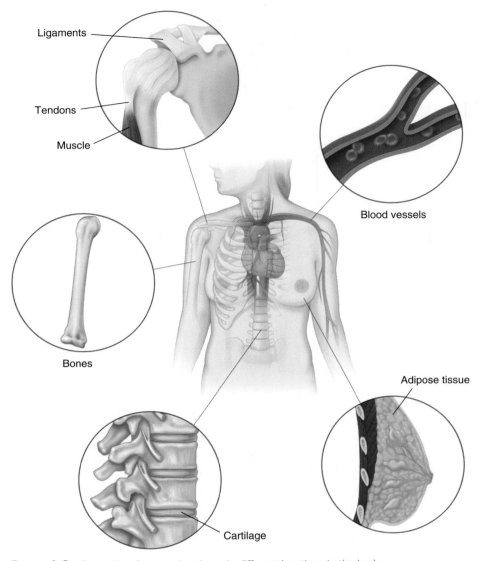

FIGURE 4-8   Examples of connective tissue in different locations in the body.

ments can be random or aligned. When the fibers are aligned in the same direction, the tissue resembles ropelike cords, as in the tendons and ligaments. Scar tissue has a random arrangement and has a patchwork-like quality. Connective tissue can be categorized into four groups: hard, fibrous, soft, and liquid. Figure 4-10 illustrates the four types of connective tissues.

Hard Connective Tissue

The hard connective tissues are very firm and not very pliable and some contain hardened minerals that further solidify their structure. The two forms of hard connective tissue in our bodies include cartilage and bones (Fig. 4-11).

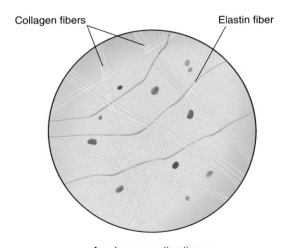

Areolar connective tissue

FIGURE 4-9   Collagen and elastin fibers in an extracellular matrix.

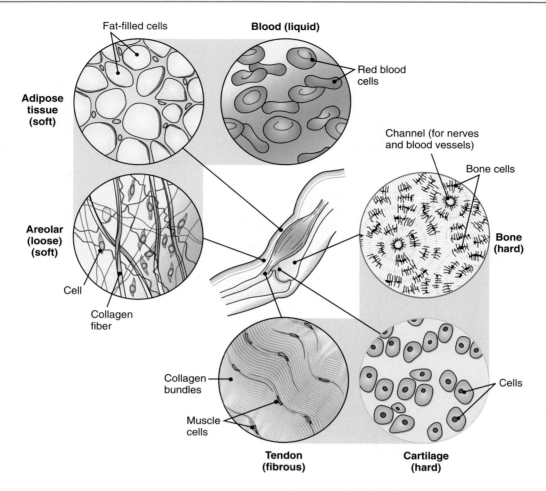

4 Types of connective tissue

FIGURE 4-10   Four types of connective tissues: soft, liquid, hard, and fibrous. (Reprinted from Cohen BJ, Wood DL. Memmler's Structure and Function of the Human Body. 9th ed. Philadelphia: Lippincott Williams & Wilkins, 2000.)

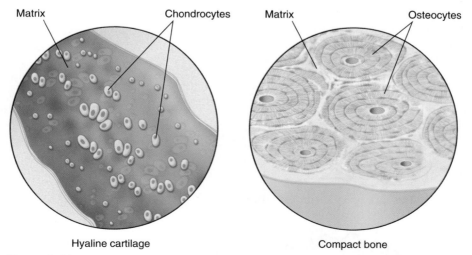

FIGURE 4-11   Hard connective tissue matrix: hyaline cartilage and compact bone.

Cartilage

Cartilage is a form of hard connective tissue that is firm, smooth, and bendable. It is composed of living chondrocytes (KON-droh-sahytz), or cartilage cells, suspended in a nonliving extracellular matrix that contains collagen and elastin protein fibers. It functions as a shock absorber that can bear mechanical stress without permanent distortion and reduce friction between moving parts, as in the knee joint. Cartilage can also be used as a material for structural support, as in the outer ear. Cartilage is avascular, which makes it slow to heal after injury. It can only receive nourishment via diffusion from capillaries in the adjacent tissues or from the synovial fluid that bathes and lubricates freely movable joints. While temporary cartilage forms the fetal skeleton and is later ossified and converted to bone, permanent cartilage remains throughout life. The three major types of cartilage are hyaline cartilage, fibrocartilage, and elastic cartilage (Table 4-2).

TABLE 4-2

Types of Cartilage

CARTILAGE	CHARACTERISTICS	EXAMPLES	
Hyaline	Strong, not very flexible	Costal cartilage	Hyaline cartilage (costal cartilage)
Fibrocartilage	Strongest	Intervertebral disks	Fibrocartilage (intervertebral discs)
Elastic	Most flexible	Outer ear	Elastic cartilage (external ear)

Hyaline cartilage is the most common form of permanent cartilage and provides strength and shock absorption but not much flexibility. It appears white or whitish blue because of its avascularity and the predominance of white collagen protein fibers. It is found where two bones come together and need some padding, for example, where the ribs contact the sternum and at the growth zones at the ends of long bones. Hyaline cartilage also provides a structural framework in the walls of large respiratory passages that go from outside the body to the lungs, including the nose, trachea, and bronchi.

Elastic cartilage has an abundance of elastic fibers, which give it a yellowish color and make it the most flexible type of cartilage. It can be bent and return to its normal shape, providing a structural framework for parts of the body that are subjected to higher amounts of movement, such as the external part of the ear, the ear canal, the eustachian tube, and the epiglottis.

Fibrocartilage has dense collagen fibers surrounding rows or groups of chondrocytes, making it extremely resilient. Providing a cushion between bones that are only slightly movable, fibrocartilage is found between adjacent vertebrae (bones in the spine) and in the sutures between the cranial bones.

Bone

Bone is the other form of hard connective tissue. Calcium and phosphate salts that accompany the dense collagen fibers in the extracellular matrix create the hardness of bone. There are three different kinds of living cells suspended in the matrix of bone: osteoblasts (AHS-tee-oh-blastz), or bone-forming cells, osteocytes (AHS-tee-oh-sahytz), or mature bone cells, and osteoclasts (AHS-tee-oh-klastz), or bone-destroying cells. Figure 4-11 shows the difference between the matrix of bone and the matrix of hyaline cartilage.

Bones are much more than a compilation of proteins and minerals. Their structure is a highly organized series of bundles of osteocytes and blood vessels. Because of its high vascularity, bone heals quickly, relative to other tissues. Bone, which is the main component of the skeletal system, has many functions:

- Bones are the main storage place for calcium and other ions.
- Bones act as a lever system for converting muscle contraction into movement.
- Blood cells are formed inside many bones.
- Bones protect soft tissue structures in the body.

Fibrous Connective Tissue

Fibrous connective tissues, sometimes called dense connective tissues, are found as tendons, ligaments, and scar tissue. Most of the protein fibers in the extracellular matrix are collagen fibers that are all aligned in the same direction, giving the fibrous connective tissues a cordlike structure that is strong and flexible.

Tendons connect muscles to bones and, as part of the muscle–tendon (musculotendinous) unit, create skeletal movement. Almost every muscle has at least one tendon attached to it, and some muscles have more than one tendon. Since the tendons themselves do not actively contract or relax, they vary in tension, depending on the activity of the muscles they attach to. For example, a tendon attached to a muscle that is working against a lot of resistance will feel tight and not very pliable, like an elastic band that has been stretched almost to its limit. A tendon attached to a muscle that is relaxed will feel looser, like a rubber band lying on a table. Specialized tendons that are broad and flat called are called aponeuroses (AP-poh-nur-OH-seez). They provide attachment for broad muscles to connect to bone or for one set of muscles to connect to another.

As a form of fibrous connective tissue, tendons have parallel collagen fibers that are dense and regular. The dense arrangement and poor blood supply make it difficult for the nutrient–waste exchange to occur. Because this exchange occurs mostly through diffusion from the surrounding tissues, injured tendons heal slowly.

Ligaments are fibrous connective tissue structures that connect bones to bones at a joint. They stabilize and strengthen the joints of the body that must withstand great mechanical force, such as the knee and the hip. As in tendons, most of the protein fibers are dense, regular, parallel strands of collagen. Ligaments are more flexible than tendons because there are more elastin fibers and the proportion of ground substance to protein is larger. Ligaments remain tight despite movement or various states of contraction and are more difficult to palpate because of their location within joints. Because of the minimal blood supply to the ligaments at their insertions, the healing process is very slow.

Scar tissue is a special kind of fibrous connective tissue that forms when tissues are injured. It is unique because, unlike those in tendons and ligaments, the collagen fibers are not arranged in a parallel pattern. Because of the abundance of dense and irregular collagen fibers, scar tissue is strong but not as pliable as normal, healthy tissue. Serving as a replacement for other injured tissue, it cannot perform the functions of tissue it replaces, and its blood supply is minimal. Extensive scarring can restrict normal movement, reduce or prevent normal circulation of blood and lymph, and impede or even prevent injured tissue from functioning properly. The structure of scar tissue depends upon where the injury occurs, but it usually contains the same components as the original tissue, accompanied by an abundance of extra collagen fibers.

Soft Connective Tissue

Soft connective tissues are also called loose connective tissues. They have more living cells and fewer protein fibers in their matrix and are highly vascular, giving them a relatively fast healing rate.

Areolar (ah-REE-oh-lahr) tissue is a form of soft connective tissue that is highly vascular, delicate, and somewhat resistant to stress. Phagocytes, living cells that engulf bacteria or cellular debris, are present in the matrix, accompanied by few collagen and elastin fibers. Found just below the skin, in membranes around blood and lymph vessels, around organs, and between muscles, areolar tissue cushions and protects the structures it surrounds.

Adipose tissue, commonly called fat, is basically areolar tissue with adipose cells suspended in the matrix instead of phagocytes. Adipose cells can synthesize fat and store it as a large droplet of oil. When the body needs a source of energy, it can use fat released by adipose cells. Besides its function as a source of energy, adipose tissue acts as a thermal insulator. Heat is not conducted well through the fat, which means that if there are different temperatures on either side of the adipose tissue, those temperatures will be maintained. Adipose tissue also provides padding and protection for organs in its locations just beneath the skin in the superficial fascia, around organs, between muscles, in the marrow of the long bone shafts, and in the breasts and hips.

Liquid Connective Tissue

Blood and lymph are sometimes called liquid connective tissues because they have living cells suspended in a nonliving matrix and they "connect" different parts of the body. Technically, however, neither blood nor lymph has an extracellular matrix that is secreted by the living cells. Moreover, blood has protein fibers present in the matrix only during the process of blood clotting. Blood flows through the blood vessels of the cardiovascular system, and lymph flows through the lymphatic vessels in the lymphatic system. Blood and lymph are described in more detail in the section on the circulatory system.

MUSCLE TISSUE

Tissues are a group of cells with similar structure and function. Muscle tissue is a group of muscle cells that are grouped together with blood vessels and packaged with connective tissue in a specific organization, more commonly called a **muscle.** These cells have an elongated shape and are sometimes referred to as muscle fibers. Muscle cells have the special ability to contract and relax, resulting in their primary function of creating movement. Skeletal, cardiac, and smooth muscle tissues are the three types of muscle tissue that have slightly different characteristics and arrangements. Some have striations (strahy-AY-shunz), which are microscopic structural features that look like stripes. Some muscle cells contain more than one nucleus, and some muscle cells form branching networks of cells. The control mechanism for muscle cells can also differ. Some are involuntary, meaning that they contract without our conscious effort, and others are voluntary, which means that we have to consciously make an effort to contract the muscle to create movement. Table 4-3 characterizes the different types of muscle tissue. This section of the anatomy and physiology chapter briefly introduces and compares the different kinds of muscle tissue. There is a comprehensive discussion of skeletal muscle tissue below in this chapter.

Skeletal Muscle

Skeletal muscle is tissue that attaches to the skeleton. The cells are long and cylindrical with multiple nuclei and heavy striations. Skeletal muscle tissue is under voluntary control, meaning that we consciously make skeletal muscles contract to move our bodies. When contracted, skeletal muscles are shortened and the muscles cells are closer together. As a result, blood vessels are constricted, and the delivery of nutrients and elimination of cellular metabolic waste is limited. Healthy muscles at their normal resting length have more space between the cells and the exchange of oxygen, nutrients, and wastes is more efficient. Skeletal muscle tissue is responsible for producing body movement and holding our bodies up against the force of gravity. Simply, gravity is the force that pulls us to the earth, and except when we are lying down, we use skeletal muscles to hold ourselves upright.

Massage deals with movement, restriction of movement, and restoration of health to the skeletal muscle system. **Understanding skeletal muscle tissue and how it functions is fundamental to massage.** Massage can relax hypertonic (tense) skeletal muscles by using the help of the nervous system to stop triggering muscles to contract. Once the muscles stop receiving signals from the nervous system to contract, they can relax, and then other massage techniques can help return skeletal muscles to their normal resting lengths. By using massage to return skeletal muscles to their normal resting lengths, there is sufficient space between muscle cells for adequate blood circulation and nutrient and waste exchange, thus enhancing the health of the tissues. Reflexive and mechanical techniques are covered in detail in the hands-on and therapeutic techniques chapters below in the text.

TABLE 4-3

Different Types of Muscle Tissue, Characteristics, Locations

TYPE OF MUSCLE CELL		CELL CHARACTERISTICS	CONTROL	FUNCTION	LOCATION
Smooth	Nucleus	Tapered at both ends Single nucleus Nonstriated	Involuntary	Slow, sustained contractions (peristalsis)	Blood vessels Intestines
Cardiac	Intercalated disks — Nucleus	Branching networks Single nucleus Light striations	Involuntary	Pumps blood out of the heart	Wall of heart
Skeletal	Nucleus	Long, cylindrical Multinucleated Heavy striations	Voluntary	Movement of skeleton	Attached to bones

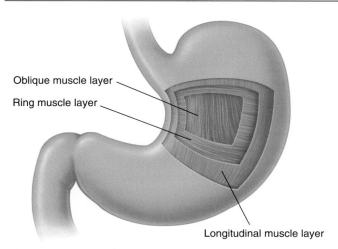

FIGURE 4-12   Layering of smooth muscle in the stomach

Cardiac Muscle

Cardiac muscle is another type of muscle tissue, which is found only in the walls of the heart. It has light striations and only one nucleus per muscle cell, but the cells branch together at tight junctions called intercalated (in-TER-kuh-lay-ted) disks. These junctions allow the electrical impulses that signal muscle contraction to move quickly across the heart. Cardiac muscle contracts involuntarily, which is why our heart continues to beat while we are asleep and cannot consciously control the contractions.

Smooth Muscle

Smooth muscle, sometimes called visceral muscle, has cells that are nonstriated and tapered at both ends. Each smooth muscle cell has only one nucleus and is involuntarily controlled. Although it provides a weaker contraction than skeletal or cardiac muscle, it can sustain contractions for a longer time. Smooth muscle tends to be arranged in layers, and the fibers of each successive layer run in a different direction than those in the previous layer. Figure 4-12 illustrates smooth muscle layering in the stomach. These layers alternate contractions to produce peristalsis, which is the wavelike pulsating contraction that propels substances along a tube in the body. For example, the digestive tract has layers of smooth muscle that push its contents in one direction, from the mouth toward the anus, via peristalsis.

NERVOUS TISSUE

Nervous tissue has a specialized structure that serves as the communication path for controlling activity within our bodies. The nervous tissues send electrochemical impulses to and from different parts of the body to receive stimuli and trigger bodily responses. The structural components that make up the brain,

spinal cord, and nerves include two kinds of nervous tissue cells called neurons (NOO-rahnz) and neuroglia (noo-ROH-glee-uh).

Neurons

A **neuron,** or nerve cell, is a specialized cell that is the basic unit of nervous tissue. A neuron has a unique structure with three basic parts: a body, a single axon, and dendrites (Fig. 4-13). The body of the neuron is similar to other cells because of its generally rounded shape that holds the nucleus and other cytoplasmic

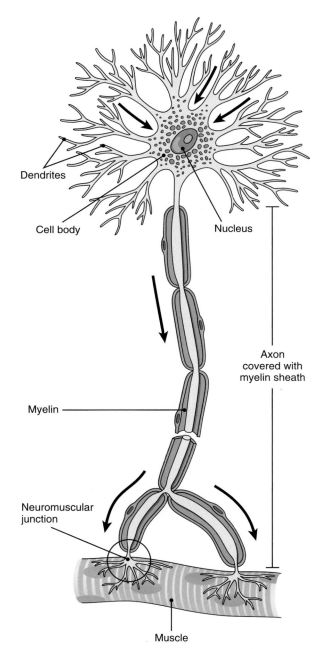

FIGURE 4-13   Basic nerve cell structure. Reprinted from Cohen BJ. Medical Terminology, 4th ed. Philadelphia. Lippincott Williams & Wilkins 2003.

organelles. Unlike other cells, the cytoplasm and cellular membrane have long branches that protrude from the body of the cell that receive and send the electrochemical impulses of nerve signal transmission. Dendrites are the processes radiating out from the cell body that receive electrochemical nerve impulses from other neurons and carry them to the cell body. Neurons usually have a lot of dendrites and can receive input from many other neurons. The axon is a long, single process radiating out from the body of the neuron that conducts nerve impulses from the cell body to another cell. The process of nerve signal transmission is like a chain of communication in which the dendrites receive the signal and pass it along to the cell body, and then the axon carries the signal from the cell body to another neuron, where it is received by the dendrites of the second neuron, and so on. Massage activates this chain of communica-

tion in a number of ways. For example, when we first touch our clients, the tactile input stimulates an electrochemical impulse to travel along the cell membrane from the dendrites, toward the cell body, out the axon, and then to another neuron. The impulse continues to travel along the neurons until it reaches the CNS, at which point the client's body responds to the initial touch. The client's response will be influenced by your professionalism, standards of care, and respect for the client's physical and conceptual boundaries, discussed in the chapter covering ethics and professionalism.

Some neurons are covered with a white, fatty material called myelin (see Fig. 4-13). It significantly increases the speed of nerve impulses along the neuron, and it functions as insulation, preventing the electrochemical impulse from short-circuiting. When myelinated nerves lose their myelin or the myelin be-

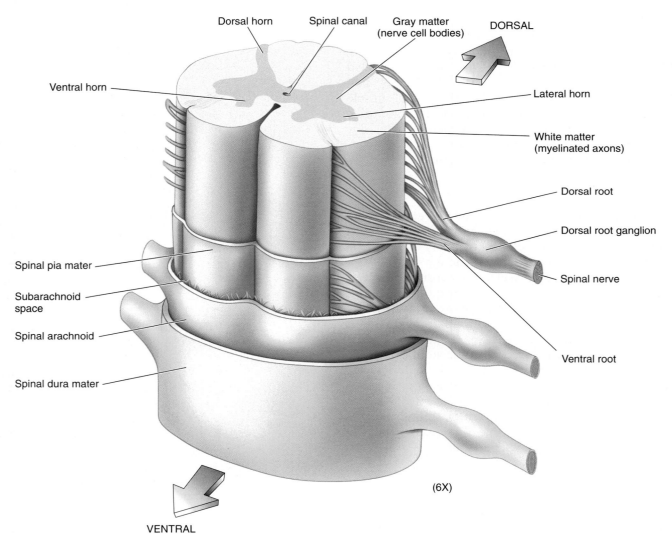

FIGURE 4-14 Cross section of the spinal cord, showing the gray matter of the nerve cell. (Reprinted from Bear MF, Connors BW, Parasido MA. Neuroscience—Exploring the Brain. 2nd ed. Philadelphia: Lippincott Williams & Wilkins, 2001.)

comes hardened, nerve transmission may become problematic. Myelinated axons appear as white fibers that when grouped together are called white matter. Groups of unmyelinated nerve cells are called gray matter. Figure 4-14 is a cross section of the spinal cord, showing the gray matter of the nerve cell bodies and the white matter made of myelinated axons.

Neuroglia

Neuroglia, also called glial (GLEE-uhl) cells, are connective tissue cells that support and protect neurons, connect them to blood vessels, produce myelin, destroy and remove pathogens and cellular debris, and help circulate the cerebrospinal fluid. They are structurally similar to neurons but cannot transmit impulses.

Membranes

Membranes are thin sheets of tissues with many different characteristics that give rise to different functions:

- Serve as a covering for the outside of the body
- Serve as a covering for organs
- Serve as an anchor for organs
- Act as a partition between structures
- Serve as a lining for tubes of cavities in the body
- Reduce friction between structures

Membranes can be fragile, tough, or transparent, and some contain cells that secrete lubricating fluids. There are two general classifications of membranes, including epithelial and connective tissue membranes.

EPITHELIAL MEMBRANES

Epithelial membranes are constructed with an epithelium that is integrated onto an underlying layer of connective tissue. The connective tissue layer, in addition to the closely packed epithelial cells, creates strong and protective membranes. There are three types of epithelial membranes: serous (SEER-us), mucous (MYOO-kus), and cutaneous (kyoo-TAY-nee-us) (Fig. 4-15).

Serous Membranes

Serous membranes are composed of a layer of simple squamous epithelial cells atop a thin layer of areolar connective tissue. The serous membranes line the ventral (anterior) body cavities and cover the organs within those cavities. Serous membranes contain cells that secrete serous fluid, a thin lubricant that al-

lows organs to move and slip past each other with minimal friction during normal body movements. Serous membranes have a layered, folded construction that forms two different layers of each membrane. The parietal (puh-RAHY-eh-tuhl) layer of a serous membrane lines a body cavity, and the visceral layer of that same serous membrane covers the organs within that body cavity.

Three types of serous membranes are found in the human body: the pleura (PLUR-uh), the pericardium (PAIR-ih-KAR-dee-um), and the peritoneum (PAIR-ih-toh-NEE-um). The pleura, or pleural membranes, are located in the thoracic cavity. The parietal layer of the pleura lines the interior walls of the thoracic cavity, and the visceral layer covers the lungs. The pericardium is also located in the thoracic cavity, but its parietal layer forms the sac that encloses the heart, and its visceral layer covers the heart muscle itself. The peritoneum is located in the abdominal cavity. The parietal peritoneum lines the abdominal cavity walls and the visceral peritoneum covers, supports, and protects the organs and structures within the abdomen.

Mucous Membranes

Mucous membranes are epithelial membranes that line tubes and spaces that are exposed to the outside of the body. These membranes are made of simple and/or stratified epithelium resting on a layer of soft connective tissue and form continuous linings in the digestive, respiratory, reproductive, and urinary systems. The primary function of most of these wet membranes is to secrete mucus, a viscous and sticky substance that moistens and protects the membranes. In the nasal passages and the bronchi in the lungs, mucus keeps the passages wet, despite exposure to external air. The mucus also traps pathogens that enter the respiratory pathway. Ciliated cells in the respiratory tract then sweep the mucus and foreign particles up and outward, away from the lungs, to protect us against infection and to get rid of pathogens that have already entered the respiratory tract. In the digestive tract, the mucus has several different functions. It acts as a protective barrier against the strong acids that break down food. When the mucus barrier breaks down, the acids can attack the organs, resulting in ulcers and irritation within the digestive tract. The mucous membranes located toward the end of the digestive tract secrete mucus that absorbs the nutrients made available as a result of our food being broken down.

Cutaneous Membrane

Cutaneous membrane, commonly called skin, has an outer layer of stratified squamous epithelial tissue

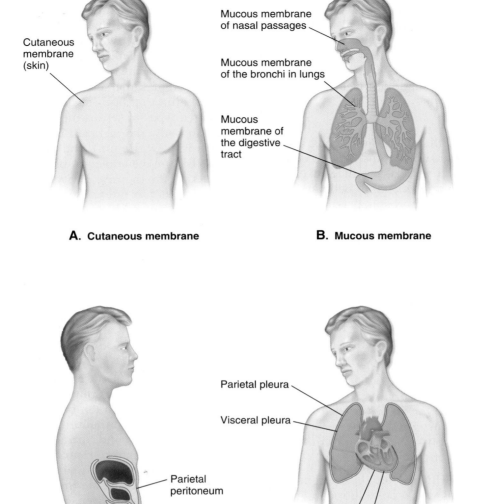

A. Cutaneous membrane

Cutaneous membrane (skin)

Mucous membrane of nasal passages

Mucous membrane of the bronchi in lungs

Mucous membrane of the digestive tract

B. Mucous membrane

Parietal pleura

Visceral pleura

Parietal peritoneum

Visceral peritoneum

Parietal pericardium

Visceral pericardium

C. Serous membranes

FIGURE 4-15   Locations of epithelial membranes. **A.** Cutaneous. **B.** Mucous. **C.** Serous.

over a layer of connective tissue. Functioning primarily to protect the body from the environment, the cutaneous membrane is the only kind that is dry. The skin is discussed in the section on the integumentary system.

CONNECTIVE TISSUE MEMBRANES

Connective tissue membranes consist of sheets of connective tissue without an attached epithelium. The different forms of connective tissue membranes include synovial membranes, meninges, connective tissue sacs around organs, and fascia.

Synovial Membranes

Synovial (sin-OH-vee-uhl) membranes line the joint cavities, tendon sheaths, and bursae, which are the small cushioning sacs located in some of the larger joints. These membranes secrete synovial fluid, a thick, clear substance that has the consistency of egg white. This slippery secretion nourishes the articular cartilage and lubricates and reduces friction in the following locations:

- At the freely movable joints
- Between muscles
- Between a tendon and ligament
- Between a muscle and a ligament

Meninges

Meninges (men-IN-jeez) consist of multiple membrane layers that cover the brain and spinal cord. The dura mater, arachnoid layer, and pia mater are the three meningeal layers that function as protective coverings. These connective tissue membranes are discussed below, in the section on the nervous system.

Connective Tissue Sacs

Connective tissue surrounds many anatomical structures in the form of connective tissue sacs. The heart is encased in a fibrous membrane sac called the pericardium, the bones are covered with periosteum, and cartilage is covered with perichondrium. These structures are discussed below in the chapter, with their respective body systems.

Fascia

Fascia (FASH-uh), sometimes called the fascial sheath, is a fibrous band or sheetlike tissue membrane that provides support and protection for the body organs. **Fascia wraps around everything in the body, stabilizing, protecting, and supporting organs and muscles.** Fascia is very pervasive, forming a sort of three-dimensional meshwork throughout the body. A restriction or adhesion in the fascia is an area where the smooth membrane has been crumpled or kinked with some sort of trauma; additional collagen fibers are deposited in the area, and a scar is created that pulls the surrounding fascia toward it. This resultant tension and pulling action can even affect anatomical structures that are a significant distance away, causing a number of problems:

- Restricted movement
- Compensation patterns
- Reduced circulation
- Muscular tension
- Pain in areas that seem completely unrelated

This situation is common following surgery. For a couple of weeks after surgery, the area that was surgically repaired is usually subjected to minimal movement to give the incision a chance to heal. The fascia has already been disrupted, and without movement, the body's healing response deposits fascia on top of the disruption, essentially fixing the disruption into place with a fascial adhesion. The three-dimensional nature of fascia creates a situation where the rest of the fascia is pulled toward the adhesion. For example, clients who have ankle surgery may complain of tightness or restricted movement in the knee. Clients who have abdominal surgery could feel tightness in the neck or shoulder. Massage therapy can reduce fascial restrictions better than many other treatments, helping to restore normal function to the body. Specific massage techniques have been especially designed to manipulate the fascia and are discussed in the chapter on therapeutic massage techniques.

Superficial fascia is a continuous sheetlike layer composed of mostly adipose connective tissue with some interspersed collagen and elastin fibers that has a number of functions:

- Provide energy from the fat stored in the adipose cells
- Provide protection for the skin
- Provide a passageway for nerves
- Provide a passageway for circulatory vessels
- Provide thermal insulation

Sometimes called the subcutaneous layer or the hypodermis, superficial fascia lies just beneath the surface of the skin. It is dense and anchors the skin firmly to underlying tissues.

Deep fascia is found in and around every skeletal muscle. It wraps almost every structure of a muscle, starting with the wrapping around a muscle cell, called the endomysium. Several wrapped fibers together form fascicles, which are wrapped in perimysium. The entire muscle, made up of several fascicles, is wrapped in the epimysium. Figure 4-16 shows the deep fascia surrounding structures of a muscle. Deep fascia contains no fat and is mostly composed of collagen fibers and some elastin, making it very strong and a little pliable. It functions to cover, separate, and protect the muscles. This tissue has a thixotropic quality, meaning that it is a gelatinous substance that without movement can thicken, contract, and become less pliable. When the deep fascia is stiff and contracted, it restricts muscle movement and circulation within the muscles. On the other hand, the thixotropic quality also means that deep fascia can be thinned to a more fluid or liquid state with mechanical manipulation. Massage therapy can provide the manipulation to thin the deep fascia and encourage movement and circulation. A special form of deep fascia, thicker than the muscular coverings and running transversely to the muscle fibers, is called a retinaculum. Found in small areas that contain numerous tendons, such as the wrist and ankle, retinacula hold the tendons down in a particular position or location.

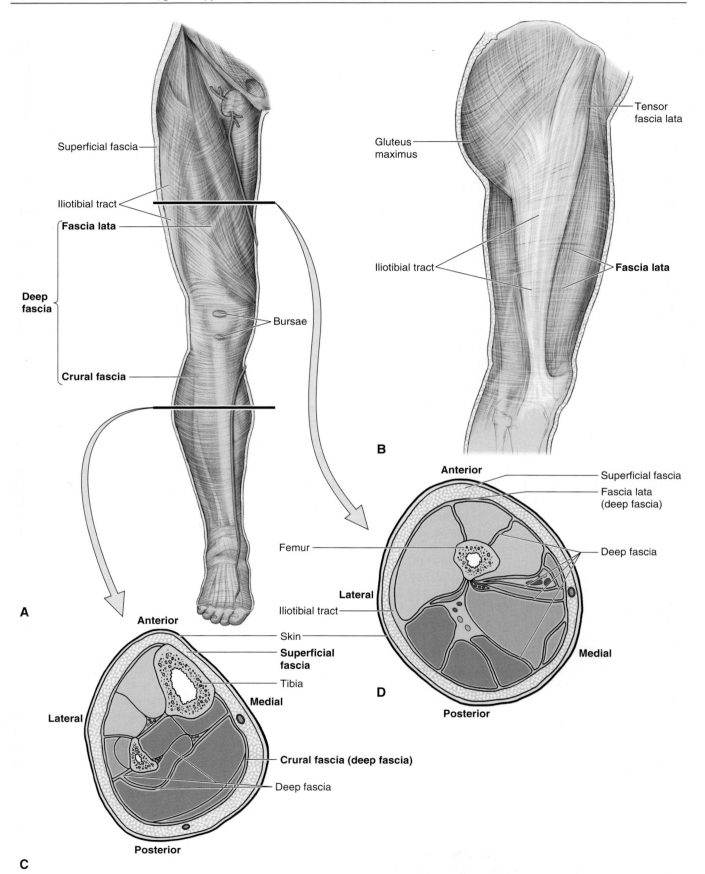

FIGURE 4-16 Deep fascia surrounding muscle. (Reprinted from Moore KL, Dalley AF II. Clinically Oriented Anatomy. 4th ed. Baltimore: Lippincott Williams & Wilkins, 1999.)

Integumentary System

The integumentary (in-TEG-yoo-MENT-ah-ree) system includes the skin, hair, nails, and the glands that reside in or near the skin. Massage therapists should know about the integumentary structures, particularly the skin, because the client's skin is the initial point of physical contact and is touched continually throughout the massage.

Functions of the Integumentary System

The main function of the integumentary system is to protect our bodies from the environment, but it also serves as a means of communication, helps regulate body temperature, provides a means of excretion, and participates in the metabolism of vitamin D.

PROTECTION

The skin is waterproof and resistant to many chemicals and bacteria. Its strength and pliability make it very tough to outside physical forces such as bumps and bruises. Essentially, it keeps the inside structures in and the outside substances out. Keratin is a protein in skin cells that makes our skin water-repellant so water cannot soak through it. Sebum, secreted by the skin, prevents our bodies from evaporating too much water through the skin and helps maintain our hydration. Acidic skin secretions help resist chemical damage and help prevent bacterial growth. Additionally, the skin protects the body from ultraviolet radiation damage. Coloration cells in the skin are called melanocytes (meh-LAN-oh-sahytz). Exposure to sunlight increases the production of melanin, creating a suntan. The darkening of the skin helps shield the cell nucleus from ultraviolet damage, like sunglasses for the DNA.

COMMUNICATION

Most essential for massage therapy is the skin's communication function. Cutaneous receptors in the skin detect touch, pressure, pain, and temperature and send their sensory signals to the brain and spinal cord for processing. These structures are made of nervous tissue and are discussed in more detail in the section covering the nervous system. In addition to the skin's function of transmitting external stimuli to the inside of our bodies, the color and texture of the skin can reveal information about the processes go-ing on inside the body. For instance, a liver dysfunction can lead to excessive amounts of liver chemicals that make the skin yellowish. Low levels of oxygen in the blood will cause the skin to look grayish.

THERMAL REGULATION

A very important function of the integumentary system is thermal regulation. The skin helps regulate body temperature via the capillaries, sweat glands, and fat. The body's thermostat recognizes a safe range for core body temperature. When the core temperature is too high, the body responds with vasodilation, or expanding blood vessels, in the skin. That allows heat to be dissipated by the large surface of the skin. When the core temperature drops too low, the body responds with vasoconstriction (blood vessel constriction) in the skin, which reduces blood flow to the skin in an effort to conserve heat in the body. Sweat glands diffuse water through the skin, and in a low-humidity environment, the water evaporates and helps the cool the body. Evaporative cooling is less effective when humidity in the air is high, because the water from our bodies cannot diffuse into the air. Subcutaneous fat, or the fat in the superficial fascia, also acts as a thermal insulator, preventing heat from being transferred into or out of the body. In cold temperatures, fat keeps body heat in the body and does not allow the cold external temperatures to affect the internal organs, which is usually a good thing. However, when it is hot, fat still keeps body heat in the body, which makes it harder for the body to dissipate heat and maintain the proper core temperature.

EXCRETION

Excretion (ehks-KREE-shun) is minor role of the integumentary system. Metabolic processes create chemical wastes that the body cannot use. The body can eliminate unwanted salts and water from the skin via perspiration. Nitrogen wastes such as urea are also excreted in minimal amounts through the skin.

VITAMIN D METABOLISM

The metabolism of vitamin D is another important function of the skin. Although we can obtain vitamin D from food sources such as milk, this is the only vitamin that can be produced by the body. When the skin is exposed to the ultraviolet rays in sunlight, a form of cholesterol is eventually transformed into vitamin D. Vitamin D is critical for the absorption of calcium for proper bone growth and normal cell growth.

Structures of the Integumentary System

The skin is the main structure of the integumentary system, but there are also some specialized structures located in or near the skin, including hair, nails, and cutaneous glands. **The skin, sometimes called the integument, is the largest organ of the body.**

SKIN

The skin has a two-layered structure consisting of the epidermis and dermis (Fig. 4-17). The skin, like all epithelial membranes, has a layer of epithelial tissue atop a layer of connective tissue. The epidermis is the epithelial layer, and the dermis is the connective tissue layer. The subcutaneous layer, also called superficial fascia or the hypodermis, is another connective tissue layer beneath the dermis and is sometimes considered part of the skin.

Epidermis

The outermost layer of our skin, the epithelial layer, is called the epidermis. It is nonvascular, like all epithelia, and is composed of five layers. From deepest to most superficial, they are the stratum germinativum, stratum spinosum, stratum granulosum, stratum lucidum, and stratum corneum. The epidermis is constantly being regenerated, which it does rapidly via cell division. Skin cells are formed in the stratum germinativum, the deepest layer that is closest to the blood vessels in the underlying dermis. The skin cells slowly progress upward and outward until they reach the external environment. As they migrate outward, they accumulate water-repelling keratin and get far-

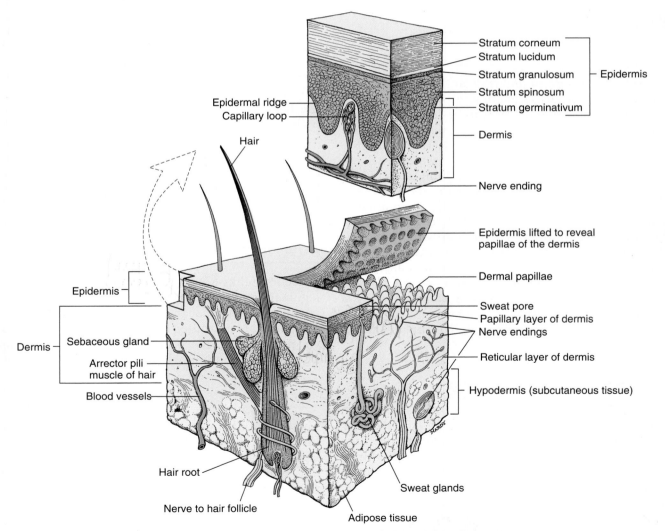

FIGURE 4-17 Cross-sectional illustration of skin. (Reprinted with permission from Stedman's Medical Dictionary, 27th ed. Baltimore: Lippincott Williams & Wilkins, 2000, p 1647.)

ther from the blood vessels that supply nutrients and oxygen. Fortunately for us, these deteriorated skin cells are sloughed off when they reach the external environment. It takes approximately 2 to 4 weeks for a cell to migrate through a layer of epidermis, meaning that in 2 to 4 weeks, a person has a completely new outer layer of skin. This process of renewal keeps our skin healthy and alive and gives us a water-repellant outer covering.

Dermis

The dermis is the layer of connective tissue beneath the epithelium. It is constructed of two layers. The superficial papillary layer is named for its dermal papillae, which are like spiked mountains that stick up into the epidermis. The papillae are highly vascular structures that provide oxygen and nutrients to the epidermis that surrounds them. Pain receptors and tactile sensory receptors reside within the dermal papillae. Beneath the papillary layer is the reticular layer. It is a dense form of connective tissue that contains blood vessels, sweat glands, sebaceous glands, and the sensory receptors for cold, heat, and pressure. The specific sensory receptors are discussed in

detail in the nervous system section, but Figure 4-18 illustrates the kinds of sensory reception in the skin. Collagen and elastin protein fibers give the dermis its toughness and elasticity. Collagen fibers are hydrophilic, meaning that they attract water molecules and hold onto them, which helps keep the skin hydrated. Elastin fibers give skin elasticity, which is noticeable in young children. As we age, the collagen and elastin wear out and diminish, giving us wrinkled, dry skin.

Subcutaneous Layer

The subcutaneous (SUB-kyoo-TAY-nee-us) layer, also known as the hypodermis or superficial fascia, lies deep to the dermis. It is connected to the dermis with numerous bundles of elastin protein fibers, so it is difficult to tell where the dermis stops and the subcutaneous layer starts. This fascia binds the skin to the underlying organs and structures, provides shock absorption, serves as a thermal insulator, and provides energy storage. It is highly vascular, has many nerve endings, and contains adipose (fat) cells. The number of fat cells in a particular person's superficial fascia varies from one area of the body to another. For ex-

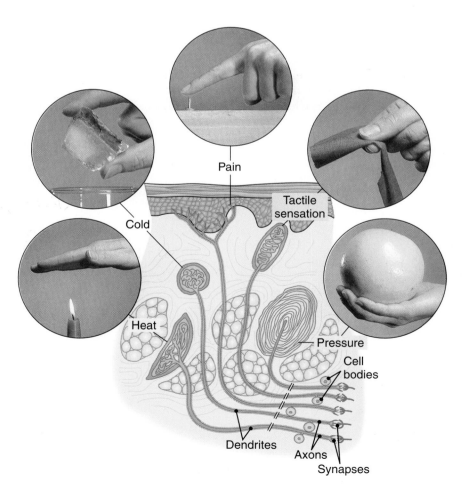

Figure 4-18 Five different kinds of sensory receptors in skin. (Reprinted from Cohen BJ, Wood DL. Memmler's Structure and Function of the Human Body. 9th ed. Philadelphia: Lippincott Williams & Wilkins, 2000.)

ample, the superficial fascia in the breasts and hips tends to have more fat cells than the superficial fascia on the hands or elbows. With age or significant weight loss, subcutaneous fat in adipose cells tends to diminish, and the skin will start to sag.

NAILS

Fingernails and toenails are special structures of the skin (Fig. 4-19A). The free edge of the nail and the body of the nail are made of hard keratin and are not alive. The nail body lies upon the nailbed, which is a vascular epidermal structure. This is the part that bleeds when someone tears a nail too far back. Nails grow from the root, and their growth rate can be affected by temperature. The general health of the body can be detected in the nails because they are the tangible, visible outcome of metabolic activity. A disease or dysfunction in the body affects homeostasis, and imbalances may show up as a difference in the quality of the nail. For example, nails that are thin and weak can be a result of poor nutrition. Nails that appear bluish can indicate poor circulation.

HAIR

Hair is present almost everywhere on the body but is more visible in some areas than in others. It is a nonliving, keratinized protein structure that grows upward from follicles in the subcutaneous layer. The follicle receives its nutrients from the blood vessels surrounding it. When fully developed, hair extends from its root at the base of a long shaft up through the skin and out into the environment (Fig. 4-19B). Hair provides animals with an additional layer of protection, as a way of regulating body temperature and as a mechanism of safety when being faced by a predator. A tiny arrector pili muscle connects the follicle to the dermis, and when it contracts, it pushes the hair out farther to make the animal appear larger (see Fig. 4-17). The same mechanism can trap air and provide a layer of thermal insulation if the hair is thick enough. In humans, however, arrector pili muscle contraction usually produces the familiar "goose bumps" on the skin. Hair serves little purpose for humans. Incidentally, what people commonly call "pores" on the face are actually the openings of hair follicles.

CUTANEOUS GLANDS

The two types of glands in the integument are sudoriferous (SOO-doh-RIF-fer-us), which produce sweat, and sebaceous (seh-BAY-shus), which secrete oil. These exocrine glands release their secretions directly to the outer surface of the skin through ducts.

Sudoriferous glands, or sweat glands, can be classified even more specifically as eccrine or apocrine sweat glands. Eccrine sweat glands are simple coiled tubular glands that open to the surface of the skin with pores. They are found all over the body and are especially abundant in the soles of the feet, palms of the hands, and forehead, where there are not many

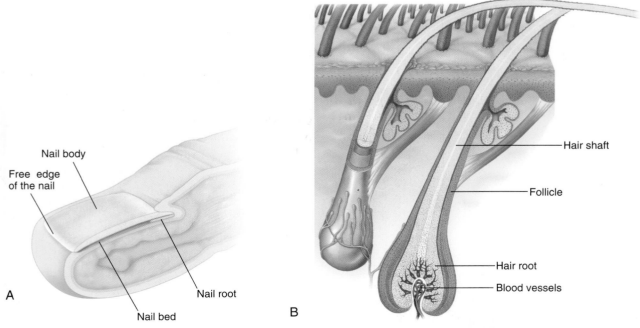

FIGURE 4-19   Structure of fingernail and hair. **A.** Nail. **B.** Hair root. (Part B provided by Anatomical Chart Co.)

hair follicles. These types of sweat glands secrete sweat, which is a thin fluid consisting mostly of water, some salts, and wastes. When sweat reaches the surface of the skin, it evaporates and helps cool the body, which is a very important mechanism of thermal regulation.

The large, branched apocrine sweat glands are found mostly in the axilla (armpit) and genital area, but they are also located in the ear canal, eyelid, and mammary areola. They produce an odorless secretion triggered by puberty, stress, pain, and excitement, and their ducts open into the upper part of the hair follicles, but their function is not fully understood. If bacteria accumulate in the secretion, they break down the apocrine secretions and an unpleasant odor is released. Some apocrine glands are highly specialized to produce milk and are found in the mammary areola.

The sebaceous glands are exocrine glands, but their ducts do not reach the surface of the skin. Instead, sebaceous glands release their secretion into the hair follicle and it travels to the skin's surface through the follicle. They secrete sebum, which is a mixture of fats, waxes, oil, and cellular debris. It is transported to the surface of the skin via the hair follicles to soften the skin, hinder evaporation, and kill bacteria.

The skin does not "breathe" or serve as an exchange for gases. It is only an avenue for transportation of perspiration and oil from the sweat and sebaceous glands.

Skeletal System

The skeletal system, sometimes called the skeleton, is made up of the bones of the body, the joints between bones, and the connective tissue cartilage and ligaments. Bones come in all shapes and sizes. Because bones are sometimes viewed simply as the hard structural support of the body, it is easy to forget that they are alive. **Bones are living tissue.** There are living processes occurring within the individual bones that contribute to the overall functions of the skeletal system. Understanding the structures and functions of the skeletal system helps massage therapists know how to evaluate and assess their clients' bodies and provide the safest and most effective treatment.

Functions of the Skeletal System

The skeleton provides the basic support and general shape to the human body. Many of the bones serve as levers that are pulled by the muscles to create move-

ment, and since muscles are the focus of the scope of practice for massage, the bones are a very important part of your anatomy education. They also provide protection for organs, act as storage sites for calcium salts, and manufacture blood cells. Bone formation, growth, and repair are processes that are responsible for converting cartilage to bone, lengthening long bones, and remodeling bones in response to the levels of calcium in the blood and mechanical stresses on the bones.

SUPPORT

The calcium salts in the extracellular matrix of bones makes them especially hard. Their hardness provides a strong internal framework for our bodies that can hold us up and firmly anchor muscles and organs.

PROTECTION

The hardness of bone also helps protect internal organs and structures. For example, the ribs protect the lungs and the heart in the thoracic cavity, and the vertebral column protects the spinal cord. The abdominal cavity has minimal protection from bones, and it is therefore the most vulnerable cavity of the body.

MOVEMENT

The skeleton provides the necessary leverage that the tendons and muscles use to create movement. Tendons attach bones to muscles, muscles contract to pull the bones, and the joints allow the bones to move.

STORAGE

Bones serve as storage sites for several different minerals as well as fat. Magnesium, phosphorus, sodium, and calcium are minerals stored in the bones. Much of the body's calcium is stored as calcium salts in the extracellular matrix of bones. Calcium is constantly being used as a necessary component for nerve conduction, muscle contraction, and blood clotting. The interior cavities of long bones store fat in the form of yellow marrow. The fat serves as a thermal insulator and a source of energy.

HEMATOPOIESIS

Blood cell formation, or hematopoiesis (HEM-ah-toh-poh-EE-sis), is another function of the skeleton. The interior cavities of some bones contain red marrow, which is a site of red blood cell formation. Red blood cells are essential for life because they carry the oxygen required for everything from cellular respiration to healing. The blood cells and components of blood are discussed in the section covering the cardiovascular system.

BONE FORMATION, GROWTH, AND REMODELING

Continuous regeneration and adjustments are made within the bones to ensure that the skeleton can support and protect our bodies adequately. This is an ongoing and dynamic process that begins prior to birth and continues throughout life as our bodies are subjected to gravity and other physical stressors. The process of bone formation converts cartilage to bone. Once all of the bones have ossified, they grow larger as we grow older. Bones undergo remodeling to maintain the proper levels of calcium in the blood and to change the shape of the bone in response to physical stressors. The continuous process of creating new bone is influenced by hormones that regulate and encourage growth, but growth will not occur without calcium and vitamin D.

Bone Formation

Ossification, the process by which cartilage is turned into hardened bone, begins with osteoblast cells in the fetus. When the fetus is only 2 or 3 months old, the osteoblasts become active, manufacturing the matrix that surrounds them. The matrix is rich in collagen, a fibrous white protein that provides strength and resilience. After it is deposited, the matrix accumulates calcium and other minerals that contribute to the hardening of the bone tissue. Once hardened, osteoblast cells are called osteocytes, or mature bone cells. Most of the hyaline cartilage has been transformed into bone by the time babies are born.

Bone Growth

A small amount of hyaline cartilage remains in bones during childhood, in the epiphyseal (ee-PIH-fih-SEE-uhl) plates, or growth zones, of long bones. Located toward the knobby end of a long bone, the epiphyseal plates are where long bones grow longer. The hyaline cartilage acts as a model for bone growth. The epiphyseal plate first grows wider, and then bony matrix is deposited on the side closer to the center of the bone. By following the hyaline model, bones maintain their shape and proportion through the normal growth process. Lengthening continues through the late teenage years, and when it stops, the epiphyseal

plates solidify and become inactive. They can then be identified on an x-ray film at the junction between the shaft (long part) of the bone and its knobby ends as thin lines called epiphyseal lines.

Bone Remodeling

Long bones increase in diameter as well but use the process of bone remodeling instead of the hyaline model. Bone remodeling is a process of moving bone material from one place to another for maintaining normal calcium levels in the blood, for bone growth, and for strengthening bone in response to physical stressors.

When there is not enough calcium in the blood, osteoclast cells in the bony matrix are activated by hormones to destroy bone tissue, a process called resorption. Bone breakdown releases calcium into the blood to maintain homeostasis. Conversely, if there is too much calcium in the blood, the body will deposit calcium salts into the bony matrix.

Bone remodeling maintains the general shape of the bones through their course of growth. To increase the width of long bones and to increase the overall size of bones other than long bones, growth follows the remodeling process. The process starts in the cavity at the center of the bone with resorption at the cavity wall. A rest period follows, and then bony matrix is deposited on the outside of the bone. The process creates a thicker, wider bone.

The rate of bone formation exceeds that of bone resorption during childhood and adolescence, allowing bones to become larger and denser. In young and middle adulthood, however, the rates tend to be fairly balanced. As a person enters old age, osteoclastic (breakdown) activity tends to exceed osteoblastic (creative) activity, resulting in weaker bones.

Structures of the Bones

The bones have structural aspects at the cellular level that are only visible with a microscope. There is also an overall structural view of the bones that we can see with our eyes, including visible structures, shapes, and exterior projections or depressions. There are two types of bone tissue that are visibly distinguishable: spongy bone and compact bone.

MICROSCOPIC STRUCTURES OF BONES

Different types of bone tissue have a different microscopic structure that contributes to their different overall appearance. Spongy bone, sometimes called cancellous bone, resembles a brittle sponge. Its airy, meshlike structure looks similar under a microscope. Compact bone, however, looks dense and ivorylike until you see the microscopic structures. The basic unit of bone tissue is the osteocyte, literally translated as bone cell. The arrangement of the osteocytes in compact bone tissue is very different from that in spongy bone tissue. The osteocytes are microscopically arranged in visibly concentric rings called lamellae (lah-MEL-lee). The rings form around a central haversian canal that can contain blood vessels, nerves, and lymph vessels. The many central canals are interconnected with blood vessels that travel through Volkmann's canals. Radiating from the central canal, out through the lamellae, are canaliculi, which transport nutrients to every osteocyte. Figure 4-20 illustrates compact and spongy bone tissue.

Microscopic osteoblasts and osteoclasts participate in bone formation, growth, and remodeling. They are discussed below in this section on the skeletal system.

VISIBLE STRUCTURES OF BONES

The bones are covered outside with a periosteum (membrane), which is a tough fibrous sheath that covers all but the joint region of a bone. It is firmly connected to the bone with hundreds of connective tissue fibers and contains a network of nerves, blood vessels, and lymphatic vessels that supply the bone. Osteoblasts, involved in bone formation, are also present in the periosteum.

Bone Shapes

The human skeleton has bones of all shapes and sizes. They are classified as short, flat, irregular, and long bones. Figure 4-21 shows the four bone shapes.

Short bones are typically shaped like cubes or elongated cubes. The carpals of the wrist are short bones. Again, the periosteum covers all but their articular surfaces. A sesamoid bone, such as the kneecap, is a special kind of short bone embedded in tendons.

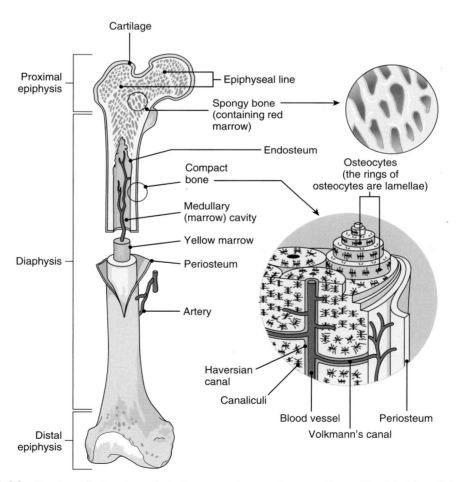

FIGURE 4-20 Structure of a long bone, including spongy bone and compact bone. (Reprinted from Cohen BJ, Wood DL. Memmler's Structure and Function of the Human Body. 9th ed. Philadelphia: Lippincott Williams & Wilkins, 2000.)

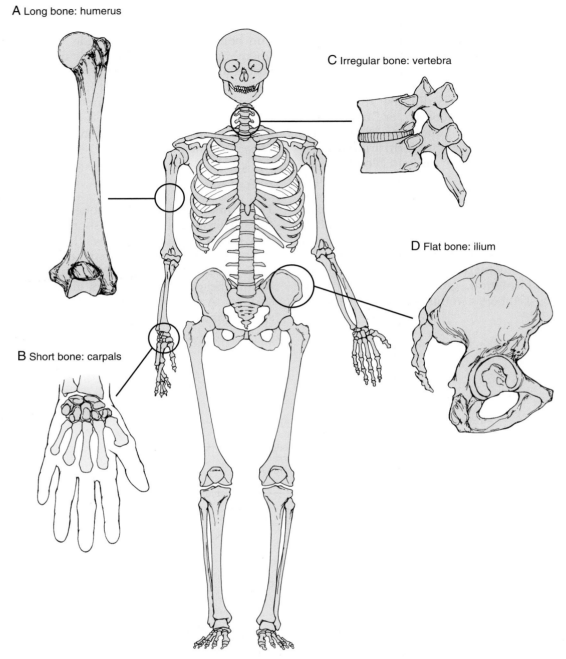

A Long bone: humerus

C Irregular bone: vertebra

D Flat bone: ilium

B Short bone: carpals

FIGURE 4-21 Four bone shapes. (Reprinted with permission from Hamill J, Knutzen K: Biomechanical Basis of Human Movement, 2nd ed. Baltimore: Lippincott Williams & Wilkins, 2003, p 39, fig 2-2.)

Flat bones are platelike and often slightly curved. The ribs and cranial bones are flat bones. Red marrow fills cavities of spongy bone of the flat bones and makes red blood cells.

The bones that do not fit into any of the other categories are called irregular bones. The vertebrae and facial bones are irregular bones.

Long bones are the ones most familiar to people. They are long and narrow with knobby ends and have a hollow inner cavity. The structure of a long bone is outlined below.

Structures of a Long Bone

Long bones are longer than they are wide, including bones such as the femur (FEE-mer) in the thigh and the humerus (HYOO-mer-us) in the upper arm. Their structure consists of a long, narrow shaft called the diaphysis (dahy-AFF-ih-sis) with two knobby ends called epiphyses (ee-PIH-fih-seez) (see Fig. 4-20 for the structure of a long bone). At the core of the compact bone diaphysis is the medullary cavity that contains bone marrow. The medullary cavity is filled with yellow marrow, which contains mostly fat. The epiphyses, the knobby ends of the long bones, are primarily made of spongy bone but are wrapped with a thin layer of compact bone. They are often part of a joint, articulating with other bones. Inside the epiphyses is red marrow that produces red blood cells. Between the epiphysis and diaphysis is an epiphyseal line that looks like a thin strip of compact bone in the midst of spongy bone. The epiphyseal line is what remains of the hyaline cartilage epiphyseal plate in a child's growing long bone.

They have a periosteum on the outside and an endosteum on the inside. The endosteum is the interior lining of the compact bone, which separates the medullary cavity from the compact bone and contains cells involved in growth and repair of the bone.

Bony Landmarks

Bones vary in outer texture. The texture can be smooth or rough and may contain projections, depressions, or hollows. These special features of bones are called bony landmarks, or bone markings, and they are the distinguishing factors for each bone. Bony landmarks are sites for muscle attachment and safe passageways for nerves and blood vessels. Several specific bony landmarks are commonly used by healthcare professionals when referring to a client's anatomy. Generally, projections stick out from the bone to offer an attachment site for muscles, tendons, aponeuroses, and ligaments. Depressions, openings, and concave portions of the bone provide smooth articulating surfaces and holes or openings that are passageways for tendons, nerves, or blood vessels. Sometimes these formations also provide muscle attachment sites. Projections and depressions are included in Table 4-4, with examples of each.

Skeleton

The skeleton normally contains 206 bones, cartilage, and joints. The bones of the skeleton can be defined as two separate groups called the axial and appendicular skeletons. Cartilage is discussed in the section covering cells and tissues, but we briefly review the skeleton-specific cartilage in this section. There are a number of joints in the body that provide different amounts and different kinds of movement.

AXIAL SKELETON

The axial skeleton makes up the axis of the body, or the central support structure. It contains 80 bones, including those of the skull, the vertebral column, and the bony thorax.

Skull

The skull is made of 8 cranial bones, 14 facial bones, 6 inner ear ossicles, and 1 hyoid bone. Its primary function is to protect the brain. It has cavities for the eyes, ears, nose and mouth, and teeth and jaws for mastication (chewing). Some of the cranial bones are paired, such as the parietal and temporal bones, but the sphenoid, ethmoid, frontal, and occipital bones are not (see Fig. 4-22). Most of the facial bones are paired, including the maxilla (upper jaw), zygomatic (cheekbones), nasal, lacrimal (tear ducts are here), palatine, and inferior nasal conchae. Unpaired facial bones include the mandible (the moveable lower jaw) and the vomer bone of the nose. There are three tiny bones, called ossicles, in each middle ear.

One facial bone is unique. Although not considered a true skull bone, the hyoid (HAHY-oyd) bone is located just superior to the larynx and deep to the base of the tongue. See Plate 4-35 in the special muscle section at the end of this chapter for an illustration of the hyoid bone. It is unique in that it does not articulate with any other bones. Instead, it acts as the attachment site for muscles involved in raising and lowering the larynx to provide speech and for moving the tongue in the process of swallowing.

Vertebral Column

The vertebral column, or spine, is made up of a series of irregularly shaped bones called vertebrae that act as a group to support the skull, protect the spinal cord, and provide passageways for the nerves. The average adult vertebral column has 26 vertebrae, separated by intervertebral disks of cartilage.

Each vertebra has specialized structures, including a body, foramen, vertebral arch, one spinous process, two transverse processes, and four articular processes (Fig. 4-23). The vertebral body resembles a hockey puck and bears weight. The foramen is a hole near the center of the vertebra through which passes the spinal cord. The vertebral arch is the part of the bone that arches around the posterior surface of the foramen, consisting of a pair of pedicles and a pair of laminae. The spinous process is the one that points out posteriorly and is most easily palpated. The transverse processes point out laterally. The four articular processes, sometimes called facets, are

TABLE 4-4

Bony Landmarks

LANDMARK	DESCRIPTION	LOCATION	EXAMPLE
Projections			
Condyle	Smooth, rounded	Articular ends of bones	Occipital condyles
Crest	Prominent ridge or border	Along an edge	Iliac crest
Epicondyle	Rough, rounded	Above or around a condyle	Lateral and medial epicondyles of humerus
Head	Rounded, knobby	End of long bone	Head of humerus, head of femur
Line	Long ridge	Shaft of bone	Linea aspera
Process	Fingerlike	Sticks out of a bone	Xiphoid process, olecranon process
Ramus	Slightly flattened, barlike	Near joint	Pubic ramus
Spine	Sharp, bladelike	Muscle attachment site	Spine of scapula, ASIS
Trochanter	Blunt, rough, bump	Muscle attachment site	Greater and lesser trochanters of femur
Tubercle	Small, rough bump	Head of bone, for muscle attachment	Greater and lesser tubercles of humerus
Tuberosity	Rough bump	Neck portion of bone, for muscle attachment	Deltoid tuberosity

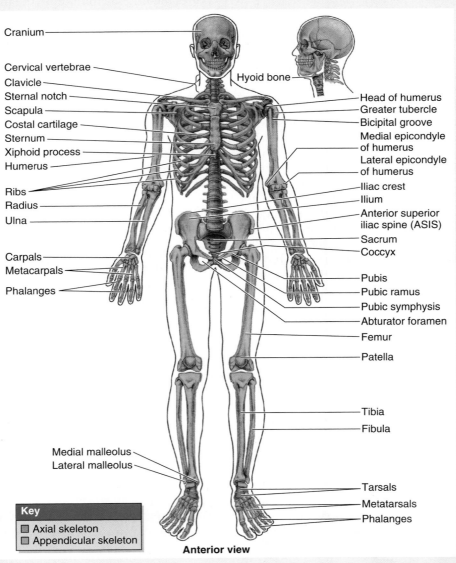

Anterior view

Key
- ☐ Axial skeleton
- ☐ Appendicular skeleton

Labels: Cranium, Cervical vertebrae, Clavicle, Sternal notch, Scapula, Costal cartilage, Sternum, Xiphoid process, Humerus, Ribs, Radius, Ulna, Carpals, Metacarpals, Phalanges, Medial malleolus, Lateral malleolus, Hyoid bone, Head of humerus, Greater tubercle, Bicipital groove, Medial epicondyle of humerus, Lateral epicondyle of humerus, Iliac crest, Ilium, Anterior superior iliac spine (ASIS), Sacrum, Coccyx, Pubis, Pubic ramus, Pubic symphysis, Abturator foramen, Femur, Patella, Tibia, Fibula, Tarsals, Metatarsals, Phalanges

TABLE 4-4

Bony Landmarks—cont'd

LANDMARK	DESCRIPTION	LOCATION	EXAMPLE
Depressions and openings			
Foramen	Hole	Through a bone	Obturator foramen, foramen magnum
Fossa	Concave	Articular bone surface	Supraspinous and infraspinous fossa of scapula
Groove	Small, concave, furrow-like	Muscle attachment site	Bicipital groove of humerus
Meatus	Short, tube-shaped passageway	Through a bone	Auditory meatus
Notch	Concave, half-moon	Cutout in a bone	Sternal notch, sciatic notch of pelvis
Sinus	Air-filled cavity	Mucus-lined areas	Cranial bone (frontal sinus)

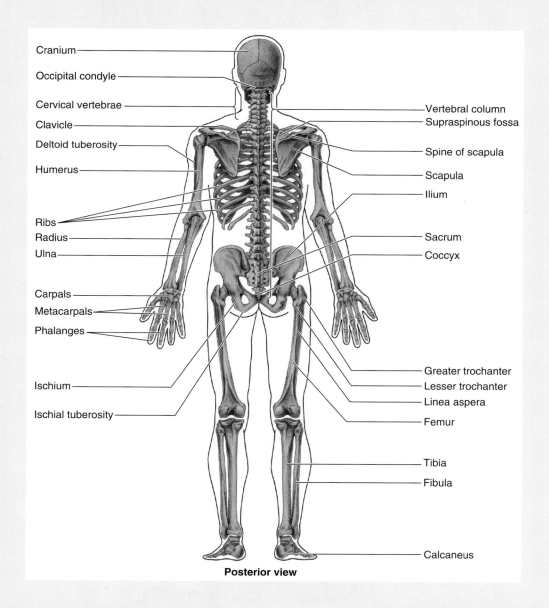

Posterior view

Images from Moore KL, Dalley AF II. Clinically Oriented Anatomy. 4th ed. Baltimore: Lippincott Williams & Wilkins, 1999.

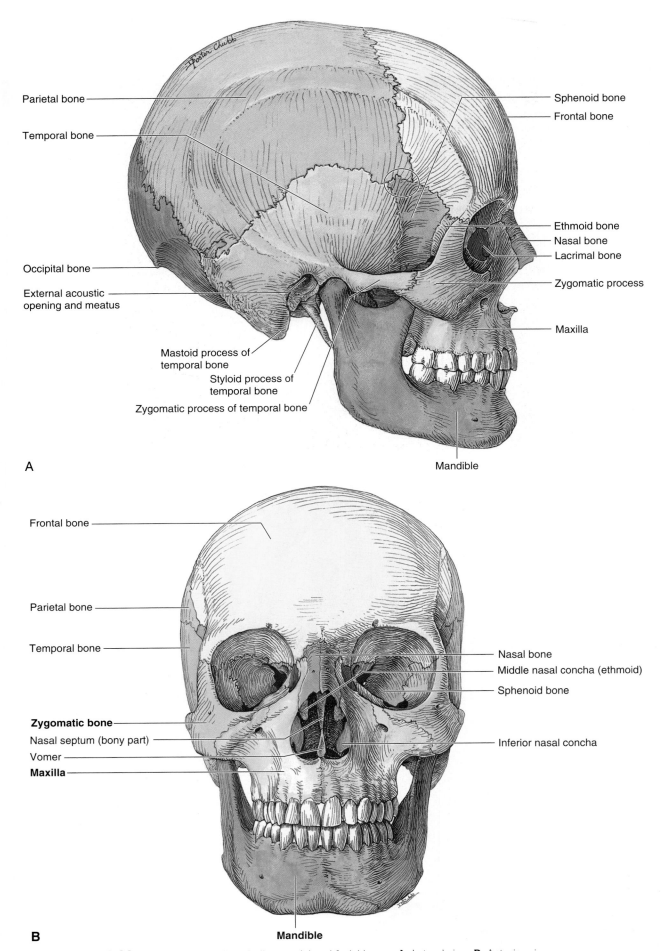

Parietal bone

Temporal bone

Occipital bone

External acoustic
opening and meatus

Mastoid process of
temporal bone

Styloid process of
temporal bone

Zygomatic process of temporal bone

Sphenoid bone

Frontal bone

Ethmoid bone

Nasal bone

Lacrimal bone

Zygomatic process

Maxilla

Mandible

A

Frontal bone

Parietal bone

Temporal bone

Zygomatic bone

Nasal septum (bony part)

Vomer

Maxilla

Nasal bone

Middle nasal concha (ethmoid)

Sphenoid bone

Inferior nasal concha

B

Mandible

FIGURE 4-22 Bones of the skull, including cranial and facial bones. **A.** Lateral view. **B.** Anterior view.

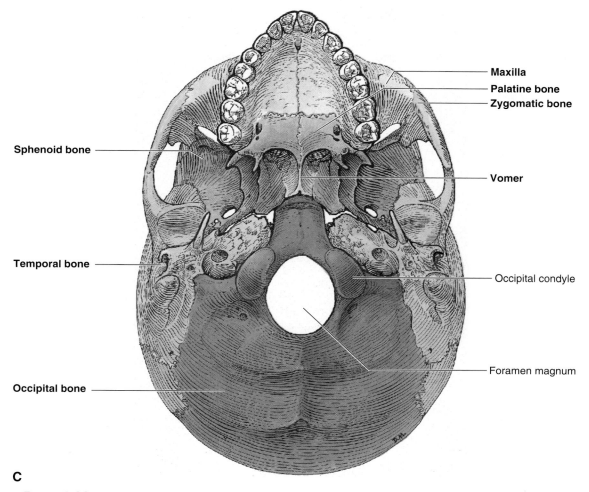

Maxilla
Palatine bone
Zygomatic bone

Sphenoid bone

Vomer

Temporal bone

Occipital condyle

Occipital bone

Foramen magnum

C

FIGURE 4-22   *(continued)* Bones of the skull, including cranial and facial bones. **C.** Inferior view.

small bumps that allow the vertebrae to articulate with each other.

Unlike adults, newborn babies are born with 33 vertebrae. The spine is the first bony structure to develop in the fetus and has concave thoracic and pelvic curves that protect the organs. Further along in fetal development, the vertebral column acquires convex curves in the cervical and lumbar regions. The convex cervical curve matures as the infant begins to hold up its head, and the convex lumbar curve matures when the baby begins to stand and walk in an upright position (Fig. 4-24). These normal spinal curves, in addition to the cartilaginous intervertebral disks, give the spine the mechanical springlike properties of strength and flexibility.

Once completely formed, the spine has five distinct sections (Fig. 4-25):

■ Cervical—7 vertebrae
■ Thoracic—12 vertebrae
■ Lumbar—5 vertebrae
■ Sacral—5 vertebrae in childhood become a single fused bone in adults
■ Coccygeal—3 to 5 vertebrae in childhood become a single fused bone in adults

The seven cervical (SER-vih-kul) vertebrae are relatively small and allow considerable neck movement. They are numbered C1 through C7, starting at the superior end. The first two vertebrae are often referred to as the atlas (C1), which allows us to nod the head "yes" and the axis (C2), which allows us to rotate the head back and forth as in shaking the head "no." A common anatomical landmark is the spinous process of C7, which protrudes on the posterior side of the neck as the most prominent bump.

The 12 thoracic (thoh-RASS-ik) vertebrae are slightly larger than the cervical vertebrae and are similarly numbered T1 through T12. They serve as attachments for the posterior ends of the 12 pairs of

Parts:

Spinous process (1)

Transverse process (2)

Articular processes (4)

Vertebral arch

Vertebral body

Functions:

Muscle attachment and movement

Restriction of movement

Protection of spinal cord

Support of body weight

(A) Superior view

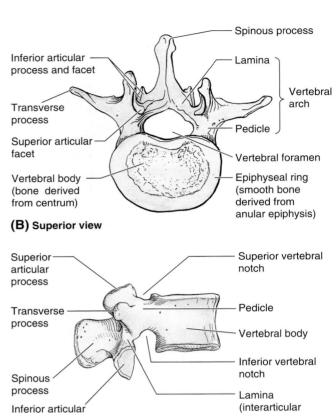

Inferior articular process and facet

Transverse process

Superior articular facet

Vertebral body (bone derived from centrum)

Spinous process

Lamina

Vertebral arch

Pedicle

Vertebral foramen

Epiphyseal ring (smooth bone derived from anular epiphysis)

(B) Superior view

Superior articular process

Transverse process

Spinous process

Inferior articular facet

Superior vertebral notch

Pedicle

Vertebral body

Inferior vertebral notch

Lamina (interarticular part)

(C) Lateral view

FIGURE 4-23 Structure of a vertebra. (Reprinted from Moore KL, Dalley AF II. Clinically Oriented Anatomy. 4th ed. Baltimore: Lippincott Williams & Wilkins, 1999.)

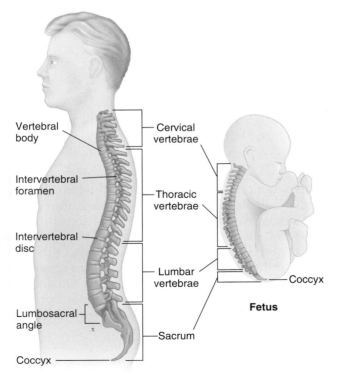

Vertebral body

Intervertebral foramen

Intervertebral disc

Lumbosacral angle

Coccyx

Cervical vertebrae

Thoracic vertebrae

Lumbar vertebrae

Sacrum

Coccyx

Fetus

Adult

FIGURE 4-24 Spinal curves of fetus and adult.

ribs. The first intervertebral foramen occurs between C7 and superior to T1, allowing the spinal nerve C8 to exit the spinal cord.

The five lumbar vertebrae, numbered L1 through L5, are even heavier and larger to support the greater mechanical stress on the lumbar region. This section bears the weight of the rest of the spine and supports the trunk.

The sacrum (SAY-krum) is a single bone composed of five vertebrae that are fused together. This bone articulates superiorly with L5 and inferiorly with the coccyx (KAHK-sikz), but it also articulates laterally with the iliac bones of the pelvis to create the posterior wall of the pelvis.

The coccyx is a single bone made of three to five vertebrae that are fused together. Commonly called the tailbone, it only articulates with the sacrum at its superior surface.

Bony Thorax

The bony thorax consists of the 12 pairs of ribs and the sternum. It functions as a protective cage for the lungs and the other organs of the thoracic cavity.

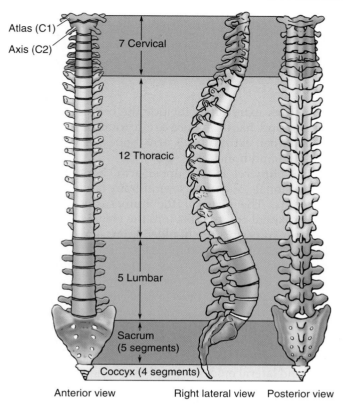

Atlas (C1)
Axis (C2)

7 Cervical

12 Thoracic

5 Lumbar

Sacrum (5 segments)

Coccyx (4 segments)

Anterior view   Right lateral view   Posterior view

FIGURE 4-25 Anterior, lateral, and posterior views of the vertebral column. (From Moore KL, Dalley AF II. Clinically Oriented Anatomy. 4th ed. Baltimore: Lippincott Williams & Wilkins, 1999.)

Like the thoracic vertebrae that they contact posteriorly, the ribs are numbered in pairs from 1 to 12 (Fig. 4-26). The first seven pairs are called true ribs because they also attach to the anterior portion of the sternum via the costal cartilage. The false ribs, pairs 8 through 10, do not have their own individual anterior attachments. Instead, they all attach to the cartilage of the seventh true rib. The last two pairs are considered floating ribs, because they have no anterior attachment. Between the ribs, in the intercostal spaces, there are muscles, blood vessels, and nerves.

The sternum is the other integral portion of the bony thorax. The sternum lies in the middle of the anterior rib cage and is the attachment site for the true ribs via the costal cartilage. The sternum has three distinct portions: the manubrium (man-OO-bree-um), the body, and the xiphoid (ZAHY-foyd) process. The manubrium is the most superior portion of the sternum and has the bony landmark called the sternal (jugular) notch at its superior end. The body, sometimes referred to as the breastbone, joins the manubrium at the sternal angle.

The xiphoid process is a spearlike projection at the inferior edge of the body of the sternum. It is often used as a starting landmark when locating hand placement for chest compressions during cardiopulmonary resuscitation (CPR). The suggested placement is approximately three finger widths superior to

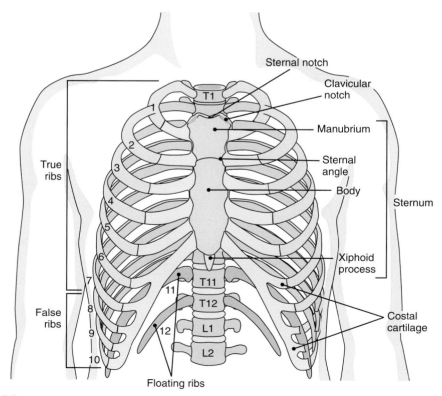

FIGURE 4-26 Bony thorax, anterior view. (Reprinted from Cohen BJ, Wood DL. Memmler's Structure and Function of the Human Body. 9th ed. Philadelphia: Lippincott Williams & Wilkins, 2000.)

the xiphoid process. Because it is sharp and can cause damage if fractured, compression or deep pressure at or near the xiphoid process should be avoided.

APPENDICULAR SKELETON

The appendicular skeleton, which appropriately includes the bones of the appendages, or upper extremities, contains 126 bones. This section contains all the bones peripheral to the axial skeleton: the shoulder girdle, the upper extremities, the pelvic girdle, and the lower extremities.

The Shoulder Girdle

The shoulder girdle, sometimes called the pectoral girdle, consists of the clavicle and the scapula (Fig. 4-27). The clavicle, also known as the collarbone, is a long bone that is frequently broken. The scapula, often called the shoulder blade, is a flat bone with many bony landmarks that are commonly used in healthcare. The spine on the posterior surface of the scapula runs transversely and is easily palpated. Above the scapular spine is the supraspinous fossa, which is a long depression that runs the length of the spine. The large, flat area of the scapula below the spine is an infraspinous fossa, which is a slight depression. The acromion process at the lateral end of the spine protrudes like a knob. It, too, can be palpated easily. Below the acromion process, on the lateral side of the scapula is the glenoid cavity, which cradles the head of the humerus in a ball-and-socket joint, a shallow landmark that cannot be palpated. Medial to the glenoid cavity is the coracoid process

that points anteriorly, like a fingertip. The coracoid process can be delicately palpated just inferior to the lateral clavicle.

Upper Extremities

The upper extremities include the bones of the arms, wrists, and hands. There are a total of 30 bones in each upper extremity: 3 arm bones, 8 wrist bones, and 19 hand bones (Fig. 4-28).

The humerus is the "upper arm" bone. Healthcare professionals reference several bony landmarks of the humerus. The head of the humerus is the ball at the proximal end that fits into the glenoid cavity of the scapula to form the shoulder joint. The greater and lesser tubercles, located more laterally on the proximal end of the humerus, provide muscle attachment sites. Between the tuberosities is the bicipital (bahy-SIP-ih-tuhl) groove, sometimes called the intertubercular groove, which is a major site for muscle attachment. The deltoid tuberosity lies midway down the humerus, on the lateral surface, and serves as the attachment site for the deltoid muscle. On the distal end, the medial and lateral epicondyles of the humerus stick out as bumps, also for muscle attachment.

The radius and ulna are the two bones that make up the forearm. The radius is on the lateral side and the ulna is more medial. An easily palpable landmark of the forearm is the styloid process of the radius, located at the lateral, distal end. This landmark is often used when locating the radial pulse, which can be found just medial and slightly anterior to the styloid process of the radius. The ulna has some major landmarks of its own. The olecranon (oh-LEK-rah-nahn) process is a bony landmark of the ulna that is often

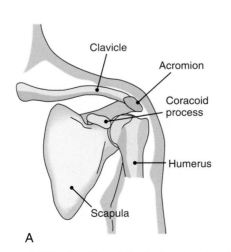

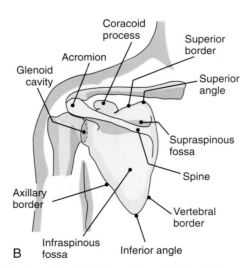

FIGURE 4-27   Shoulder girdle. **A.** Anterior view. **B.** Posterior view. (Reprinted from Cohen BJ, Wood DL. Memmler's Structure and Function of the Human Body. 9th ed. Philadelphia: Lippincott Williams & Wilkins, 2000.)

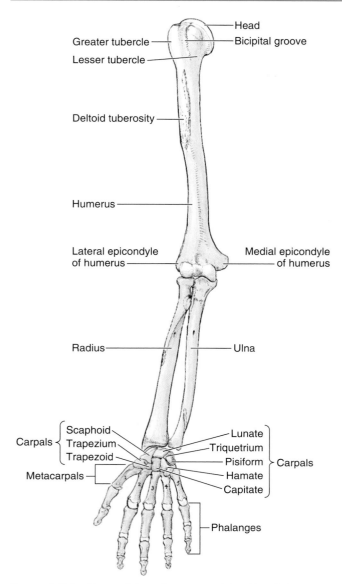

Greater tubercle
Lesser tubercle
Head
Bicipital groove

Deltoid tuberosity

Humerus

Lateral epicondyle
of humerus

Medial epicondyle
of humerus

Radius

Ulna

Carpals {
Scaphoid
Trapezium
Trapezoid
}

Metacarpals

Lunate
Triquetrium
Pisiform
Hamate
Capitate
} Carpals

Phalanges

FIGURE 4-28 Bones of the wrist, arm, and shoulder girdle. (Reprinted from Agur AMR, Ming JL. Grant's Atlas of Anatomy. 10th ed. Baltimore: Lippincott Williams & Wilkins, 1999.)

mistaken for part of the humerus. It is very easily identified as the point of the elbow, sometimes feeling sharp, depending on the amount of subcutaneous fat in the area. The styloid process of the ulna is the bump located at the distal end, next to the wrist, on the posterior (dorsal) surface. It is most easily seen and palpated with the forearm in a prone position, palm down.

The wrist comprises eight carpal bones: capitate, hamate, lunate, pisiform, scaphoid, trapezium, trapezoid, and triquetral. The carpals are short bones that fit together like puzzle pieces (see Fig. 4-28).

The hand is made up of five metacarpals and the phalanges (see Fig. 4-28). They are numbered 1 through 5, with the thumb being the first and the

"pinky" being the fifth. The phalanges consist of 14 bones, with 2 in the thumb and 3 in each of the others.

Pelvic Girdle

The pelvic girdle consists of three bones that are fused together: the ilium (ILL-ee-um), the ischium (ISH-ee-um), and the pubis (PYOO-bis) (Fig. 4-29). There are two major bony landmarks on the pelvic girdle that cannot be palpated. One is the acetabulum, literally translated to "vinegar bowl." Created at the intersection of the three fused bones, the acetabulum (ASS-sih-TAB-yoo-lum) is the cuplike socket that cradles the head of the femur. Another important bony landmark that cannot be palpated is the obturator foramen. This is a large hole encircled by the ischium and pubis that allows nerves and blood vessels to pass through.

The individual bones of the pelvis each have some identifiable, easily palpated landmarks. The posterior side of the ilium has a transverse ridge called the iliac crest, just inferior to the waist. The front of each hip has a prominent bump called the anterior, superior iliac spine (ASIS), commonly known as the "hip bone." The ischia have the ischial tuberosities that are sometimes called the "sit bones" because these protruding landmarks can be felt and may become uncomfortable when one sits on a hard surface. The pubic bones are joined anteriorly at the cartilaginous pubic symphysis. During the late stages of pregnancy, the cartilage softens to allow the pelvic girdle to expand for childbirth.

The male pelvis differs from the female pelvis in several ways. From the superior view, looking down through the pelvis, the opening within the female pelvis is circular, and the male's is shaped more like a heart. In the anterior view, the female pelvis has a less significant pubic arch than the male pelvis. The more pronounced arch in the male pelvis narrows the entire structure compared with the female pelvis, which is wider and gives women wider hips. The sacrum is fairly straight in the female and more curved in the male. (Compare Figs. 4-29 and 4-30.)

Lower Extremities

The lower extremities of the appendicular skeleton consist of the thigh, knee, lower leg, ankle, and foot. There are a total of 30 bones in each lower extremity (Fig. 4-31).

The femur, or thighbone, is the largest bone in the body. Its major proximal landmarks include the head and neck, which fits into the acetabulum to create the hip joint, and the trochanters, which serve as sites for muscle attachment. The greater trochanter is the large, lateral protrusion that is easily palpated. The

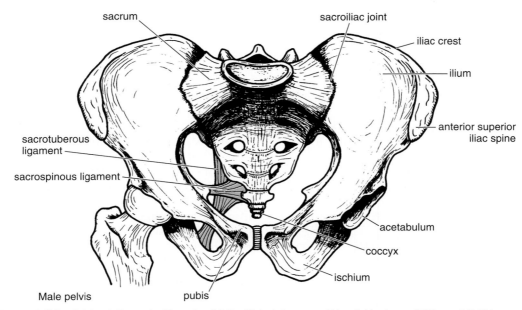

FIGURE 4-29 Pelvic girdle, male. (From Snell MD. Clinical Anatomy. 7th ed. Lippincott Williams & Wilkins, 2003.)

lesser trochanter is the smaller and more distal of the two, located medially, and is quite difficult to palpate. The lateral and medial epicondyles of the femur are located at the distal end, near the knee, just above the condyles that articulate with the tibia of the lower leg. The patella (puh-TEL-luh), also called the "kneecap," is a sesamoid bone embedded in the tendon of the quadriceps femoris muscle. The linea aspera (LIN-ee-uh ASS-per-uh) is a protruding line found on the posterior shaft of the femur that serves as a site for muscle attachment.

The tibia and fibula are the bones of the lower leg. The tibia is the larger and more medial of the two and is the weight-bearing bone. It has an anterior ridge that runs vertically, a tibial tuberosity on the anterior surface of the proximal end, and the medial malleolus (inner ankle bone) at the distal end. The tibia is part of the knee joint, along with the femur and the patella. The fibula is the smaller, more lateral bone of the lower leg that does not bear weight and is not part of the knee joint. Its landmarks are located on the lateral aspect of the lower leg. The head of the fibula is

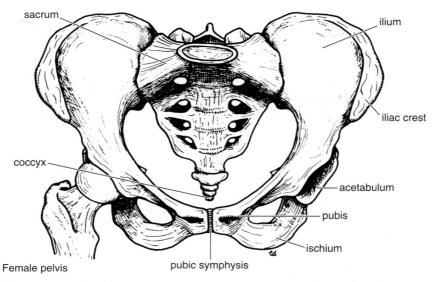

FIGURE 4-30 Pelvic girdle, female. From Snell MD. Clinical Anatomy. 7th ed. Lippincott Williams & Wilkins, 2003.)

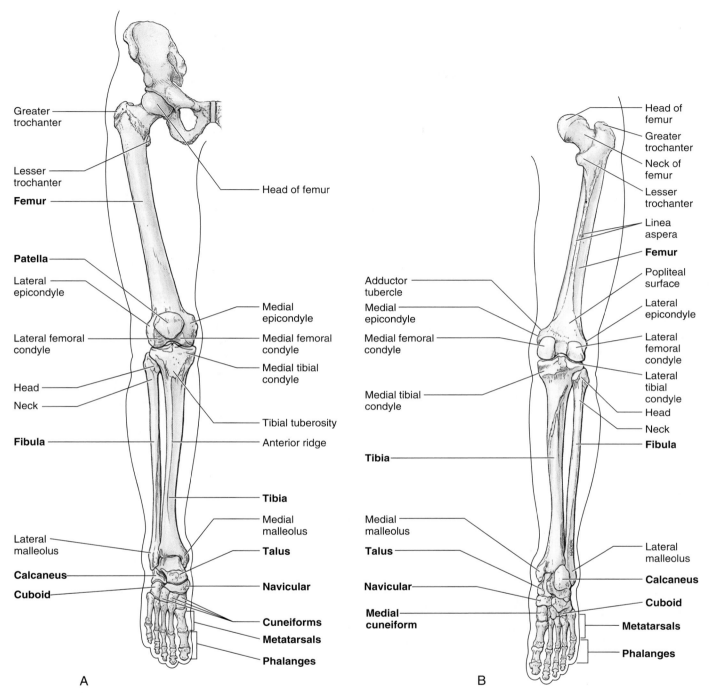

FIGURE 4-31 Bones of the lower extremity. **A.** Anterior view. **B.** Posterior view. (From Moore KL, Dalley AF II. Clinically Oriented Anatomy. 4th ed. Baltimore: Lippincott Williams & Wilkins, 1999.)

on the proximal end, and the lateral malleolus (outer ankle bone) is located at the distal end.

The seven tarsals that make up the ankle joint are the calcaneus (the largest of the seven, also known as the "heel"), talus, navicular, medial cuneiform, intermediate cuneiform, lateral cuneiform, and cuboid.

The structure of the foot is similar to that of the hand. The foot has five metatarsals that form the instep and the ball of the foot; the metatarsal behind the "big toe" is metatarsal 1 and behind the "baby toe" is metatarsal 5. The toes are made up of 14 phalangeal bones.

CARTILAGE

Cartilage is essential for bone formation early in life, and it provides cushion and support for various body structures. The three types of cartilage are elastic, hyaline, and fibrocartilage.

Hyaline cartilage is the most abundant in the body. It is translucent and pearly blue, and no nerves are found within hyaline cartilage. It is firm but elastic, providing flexibility and support and allowing smooth, efficient movement at the joints. Examples of hyaline cartilage include the temporary cartilage in infants and children, the costal cartilages of the ribs, and articular cartilage. Figure 4-32 illustrates the location of articular cartilage.

Fibrocartilage, sometimes called white fibrocartilage, has much collagen that provides strength and structure but little flexibility. It is found in the intervertebral disks of the spinal column and the temporomandibular joint (TMJ).

Elastic cartilage, also referred to as yellow cartilage, is more opaque and flexible than the other types. It consists of many elastin fibers within the collagen, giving strength to flexible structures. For example, the external ear is made up of elastic cartilage, as is the larynx.

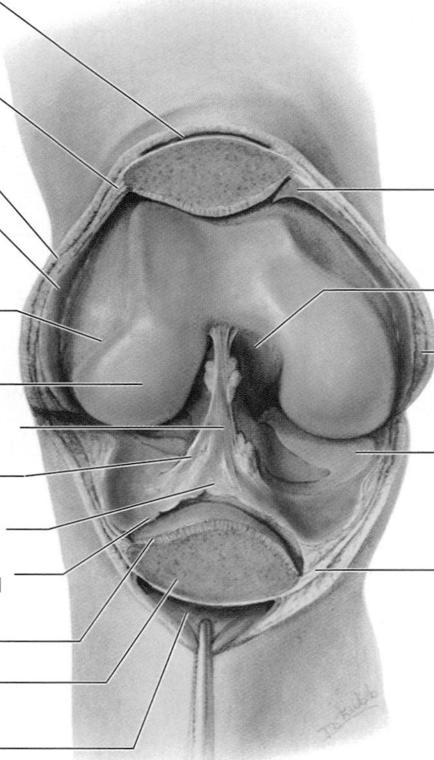

JOINTS

Bones can fit together in various ways to create movement, sometimes called articulation, and provide stability between the bones. There are three main types of joints that can be classified according to the amount of movement that can occur at the joint or by the material found between the bones of the joint. The joints that are nearly immovable are called synarthrotic (SIHN-ahr-THRAH-tik) or fibrous joints. The joints that are slightly moveable are amphiarthrotic (AM-fee-ahr-THRAH-tik) or cartilaginous joints. The joints that are freely moveable are called diarthrotic (DAHY-ahr-THRAH-tik) or synovial joints (Table 4-5).

Synarthrotic Joints

Joints in which bones are held together with fibrous connective tissue are synarthrotic, allowing very little, if any, movement to occur. The sutures of the skull are synarthrotic joints that allow very little movement. Understanding that bones are living tissue and remodel according to the stresses placed upon them, it is simple to see how fibrous sutures are moveable, even if only slightly.

Amphiarthrotic Joints

Some joints have cartilage between the bones and are slightly moveable, or amphiarthrotic. The pubis symphysis and the joints between the vertebral bodies are examples of amphiarthrotic joints.

Diarthrotic Joints

The most prolific joints in the body are freely moveable diarthrotic joints, such as the knee, the shoulder, and the elbow. Diarthrotic joints have several components:

- Articular cartilage—hyaline cartilage that covers the articular surfaces of the bones to reduce friction
- Bursae—synovial membrane-lined sacs full of synovial fluid that cushion the movement of tendons over bones (not present in all synovial joints)
- Joint capsule—a fibrous connective tissue sac that encloses the joint cavity
- Joint cavity—a space between the bones of the synovial joint that contains a lubricating, cushioning fluid

Labels (left side, top to bottom): Prepatellar bursa; Fibrous capsule; Iliotibial tract; Synovial membrane; Junction of membrane with cartilage; **Articular cartilage**; Infrapatellar fold; Alar fold; Infrapatellar fatpad; Infrapatellar synovial fold; Articular cartilage; Patella; Prepatellar bursa (opened)

Labels (right side, top to bottom): Synovial fold; Intercondylar fossa; Tibial collateral ligament; Medial meniscus; Fibrous capsule

FIGURE 4-32 Knee joint showing articular cartilage. (Reprinted from Moore KL, Dalley AF II. Clinically Oriented Anatomy. 4th ed. Baltimore: Lippincott Williams & Wilkins, 1999.)

TABLE 4-5

Types of Joints

TYPE OF JOINT	CHARACTERISTICS	LOCATION	
Synarthrotic	Nearly immovable, fibrous	Skull sutures	Coronal suture Lambdoidal suture
Amphiarthrotic	Slightly moveable, cartilaginous	Pubic symphysis, between vertebrae	Pubic symphysis
Diarthrotic (synovial)	Freely moveable, joint capsule with synovial fluid	Shoulder, hip, knee, elbow	
Ball and socket	Provides the greatest range of motion and allows movement in many directions (circumduction)	Glenohumeral joint (shoulder), acetabulum (hip joint)	Clavicle Head of humerus Scapula
Condyloid	Allows movement in two planes (flexion, extension, lateral movement)	Metacarpophalangeal joints, between occiput and C1 (atlas)	Metacarpal Phalanx

(continued)

TABLE 4-5

Types of Joints—cont'd

TYPE OF JOINT	CHARACTERISTICS	LOCATION	
Gliding	Bones slide past each other (side to side movement)	Between carpals, between tarsals	
Hinge	Allows movement in one plane (flexion, extension)	Elbow joint, knee joint, between phalanges	
Pivot	Allows rotational movement	Between C1 (atlas) and C2 (axis), between radius and ulna	
Saddle	Allows movement in many directions	Carpometacarpal joint of the thumb	

- Ligaments—fibrous connective tissue bands that hold the bones of the joint together and stabilize the joint
- Synovial membrane—the lining of the joint capsule that secretes synovial fluid, a thick, colorless, lubricating fluid similar in consistency to egg white. These freely moveable joints are often called synovial joints because the joint cavity is filled with synovial fluid, which is produced on demand in response to movement of the joint.

Types of Synovial Joints

There are six different types of synovial joints, grouped by their mechanical structure: gliding, hinge, pivot, condyloid (KAHN-dih-loyd), saddle, and ball-and-socket. The mechanical structure determines the kind of movement possible at a joint and the degree to which a joint can safely move, also known as its range of motion.

Gliding joints are found at the interphalangeal, intercarpal, and intertarsal joints and at the joints between superior and inferior vertebral facets. The bones slide across each other, creating movements such as inversion and eversion at the ankle. Hinge joints are held together with strong, collateral ligaments. The elbow, knee, fingers, and toes are hinge joints allowing movements of flexion and extension. Pivot joints are limited to rotation, allowing one bone to pivot within the annular (ring-shaped) ligament of another. The proximal radioulnar pivot joint creates pronation and supination of the forearm. There is also a pivot joint between the atlas (C1) and axis (C2). Condyloid joints have a convex (rounded) surface fitting in a concave (dented) surface that allows flexion, extension, adduction, and abduction but not axial rotation. The metacarpophalangeal joints and the joint between the occiput and the atlas are condyloid joints. Sometimes considered condyloid joints, ellipsoid joints differ because their convex and concave surfaces are oval instead of round. The radiocarpal joint is an example of an ellipsoid joint whose movements include flexion, extension, adduction, and abduction. Saddle joints have two opposing surfaces, each shaped like a saddle. This kind of joint allows flexion, extension, adduction, and abduction but not axial rotation. The carpometacarpal joint of the thumb and the calcaneocuboidal joint of the ankle are both saddle joints. The ball-and-socket joint is multiaxial, meaning that movement can occur in several different planes. Ball-and-socket joints include the shoulder and the hip, allowing flexion, extension, adduction, abduction, rotation, and circumduction.

Many different movements occur at joints, some of which are mentioned above. The shoulder area also allows other ranges of motion, but these are movements of the shoulder as a whole or movements of the scapula bone rather than articulations of the ball-and-socket joint. There are many body movements, most of them occurring at joints, as Table 4-6 illustrates. Terminology is important when referring to movement. For example, "bending the arm" is an unclear statement because "the arm" includes dozens of bones and joints. A more accurate description is flexion of the elbow. Likewise, "straightening the leg" is a description of knee extension, and "straightening the back" is the act of extending the spine.

Massage therapists should know the major joints of the body, the normal movements for each of those joints, and which muscles provide those movements. (See the special muscle section at the end of this chapter.) With this understanding you can recognize a client's limited range of motion in a joint and thus avoid hurting the client.

Muscular System

Muscles comprise almost half of an average person's body weight. Muscle tissue, like nervous tissue, does not reproduce, meaning that people are born with all of their muscle cells. These cells can get larger or smaller, and can die, but we do not grow additional muscle tissue. Because muscle cells have an elongated shape, they are often referred to as muscle fibers.

Types of Muscle Tissue

Classified by structure, function, and location, there are three types of muscle tissues: cardiac, smooth, and skeletal. These different types of muscle tissues all share the following features:

- Contractility—the elongated muscle fibers contract better than a square or round cell, thus creating tension
- Excitability—the fibers are capable of a forceful response to a nervous impulse
- Extensibility—muscles can be stretched beyond their normal resting length
- Elasticity—after being stretched or contracted, muscles can return to their original length

CARDIAC MUSCLE

Cardiac muscles are only found in the walls of the heart and are responsible for pushing blood into the blood vessels. The muscle cells are striated, each cell

TABLE 4-6

Body Movements

MOVEMENT	ILLUSTRATION	MOVEMENT	ILLUSTRATION
Extension—Increases the angle at a joint		Finger	
Spine		Knee	
Neck		Hip	
Shoulder		**Flexion**—Decreases the angle at a joint	
Elbow		Spine	
Wrist		Neck	
Thumb		Shoulder	

TABLE 4-6

Body Movements—cont'd

MOVEMENT	ILLUSTRATION	MOVEMENT	ILLUSTRATION
Elbow		**Lateral flexion**—Curves the spine to the left or to the right Spine	
Wrist		Neck	
Thumb		**Dorsiflexion**—Lifts the toes of the foot superiorly and lowers the heel	
Finger		**Plantarflexion**—Lowers the toes of the foot and raises the heel	
Hip		**Hyperextension**—Joint is extended past anatomical position Spine	
Knee		Neck	

(continued)

TABLE 4-6

Body Movements—cont'd

MOVEMENT	ILLUSTRATION	MOVEMENT	ILLUSTRATION
Pronation—Turns the palm of the hand down Forearm		**Adduction** (commonly clarified as A-D-duction)—Takes a structure toward the body or brings fingers together Shoulder	
Supination—Turns the hand palm up Forearm		Wrist (medial deviation)	
Abduction (commonly clarified as A-B-duction)—Takes a structure away from the body or separates fingers Shoulder		Thumb	
Wrist (lateral deviation)		Finger	
Thumb abduction		Hip	
Finger abduction		**Eversion**—Turns the sole of the foot laterally, combining dorsiflexion and abduction	
Hip abduction			

TABLE 4-6

Body Movements—cont'd

MOVEMENT	ILLUSTRATION	MOVEMENT	ILLUSTRATION
Inversion—turns the sole of the foot medially, combining plantarflexion and adduction Inversion		**Rotation**—Twisting or turning of a bone along its own axis Spine	
Lateral deviation—The wrist angle is decreased as the hand moves laterally Jaw Wrist (see abduction)		Neck	
Medial deviation—The wrist angle is decreased as the hand moves medially Wrist (see adduction)		Lateral rotation of the humerus	
Circumduction—A fluid circular movement that combines flexion, extension, abduction, and adduction Shoulder		Medial rotation of the humerus	
Hip		Lateral rotation of the femur	
Opposition—Movement of the thumb toward the "pinkie finger" Thumb		Medial rotation of the femur	

(continued)

TABLE 4-6

Body Movements—cont'd

MOVEMENT	ILLUSTRATION	MOVEMENT	ILLUSTRATION
Depression—Opens the jaw or lowers the entire scapula		**Protraction**—Moves the mandible or scapula anteriorly	
Mandible		Mandible	
Scapula		Scapula	
Elevation—Closes the jaw or lifts the entire scapula or femur		**Retraction**—Moves the mandible or scapula posteriorly	
Mandible		Mandible	
Scapula		Scapula	
Pelvis		**Inhalation**—Expands and lifts the bony thorax	
		Exhalation—Contracts and lowers the bony thorax	

has only one nucleus, they have a branching structure, and they contract involuntarily. Between cardiac muscle cells are intercalated disks. They are unique to cardiac muscle tissue and allow the electrical impulses that stimulate contraction to be conducted along the network of fibers, creating contractions that are strong and rhythmic (Fig. 4-33). These cardiac muscle contractions forcibly pump blood out of the heart with a rush that can be felt, referred to as the pulse.

SMOOTH MUSCLE

Smooth muscles are found in the walls of hollow organs, such as the stomach and intestines. They have no striations, each cell has only one nucleus, and they contract involuntarily (Fig. 4-34). Smooth muscle contracts as nerve impulses move from one fiber to the next, creating sequential, strong, slow contractions. Arranged in sheetlike layers in which one runs along the length and the other encircles the tube like a belt, the layers take turns, alternating contraction and relaxation. These coordinated contractions result in a wavelike movement called peristalsis that squeezes the organ to move substances through the system, such as food through the digestive tract (Fig. 4-12 illustrates smooth muscle layering).

SKELETAL MUSCLE

Skeletal muscles attach to the skeleton. Made up of masses of muscle fibers wrapped in connective tissue that are organized in bundles, the muscle cells are long and thin (some are almost a foot long). They are striated, and each muscle fiber has more than one nucleus. The more bundles of fibers there are, the thicker that particular muscle is. The contraction of

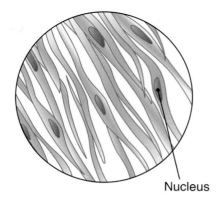

FIGURE 4-34 Smooth muscle cells. (Reprinted from Cohen BJ, Wood DL. Memmler's Structure and Function of the Human Body. 9th ed. Philadelphia: Lippincott Williams & Wilkins, 2000.)

an entire skeletal muscle can be fast and forceful. Contraction is controlled voluntarily, meaning that we can consciously make skeletal muscles contract. There are, however, nervous system reflexes that create involuntary skeletal muscle contractions, usually in response to a potentially dangerous situation. When you touch a burning hot surface, reflexes will contract a series of muscles to pull your arm away before you think about it.

In Western massage and bodywork, the best massage therapists are, in essence, muscle specialists. Just knowing the names of the muscles is not sufficient for a professional massage therapist. You should also know the attachment points of muscles, the actions of the muscles, how skeletal muscles work on a microscopic level, as well as how they work to create movement of the skeleton. Since skeletal muscles are the most relevant to massage therapy, they are the focus of this text (Fig. 4-35).

Functions of the Muscles

The primary function of the muscular system is to create movement, but muscles also produce heat, support the skeleton and maintain posture, and provide some protection from external forces.

MOVEMENT

All muscle cells have the ability to contract, bringing the ends of the cell closer together. On a cellular scale, this movement is amplified by the many bundles of muscle cells to create movement of entire muscles. Cardiac and smooth muscles in the walls of organs squeeze contents out or push contents through organs.

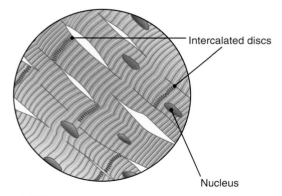

FIGURE 4-33 Cardiac muscle cells. (Reprinted from Cohen BJ, Wood DL. Memmler's Structure and Function of the Human Body. 9th ed. Philadelphia: Lippincott Williams & Wilkins, 2000.)

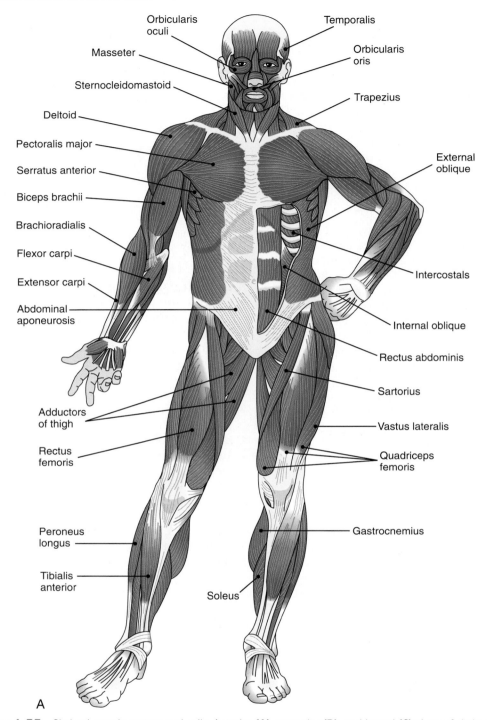

FIGURE 4-35 Skeletal muscle system and cells. Anterior **(A)**, posterior **(B)**, and lateral **(C)** views of skeletal muscle system. **D.** Skeletal muscle cells. (A, B, and D reprinted from Cohen BJ, Wood DL. Cohen BJ, Wood DL. Memmler's Structure and Function of the Human Body. 9th ed. Philadelphia: Lippincott Williams & Wilkins, 2000.)

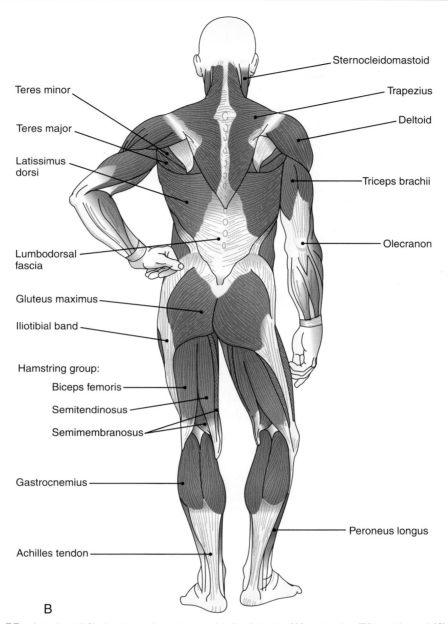

Teres minor

Teres major

Latissimus dorsi

Lumbodorsal fascia

Gluteus maximus

Iliotibial band

Hamstring group:

Biceps femoris

Semitendinosus

Semimembranosus

Gastrocnemius

Achilles tendon

Sternocleidomastoid

Trapezius

Deltoid

Triceps brachii

Olecranon

Peroneus longus

B

FIGURE 4-35 *(continued)* Skeletal muscle system and cells. Anterior **(A)**, posterior **(B)**, and lateral **(C)** views of skeletal muscle system. **D.** Skeletal muscle cells. (A, B, and D reprinted from Cohen BJ, Wood DL. Cohen BJ, Wood DL. Memmler's Structure and Function of the Human Body. 9th ed. Philadelphia: Lippincott Williams & Wilkins, 2000.)

(continued)

The main function of skeletal muscles is to move bones and sometimes to move connective tissue structures such as the lips. Most muscles attach indirectly to bone, meaning that their connective tissue covering continues past the muscle and blends into a tendon or aponeurosis, which then attaches to the bone. If muscles attach directly to a bone, their connective tissue covering fuses with the connective tissue that covers the bone.

Each skeletal muscle has two kinds of attachments: origin and insertion. **The origin of a muscle is the attachment on the bone or connective tissue structure that is more stationary during muscle contraction. The insertion of a muscle is the point of attachment that moves most during contraction, often at the distal end. All muscles have at least one of each of these two attachments.** If muscle inserts into a bone, the bone will be pulled toward the origin of the contracting muscle. If

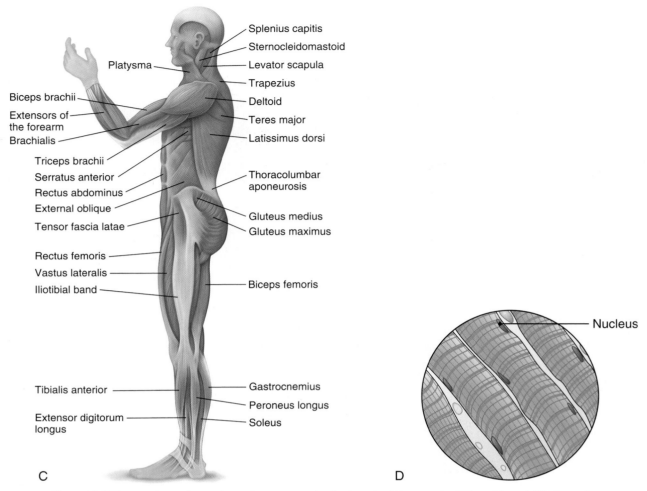

Splenius capitis
Sternocleidomastoid
Platysma
Levator scapula
Trapezius
Biceps brachii
Deltoid
Extensors of
the forearm
Teres major
Brachialis
Latissimus dorsi
Triceps brachii
Serratus anterior
Rectus abdominus
Thoracolumbar
aponeurosis
External oblique
Tensor fascia latae
Gluteus medius
Gluteus maximus
Rectus femoris
Vastus lateralis
Iliotibial band
Biceps femoris
Tibialis anterior
Gastrocnemius
Peroneus longus
Extensor digitorum
longus
Soleus

Nucleus

C

D

FIGURE 4-35 *(continued)* Skeletal muscle system and cells. Anterior **(A)**, posterior **(B)**, and lateral **(C)** views of skeletal muscle system. **D.** Skeletal muscle cells. (A, B, and D reprinted from Cohen BJ, Wood DL. Cohen BJ, Wood DL. Memmler's Structure and Function of the Human Body. 9th ed. Philadelphia: Lippincott Williams & Wilkins, 2000.)

a muscle inserts into a connective tissue structure, such as the lips, the lips will be pulled toward the origin of the contracting muscle (Fig. 4-36 illustrates origin and insertion).

In addition to moving the skeleton and connective tissue structures, muscles also help move blood and lymph. Muscles become shorter and wider when they contract, which you see in a bodybuilder who strikes a pose. As the muscles contract, they constrict the blood and lymph vessels, squeezing the fluids out. As the muscles relax, the vessels are opened up to allow more fluid to pass through.

HEAT PRODUCTION

The core temperature of the body is maintained in a safe range of 96.8 to 98.6° F. Skeletal muscles release heat in the process of contraction, and the heat gen-

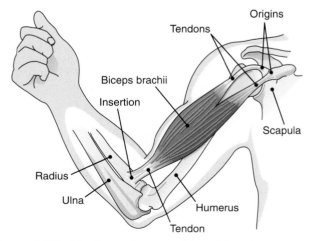

Origins
Tendons
Biceps brachii
Insertion
Scapula
Radius
Ulna
Humerus
Tendon

FIGURE 4-36 Muscle attachments: origin and insertion. (Reprinted from Cohen BJ, Wood DL. Memmler's Structure and Function of the Human Body. 9th ed. Philadelphia: Lippincott Williams & Wilkins, 2000.)

erated helps maintain the body's core temperature. Shivering, for example, involves the body making small, involuntary muscle contractions to release chemical energy or heat.

PROVIDE SUPPORT

Skeletal muscles support and maintain posture by holding the body upright against gravity and by stabilizing joints. The skeleton is only a collection of bones, joints, cartilage, and ligaments. Even standing still, our muscles work continuously to hold the skeleton up in a balanced, stable position.

PROTECTION

The muscles protect structures that are deep to them. Our organs and bones would be much more vulnerable to trauma without the muscles surrounding them.

Structures of Skeletal Muscle

The structural aspect of skeletal muscle can be studied from a microscopic, cellular level as well as an overall view of a whole muscle. The basic muscle cell, or muscle fiber, is made up of several different components that influence the overall look of a whole muscle.

MICROSCOPIC STRUCTURES OF A SKELETAL MUSCLE CELL

The microscopic anatomy and physiology of skeletal muscle cells illustrates how they create movement. Muscle cells consist of a bundle of myofibrils, also called fibrils, encased in a plasma membrane called the sarcolemma (SAHR-koh-LEM-muh). The myofibrils are made of thick myofilaments called myosin (MAHY-oh-sin) and thin myofilaments called actin. Because bunches of dark myosin filaments alternate with bunches of light actin filaments, the muscle fibers appear to have shaded bands, or stripes, which is why they are called striated muscle tissue. Multiple chains of these bands, called sarcomeres (SAHR-koh-meerz), are the contractile units of the muscle fiber.

Sliding Filament Theory

Although it has not been proven, the sliding filament mechanism is a widely accepted theory of how muscle contraction occurs. This theory suggests that the actin and myosin myofilaments remain the same length, but that the overall length of the sarcomere shortens because the myofilaments slide together. Calcium molecules first uncover sites on the actin where the myosin can attach. Once those sites are exposed, the myosin's cross bridges latch onto the actin filaments like Velcro. Temporarily connected, the actin filaments are pulled closer together, overlapping the myosin filaments. Figure 4-37 illustrates the sliding filament mechanism. The overlapped filaments create a shorter sarcomere, resulting in a shorter fibril. When many fibrils shorten, the whole muscle cell shortens. Clearly, calcium is necessary for muscle contraction, which is one of the reasons calcium should be included in a balanced diet.

Muscular Control Mechanism

The sliding together of the myofilaments begins with a nerve impulse from the CNS via a somatic motor neuron. One somatic motor neuron can stimulate hundreds of muscle cells, but each muscle cell is controlled by only one somatic motor neuron. The more muscle fibers one nerve must supply, the less precise the movements. One motor neuron and all of the muscle cells it stimulates is called a **motor unit** (Fig. 4-38). The extension of this neuron that communicates to the fibril is called an axon (AK-sahn) and branches out with axonal terminals, like tree roots, as it nears the muscle cells. Each axonal terminal meets a separate cell at the synaptic cleft, which is a fluid-filled indentation on the sarcolemma. The synaptic cleft between a motor neuron and a muscle cell is also called a motor endplate. There is no direct contact between the axonal terminal and the synaptic cleft, and this gap is called the neuromuscular junction. Figure 4-39 illustrates the neuromuscular junction.

The axonal terminal releases a chemical neurotransmitter called acetylcholine (ah-SEE-tuhl-KOH-leen) that is received by the synaptic cleft and triggers muscle contraction. (The series of events that occurs at the neuromuscular junction is described in detail below in the nervous system section.) As soon as the acetylcholine causes the muscle fiber to contract, it is broken down by a chemical in the synaptic cleft to prevent an unwanted sustained contraction. If more nerve impulses are conducted to the same muscle cell, it can sustain a prolonged contraction.

A minimal amount of current, called the threshold stimulus, is necessary to stimulate the contraction of a muscle cell. When the threshold is reached, the muscle cell reacts with complete contraction. All the muscle cells in a motor unit respond as one when stimulated. This response is commonly called "the all-or-none principle," meaning the muscle cells contract completely or not at all. The all-or-none principle may seem counterintuitive, since we know muscle

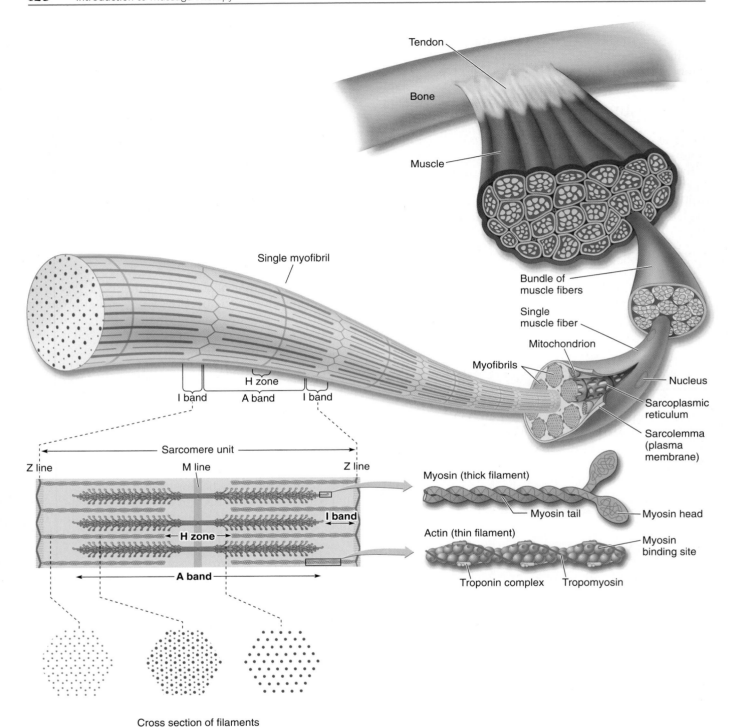

FIGURE 4-37 Sliding filament mechanism. (Reprinted with permission from McArdle WD, Katch FI, Katch VL: Exercise Physiology: Energy, Nutrition, and Human Performance. 5th ed. Baltimore: Lippincott Williams & Wilkins, 2001, fig 18.2B-D.)

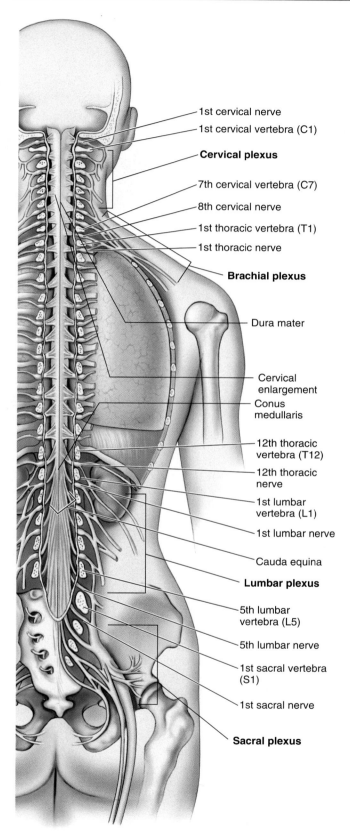

though they are part of the PNS, ganglia are located very close to the spinal cord, within the vertebral canal.

CLASSIFICATION BY FUNCTION

There are many types of nerves that monitor, integrate, and respond to external and internal stimuli and changes occurring within the body. Functional classification of nerve cells separates them into two separate groups. **Sensory (afferent) neurons** receive sensory input and transmit that information to the CNS. **Motor (efferent) neurons** carry messages away from the CNS to the muscle or organs that must react. Groups of sensory neurons form sensory nerves, and groups of motor neurons are called motor nerves. Most nerves, however, are mixed nerves, which have both sensory and motor neurons that carry information to and from the CNS.

Sensory Neurons

Sensory neurons, or dendritic end organs, are classified by their location, sensitivity, or structure. They send signals to the CNS in response to external or internal stimuli. Exteroceptors respond to stimuli from the external environment, such as touch, pressure, temperature, smell, sight, and hearing. These are mostly found in the skin and near the surface of the body. **Proprioceptors** (PROH-pree-oh-SEP-torz) are sensory nerve cells sensitive to body position, muscle tone, and equilibrium. They are located in the muscles, tendons, joints, and inner ear. Interoceptors, also called visceroceptors, detect stimuli such as pressure within the organs and blood vessels.

The integument contains several different exteroceptors that constantly monitor our surroundings (Fig. 4-48). The closer these exteroceptors are to the surface of our skin, the more sensitive they are.

- Nociceptors, also called free nerve endings, located in the lower layer of the epidermis, detect pain.
- Merkel cells, found in the lower layer of the epidermis, detect very light touch.
- Meissner's corpuscles, found in the upper part of the dermis in the lips, hands, feet, and genital organs, detect very light touch.
- Krause end bulbs, found in the dermis and subcutaneous layer, are sensitive to cold, pressure, and vibration.
- Ruffini end organs, located in the dermis, detect heat and strong or continuous pressure.
- Pacinian corpuscles, found in the deep dermis, sense vibrations and deep pressure.

FIGURE 4-47 Nerve plexuses. (Reprinted with permission from Bear MF, Connors BW, Paradiso MA: Neuroscience: Exploring the Brain. 2nd ed. Baltimore: Lippincott Williams & Wilkins, 2001, p 230.)

Labels in figure:
- 1st cervical nerve
- 1st cervical vertebra (C1)
- **Cervical plexus**
- 7th cervical vertebra (C7)
- 8th cervical nerve
- 1st thoracic vertebra (T1)
- 1st thoracic nerve
- **Brachial plexus**
- Dura mater
- Cervical enlargement
- Conus medullaris
- 12th thoracic vertebra (T12)
- 12th thoracic nerve
- 1st lumbar vertebra (L1)
- 1st lumbar nerve
- Cauda equina
- **Lumbar plexus**
- 5th lumbar vertebra (L5)
- 5th lumbar nerve
- 1st sacral vertebra (S1)
- 1st sacral nerve
- **Sacral plexus**

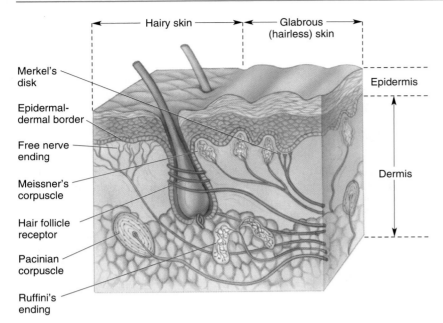

Hairy skin — Glabrous (hairless) skin

Merkel's disk

Epidermal-dermal border

Free nerve ending

Meissner's corpuscle

Hair follicle receptor

Pacinian corpuscle

Ruffini's ending

Epidermis

Dermis

FIGURE 4-48 Sensory receptors of the integument. (Reprinted with permission from Bear MF, Connors BW, Paradiso MA: Neuroscience: Exploring the Brain. 2nd ed. Baltimore: Lippincott Williams & Wilkins, 2001, p 398, fig 12.1.)

For a massage therapist, the proprioceptors and exteroceptors are the most important of all the sensory receptors. In the muscle, the muscle spindles are complex proprioceptors that respond to tension in the muscle fibers (see Fig. 4-40). Between the collagen fibers in tendons are Golgi (GOHL-jee) tendon organs that respond to tension on the tendon. Both muscle spindles and Golgi tendon organs provide information to the CNS regarding the length and tension of a muscle and its tendon(s). Within a joint capsule are Ruffini end organs and Pacinian corpuscles. Both respond to pressure within a joint, essentially sensing the position of the joint by sensing different amounts of pressure at different places.

The muscle spindles and Golgi tendon organs respond as muscles move a joint through its range of motion, but joint proprioceptors are active when a joint is at the ends of its range. All of the proprioceptors act as a group to provide a sense of joint position, body position, effort, heaviness, and timing of movement; together this is sometimes called a kinesthetic sense. Manipulating the muscle spindles and Golgi tendon organs with advanced massage techniques can encourage muscles to shorten or lengthen. One of these techniques, appropriately called proprioceptive neuromuscular facilitation (PNF), is discussed in the chapter covering therapeutic techniques.

Motor Neurons

Motor neurons send signals from the CNS to create bodily response. The skeletal muscles can be effec-

tors, or endpoints, for nervous signals, under voluntary control. The motor neurons can also control involuntary activity of the organs, glands, and smooth and cardiac muscle.

Mixed Nerves

Most of the nerves of the body are mixed nerves that contain both sensory and motor nerve cells. They can monitor for input, integrate the information received, and stimulate the body to respond to the input. The sciatic (sahy-AT-ik) nerve in the leg is an example of a mixed nerve that can receive and send information.

Nerve Impulses

Nerve cells have two primary functions: irritability and conductivity. A neuron's irritability allows it to respond to a stimulus and translate that perception into a nerve impulse. Its conductivity allows the neuron to communicate that nerve impulse to another neuron, a muscle, or a gland.

IRRITABILITY

The neuron's irritability is the result of a chemical process of depolarization. The mechanism is sometimes referred to as the sodium–potassium pump because it involves sodium and potassium ions. There are several steps to creating a nerve impulse from a stimulus. Following is the series of events that takes place in response to a stimulus, such as a sharp thorn poking your finger:

1. Resting state—A nerve membrane at rest is in a polarized state, meaning that the positive and negative charges on either side of the membrane are not balanced. There are more sodium ions (Na^+) outside the neuron than there are potassium ions (K^+) inside, creating an overall negative charge inside the membrane.

2. Excitation—When the thorn is perceived by a pain receptor, a neurotransmitter chemical is usually released to alter the permeability of the membrane.

3. Depolarization—The membrane becomes more permeable to sodium ions, and they diffuse into the cell, rushing from the high sodium concentration outside the cell to the lower sodium concentration inside. With the extra supply of sodium ions inside, the membrane becomes depolarized; that is, the negative and positive charges on either side of the membrane are balanced.

4. Repolarization—Almost as soon as the sodium has rushed in, the permeability of the membrane reverts, preventing any more sodium from entering. The cell membrane becomes more permeable to potassium, which quickly rushes out of the cell, restoring the positive charge outside the cell and the negative charge inside. The sodium–potassium pump uses ATP to move sodium ions out and potassium ions in to return the cell to its resting state, ready to receive another stimulus.

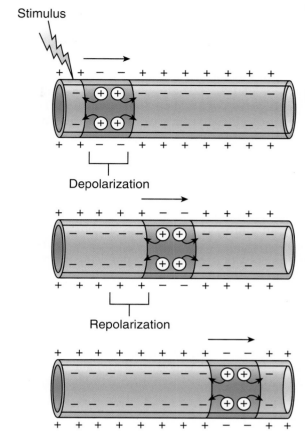

FIGURE 4-49 Action potential (nerve impulse). (Reprinted from Cohen BJ, Wood DL. Memmler's Structure and Function of the Human Body. 9th ed. Philadelphia: Lippincott Williams & Wilkins, 2000.)

This process is called the action potential, also known as the nerve impulse (Fig. 4-49). There is a threshold stimulus that acts as a switch for the impulse. If a stimulus is not strong enough and does not reach the threshold stimulus, the nerve impulse will not occur at all. Stimuli above the threshold stimulus will trigger the nerve impulse over the entire nerve cell. The permeability of the entire membrane is altered at the same time, so the whole nerve cell either responds to the stimulus or does not. This is called the all-or-none response.

The PNS is equipped with Schwann cells that are strung like beads along the nerve cell. The Schwann cells insulate the nerve membrane and in between the Schwann cells are gaps called nodes of Ranvier. The myelin provides insulation to the axon, like the plastic coating around electrical wires, preventing the nerve impulse from spreading out and short-circuiting. The nerve impulse is forced to jump from node to node instead of traveling along the entire surface of the membrane. By jumping over the Schwann cells, the impulse can travel much faster and trans-

mission speed increases. The CNS does not have any Schwann cells, but it is equipped with oligodendrocytes that form the myelin sheath on some of the neurons that need insulation. The myelin insulation is especially helpful when there are hundreds of neurons transmitting hundreds of nerve impulses through one nerve. The pain receptors in the integument are unmyelinated, but they do not need insulation from impulses of other neurons.

Once the impulse reaches the end of the axon, it can be terminated or conducted, depending on the strength of the action potential. If it is conducted, it will either stimulate an action potential in another nerve cell or stimulate activity of a gland or organ.

Alcohol, cold temperature, continuous pressure, and anesthetics are some factors that can reduce the speed of the action potential. These factors either reduce the membrane's permeability to sodium or prevent oxygen and other nutrients from reaching the nerve. Without oxygen, cells suffer and eventually die.

CONDUCTIVITY

If the electrical impulse at the end of the axon is strong enough, the impulse will be conducted from one neuron to another neuron or an effector (muscle, organ, or gland). The impulses are conducted in a tiny but active gap called the synapse (SIHN-aps). The nerve cell that needs to transmit the impulse is called the presynaptic cell, and the cell that will receive the impulse is called the postsynaptic cell.

The electrical nerve impulse on the presynaptic cell triggers the axonal terminal to release a neurotransmitter chemical into the synapse. Approximately 30 different neurotransmitters are made in the brain and stored in vesicles at the axonal terminals all over the body. Some of the neurotransmitters are epinephrine (adrenaline), norepinephrine (noradrenaline), dopamine, serotonin, and acetylcholine. Acetylcholine, discussed in the muscular system, is the neurotransmitter released at the neuromuscular junction. Once the vesicles release the neurotransmitter into the synapse, special receptor sites on the postsynaptic cell receive the neurotransmitters.

The receptor site is activated and starts the action potential along the postsynaptic cell. The neurotransmitter is immediately deactivated in the dendrite of the postsynaptic cell to prevent conduction of multiple nerve impulses.

The synapse is designed such that the axon produces the neurotransmitters and the dendrites have specific receptor sites. In other words, a specific neurotransmitter must be received by the dendrite to complete the conduction. This design ensures a specific, one-way communication along the path (Fig. 4-50). Although most synapses are chemical (neurotransmitters and receptors), electrical synapses occur in cardiac or smooth muscle tissue where rhythmic, sequential muscle contractions are required.

Nervous System Organization

The nervous system is structurally organized in two distinct systems: the CNS and the PNS. The CNS consists of the brain and spinal cord. The PNS includes everything in the nervous system outside the brain and spinal cord: the nerves that exit the brain, called cranial nerves, and the nerves that exit the spinal cord, called spinal nerves.

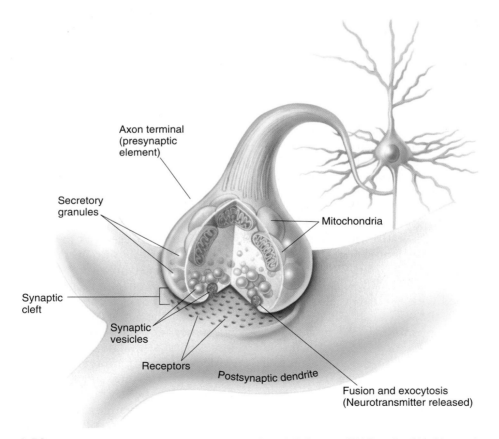

FIGURE 4-50 Synapse. (Reprinted with permission from Bear MF, Connors BW, Paradiso MA: Neuroscience: Exploring the Brain. 2nd ed. Baltimore: Lippincott Williams & Wilkins, 2001, p 102, fig 5.2.)

Central Nervous System

The brain and the spinal cord are the structures that make up the CNS. This is the body's main control center for all of the body's functions, receiving sensory input from everywhere in the body, processing the information, and directing the body to make appropriate responses. Within the brain are four ventricles, or cavities, and outside the brain and spinal cord are three distinct layers of connective tissue coverings.

THE BRAIN

The four main sections of the brain are the cerebrum (seh-REE-bruhm), the cerebellum (SAIR-eh-BEHL-uhm), the brainstem, and the diencephalon (DAHY-ehn-SEHF-uh-lahn) (Fig. 4-51).

The cerebrum is the largest portion, divided into two halves by a deep fissure called the longitudinal fissure. Each cerebral hemisphere is divided into four different sections, called the parietal, occipital, temporal, and frontal lobes. The central fissure divides the brain into anterior and posterior sections, and just posterior to the central fissure is the parietal lobe. It is responsible for processing sensory input such as pain, pressure, and temperature. The occipital lobe, the most posterior section of the cerebrum, processes visual input. The temporal lobe is located laterally and is responsible for hearing and the sense of smell. Anterior to the central fissure is the frontal lobe, which processes voluntary movement of our skeletal muscles, including speech. The cerebral hemispheres are connected by a mass of nervous tissue called the corpus callosum, which helps us coordinate movements that require the left and right side of our bodies to work together in activities such as crawling and walking.

The cerebellum is a cauliflower-like structure toward the back and base of the brain. It acts as the center for equilibrium and helps us maintain our balance. The cerebellum also controls coordination of skeletal muscles and allows movements to be fluid instead of jerky. Maintaining muscle tone, as discussed in the muscular system section of this chapter, is another function of the cerebellum.

The brainstem, located at the central base of the brain, consists of the midbrain, pons, and medulla oblongata. The brainstem controls such activities as hearing, vision, breathing, sleep cycles, and organ activity.

The diencephalon sits above the brainstem, deep within the cerebrum, and includes the hypothalamus and thalamus. The hypothalamus plays a significant role in homeostasis. It regulates hunger, thirst, pain, sexual behavior, body temperature, and emotions. The activity of the thalamus is less specific, processing sensory input and redirecting it to the cerebrum and determining sensations as pleasant or distasteful.

THE SPINAL CORD

The spinal cord runs through the bony vertebral column, starting at the base of the brainstem and ending around the first or second lumbar vertebra. The spinal cord acts as a telegraph wire for sending signals to and from the brain. The inner core of the spinal cord is gray matter, nerve cell bodies without myelin covering. The outer periphery is white matter made of myelinated axons and dendrites (see Fig. 4-14).

REFLEX ARCS

The spinal cord acts as the control center for reflexes, which are instantaneous, automatic responses that require very few nerve cells. The communication path allows the body to respond automatically and predictably to stimuli that are potentially dangerous. Reflex arcs are the specific nerve cell paths from stimulus to response, or receptor to effector. Receptors are located at the end of dendrites to detect stimuli. The information from a stimulus travels along a sensory neuron to the CNS. In the CNS, the impulses are coordinated and processed into an automatic, involuntary response. Once the response is determined, the motor neuron carries the signal away from the

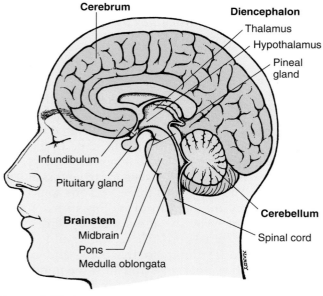

FIGURE 4-51 Brain. (Reprinted with permission from Neil O. Hardy, Westpoint, CT.)

CNS to the effector. The effector is the muscle, organ, or gland that reacts or responds according to the information received. Motor reflexes, or somatic reflexes, activate skeletal muscles. Autonomic reflexes stimulate organs and glands to react. Figure 4-52 illustrates a reflex arc.

The simplest reflex arc only requires two neurons—one sensory and one motor. A nerve impulse travels along a sensory receptor to the spinal cord and back out to the effector along a motor neuron. Also called a spinal reflex, this reflex arc does not travel to the brain for coordination.

Stretch Reflexes

Stretch reflexes are protective muscle contractions that occur when the tissues are stretched too far and/or too fast. They prevent the muscle from being torn. The familiar patellar tendon reflex, also called the "knee jerk reaction," is actually a stretch reflex. The tendon that lies just inferior to the patella is the tendon for the quadriceps femoris muscles that extend the knee joint and flex the hip joint. When the tendon is tapped, the muscle spindles in the quadriceps femoris sense that the muscle is being pulled too quickly. The proprioceptors send an impulse to the spinal cord, and the spinal cord sends an impulse back along a motor neuron to the quadriceps femoris, causing it to contract quickly in a protective mechanism. Stretch reflex contraction of the quadriceps femoris quickly extends the knee with a kicking action.

This stretch reflex comes into play in massage therapy when you move a client's body. If a muscle is being stretched too fast and beyond its comfort zone, it can respond with a protective contraction that the client feels as a cramp. Therefore, always move the client's body carefully and knowledgeably to prevent protective muscle cramps.

Tendon Reflexes

Tendon reflexes occur when a muscle and its tendon are subjected to slow and gentle tension. The nerve impulse travels to the CNS, which determines that the muscle is not in danger of being torn and sends a nerve impulse that reflexively lengthens the muscle, allowing the stretch to go a bit further. Because the tendon reflex causes the opposite result from the stretch reflex, it is also important to a massage therapist. It can be used to encourage clients' tissues to stretch and create more space for circulation.

Protecting the body is the purpose of reflexes. When a stretch is potentially harmful to the muscle tissue, the body reflexively responds to the stretch with a reflexive contraction. A stretch that does not threaten the integrity of the tissues initiates the tendon reflex, which relaxes the muscle. The tendon reflex allows the connective tissue to stretch farther; the stretch reflex does not. For that reason, athletes can stretch more effectively by slowly and steadily increasing the stretch instead of by bouncing. Bouncing can induce the stretch reflex.

Flexor Reflexes

The flexor reflex, or withdrawal reflex, is another type of spinal reflex. Usually in response to a harmful or painful stimulus, the flexor reflex is activated by stepping on a tack or touching a hot pan. Unlike the stretch reflex that is activated by proprioceptors, the flexor reflex is activated by sensory receptors in the integument. The body uses three neurons to accomplish the safety mechanism of pulling away. A sensory neuron receives the input that is sent as an impulse to the spinal cord. There, the input is determined a potential threat to the body, and an interneuron in the spinal cord transmits the impulse to a motor neuron. The impulse travels along the motor neuron to the appropriate muscles that must contract to move the body out of harm's way.

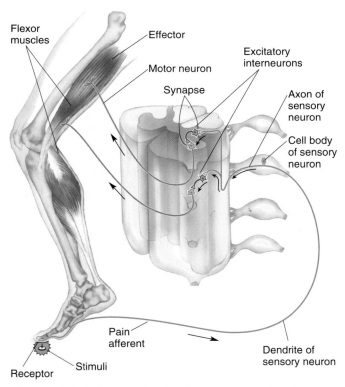

FIGURE 4-52 Reflex arc. (Reprinted with permission from Bear MF, Connors BW, Paradiso MA: Neuroscience: Exploring the Brain. 2nd ed. Baltimore: Lippincott Williams & Wilkins, 2001, p 459, fig 13.24.)

VENTRICLES

Enclosed inside the brain are four ventricles, or cavities. There are networks of blood capillaries in the ventricles that filter the blood and add cellular secretions to produce cerebrospinal fluid (CSF). The fluid is constantly generated and circulated throughout the CNS to provide nutrients and remove waste to the brain and spinal cord. It also acts as a cushion against impact and other trauma. The CSF eventually returns to the venous blood through the connective tissue covering of the brain.

MENINGES

The brain and spinal cord are supplied with three layers of connective tissue coverings called meninges (Fig. 4-53). The dura mater (DUHR-uh MAH-ter) is the toughest and outermost layer that provides a strong, protective covering for the structures of the CNS. The dura mater covering the spinal cord is sometimes referred to as the dural tube. The arachnoid mater (ah-RAK-noyd MAH-ter) is the middle layer with a structure like a spider web that allows CSF to flow through the meninges. The pia mater (PEE-ah MAH-ter) lies closest to the brain. It is delicate and carries most of the blood supply for the brain.

Peripheral Nervous System

The PNS consists of all the nerve tissue outside the CNS. Its function is to transmit information to and from the CNS. Again, nerves are made up of organ-

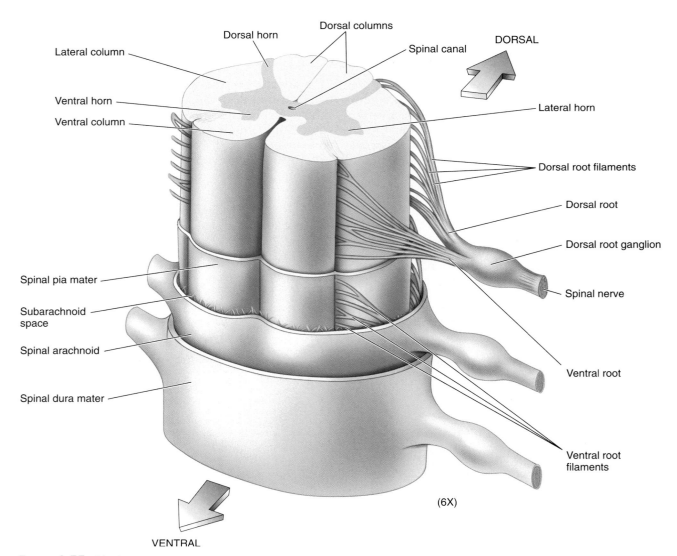

FIGURE 4-53 Meninges.

ized bundles containing nerve cells, connective tissue coverings, and blood vessels. The nerves that branch out from the brain are called cranial nerves, and the nerves that branch out from the spinal cord are called spinal nerves. Functionally, the PNS can be divided into the somatic and autonomic nervous systems. The somatic nervous system is responsible for voluntary skeletal muscle contractions, which are discussed above in this section. The autonomic nervous system controls the involuntary smooth muscles of the organs, the cardiac muscles in the heart, and the activity of glands. The cranial and spinal nerves of the autonomic nervous system are separated into the sympathetic and parasympathetic divisions, each with its own set of responses.

The PNS can be classified structurally, by the location of the nerves. There are cranial nerves, spinal nerves, and nerves in the extremities.

There are 12 pairs of cranial nerves originating from the brain (Fig. 4-54). The cranial nerves are identified by names and roman numerals, starting at the superior end. Most of them serve the head and neck region, but the vagus nerve (cranial nerve X) extends to the thoracic and abdominal cavities.

The 31 pairs of spinal nerves extend out from the spinal cord. They are identified according to where they exit the spinal cord, named for the closest vertebrae. For example, C8 exits the spinal cord just inferior to the 7th cervical vertebra (Fig. 4-55). Spinal nerves are mixed nerves, carrying sensory and motor neurons. Each spinal nerve is connected to the spinal cord by two roots. The dorsal root contains the sensory neurons that transmit nerve impulses to the spinal cord. The ventral root is made of the motor neurons that transmit the nerve impulses from the spinal cord out to the effectors.

The nerves in the extremities are located in the anterior and posterior arms and legs as shown in Figure 4-56. These are important for massage because they innervate the skeletal muscles of the body.

The PNS can also be classified by functions of the different tissues. The PNS is responsible for receiving sensory input and delivering nerve impulses that control bodily activities. The functions of the PNS can be separated into voluntary and involuntary activities. Voluntary activity is controlled by the somatic (soh-MAT-ik) nervous system. It serves all the skeletal muscles, allowing us to move muscles when we want to. Involuntary activities, including those of organs and glands, are controlled by the autonomic nervous system.

SOMATIC NERVOUS SYSTEM

The effectors of the somatic nervous system are our skeletal muscles, which are discussed in the section above on the muscular system. Recall that a motor unit is one motor neuron and all of the muscle cells that it controls. Precision movement is created by motor units with very few muscle cells. Strength is a

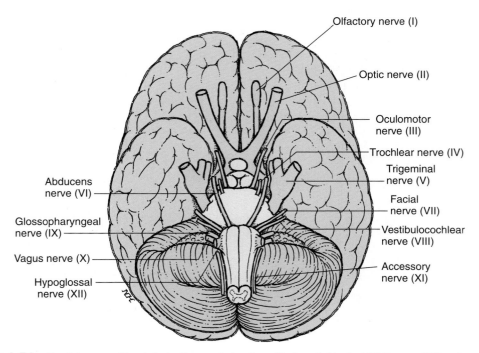

FIGURE 4-54   Cranial nerves. (Reprinted with permission from Stedman's Medical Dictionary, 27th ed. Baltimore: Lippincott Williams & Wilkins, 2000, p 1194.)

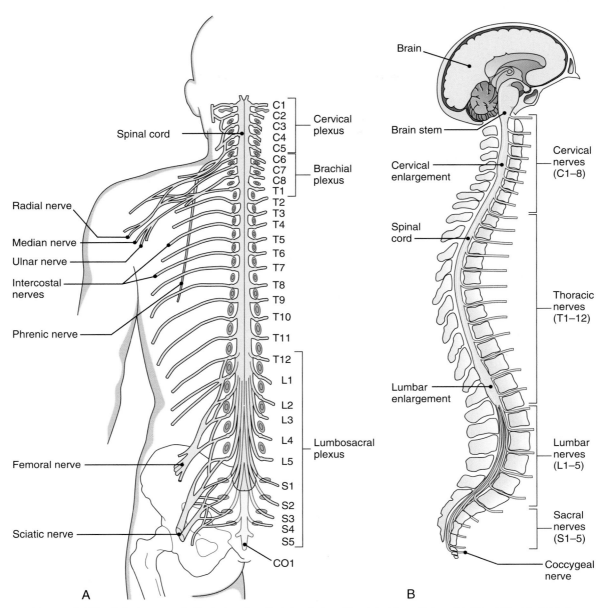

FIGURE 4-55 Spinal nerves. **A.** Posterior view. **B.** Lateral view. (Reprinted from Cohen BJ, Wood DL. Memmler's Structure and Function of the Human Body. 9th ed. Philadelphia: Lippincott Williams & Wilkins, 2000.)

function of the quantity of actin and myosin filaments within a muscle cell.

Neurological Memory

"Practice makes perfect," as the old saying goes. This is the basis for neurological memory. Repetition of a movement or holding the body's position in space reinforces the body's ability to produce that movement or position over time. The same activity, practiced over and over, creates a worn path in the brain and nervous system, sometimes called a nerve track. Very similar to a reflex arc, this figurative "groove" in-

volves chemical and anatomical changes that reinforce learning. An association area of the brain handles the ability to remember movements and positions, but the nerve track promotes this ability. One theory of neurological memory suggests that the neurons that store the memories grow in size. Another theory is that the repetition increases the neuron's output of memory-enhancing proteins. The repetitions may also strengthen the connections between neurons, facilitating the transmission of impulses along a specific path.

The reinforcement of nerve tracks occurs with repetition, so repeating an activity correctly will reinforce the correct

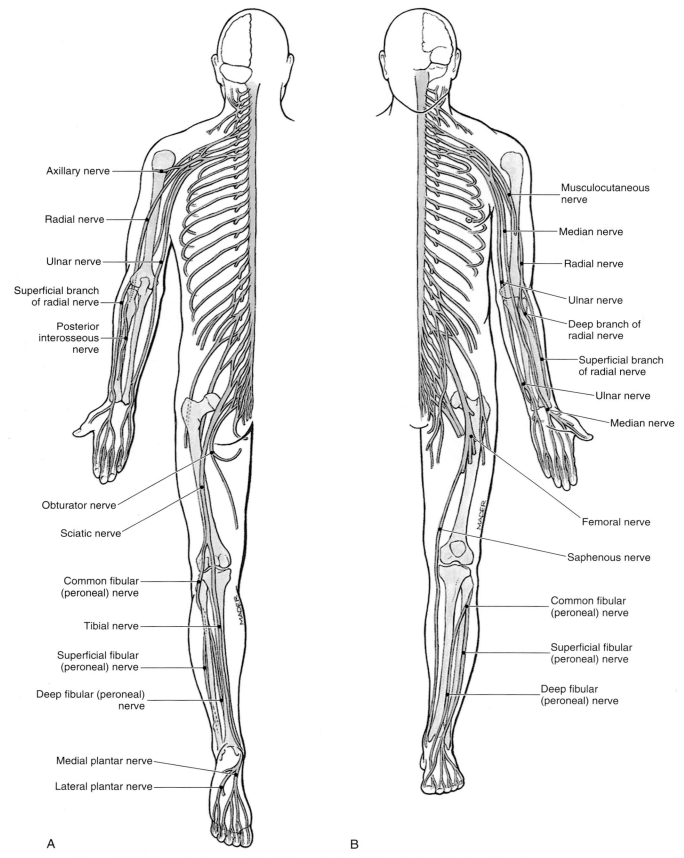

Axillary nerve

Radial nerve

Ulnar nerve

Superficial branch
of radial nerve

Posterior
interosseous
nerve

Obturator nerve

Sciatic nerve

Common fibular
(peroneal) nerve

Tibial nerve

Superficial fibular
(peroneal) nerve

Deep fibular (peroneal)
nerve

Medial plantar nerve

Lateral plantar nerve

A

Musculocutaneous
nerve

Median nerve

Radial nerve

Ulnar nerve

Deep branch of
radial nerve

Superficial branch
of radial nerve

Ulnar nerve

Median nerve

Femoral nerve

Saphenous nerve

Common fibular
(peroneal) nerve

Superficial fibular
(peroneal) nerve

Deep fibular
(peroneal) nerve

B

FIGURE 4-56   Nerves in the extremities. **A.** Posterior view. **B.** Anterior view. (Reprinted from Agur AMR, Ming
JL. Grant's Atlas of Anatomy. 10th ed. Baltimore: Lippincott Williams & Wilkins, 1999.)

movement, and repeating an activity incorrectly will rein-force the incorrect movement. Unlearning an incorrect process and relearning it correctly is much more difficult than simply learning it properly from the beginning. For example, consider how children learn to hold a crayon or pencil. Those who learn to hold a pencil "incorrectly" will probably hold a pencil the same way for the rest of their lives despite efforts to hold it the "right" way. Once a nerve track is established, the body tends to respond predictably with the same pattern, just like in a reflex response. Repatterning undesirable actions or behaviors requires effort and repetition of the desired action or behavior.

This concept is commonly seen in massage clients. When people get hurt, they tend to favor the injury and acquire compensation patterns. Consider a person who stepped on a piece of glass and cut her foot. She might favor the injured foot with a limp or an abnormal posture, and her muscles and body will acquire a new "normal" position in space. The longer a client maintains the new position, the more the brain and nervous system reinforce the nerve track, and the more difficult it is for the client to return to the "normal" posture. Theoretically, a client who has an acute injury can return to a balanced posture more quickly than one who has allowed an injury to go untreated for months or years. Understanding this concept of neurological memory and educating your clients about it can help them understand that it may take more than one massage session to rid them of their aches and pains.

AUTONOMIC NERVOUS SYSTEM

The autonomic nervous system (ANS) controls the smooth muscles, cardiac muscles, organs, and glands, allowing them to function without our conscious effort. The ANS is divided into two systems that work together to maintain homeostasis: the sympathetic and parasympathetic divisions. When one of these two systems is too active or not active enough, homeostasis is disrupted, and the whole body suffers.

Sympathetic Nervous System

The sympathetic nervous system is the stimulatory division of the ANS. It is also known as the thoracolumbar division because it includes spinal nerves T1 through L2. It regulates the "fight or flight" response to stress when the body reacts to real or perceived threats. Even a thought or perception of a threat can stimulate the sympathetic nervous system to release its neurotransmitters, including epinephrine (adrenaline) and norepinephrine (noradrenaline). The sympathetic nervous response occurs to some degree with stress. When stimulated, the sympathetic nervous system affects many structures and organs, preparing them for an emergency situation. For example, the heart pumps faster to provide more oxygen, the skeletal muscles contract, the pupil of the eye dilates to allow more light in, the sweat glands are stimulated to perspire, and digestive activity slows down (Table 4-7).

TABLE 4-7
Autonomic Nervous System Responses

SYMPATHETIC	EFFECTOR	PARASYMPATHETIC
Dilation	**Pupils of the eyes**	Constriction
Inhibition	**Digestive glands**	Stimulation
Vasoconstriction	**Blood supply to digestive system**	Vasodilation
Decrease peristalsis	**Smooth muscles of digestive system**	Increase peristalsis
Increase strength and rate of contractions	**Heart**	Decrease strength and rate of contractions
Dilation	**Bronchioles**	Constriction
Stimulates epinephrine and norepinephrine release	**Adrenal gland**	(none)
Decrease activity	**Kidneys**	(none)
Relaxation	**Urinary bladder**	Contraction for urination
Release more glucose	**Liver**	(none)
Ejaculation	**Penis**	Erection
Vasodilation	**Blood supply to skeletal muscles**	(none)
Vasoconstriction	**Blood supply to skin**	(none)
Stimulates perspiration	**Sweat glands in skin**	(none)

Parasympathetic Nervous System

The parasympathetic nervous system is the relaxing, restorative division of the ANS. It is also known as the craniosacral (KRAY-nee-oh-SAY-kruhl) system because the motor pathways arise from the cranial nerves and sacral portions of the spinal nerves. The primary neurotransmitter of the parasympathetic nervous system is acetylcholine. When the parasympathetic nerves are triggered, the organs and glands have a response opposite to the sympathetic nervous response—the heart slows down, the skeletal muscles relax, the pupils constrict, sweat glands are not activated, and normal digestion occurs (Table 4-7). Typically, massage evokes the **parasympathetic response,** helping the body to rest and digest.

These divisions of the nervous system are not intended to work full time and our bodies are not supposed to be flooded with their neurotransmitters all the time, either. Too much stress or too much excitement overworks the sympathetic nervous system and can result in exhaustion. Likewise, too much rest or not enough activity can overwork the parasympathetic nervous system. The body works best when structures and functions are balanced, including the activity of the ANS.

Circulatory System

People often associate the circulatory system with the heart, but, it also includes all the blood vessels, lymphatic vessels, the fluids they transport, and some related organs. The major function of this system is transportation, but some of its structures also provide immunity, protect us from blood loss, and help regulate core body temperature. It provides a link between the external environment and the internal fluid environment of the body by carrying nutrients and gases to all cells, tissues, organs, and organ systems and removing metabolic wastes. This exchange is necessary to maintain homeostasis within the body. Massage promotes the mechanical movement of fluids and thereby enhances the delivery of vital ingredients and removal of wastes.

The circulatory system can be separated into the cardiovascular and lymphatic systems. The cardiovascular structures include the blood, blood vessels, and heart. The spleen, liver, bone marrow, and thymus gland also have circulatory functions, producing and storing blood and differentiating immune cells. Lymphatic structures include the lymph, lymph vessels, and lymph nodes.

Functions of the Cardiovascular System

The primary function of the cardiovascular system is to transport blood and all of its components. In addition to its important blood delivery service to all the cells of our bodies, the cardiovascular system has some other important functions. It carries cells that protect us from infection and diseases, provide immunity from disease, and prevent blood loss. The cardiovascular system is also involved in regulating our core body temperature and maintaining the correct acidity of our blood, measured as pH.

TRANSPORTATION

The cardiovascular system is the delivery system within the body. Using the blood as a transport mechanism, the cardiovascular system carries oxygen, carbon dioxide, hormones, and nutrients to and from all parts of the body. There is a certain pathway for taking blood from the heart to the lungs to pick up oxygen, a separate path that delivers oxygenated blood from the heart to the cells of the body, and yet another pathway for returning deoxygenated blood to the heart.

PROTECTION

The cardiovascular system uses the blood to carry leukocytes (LOO-koh-sahytz), antibodies, and platelets throughout the body. The leukocytes, also called white blood cells, along with the antibodies fight pathogens and destroy foreign substances. Their ability to protect us from infection and disease is called immunity.

Platelets in the blood activate hemostasis, a clotting process that the body uses to automatically stop bleeding. By forming a blood clot, our bodies protect us from losing too much blood. When the clotting mechanism takes place on the integument, it forms a scab that protects us from having bacteria in the external environment enter the body through the open wound.

The mechanism of hemostasis starts when blood vessels within a tissue are injured. Blood platelets contact the injured tissue and burst open, releasing chemicals that attract more platelets to the area. They stimulate localized vasoconstriction to minimize blood flow in the area, and they clump together to form a platelet plug or clot to seal the hole in the blood vessel. Fibrinogen, a protein suspended in the blood, is converted into strands of fibrin, which tangle together at the injury site. As circulation continues, red blood cells and platelets are caught in the tangle, further reducing blood flow in the area. Leukocytes also get caught, which remove cellular debris and fight infection. As the platelet plug shrinks, the fibrin strands contract and pull the edges of the wound together to provide a framework for tissue repair.

REGULATION

The cardiovascular system also helps maintain body temperature by constriction and dilation of the blood vessels. A thermostat in the brain maintains the body's temperature normal temperature at approximately 98.6°F. When external temperatures, muscular exertion, or fever create excessive heat, vasodilation (dilation of the blood vessels) in the skin allows more warm blood to flow near the skin's surface, where heat can dissipate. Conversely, the vessels constrict (vasoconstriction) in the skin when the external environment is excessively cold, in an effort to preserve body heat. The brain needs blood to function properly and has priority over all other organs, regardless of the body's temperature or activity. In extreme situations, more blood will be sent to the brain and less to the rest of the body. Body heat is dissipated from the head, despite the body's core temperature. Thus, wearing a hat in colder temperatures helps keep fingers and toes warmer.

The acidity or alkalinity of a substance is measured as pH. Neutral pH, or pH balanced, indicates a substance that is neither acidic nor alkaline and has a pH of 7. When the pH is below 7, the solution is considered acidic, and above 7 it is considered basic, or alkaline. The interstitial fluids (also called extracellular fluids or tissue fluids) are kept at pH 7.4, which means that tissue fluids are slightly basic, or alkaline. The blood has hemoglobin and plasma proteins that act as buffers, or chemicals that stabilize pH levels.

Structures of the Cardiovascular System

The cardiovascular system consists of the blood, the heart, the blood vessels, and the capillaries. These structures create separate pathways for blood, including the pulmonary circuit and the systemic circuit.

BLOOD

A single drop of blood contains over 250 million separate blood cells. Blood is a liquid connective tissue whose cells are suspended in an extracellular fluid matrix called plasma. Suspended in the blood plasma are various components including red blood cells, white blood cells, platelets, and proteins.

Blood Plasma

Plasma is a clear, straw-colored matrix that is similar in composition to cytosol. Mostly water, it also contains proteins, glucose, salts, vitamins, hormones, antibodies, and wastes. It acts as the transport system for delivering gases and nutrients throughout the body. Fibrinogen is a protein manufactured in the liver that resides in the plasma to help with hemostasis. Alpha and beta globulins are plasma proteins that act as transport molecules for lipids and hormones; they are also made in the liver. Gamma globulins, or immunoglobulins, are antibodies that float in the plasma. They are made in the lymphoid tissues and serve as the basis for the immune system.

Erythrocytes

Erythrocytes (ee-RITH-roh-sahytz), also called red blood cells or rbcs, are biconcave, rounded structures with a central depression (Fig. 4-57). Erythrocytes are the only cells that do not have a nucleus. Instead, these cells are full of hemoglobin molecules that transport oxygen and iron and buffer the pH of fluids throughout the body. Erythrocytes are enclosed by a highly permeable, elastic membrane that allows gases to diffuse through. Oxygen moves in and out of red blood cells via diffusion. The high concentration of oxygen in the lungs causes oxygen to diffuse into the blood cells and onto the hemoglobin molecule. As the blood cells move through the body, oxygen diffuses out of the red blood cells to tissues with lower concentrations of oxygen.

A tiny drop of blood contains over five million red blood cells that circulate through the body 300,000 times in about 4 months before they break down and disintegrate. Homeostasis is maintained via hematopoiesis in the red bone marrow, which generates approximately three million new red blood cells each second.

Leukocytes

Leukocytes are sometimes called white blood cells because they have a clear, colorless appearance (Fig. 4-57). They differ from erythrocytes because they are larger, they have a nucleus, they do not carry hemoglobin, and they have the special ability to squeeze through the cells in the capillary membranes to reside in the interstitial fluids (Fig. 4-58). There are five different kinds of leukocytes—neutrophils, basophils, eosinophils, lymphocytes, and monocytes—and they

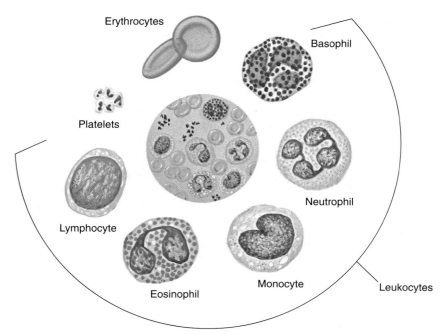

FIGURE 4-57   Erythrocytes, leukocytes, platelets. (Reprinted with permission from Brunner and Suddarth's Textbook of Medical-Surgical Nursing. 9th ed. Baltimore: Lippincott Williams & Wilkins, 2000, p 732, fig 30-2.)

all function to defend the body against disease and foreign substances by destroying pathogens.

A tiny drop of blood only contains about five thousand leukocytes, in contrast to five million erythrocytes. They are manufactured in the red bone marrow, lymph nodes, spleen, thymus, and tonsils. The white blood cells circulate within the tissues for a day or less or may reside in the tissues for months, depending upon the severity of the infection or injury. In response to an injury or infection, leukocytes are produced at a higher rate and are much more abundant, so white blood cell counts can be useful tools for determining the presence of infection.

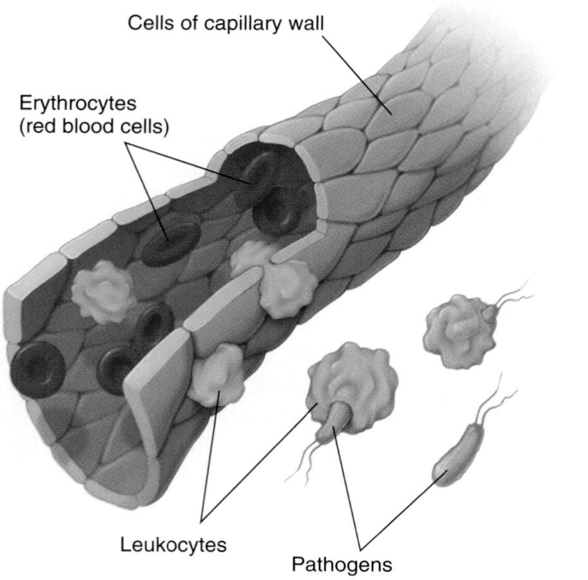

Platelets

Platelets, also called thrombocytes, are nonnucleated cell fragments that are half the size of red blood cells (Fig. 4-57). Formed in the red bone marrow from large cells that burst, there are 150,000 to 400,000 platelets in a tiny drop of blood. Their main function is to aid in blood clotting, also known as hemostasis, and they can respond within 15 seconds to 2 minutes of the injury.

THE HEART

The heart is the main structure of the cardiovascular system. It is about the size of a fist and is located between the lungs in the middle of the thoracic cavity. The heart has four separate chambers separated by muscle walls and valves. The two upper chambers are called atria (AY-tree-uh) and are encased by thin walls of cardiac muscle. The left and right atria are receiving chambers for incoming blood and are not directly involved in the pumping action. The two ventricles have thicker walls and are located below the atria. The ventricles are the discharging chambers re-

FIGURE 4-58   Leukocytes passing through membrane wall.

sponsible for pumping blood from the heart to deliver it to the rest of the body (Fig. 4-59).

The myocardium, or cardiac muscle tissue, varies in thickness and is arranged in spiral bundles that wrap around the heart chambers. The spiral bundles contract with a wringing action that squeezes blood out of the chambers. Cardiac muscle tissue contracts spontaneously and independently and, unlike skeletal muscle, can contract even if all the nerve connections are severed. Cardiac muscle fibers contain electrical impulses that exchange charges back and forth to create a rhythmic contraction. These rhythmic contractions allow the heart to push approximately 6000 quarts of blood through the body each day. The ANS controls the heart rate, which varies depending on the demands of the body for oxygen. The heart rate accelerates when the sympathetic nervous system is in control, and it decelerates under the parasympathetic response.

The valves in the heart are one-way gates that allow blood to flow in only one direction. Atrioventricular valves (AV valves) sit between the atrium and ventricle and are forced shut when the ventricle contracts, to prevent blood from leaking into the atria. The semilunar valves are located at the exits of the ventricles. When the ventricle contracts, the semilunar valves are forced open and allow blood to only flow out of the heart. When the ventricle relaxes, the semilunar valves prevent the blood from leaking back into the ventricles.

Blood follows a specific path through the heart:

1. Deoxygenated blood collects in the right atrium.
2. The right atrium contracts to push the blood through an AV valve into the right ventricle.
3. The ventricle, full of deoxygenated blood, contracts to push the blood through a semilunar valve into the pulmonary artery in the lungs.
4. The blood is oxygenated in the lungs and goes out through the pulmonary veins into the left atrium.

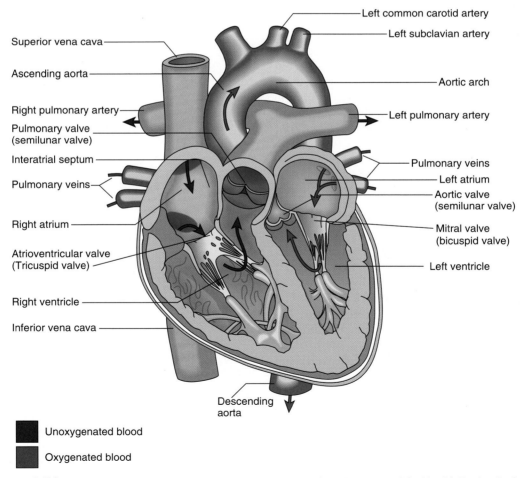

FIGURE 4-59   Heart and its chambers. (Reprinted with permission from Brunner and Suddarth's Textbook of Medical-Surgical Nursing. 9th ed. Baltimore: Lippincott Williams & Wilkins, 2000, p 533, fig 23-1.)

5. The left atrium contracts and forces blood through an AV valve into the left ventricle.

6. The left ventricle contracts and forces blood through a semilunar valve into the aorta, where it enters the arterial system and is delivered to the body.

BLOOD VESSELS

The blood vessels transport blood from the heart to the rest of the body. The arteries, veins, and capillaries are collectively called the blood vessels. The largest blood vessel is the aorta (ay-OR-tuh), which measures about an inch across where it leaves the heart to provide blood to the entire body. The smallest blood vessels are the capillaries, which are less than a tenth of a millimeter in diameter. Their small size limits the passage of molecules to a single file.

Arteries

The **arteries** are tubes that carry blood away from the heart. The strong mechanical pumping force of the heart pushes the blood through the aorta and into its branches called arteries. As an artery travels further from the heart, it branches out, becoming smaller and thinner with distance. Arterioles are small arteries that are far from the heart, delivering the oxygenated blood to the capillaries. Figure 4-60 shows the arteries of the body. Gravity also helps the arteries move blood to different parts of the body. "Artery" is derived from the Greek word *arteria*, meaning air pipe. Originally, when they were discovered in corpses, the arteries were empty and assumed to transport air. Although it has since been determined that they carry blood, the name has not changed.

Arteries are constructed with three layers of tissues (Fig. 4-61). The interior layer, called the tunica intima, or endothelium, is a layer of simple squamous epithelium that is very smooth and slippery. The middle layer, called the tunica media, is a layer of smooth muscle and elastic connective tissue. The smooth muscles work to hold the arteries taut between heart contractions. In other words, the smooth muscles help maintain blood pressure. The outer layer of arteries is made of fibrous connective tissue called the tunica externa. It protects the arteries from damage and keeps the larger arteries from bursting as a result of the high blood pressure exerted by the force of the heart contraction.

Veins

Veins transport blood from the capillaries of the body back to the heart (Fig. 4-62). The smallest veins, called

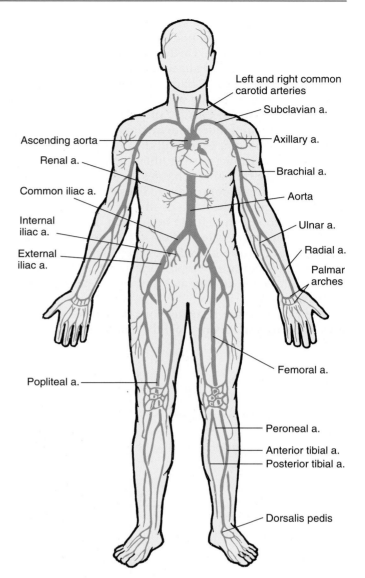

Figure 4-60   Arterial system. (Reprinted with permission from Stedman's Medical Dictionary, 27th ed. Baltimore: Lippincott Williams & Wilkins, 2000, p 145.)

venules, receive the blood from the capillaries immediately after the blood has delivered its oxygen to the tissues and immediately after the blood has picked up oxygen in the lungs. The largest veins are the superior vena cava and inferior vena cava, which are the last collection point of deoxygenated blood before it goes into the heart. Much of the blood is moving against gravity, without a strong heart to pump it.

To compensate for the disadvantages and prevent blood from going the wrong direction, venous blood flow is aided by valves and skeletal muscle contractions. The valves are one-way gates that allow blood to flow in one direction only, similar to doors that only open outward. There are more valves in areas

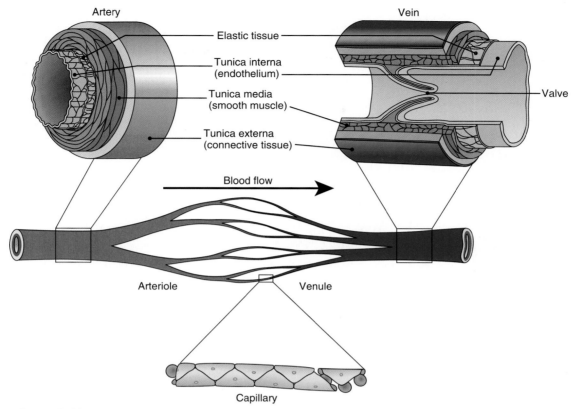

FIGURE 4-61 Comparison of arterial, venous, and capillary walls. (Reprinted from Cohen BJ, Wood DL. Memmler's Structure and Function of the Human Body. 9th ed. Philadelphia: Lippincott Williams & Wilkins, 2000.)

where blood typically must fight gravity to return to the heart, such as the legs. As the skeletal muscles contract, they squeeze the veins, and blood can only flow toward the heart. Figure 4-63 shows how the skeletal muscles work with the valves to encourage venous blood flow.

Veins are constructed with the same three layers as the arteries and are similar in size to the arteries but have thinner walls (see Fig. 4-61). The tunica media, or smooth muscle layer, is thinner because veins do not regulate blood pressure. The tunica externa is thinner because blood pressure is much lower in the veins, and they are not in danger of bursting.

Capillaries

Capillaries are the smallest, finest branches of the blood vessels where gases and fluids are exchanged. The capillary walls are composed of only one layer of cells (Fig. 4-61). All transfers between blood and tissue cells occur at the capillary membranes via diffusion, osmosis, or filtration. Diffusion is a passive transport mechanism that allows molecules to pass through semipermeable membranes without assis-

tance. Respiratory gases diffuse through the capillary walls and tissue cells. Osmosis allows water molecules, which are not fat soluble and cannot diffuse through the lipid bilayer, to use channel proteins to move through a membrane to balance concentrations on either side. Osmosis carries fluid from the interstitial spaces through the membrane and into the blood in the capillaries, where the concentration of solutes is higher. Filtration is the passive transport mechanism that takes water and dissolved substances through a membrane in an effort to balance concentrations on either side of the membrane. Filtration occurs in the kidneys (discussed later in this chapter).

BLOOD CIRCUITS

The blood vessels can be separated into two separate pathways, called the pulmonary and systemic circuits. The pulmonary circuit takes blood to the lungs for gas exchange and returns it to the heart. The systemic circuit transports blood through the rest of the body.

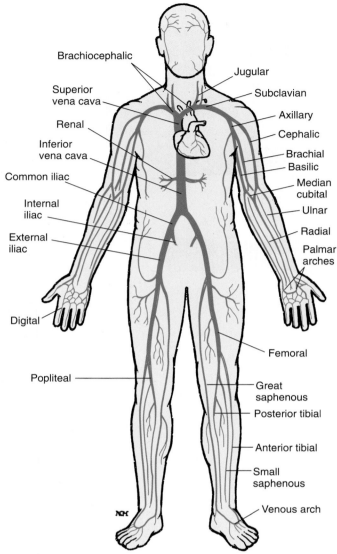

FIGURE 4-62 Venous system. (Reprinted with permission from Stedman's Medical Dictionary, 27th ed. Baltimore: Lippincott Williams & Wilkins, 2000, p 1936.)

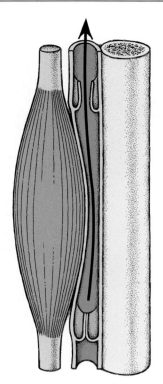

FIGURE 4-63 Skeletal muscle "pump" for venous blood flow. Skeletal muscle contraction squeezes the veins and their valves, causing venous blood to be forced through the one-way valves. (Image from Neil O. Hardy, Westpoint, CT.)

at the capillaries diffuses out, into the tissues. Carbon dioxide diffuses from the tissues into the blood in the capillaries. The deoxygenated blood is then returned to the heart through the systemic veins.

Functions of the Lymphatic System

The lymphatic system is a component of the circulatory system that has drainage, transportation, and immune functions. The system consists of lymphatic fluid, lymphatic vessels, lymph nodes, spleen, tonsils, and the thymus gland.

DRAINAGE

Interstitial fluid contains chemicals and metabolic wastes that have been transported out of the cells. The interstitial fluid can either diffuse back through the capillary walls into the blood or it can be drained via the lymphatic system. This mechanism is important for maintaining blood volume and blood pressure.

Pulmonary Circuit

The pulmonary arteries carry deoxygenated blood from the right ventricle to the lungs. There, carbon dioxide diffuses out of the blood and into the lungs, where it is exhaled into the external environment. Oxygen in the air we inhale diffuses from the lungs into the blood, and the pulmonary veins carry the oxygenated blood to the left atrium of the heart.

Systemic Circuit

The systemic arteries carry oxygenated blood to the capillaries throughout the body. Oxygen in the blood

TRANSPORTATION

The interstitial fluids that are drained by the lymphatic system carry substances that must be transported via the bloodstream. Fatty acids and vitamin A are end products of digestion found in the small intestine that are absorbed into the lymphatic system and eventually added to the bloodstream to nourish cells throughout the body.

IMMUNITY

The lymphatic system helps us fight bacteria and other foreign substances. Leukocytes, or white blood cells, which are critical to immunity are made in the lymphatic tissue. The fluid that is drained from the interstitial spaces by the lymphatic system carries the leukocytes known as lymphocytes and monocytes. As the fluid is transported to the heart to be added to the blood, it is filtered in lymph nodes where antibodies and macrophages destroy or inactivate pathogens that cause illness.

Structures of the Lymphatic System

The lymphatic system includes the lymph, lymph vessels, lymph nodes, spleen, tonsils, and thymus gland.

LYMPH

Lymphatic fluid, or lymph, is the fluid that travels through the lymphatic system. Remember that in the capillaries, blood plasma seeps through the capillaries to fill the interstitial space, or the space between cells. There, it acquires cellular debris and foreign substances that are eliminated by the surrounding cells. The interstitial fluid that is drained into the lymphatic system is the basic component of lymph. The additional components include the lymphocytes, monocytes, proteins, and cellular waste.

LYMPH VESSELS

The interstitial fluids are first collected by the lymph capillaries throughout the body. The lymph capillaries join to form larger lymphatic vessels that carry the lymph back to the heart. The lymph from the upper right quadrant of the body exits the lymphatic system at the right lymphatic duct, which drains into the right subclavian vein. The lymph from the rest of the body drains out of the lymphatic system through the thoracic duct and into the left subclavian vein. The subclavian veins join together and empty lymph and deoxygenated blood into the heart (Fig. 4-64 illustrates the lymph vessels).

Lymph vessels have the same basic structure as veins but are more delicate and smaller. Being a one-way system without a mechanical pump behind it, the lymphatic system puts little pressure on the walls of the vessels, so the layers of muscle and fibrous connective tissue covering are thin. Like venous blood, lymph does not have a pump behind it to force it through the lymph vessels, and much of the lymph travels against gravity. Skeletal muscle movements encourage lymph through the lymph vessels and valves, similar to the mechanism that encourages venous flow (Fig. 4-63). The flow of lymph through the vessels is also aided by the contraction of the diaphragm muscle during inspiration, which creates a vacuumlike suction that pulls blood and lymphatic fluid upward and toward the heart.

LYMPH NODES

Lymph nodes are oval, bean-shaped structures that produce lymphocytes and filter the lymphatic fluid. Thousands of lymph nodes can be found in groups along the lymph vessels, and large concentrations of lymph nodes are found in the cervical, inguinal, and axillary regions (Fig. 4-64). Lymph nodes contain lots of macrophages and lymphocytes and have a structural framework of reticular connective tissue that creates a meshwork for filtering lymph. Pathogens and toxins in the lymph are destroyed or inactivated and filtered out with a series of fibrous traps. The clean lymphatic fluid flows out of the node and continues on its path toward the heart.

SPLEEN, TONSILS, AND THYMUS GLAND

The largest lymph organ is the spleen, which is approximately the size of the heart. The spleen produces lymphocytes, filters the blood, and removes old, worn-out erythrocytes from the blood. In the process of removing erythrocytes, iron is extracted for future use. The spleen also functions as a storage container for extra blood, releasing it when necessary. It acts as a conference center for immune cells and blood cells, providing a meeting place and activity center for them. Macrophages bring antigenic cells, cells with chemical antigens on their surface

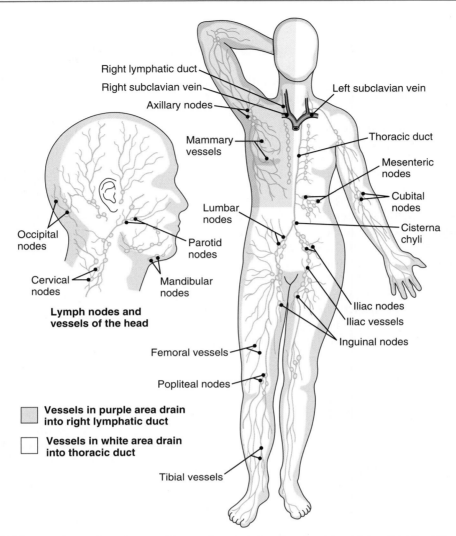

Right lymphatic duct
Right subclavian vein
Axillary nodes
Mammary vessels
Left subclavian vein
Thoracic duct
Mesenteric nodes
Cubital nodes
Lumbar nodes
Cisterna chyli
Occipital nodes
Parotid nodes
Cervical nodes
Mandibular nodes
Iliac nodes
Iliac vessels
Inguinal nodes

Lymph nodes and vessels of the head

Femoral vessels
Popliteal nodes

Vessels in purple area drain into right lymphatic duct

Vessels in white area drain into thoracic duct

Tibial vessels

FIGURE 4-64   Lymph vessels and areas with many lymph nodes. (Reprinted from Cohen BJ, Wood DL. Memmler's Structure and Function of the Human Body. 9th ed. Philadelphia: Lippincott Williams & Wilkins, 2000.)

that stimulate the immune response, to the spleen to be destroyed. Bacteria, pollen, and viruses have antigens on their surfaces that activate the immune response. To destroy antigenic cells, the spleen can activate the production of antibodies, proteins that recognize and bond to specific antigens. The antigen is rendered inactive once an antibody bonds to it. The process of inactivating foreign substances is called the immune response.

Tonsils are small masses of lymph tissue on either side of the soft palate at the back of the throat. These areas of moist epithelium are in contact with the external environment, so the tonsils help prevent bacteria and other pathogens from entering the throat. They differ from other lymphoid organs because they do not filter the lymph.

The thymus gland in children is located deep to the sternum, but as we age, the thymus gland shrinks and only a small amount of tissue remains in adults, superior to the heart. It is the site where some lymphocytes mature.

Respiratory System

The respiratory system allows us to breathe, which is an activity controlled by the CNS. Awake or asleep, breathing continues as long as we are alive. The nervous system controls contractions of the diaphragm muscle, which pulls air into the respiratory system. In the lungs, oxygen diffuses from the air we breathe into the blood in the capillaries, and the circulatory system delivers the oxygen throughout the body.

Functions of the Respiratory System

The respiratory system moves air in and out of the lungs, which is also known as ventilation. In addition to ventilation, the respiratory system cooperates with the circulatory system to perform respiration, which provides oxygen to the body and removes carbon dioxide. The respiratory system also allows us to maintain the proper pH level for interstitial fluids and produce speech, and it provides body defenses by coughing and sneezing unwanted particles out of the airway.

VENTILATION

Ventilation moves air in and out of the lungs, and respiration takes the carbon dioxide out of the body and brings oxygen in. The gas exchange must occur in both directions to maintain homeostasis.

Inhalation

Inhalation, also known as inspiration, draws air into the lungs. It occurs as the diaphragm and external intercostals muscles contract. The floor of the thoracic cavity is pulled downward as a result of the diaphragm contraction, and the walls of the thoracic cavity are widened by the contraction of the external intercostals. The parietal pleural membranes are attached to the walls of the thoracic cavity and expand along with it, pulling air from the external environment into the respiratory pathway.

Exhalation

The ventilation process that moves air out of the lungs is called exhalation, or expiration. Normal exhalation is a passive process that mostly results from the relaxation of the diaphragm and external intercostals. Some activities require additional, forced exhalation, such as speaking, singing, or blowing. The internal intercostal muscles can be contracted to reduce the size of the thoracic cavity, and the abdominal muscles can be contracted to push the floor of the thoracic cavity upward.

Respiration

The exchange of oxygen and carbon dioxide that occurs in the respiratory system is called external respiration because the gas exchange occurs between our tissues and the external environment. As discussed above, internal respiration, or cellular respiration, occurs within the cells and tissues. Inhalation and exhalation are equally important for maintaining proper chemical levels in the blood. The respiratory and circulatory systems cooperate to provide a transport mechanism for the blood gas exchange.

The nervous system and chemical signals can trigger increased ventilation to provide more gas exchange via external respiration. The brain and motor nerves control the muscles that set the rate and depth of respiration. If you think about how you breathe when we cry, laugh, or exercise, you will see how emotions and physical activity affect our breathing patterns. Emotions are associated with chemicals produced in the brain, and those chemicals can stimulate or alter respiration.

The proprioceptors of the nervous system play an important part in respiratory activity. Muscle spindles sense tension in the muscle fibers. Low levels of oxygen can cause the respiratory muscles to contract insufficiently, which can be detected by the muscle spindles. To maintain homeostasis, the CNS will increase ventilation to increase external respiration.

MAINTAINING PH BALANCE

The proportion of oxygen to carbon dioxide in the blood affects the pH. Too much carbon dioxide lowers the pH and makes blood more acidic than normal. Acidic fluids can destroy the cellular membrane and are harmful to the health of the cells and tissues. When the pH is too low, the body will try to raise the pH by raising oxygen levels in the tissues. The heart rate can increase, to speed up the delivery of oxygenated red blood cells, and ventilation can increase, to expose the lungs to more oxygen. When the pH is too high and the fluids are too basic, the body can respond by reducing respiratory activity to build up carbon dioxide and acidify the fluids. The cooperation between the respiratory and circulatory systems is an obvious example of how interdependent the body systems are from the cellular level all the way up to the organism level.

PRODUCE SPEECH

The larynx (LAIR-inks), or voice box, is part of the respiratory system where sounds can be created. Specifically, the vocal cords vibrate as air passes over them, creating sound. By combining movement of the tongue, lips, and cheeks and the speed of exhalation, we can control our voices to create precise sounds.

BODY DEFENSES

There are some reflexive activities of the respiratory system that protect us from irritating objects in the airway. Irritation of the mucous membrane at the back of the throat or farther down the respiratory pathway can cause a cough, our body's attempt to eliminate unwanted material through the mouth. When the mucous membrane of the nasal passages is irritated, our body sneezes reflexively in an attempt to expel unwanted material through the nose.

Structures of the Respiratory System

The structures of the respiratory system include the nose, nasal cavity, pharynx (FAIR-inks), larynx, trachea (TRAY-kee-ah), bronchi (BRAHN-kahy), bronchioles, alveoli (al-VEE-oh-lahy), and lungs (Fig. 4-65). These structures can be separated into two groups, the upper and lower respiratory tracts.

UPPER RESPIRATORY TRACT

The upper respiratory tract includes the nose, nasal cavity, pharynx, larynx, and the upper part of the trachea. Cartilage, mucus, and ciliated cells are present in all of the structures of the upper respiratory tract. Cartilage maintains the shape of the structures to prevent the airway from collapsing and stopping air flow. The mucus traps foreign particles that are then swept toward the external environment by ciliated cells. The lungs are a good breeding ground for infection because they are moist and warm, so it is very important to have the cells that secrete mucus and the ciliated cells functioning properly.

Nose and Nasal Cavity

The first part of the respiratory tract to receive air from the external environment is the nose and the nasal cavity. The cartilage in the nose holds it open to allow air to enter easily. There, the mucous secretions moisten the air to keep the lungs from drying out. The capillaries lying just beneath the surface of the epithelium warm the air, again for the benefit of the delicate tissues of the lungs. There are olfactory cells within the nasal cavity that are the sensory receptors for smell.

Pharynx

As the incoming air leaves the nasal cavity, the air is received by the pharynx. The pharynx acts as a passageway for both the respiratory and digestive systems. Eustachian tubes connect the upper part of the pharynx to the middle ear, equalizing air pressure on either side of the ear's tympanic membrane. The tonsils, also called adenoids, are made of lymphatic tis-

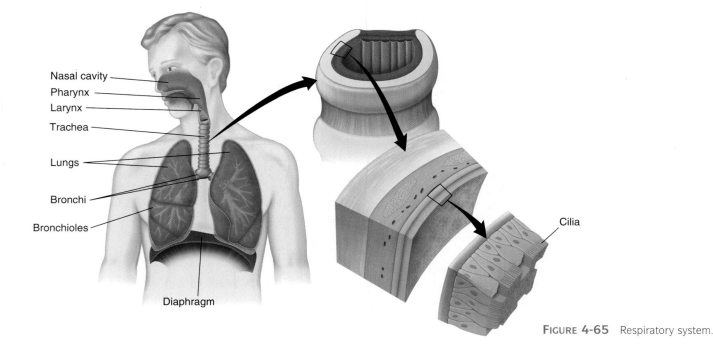

Nasal cavity
Pharynx
Larynx
Trachea
Lungs
Bronchi
Bronchioles
Diaphragm
Cilia

FIGURE 4-65 Respiratory system.

sue in the pharynx and are discussed in the circulatory system section above. If the lymphatic activity is high enough, the tonsils can enlarge, and the air passage can actually be obstructed.

Larynx

The larynx, or voice box, is made of cartilage and lies just inferior to the pharynx. The thyroid cartilage, commonly referred to as the Adam's apple, is part of the larynx. The epiglottis is a little structure in the larynx that prevents food from going down the airway. The vocal cords are connected to the larynx's cartilage, and as air moves by them, they vibrate and create sound.

Upper Trachea

The trachea is a tubelike structure that connects the larynx to the bronchi in the lungs. The trachea has cilia that sweep foreign particles caught in mucus up toward the external environment. These unwanted particles are coughed out, spat out, or swallowed.

LOWER RESPIRATORY TRACT

The structures of the lower respiratory tract include the lower part of the trachea, the bronchi, bronchioles, alveoli, and lungs.

Lower Trachea

At the inferior end of the trachea, the airway splits into two separate paths. Rings of hyaline cartilage hold the trachea open, and mucus and cilia cooperate to remove foreign matter from the respiratory path.

Bronchi

The left and right branches of the airway following the trachea are called the bronchi. The bronchi enter the lungs and each of the bronchi branches into finer and finer airways. Bronchioles are the smallest airways inside the lungs, and they do not contain any cartilage. Their walls are mostly made of smooth muscles that are controlled by the ANS. Although the air that reaches the bronchi is usually warm, moist, and particle-free, mucus and cilia are still present to sweep foreign particles out to the environment.

Alveoli

At the ends of the tiny bronchioles, air enters the pulmonary alveoli, which resemble clusters of grapes. They have thin walls of simple squamous epithelium that allow gases to be exchanged with the blood in the capillaries that wrap around them. Diffusion allows oxygen to move into the capillaries and carbon dioxide to move into the alveoli (Fig. 4-66). Surfac-

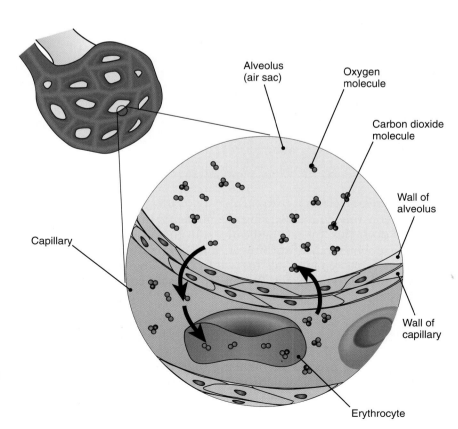

FIGURE 4-66 Alveoli and gas exchange. (Reprinted from Cohen BJ, Wood DL. Memmler's Structure and Function of the Human Body. 9th ed. Philadelphia: Lippincott Williams & Wilkins, 2000.)

tants are secreted by cells in the alveoli to reduce surface tension and allow the alveoli to expand without stress.

Lungs

The left and right lungs are separated by the section of the thoracic cavity that holds the heart and large blood vessels and is called the mediastinum (MEE-dee-ah-STAHY-num). The tops of the lungs are just inferior to the clavicles, and the bottoms of the lungs rest on the diaphragm. The lungs are enveloped in a serous membrane called the visceral pleura, and the thoracic cavity is lined with a serous membrane called the parietal pleura. The serous fluid that these membranes secrete provides lubrication to prevent friction between the two membranes and also helps keep the separate layers of membranes together. The concept is similar to how water between two layers of plastic wrap keeps the layers close together while allowing them to slip past each other easily.

Digestive System

The digestive system is the pathway for food from the moment it enters the mouth until it is eliminated at the anus. The nervous system sends motor signals to the structures of the digestive system to take the food we eat and transform it into a substance that can release the nutrients. The capillaries absorb the nutrients and deliver them throughout the body by way of the blood. The organ systems must work together for our bodies to function normally.

Functions of the Digestive System

Our digestive system is responsible for taking the food we consume and delivering the nutrients to the body. It does this by mechanically and chemically breaking down food, absorbing it, and eliminating the indigestible remains, all the while propelling it through the digestive tract by smooth muscle contractions called peristalsis.

DIGESTION

Digestion is the process of breaking food down by mechanical and chemical activity. When food enters the mouth, we chew it up and mechanically grind the food into smaller pieces. Saliva, secreted by three pairs of salivary glands and delivered to the oral cav-

ity through ducts, contains a digestive enzyme that can chemically break down some foods. The stomach contains acids and enzymes to chemically break down food particles even more.

Several muscles are involved in the process of digestion. The process of chewing requires muscles to move the mandible, or lower jaw. The muscles of the tongue push food around the mouth to be chewed completely. Both skeletal and smooth muscles create peristalsis.

ABSORPTION

Food that has been completely broken down into a substance called chyme (KAHYM) can release the nutrients. The nutrients are absorbed into the blood and lymph in the intestines. From there, the nutrients can be delivered throughout the body via the circulatory vessels.

ELIMINATION

Since we cannot digest every component of food we eat, such as cellulose from plants, the digestive system eliminates the parts we cannot digest. The indigestible material, along with water and bacteria in the digestive tract, is called fecal matter. The fecal matter is propelled through the digestive tract and eliminated through the anus to the external environment, at which point it is called feces.

PERISTALSIS

The smooth muscles of the digestive tract, as discussed in the muscular system section, are layered structures capable of long, sustained contractions. The rhythmic contractions of the layers propel the contents of the digestive system through the digestive tract from oral cavity to anus.

Structures of the Digestive System

The digestive system can be broken into two sets of structures: the alimentary canal and the accessory organs. The alimentary (AL-ih-MEN-tah-ree) canal is the passageway that includes the oral cavity, pharynx, esophagus, stomach, small intestine, and large intestine. The accessory digestive organs include the pancreas, liver, gallbladder, and salivary glands that produce chemicals necessary for digestion. Figure 4-67 shows the structures of the alimentary canal and the accessory digestive organs.

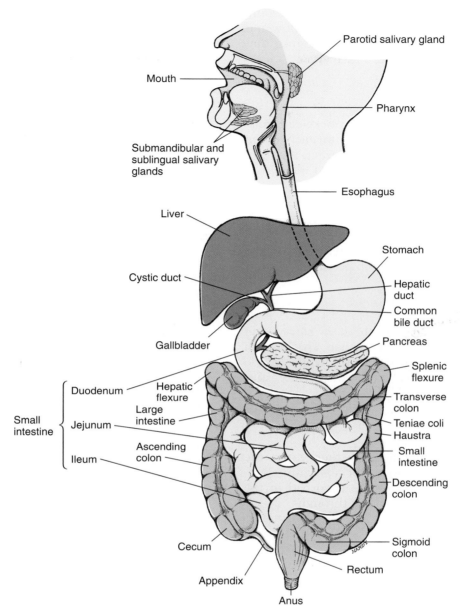

FIGURE 4-67 Structures of the digestive system. (Reprinted with permission from Stedman's Medical Dictionary, 27th ed. Baltimore: Lippincott Williams & Wilkins, 2000, p 500.)

THE ALIMENTARY CANAL

The alimentary canal, or digestive tract, is where food is broken down and eventually absorbed. It includes the oral cavity, pharynx, esophagus, stomach, small intestine, and large intestine. The canal is constructed of four layers, including the mucous membrane, submucosa, external muscle layer, and serous membrane. The deepest layer is the mucous membrane. It secretes mucus to lubricate the passage of food through the canal and secretes digestive enzymes to encourage the breakdown of food. Just outside the mucous membrane is the submucosa, which is a layer of connective tissue filled with blood vessels

and lymph vessels. The external muscle layer is made of smooth muscle for most of the length of the canal, but the esophagus contains skeletal muscle. The outermost layer of the alimentary canal is fibrous connective tissue above the diaphragm, but below the diaphragm, the outer layer is a serous membrane called the visceral peritoneum.

Oral Cavity

The oral cavity contains the teeth and tongue, which begin the process of digestion. Teeth grind food into smaller pieces while the tongue circulates the food to make sure everything gets evenly chewed. The salivary glands are located below the tongue, above and behind the temporomandibular joint, and below and behind the joint. The saliva contains enzymes that chemically break down food even further.

Pharynx

The pharynx has overlapping layers of skeletal muscle whose fibers run perpendicular to each other. When these muscles rhythmically contract, they create peristalsis, wavelike contractions that move substances through a tube.

Esophagus

The esophagus is a tube that runs from the pharynx to the stomach, moving the food with peristaltic action.

Stomach

Once food reaches the stomach, it is stored and chemically broken down even further. The smooth muscles churn the food mechanically while gastric juice continues the chemical breakdown. The resulting chyme exits the stomach.

Small Intestine

The chyme formed in the stomach then enters the small intestine, the major organ for absorption. Nutrients, water, and electrolytes are absorbed in the small intestine as the chyme passes through.

Large Intestine

The chyme leaves the small intestine and enters the large intestine, where more water and minerals are absorbed. Bacteria in the large intestine feed on fecal material and release gas as a byproduct. The remaining fiber and other indigestible wastes are eliminated at the exit of the large intestine, the anus.

ACCESSORY DIGESTIVE ORGANS

The accessory organs of the digestive system include the pancreas, liver, gallbladder, and salivary glands. They secrete enzymes and hormones that are required for digestion. The pancreas also produces the hormones insulin and glucagon, which are critical for the regulation of blood sugar levels. The liver makes bile, which breaks fats into smaller pieces that are more easily digested, and it detoxifies and excretes wastes and toxins. Fats and glycogen for energy are stored in the liver, as are many vitamins, and

iron for hemoglobin formation. The gallbladder is a small organ just below the liver that acts as a sort of holding tank for bile that is not being used. When the body must process large amounts of fat, the gallbladder releases bile to emulsify it. The salivary glands, located anterior to the ears (parotid gland), under the tongue (sublingual gland), and just under the lower jaw (submandibular gland), all produce saliva, which chemically breaks down starches, inhibits bacterial growth, and eases the processes of chewing and swallowing.

Urinary System

The urinary system is primarily responsible for forming and excreting urine; however, in doing so, it also performs many regulatory functions. There are nitrogen-based wastes produced during cellular metabolism that are only eliminated with the passive transport mechanism of filtration. The CP mechanism for creating ATP in muscles generates some of the wastes that are removed by the kidneys, demonstrating the interdependence of the muscular system, circulatory system, and urinary system.

Functions of the Urinary System

The structures of the urinary system accomplish several tasks. They filter the blood to remove chemical wastes and excrete the wastes in the form of urine. The system regulates the volume of blood, pH of body fluids, and red blood cell formation in red bone marrow.

URINE FORMATION

The urinary system goes through a series of steps to eliminate chemical wastes in the form of urine. First, the passive transport mechanism of filtration occurs in the capillaries that serve the kidneys. The blood traveling through the kidneys is under a high pressure that forces water and dissolved substances through the capillary walls. Second, the filtrate, or the solution that comes through the membrane, undergoes reabsorption. All of the dissolved material is not waste, so the body reabsorbs the substances that are useful, such as amino acids to build proteins, ions to use in cellular functions, glucose to use for creating ATP, and water to keep cells and tissues hydrated. Most of the substances must be actively transported out of the kidney and back into the blood capillaries, but water passes through via osmosis. The third step of urine formation removes some additional ions and creatinine from the capillaries as a secretion of the kidney.

EXCRETION

Once the urine has been produced, it is excreted from the body by the other structures of the urinary system. The urine travels from the kidneys through a pair of tubes called the ureters (YOO-rih-terz) to the urinary bladder. Urine is stored in the bladder temporarily, and is carried to the external environment through a tube called the urethra (yoo-REETH-rah).

REGULATION

In the process of making urine, the complex structure and functions of the kidney also regulate blood volume, chemical content of blood, pH of body fluids, and red blood cell formation.

Blood Volume

The reabsorption activity of the kidney moves water from the kidney back into the blood capillaries via osmosis. The amount of water reabsorbed in the kidneys is a homeostatic mechanism that keeps the blood volume stable after water is lost through the skin as perspiration, out the lungs as water vapor, or out the digestive tract in the feces.

Chemical Balance

Once the blood has been filtered in the kidneys, the filtrate contains ions and other molecules that are necessary for cellular metabolism. Reabsorption of molecules is another homeostatic mechanism for regulating chemical balance in the blood and body fluids.

pH Balance

As mentioned in the respiratory system section, the pH of blood is normally kept at 7.4. The body constantly creates byproducts of cellular metabolism that affect pH levels, but homeostatic mechanisms maintain a stable pH in body fluids. The kidneys are the primary structures for regulating pH, although respiratory activity can also change pH levels. The kidneys can excrete bicarbonate ions to lower pH, and they can reabsorb bicarbonate ions to raise pH.

Red Blood Cell Formation

The kidneys are the primary structures that secrete erythropoietin, a hormone that stimulates red blood cell formation in the red marrow of bones. A small amount is present in the blood all the time, but when oxygen levels in blood are low, the kidneys secrete extra erythropoietin to increase the production of red blood cells.

Structures of the Urinary System

The urinary system includes the kidneys, ureters, urinary bladder, and urethra (Fig. 4-68).

KIDNEYS

Our two kidneys are located against the posterior wall of the abdominal cavity, on either side of the spine, at the level of the superior lumbar vertebrae. Each kidney is the shape of a kidney bean and measures about 5 inches long, 2½ inches wide, and 1 inch thick. These organs are suspended in the abdominal cavity by a fatty mass called the adipose capsule and are not well protected by bones, which is why they are such vulnerable organs. Losing weight too rapidly can reduce the size of the adipose capsule and change the position of the kidneys. If they shift inferiorly, the ureters can develop kinks, and eventually, if the urine cannot flow down to the urinary bladder, the urine can back up and damage the kidneys.

The functional part of the kidney is called the nephron, of which there are over a million in each kidney. They filter the blood, reabsorb water, secrete ions and creatinine that were originally removed from the blood, and maintain the high fluid pressure necessary for filtration. Adequate amounts of water must be consumed for the urinary system to function properly.

URETERS

The ureters are tubes about a foot long and ¼ inch in diameter that carry urine away from the kidneys. They have an inner lining of mucous membrane, but their outer walls are made of overlapping layers of smooth muscle. Gravity and the peristaltic contractions of the ureters propel urine through the ureters toward the urinary bladder.

URINARY BLADDER

The urinary bladder is a storage site for urine, located just behind the pubic symphysis. It is made of three layers of smooth muscle and has a mucous

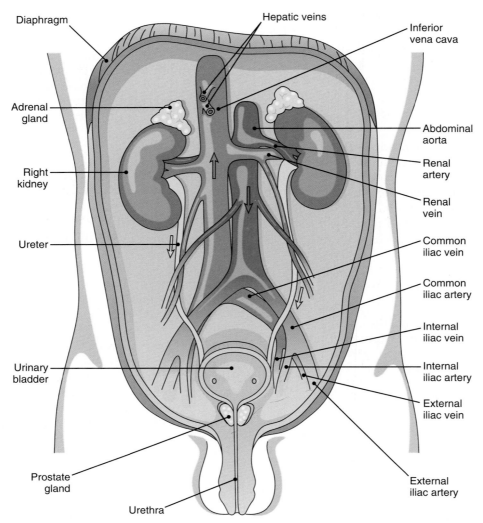

FIGURE 4-68 Structures of the urinary system. (Reprinted from Cohen BJ, Wood DL. Memmler's Structure and Function of the Human Body. 9th ed. Philadelphia: Lippincott Williams & Wilkins, 2000.)

membrane lining of transitional epithelium. It can expand from its normal size of about 2 inches long to a distended size of about 5 inches long when full of urine.

URETHRA

From the urinary bladder, the urethra carries urine to the exterior of the body for elimination, called excretion. An involuntary smooth muscle sphincter at the exit of the urinary bladder closes the urethra when urine is being stored. There is also a voluntary skeletal muscle sphincter farther down the urethra that we control. When we contract the skeletal muscle sphincter, urine flow is stopped, and when we relax the sphincter, urine is excreted through the urethra to the external environment.

Endocrine System

The endocrine system is a regulating control system of the body. It is made up of several ductless glands and some organs that are involved in other systems. Endocrine system hormones are secreted directly into the blood or lymph and circulate through the body. The hormones have specific effects on their target tissues to keep metabolic and developmental processes of the body functioning normally. They work both antagonistically and cooperatively to maintain homeostasis.

Functions of the Endocrine System

The endocrine system produces hormones that increase or decrease cellular activities. They regulate growth, metabolism, reproduction, and behavior. Some hormones have several target tissues, and others only have one kind of target tissue.

Structures of the Endocrine System

The major endocrine structures are the pituitary (pih-TOO-ih-tair-ee), thyroid (THAHY-royd), parathyroid, adrenal (a-DREE-nul), pineal (PAHY-nee-ahl), and thymus glands, as well as parts of the hypothalamus, pancreas, ovaries, testes, and placenta (Fig. 4-69).

PITUITARY GLAND

The pituitary gland is often called the master gland of the body (Fig. 4-70). Located at the base of the brain, it secretes six different hormones that stimulate other glands and organs to act. In addition to its six secre-

tions, it stores and releases the two hormones secreted by the hypothalamus:

- Growth hormone (GH) primarily stimulates muscles and long bones to grow.
- Prolactin (PRL) is similar to GH, but only activates milk production in the breasts.
- Thyroid-stimulating hormone (TSH) regulates the thyroid gland.
- Adrenocorticotropic hormone (ACTH) regulates the adrenal gland.
- Follicle-stimulating hormone (FSH) promotes the maturation of eggs and development of sperm production.
- Luteinizing hormone (LH) signals the ovary to release an egg or the testes to produce testosterone.
- Oxytocin, secreted by the hypothalamus stimulates contractions of the uterus and the milk "letdown" reflex of new mothers.
- Antidiuretic hormone (ADH), secreted by the hypothalamus, promotes water retention in the kidneys.

THYROID GLAND

The thyroid gland is slightly larger than the other glands and is located in the anterior neck area in two lobes on either side of the trachea. Its hormones, in-

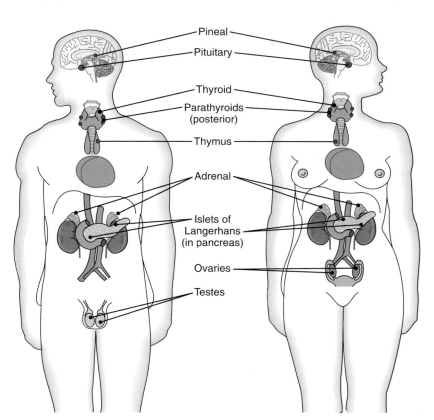

FIGURE 4-69 Structures of the endocrine system. (Reprinted from Cohen BJ, Wood DL. *Memmler's Structure and Function of the Human Body.* 9th ed. Philadelphia: Lippincott Williams & Wilkins, 2000.)

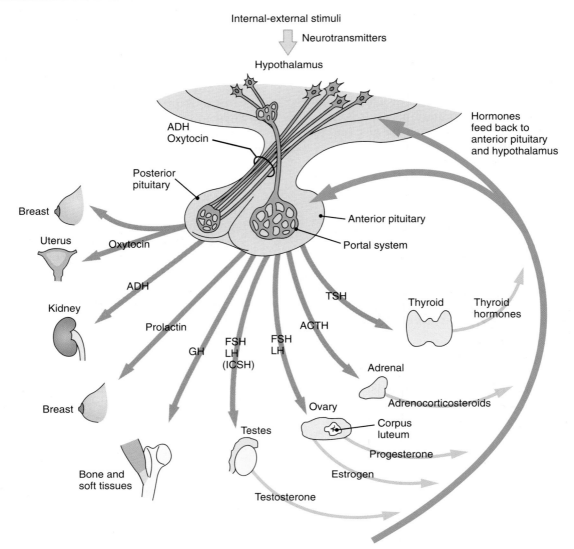

FIGURE 4-70 Pituitary gland activity. (Reprinted from Cohen BJ, Wood DL. Memmler's Structure and Function of the Human Body. 9th ed. Philadelphia: Lippincott Williams & Wilkins, 2000.)

cluding thyroxin, triiodothyronine, and calcitonin, regulate metabolism and reduce blood calcium levels by triggering calcium from the blood to be deposited in the bones. The thyroid requires iodine to produce its hormones; without enough dietary iodine, the thyroid overworks and become enlarged, creating a goiter. Since iodine was added to table salt, goiters are fairly rare.

PARATHYROID GLAND

The parathyroid gland sits just posterior to the thyroid and is about the size of a pea. Its hormone, aptly called parathyroid hormone, increases calcium levels in the blood. It does so by triggering the bones to release calcium into the blood when calcium is needed.

ADRENAL GLANDS

The adrenal glands sit on the superior surface of kidneys. The hormones they secrete include epinephrine (adrenaline), norepinephrine (noradrenaline), glucocorticoids, and mineralocorticoids. The adrenal hormones promote sodium and water conservation; they also help cope with long-term stress, reduce inflammation and edema, and reduce pain. In addition, adrenaline and noradrenaline initiate the alarm response of the sympathetic nervous system.

PINEAL GLAND

The tiny pineal gland hangs from the roof of the third ventricle in the brain and is responsible for producing melatonin. Although not proven, melatonin is commonly known to help the body recognize and move through sleep/wake cycles. When nerves in the eyes are exposed to light, the pineal gland is triggered to produce less melatonin. As night falls and environmental light diminishes, the pineal gland produces more melatonin.

THYMUS GLAND

The thymus gland, discussed in the circulatory system section, is located posterior to the sternum and decreases in size as we get older. It produces thymosin, which triggers leukocytes to mature into T lymphocytes, special immune cells that help the body recognize foreign substances.

OTHER ENDOCRINE ORGANS

Parts of the hypothalamus, pancreas, ovaries, testes, and placenta are considered components of the endocrine system because of their secretions.

The hypothalamus sits just above the pituitary gland and controls its hormone release, giving them a close, cooperative relationship. It produces antidiuretic hormone (ADH) and oxytocin but immediately stores them in the pituitary gland. Once it stimulates the pituitary gland to release them, ADH causes the kidneys to reabsorb more water instead of excreting it in the urine, and oxytocin stimulates uterine contractions during childbirth and the initial milk letdown in the breasts.

The pancreas secretes glucagon and insulin for metabolizing carbohydrates. The ovaries produce the hormones estrogen and progesterone, and the testes produce testosterone. These hormones are responsible for sexual maturation and development.

The placenta develops in the uterus during pregnancy. It is the organ that serves as the intermediary between the mother and the fetus, made of tissue from both. It provides fetal nutrition, eliminates fetal wastes, and produces estrogen and progesterone. These hormones help maintain the pregnancy by preventing contractions that can cause miscarriage, and they prepare the mother's body for breastfeeding.

Reproductive System

The reproductive system is relatively inactive in humans until puberty; then the overall function is to produce offspring. The female reproductive system is slightly more complex than the male reproductive system, and the structures perform very different activities.

Functions of the Female Reproductive System

The primary goal of the female reproductive system is to reproduce. To reach that goal, the system must produce sex hormones, produce and release ova (OH-vah), incubate the growing fetus in a safe, nurturing environment, deliver the infant, and nourish the infant.

SEX HORMONES

The hormones produced by the female reproductive system include estrogen and progesterone. They are released by the ovaries in varying amounts during the menstrual cycle. Estrogen promotes the maturation and release of eggs from the ovary and stimulates the lining of the uterus to develop more blood vessels. There are some physical changes that occur with the increased production of hormones during the teen years: the breasts enlarge, the reproductive organs enlarge, more body hair grows in the axillary and pubic areas, increased amounts of fat are deposited in the subcutaneous layer, the pelvis widens, and the menstrual cycle begins.

OVA

The eggs produced by the female reproductive system are referred to as ova. They start out as immature cells in the ovary and mature over time. Ovulation is the release of a mature egg from the ovary, stimulated by estrogen.

MATERNAL REPRODUCTIVE SYSTEM FUNCTIONS

Once an egg has been fertilized and has been implanted in the uterine lining, the female reproductive system is responsible for incubating the growing fetus in a safe, nurturing environment, delivering the baby, and nourishing the baby. The progesterone produced by the ovaries causes even more blood vessels to form in the uterine lining and inhibits contractions of the uterus to prevent miscarriage.

Delivering the baby, also called parturition or birth, is also a responsibility of the female reproductive system. During pregnancy, the smooth muscles of the uterus increase in size to expand with the growing fetus and to accomplish the delivery. Remember that new muscle cells are not created; they can only increase in size. In a normal pregnancy, the full-term fetus is squeezed out of the uterus by strong, smooth muscle contractions and through the vagina to the external environment. The smooth muscles work very hard to deliver the baby, and most women are encouraged to contract their abdominal muscles to reduce the size of the abdominal cavity and help push the baby out.

The mammary glands in the breasts are specialized sweat glands, as discussed in the integumentary system section. Once the baby is born, progesterone stimulates the initial milk letdown in the breasts, and oxytocin stimulates the release of milk to feed the baby.

Structures of the Female Reproductive System

The many structures of the female reproductive system include the ovaries, fallopian tubes, uterus, vagina, and mammary glands. The female reproductive organs are located in the lower abdomen, except for the mammary glands, located in the breasts (Fig. 4-71 shows frontal and sagittal section views of these structures).

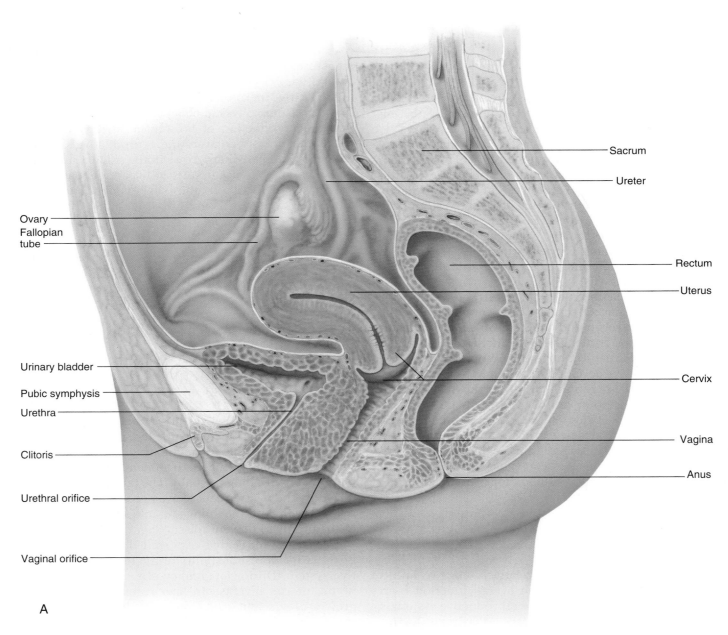

A

FIGURE 4-71 Structures of the female reproductive system. **A.** Sagittal view. (A and B provided by Anatomical Chart Co. C from Pillitteri A. Maternal and Child Health Nursing. 4th ed. Philadelphia: Lippincott Williams & Wilkins, 2002.)

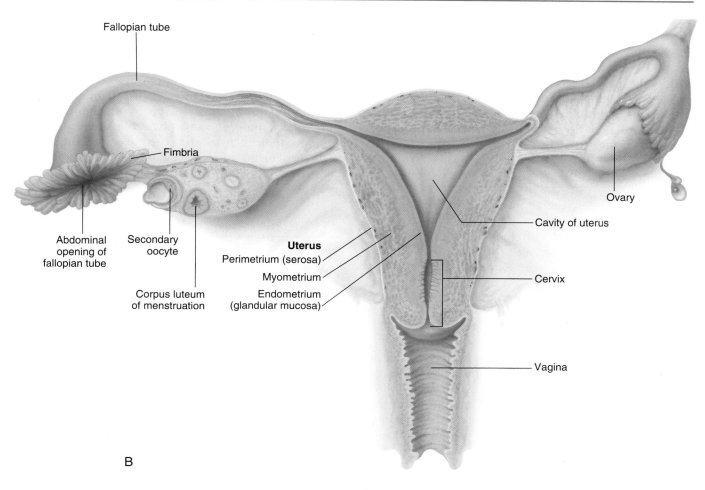

B

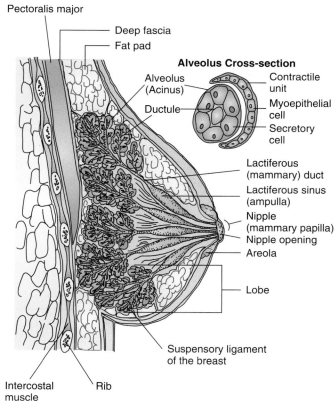

C

FIGURE 4-71 *(continued)* Structures of the female reproductive system. **B.** Frontal view. **C.** Breast (mammary gland). (A and B provided by Anatomical Chart Co. C from Pillitteri A. Maternal and Child Health Nursing. 4th ed. Philadelphia: Lippincott Williams & Wilkins, 2002.)

OVARIES

The ovaries are the primary female sex organs that secrete the sex hormones, estrogen and progesterone. Within the ovaries are immature egg cells that develop over time in response to sex hormones. Luteinizing hormone, secreted by the pituitary gland, stimulates the ovaries to typically release one egg per menstrual cycle.

FALLOPIAN TUBES

The fallopian tubes receive the eggs from the ovaries and transport the eggs to the uterus. Incidentally, fertilization usually occurs in the fallopian tubes. To transport the egg, the smooth muscles of the fallopian tubes use peristalsis to encourage the egg to move toward the uterus, and ciliated cells along the lining of the tubes rhythmically sweep toward the uterus.

UTERUS

The uterus is the organ that serves as the incubator for the growing fetus. It is constructed with three layers. The inner layer is a lining of mucous membrane called the endometrium. The thick middle layer, the myometrium, is made of smooth muscle that expands to accommodate the growing fetus, and rhythmically contracts to deliver the baby. The outer layer of the uterus is a serous membrane called the perimetrium.

VAGINA

The vagina is a muscular tube that connects the uterus to the external environment. It provides a pathway for sperm and becomes the infant's birth canal during delivery.

MAMMARY GLANDS

The mammary glands are modified sweat glands that produce milk and release it through the nipple to provide nourishment to the infant. The initial letdown of milk is triggered by progesterone, and the continued production of milk is stimulated by oxytocin, a hormone created in the hypothalamus.

Functions of the Male Reproductive System

The functions of the male reproductive system are to produce the male sex hormone, produce sperm that can fertilize a female's egg, and deliver that sperm to the female.

SEX HORMONE

Testosterone is the male sex hormone produced in the testes. It stimulates development and maturation of the male reproductive system and also results in some secondary sex characteristics of males. When testosterone production increases during the teen years, males undergo some physical changes that accompany their growth: the voice deepens, the bones thicken, skeletal muscles enlarge, and more body hair grows, especially in the axillary, facial, and pubic areas.

SPERM

Millions of immature sperm are produced daily in the testes, are pushed through the testes with peristaltic smooth muscle contractions, and arrive at the epididymis to mature. Mature sperm contain mitochondria to produce ATP, chemical energy. They are equipped with a flagellum that they use to propel themselves through the ducts and into the female, which they can do only with energy from ATP.

Structures of the Male Reproductive System

The male reproductive system includes the testes, ducts, accessory organs, and external genitalia (Fig. 4-72 shows frontal and sagittal views).

TESTES

There are two testes, each about 1½ inches long and 1 inch wide. Outside, they are encased in a fibrous connective tissue. Inside, they contain structures that form sperm and testosterone. The epididymis, where the sperm mature, is the beginning of the delivery system for the sperm, and it starts in the testes.

DUCTS

Mature sperm travel through a series of ducts in their quest for an ovum:

1. Epididymis
2. Ductus deferens (vas deferens)
3. Urethra

Smooth muscles in the ducts propel the sperm toward the external environment with peristalsis.

Sagittal section

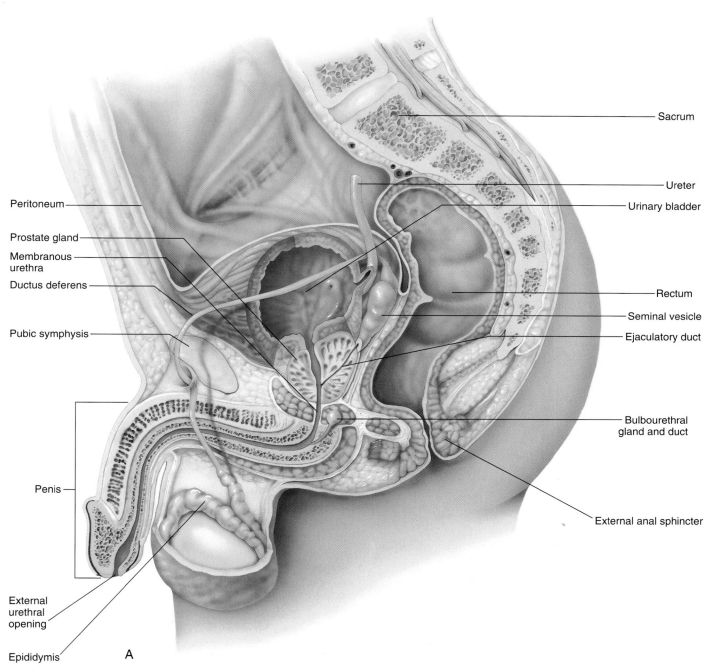

Sacrum

Ureter

Urinary bladder

Peritoneum

Prostate gland

Membranous
urethra

Ductus deferens

Pubic symphysis

Penis

External
urethral
opening

Epididymis

Rectum

Seminal vesicle

Ejaculatory duct

Bulbourethral
gland and duct

External anal sphincter

A

FIGURE 4-72   Structures of the male reproductive system. **A.** Sagittal view. (Assets provided by Anatomical
Chart Co.)

(continued)

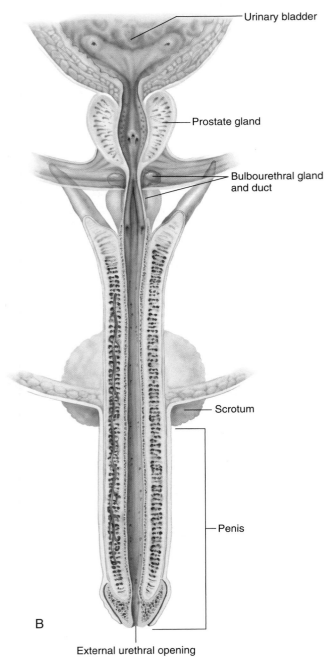

B

FIGURE 4-72 *(continued)* Structures of the male reproductive system. **B.** Frontal view. (Assets provided by Anatomical Chart Co.)

Labels on figure: Urinary bladder · Prostate gland · Bulbourethral gland and duct · Scrotum · Penis · External urethral opening

ACCESSORY MALE REPRODUCTIVE ORGANS

The accessory organs of the male reproductive system produce everything in the semen except the sperm. The seminal vesicles, bulbourethral glands, and prostate gland all secrete fluids containing sugar, vitamins, or hormones. These components of semen nourish and activate the sperm as well as cleanse the urethra prior to sperm delivery. The prostate gland wraps around the beginning part of the urethra. It has smooth muscle walls that contract during ejaculation, and the force of the contraction aids the expulsion of semen.

EXTERNAL GENITALIA

The penis is an external genital organ that is responsible for delivering sperm into the female reproductive tract. There are three areas of spongy tissue that fill with blood during sexual arousal and cause the penis to become erect. The parasympathetic nervous system can trigger erections unrelated to sexual stimulation.

The scrotum holds and protects the testes, maintaining their temperature below normal body temperature to avoid overheating the sperm. Muscles raise and lower the testes, as a protective mechanism; the wrinkled scrotal skin allows movement.

Body System Conditions

To maintain homeostasis physiologically or structurally, the body continually adjusts to changes in its environment on the basis of a myriad of stimuli and processes that occur constantly. When an imbalance occurs, the overall health of the tissues or body may be compromised. Massage can contribute to the homeostatic balance by enhancing the flow of body fluids with mechanical effects and can have reflexive effects that affect chemical activity in the body. Because massage helps facilitate these changes, it is important for you to understand how a certain symptom, condition, or more advanced pathology affects the body to determine whether massage is appropriate or not.

There are conditions that affect homeostasis or structural balance that may be considered precursors to, or symptoms of, a disease process (pathology). For example, increased muscle tension and pain in and of itself is not necessarily pathological, but it is sometimes a precursor to, or symptom of, fibromyalgia, a chronic muscular pain condition. Since massage therapy affects many body systems, you must understand some of the more common body conditions and their symptoms, especially with regards to the musculoskeletal system.

This section is meant to be an introduction to pathology to understand the process of determining if massage is appropriate or if the client should first be referred to a healthcare professional for further evaluation. If you question whether massage should or should not be applied, withhold massage treatment until the appropriate healthcare professional can examine and diagnose the condition. **Remember the rule: when in doubt, refer out.** It is not within your scope of practice as a massage therapist to diagnose or prescribe, so suggesting a client see another healthcare professional must be done sensitively and carefully. Use a gentle approach in making the client aware of the possible symptom or condition and explain that a more thorough examination is in everyone's best interest. If the client asks you about a condition that you think may require a diagnosis, you can simply say, "I cannot diagnose any medical conditions, but massage may not be helpful. I recommend that you see your healthcare professional for further evaluation before we continue treatment." However, if you happen to notice a condition or a set of symptoms that may require a diagnosis, you can carefully encourage the client to recognize and discuss the symptoms. Once the client is aware of the symptoms or condition, you could gently encourage him or her to get a diagnosis to put everyone's mind at rest. Referring clients out for conditions that massage does not treat instills confidence and respect in your professionalism to the client and the healthcare professional. It also helps you maintain the client-centered philosophy.

Terminology

Throughout this section, the following terms are used frequently:

- **Acute**—refers to a condition that developed very quickly and severely or has been present for 1–3 days
- **Subacute**—the period from about 3 days to 3 weeks after a condition started
- **Chronic**—refers to a condition that develops slowly, recurs, or persists longer than 3 weeks
- **Contraindication**—a condition in which massage is inappropriate and should be avoided
- **Indication**—a condition for which massage could be beneficial and is recommended

For each condition or pathology included in this section, there is a brief description of the condition or pathology, some symptoms that can help identify it, and an explanation of whether massage is commonly indicated (recommended) or contraindicated (inappropriate). Some conditions are considered **local contraindications** for massage, meaning that massage should be avoided in the affected area. If there is a local contraindication such as bruise or open wound, massage is appropriate for all areas except the one affected. There are also **systemic contraindications,** which are health conditions in which massage should be avoided altogether because massage could worsen the condition or spread disease. Any time fever is present, such as in the acute stages of a cold, massage is systemically contraindicated.

Treatments

When appropriate, some common medications and treatments for the symptom or condition are identified. These treatments and medications are typically prescribed by the appropriate healthcare professional, not the massage therapist. In this text, a healthcare professional is a practitioner who can diagnose and prescribe, such as a medical doctor (MD), osteopath (DO), or chiropractor (DC). **Diagnosing and prescribing are not in the massage therapist's scope of practice.** Treatments and medications are mentioned because a client may be using them when they come for massage treatment. They are mentioned as information only. Generally, if a medication is taken internally and is delivered through the bloodstream, massage techniques such as effleurage and petrissage, which increase blood flow, may increase the effect of the medication in the body. It is always good to know about the client's health and treatment regimens that may be affected by massage.

This introduction to body system conditions is meant to serve as a foundation for understanding the process of assessing the appropriateness of massage; you may need to consult more expanded resources on pathology and medications. See suggested readings and web sites at the end of the chapter for more resources.

Integumentary (Skin) Conditions

Skin is the first point of contact in massage. Often you may see a change in the appearance of the skin or you may feel changes in the skin before the client does. If the skin is compromised in any way, as happens with a scratch or cut, it cannot function effectively as a protective barrier. There is an increased possibility of infection, so the area should be avoided and is a local contraindication for massage. If you suspect a condition is more serious, refer the client to his or her healthcare professional for further evaluation. All treatments other than massage are mentioned because clients may already be using them when they come to you for massage therapy. A few common conditions that you may encounter in your practice include open wounds or sores, acne, superficial scar tissue, and fungal infections.

OPEN WOUNDS OR SORES

An open wound or sore is any injury to the skin that breaks the surface and leaves it open for bacteria to enter and possible infection to occur. Types of open wounds or sores include cuts, holes, abrasions, blisters, and ulcers. You can recognize these conditions by a crust or scab at the site of the injury except in the case of ulcers, which remain open.

> ⚠ *Massage is locally contraindicated for the affected area of a wound. If the client has a related systemic condition such as diabetes, massage is a systemic contraindication unless you obtain medical clearance from the client's healthcare professional.*

Typically, open wounds are covered with a bandage and treated with topical medications that often contain antibiotics, analgesics, or antihistamines.

ACNE

Acne is a bacterial infection of the oil (sebaceous) glands that can be influenced by overactive oil glands and liver congestion due to a high-fat diet, smoking, drugs (medications), and chemical pollutants. Acne is commonly recognized as raised, white or black and sometimes reddened, inflamed pimples often found on the face, neck, and upper back.

> ⚠ *Massage is locally contraindicated for acne because it can increase the possibility of spreading infection, and the lubricant can make acne worse.*

Treatment for acne may include topical or oral medications, depending upon the severity of the condition.

SUPERFICIAL SCAR TISSUE

Superficial scar tissue is new tissue growth that occurs during the acute stage of an injury to the skin. It is made of randomly structured, dense, fibrous tissue that has a decreased blood supply, may have decreased sensory neurons, and has no hair follicles or pigmentation (Fig. 4-73).

> ⚠ *Massage is locally contraindicated during the acute stage of a skin injury because bacteria could enter any break or tear in the skin.*

Once the scar has formed, massage on and around the scar tissue can increase the speed of healing by increasing circulation to the area, which prevents fascial restriction and increases mobility of the tissue. You should be aware that the scar tissue may have re-

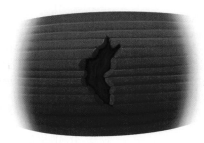

A Injured muscle tissue

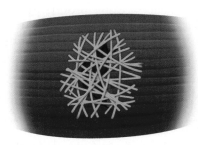

B Random arrangement of deposited scar tissue

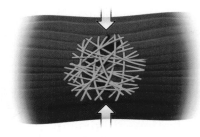

C Structural weak spot

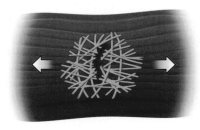

D New injury at site of scar tissue

FIGURE 4-73   Scar tissue.

duced sensation, and you will need to be especially sensitive to the client's feedback.

 In the subacute and chronic stages of a skin injury, massage is indicated and can be very beneficial.

Soft tissue work is the recommended treatment for superficial scar tissue and may be initially applied by a physical therapist or a massage therapist.

FUNGAL INFECTIONS

Fungal infections are contagious conditions of the skin that can be caused by several types of fungi and a compromised immune system and result in lesions, or tinea. Ringworm and athlete's foot are some examples of fungal infections. Fungal infections are recognized as red, circular lesions and itchy patches that thrive in warm, moist places. Touching or scratching the lesions will spread the infection.

 Massage is locally contraindicated if the area is small and minimal lesions are present, such as on the feet in athlete's foot. If the affected area is large, massage is systemically contraindicated until the infection is healed.

Treatment for this condition usually includes topical fungicides and/or oral medications.

Skeletal System Conditions

One benefit of massage is increased circulation of blood and lymph because it increases nutrient delivery to, and waste removal from, body tissues. The bones and joints benefit from these effects as well, leading to healthier bones and better healing of fractures and other bone injuries. Massage enhances the circulation to the bones and joints and expedites the removal of debris and waste from the cells and any injured areas, facilitating the body's natural healing process.

The joints of the skeleton also benefit from massage. Joint movement techniques used in a massage session are additionally beneficial for the restoration of range of motion. Passively or actively moving the joint produces synovial fluid and provides nourishment to the area. These techniques are covered in the therapeutic techniques chapter.

The mechanical design of the joints enforces limits on a joint's range of motion, as does the condition of soft tissue structures surrounding the area. Tight muscles, injured tendons and ligaments, and abnormalities in other connective tissue structures generally create dysfunction and compensation patterns in the movement of the bones and joints of the skeleton. Generally, if the muscles and soft tissue are brought back into balance, then the bones and joints may return to, or more easily retain, their most functional alignment. All treatments other than massage are typically prescribed by the client's healthcare professional, who can prescribe treatments within his or her scope of practice. Again, it is not in the massage therapist's scope of practice to diagnose or prescribe. These treatments are mentioned because clients may already be using one or more of the following treatments when they come to you for massage therapy. Some of the conditions you may see in your clients include postural deviation, fracture, sprain, or osteoarthritis.

POSTURAL DEVIATIONS

Postural deviations are overdeveloped curves in the spine. In the thoracic section, an overdeveloped curve looks like a hunched posture and is called kyphosis. Someone with an excessive lumbar curvature, or lordosis, often stands with "locked" knees and a protruding pelvis. When the spine curves from side to side instead of running vertically, the condition is called S- or C-curve scoliosis (Fig. 4-74). These curves can have functional or structural causes. Functional postural deviations occur when the soft tissue structures, muscles, tendons, and ligaments pull the spine out of alignment. Structural deviations are congenital, meaning that the person was born with the bones

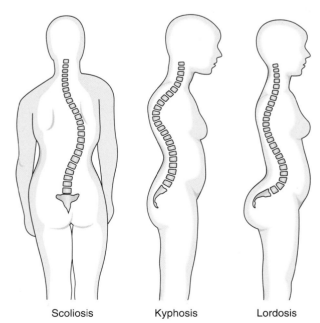

Scoliosis   Kyphosis   Lordosis

FIGURE 4-74 Postural deviations. (Reprinted from Cohen BJ, Wood DL. Memmler's Structure and Function of the Human Body. 9th ed. Philadelphia: Lippincott Williams & Wilkins, 2000.)

already in the deviated formation, or result from untreated functional conditions that may have been caused by an injury. Deviations can be recognized by the extreme visible curves apparent by visual or palpable assessment. X-ray images can detect minor curves, but these tests are ordered by a healthcare professional such as a chiropractor, osteopath, or medical doctor.

> ⚠️ *Massage is indicated for scoliosis to reduce muscle and soft tissue tension and pain, but massage will not make the bones realign.*

Treatment for postural deviation may include physical therapy for exercises, chiropractic care for relieving pressure in the spine, and more dramatically, braces or surgical rods for severe scoliosis.

FRACTURES

A fracture is any type of cracked or broken bone (Fig. 4-75). A fracture can be recognized by increased pain and decreased function and the joint closest to the injury. Some conditions mask the symptoms of a fracture, such as a sprained ankle ligament or shin splints, but a healthcare professional can officially diagnose a fracture using an x-ray or bone scan.

> ⚠️ *Massage is locally contraindicated during the acute stage of a fracture, but massage to the rest of the body will enhance circulation and encourage healing. A few days after the fracture occurs, massage can be beneficial for healing and is locally indicated.*

Treatment for fractures includes immobilization, casting, and in more severe injuries surgery to repair the fractured bone(s) with pins or plates.

SPRAINS

A sprain refers to a sprained ligament, which connects bone to bone and stabilizes a joint. Sprains occur when ligaments are suddenly overstretched or torn because of trauma or an exceeded range of motion. When torn, their ability to maintain the stability of the joint is obviously compromised. In the acute stage (24 to 72 hours), the symptoms include pain, redness, heat, swelling, and decreased mobility at the affected joint. Swelling, in particular, is a part of the body's healing mechanism, limiting movement to prevent further injury. These symptoms decrease as healing progresses; however, pain remains during all stages. You should suggest that the client see his or her healthcare professional to rule out fracture prior to massage treatment. A severe sprain may be medically diagnosed as a rupture or separation of the ligament from the bone.

> ⚠️ *Massage is locally contraindicated during the acute stage of a severe sprain, but the client's entire body will benefit from the relaxing and restorative qualities of massage therapy. Massage is indicated in the subacute stage, when it can enhance healing, decrease swelling and adhesion, as well as create helpful scar tissue and restore range of motion to the affected joint.*

Treatment for sprains includes immobilization via a splint or support bandage, ice and compression to reduce swelling, and elevation to keep excess lymphatic fluid from accumulating in the injured area.

OSTEOARTHRITIS

Osteoarthritis literally means inflammation of the bone and joint. More specifically, it is a condition that occurs when repetitive wear and tear of synovial joint

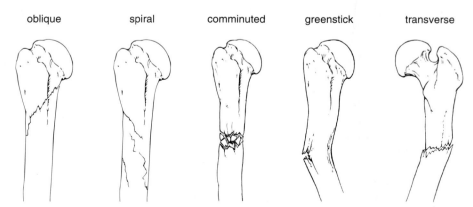

FIGURE 4-75 Types of fractures. (Reprinted from Cohen BJ. Medical Terminology: An Illustrated Guide. 4th ed. Baltimore: Lippincott Williams & Wilkins, 2004.)

structures result in irritation and inflammation. Fingers, thumbs, knees, and hips are common joints affected in this condition. Massage therapists may develop this condition over time because of repetitive use of fingers and thumbs. Clients with this condition complain of stiffness and pain in the affected joints that may be accompanied by signs of inflammation such as redness and heat. Occasionally, muscles around the affected joint will become tense, effectively "splinting" the area to decrease mobility. Chronic muscle tension can result in the formation of trigger points in the muscle, which are explained in the muscular system conditions.

> *Massage is locally contraindicated in the acute stage of osteoarthritis when inflammation is present, but massage is indicated in all other stages to relieve pain and stiffness as well as to increase joint mobility.*

Massage can also help treat trigger points in the surrounding muscles that are splinting the joint. Treatment for osteoarthritis may include pain or antiinflammatory medications, nutritional supplements such as glucosamine and chondroitin, or dietary modifications.

Muscular System Conditions

There are many indications for massage therapy for clients with muscle or movement dysfunction. Abnormal posture is often accompanied by muscles that are out of balance. When one muscle of a pair of antagonistic muscles is hypertonic, they are considered to be out of balance. The hypertonic muscle pulls the joint into an abnormal resting position and the body must compensate for the imbalance. Muscles that get out of balance are in a less than optimal state or have a reduced functional activity, and vice versa. Any deviation from normal, healthy function or movement indicates that a muscle or series of muscle groups have abnormal stresses placed upon them. One goal of massage therapy is to bring the muscles and surrounding soft tissue back into balance to create the most functional movement for the client. You should understand muscular system symptoms, conditions, or states of dysfunction. All treatments other than massage are typically prescribed by the client's healthcare professionals who can diagnose and prescribe within their scope of practice. Again, it is not in the massage therapist's scope of practice to diagnose or prescribe, but these treatments are mentioned because clients may already be using one or more of the following treatments when they come to you for massage therapy. You will most likely see hypertonic muscles, spasms (cramps), trigger points, fibromyalgia, strain, and tendinitis in your massage practice.

HYPERTONIC MUSCLES

Muscles that are too tight are referred to as hypertonic, meaning that they have contracted and have not completely relaxed. Exercise, for example, puts muscles through repetitive contractions, and when the exercise is finished, the muscles may not "remember" their original resting length. Because they are so used to contracting, they may assume a new, shorter resting length and are considered hypertonic. When muscles are hypertonic, circulation within them is reduced, so they receive less oxygen than they need, a condition called ischemia (iss-KEE-mee-ah). The symptoms can include pain, discomfort, restrictions in functional movement, and compensation patterns. This is an interconnected pattern commonly called the pain–spasm cycle (Fig. 4-76):

1. Pain causes a person to tense up, resulting in hypertonicity.
2. Hypertonicity causes ischemia.
3. Ischemia causes pain.
4. Pain causes hypertonicity, and so on . . .

> *Massage is beneficial for all of the symptoms of hypertonic muscles, including pain, the shortened muscle length, and ischemia.*

Therapeutic techniques can be used to reflexively trigger the muscles to lengthen. People commonly treat hypertonic muscles with or without a professional diagnosis by using ice packs or heat packs,

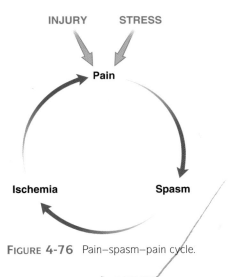

FIGURE 4-76 Pain–spasm–pain cycle.

soaking in hot tubs, analgesics (pain relievers), muscle relaxants, and self-massage. Pain relievers can be helpful because they can break the pain–spasm cycle by reducing pain, which allows more movement of the muscle, which increases the circulation to the muscle. Ice is also very helpful because in addition to its analgesic properties that break the pain cycle, the homeostatic mechanism of our body will flood the area with warm blood to maintain a stable core body temperature. Circulation increases healing.

MUSCLE SPASMS

Muscle spasms and cramps occur when a skeletal muscle contracts involuntarily and does not relax immediately. Spasms are muscle contractions that result in decreased movement at the related joint and can last for weeks. A cramp is a spasm that is accompanied by intense pain. Spasms and cramps are caused by ischemia (decreased oxygen), muscle splinting after an injury, and low levels of calcium and magnesium in the blood.

> *Massage to the muscle bellies is contraindicated in the acute stage of muscle spasm to prevent further injury; however, it is acceptable to manipulate the tendons of that muscle and the antagonistic muscles to reflexively relax the affected muscle.*

Reflexive techniques are covered in the chapter on therapeutic techniques.

> *In the subacute and chronic stages of a muscle spasm, massage is indicated because it can decrease pain and hypertonicity as well as increase circulation, resulting in more oxygen and nutrients delivered to, and removal of waste from, the area.*

This helps break the pain–spasm cycle. Sometimes spasms are referred to as muscle guarding or splinting. In this phenomenon, the body responds to pain by holding a muscle contraction to minimize movement in an attempt to protect an area from further injury.

> *Massage is locally contraindicated for situations of splinting or protective guarding.*

As part of the body's own healing mechanism, splinting serves an important purpose, and if the muscles that are acting as splints are relaxed, further injury could result. Treatment for spasms is also commonly

used with or without a professional diagnosis or prescription and may include heat packs, ice packs, analgesics, muscle relaxants, self-massage, and nutritional supplements such as calcium, magnesium, and potassium.

TRIGGER POINTS

Trigger points (TrPs) are spasms that occur on the cellular level, at the motor end unit, or the point of communication between axonal terminals and the muscle cells. When very few muscle cells are in spasm, they become hyperirritable and refer pain to another part of the body because of the neuron involvement. There are several factors that contribute to the formation of trigger points:

- Decreased circulation to a hypertonic muscle
- Insufficient hydration of the muscle cells and tissues, which creates homeostatic imbalance that can affect the action potential
- Mechanical stress on a muscle caused by bony misalignments, excessive pressure from a purse or backpack strap
- Inadequate sleep, which can overwork the sympathetic nervous system to stay alert
- Increased stress, which can also affect homeostasis with overactivity of the sympathetic nervous system

Trigger points are not pathological, but can be a symptom of a pathological condition. For example, TrPs are often a symptom of fibromyalgia, a chronic muscle pain condition.

> *Massage is indicated for trigger points to relieve them and allow the muscle to relax, as well as to increase circulation to the muscle tissue.*

All treatments other than massage are typically prescribed by the client's healthcare professional whose scope of practice includes prescription. Again, it is not in the massage therapist's scope of practice to diagnose or prescribe. Treatment may include heat packs, ice packs, injections of pain medication, oral pain medication, and muscle relaxants. These treatments are only mentioned because clients may already be using one or more of the treatments when they come to you for massage therapy.

FIBROMYALGIA

Fibromyalgia is a chronic muscle pain syndrome sometimes called fibrositis, myofibrositis, or fibromyositis. A syndrome is not a pathological condition, but is diagnosed when a client has a certain set of symptoms. Fibromyalgia is diagnosed by a healthcare professional when the patient has 7 to 10 specific trigger points or tender points (localized areas of pain in a muscle), widespread pain, decreased stamina, and minimal pain tolerance. Pain is the predominant symptom in this condition, present in the muscles and soft tissues to varying degrees. The soft tissue hypersensitivity can elicit pain with any kind of movement or light touch. Typically, the higher the stress level and the more compromised the internal healing environment, the more hypersensitive the client and client's tissues are. Any time you treat clients with fibromyalgia, you should carefully consider their stress level and internal healing environment, which can affect their pain tolerance.

 Massage is indicated for fibromyalgia as long as you do not overtreat the client.

Due to the increased sensitivity to pain, decreased circulation to the muscles, tender points, and trigger points, sometimes massage can create more stress on the body and worsen the condition. There is a fine line between appropriate treatment and overtreatment. Over time, you will easily detect changes in the muscles and surrounding soft tissue through palpation in a massage and will be able to judge the appropriateness of the treatment. **Less is often more** when treating this particular condition, which can be managed by using less pressure or treatments of shorter duration.

All treatments other than massage are typically prescribed by the client's prescribing healthcare professional and are only mentioned to make you aware of what your clients may bring into your treatment room to know whether you need to adjust the treatment. With fibromyalgia, there are no rules, and people tend to respond differently to the same treatment, but ice may increase symptoms and should generally be avoided. Treatments for this condition may include pain, sleep and/or antidepressant medications, and muscle relaxants as well as changes in nutritional habits, nutritional supplementation, exercise, stretching, acupuncture, and anything to reduce the client's stress level, which includes massage.

MUSCLE STRAIN

A muscle strain involves torn muscle cells and is characterized by mild-to-severe localized pain, stiffness, and inflammation (heat, redness, and swelling). Inflammation increases with the severity of the injury. Resisted movement, in which the client is mov-

ing against a counterforce, and stretching will also elicit pain in a strained muscle. A muscle that undergoes excessive stretch or excessive contraction can suffer a muscle strain.

During the acute and subacute periods following a muscle strain, massage is locally contraindicated. If the strain is determined by a physician to be very severe, such as a rupture of the entire muscle, massage is locally contraindicated until the physician has determined that the muscle has healed.

The body starts the healing process in the acute phase of a muscle strain by depositing a dense network of collagen fibers at the injury site in random arrangements. Because this network is not aligned with the muscle fibers, the surrounding layers of tissue cannot slip past each other as easily, and the layers have a tendency to stick to each other and create fascial adhesions. Thus, gentle movement is beneficial for a healing muscle strain because it prevents the buildup of fascial adhesions. Even so, the client should be cautious about exerting the injured muscle during the subacute period because the new collagen fiber network lacks strength and the risk of reinjury is higher. Once the adhesions have settled in and bound tissue layers together are left untreated, scar tissue will form.

Massage is indicated for muscle strains to help break up adhesions and scar tissue, to reduce edema (swelling), and to restore range of motion to the joint nearest the strain.

Treatment for strains may or may not have a professional diagnosis, but can include ice or heat, medications to reduce inflammation, analgesics, and muscle relaxants if muscle guarding occurs with the injury.

TENDINITIS

Tendinitis involves injury and inflammation of the tendon, usually at the union of the muscle and tendon (musculotendinous juncture) or where the tendon attaches to the bone (tenoperiosteal juncture). Tendons have a limited blood supply that is further compromised by compression, repetitive movements, and constant twisting. In the acute stage, tendinitis is recognizable by pain, stiffness, and inflammation as well as decreased movement. In the subacute stage, adhesions begin to form from a random collagen matrix.

> ⚠ *Although massage is locally contraindicated in the acute stage of tendinitis systemic massage is indicated. Local massage is indicated in the subacute stage to increase circulation to the surrounding tissues, reduce edema, break up fascial adhesions or scar tissue, and reestablish range of motion to the joint affected.*

Treatments for tendinitis may include ice, heat, rest or inactivity of the affected tendon, pain medication, antiinflammatory medications, or applications of ultrasound.

Nervous System Conditions

Massage affects the nervous system in several ways, depending on the technique and the speed of its application. If the goal is to stimulate the client's system, you could apply techniques using a faster pace to evoke the sympathetic nervous response. Conversely, if the goal is to relax the body, the techniques could be applied more slowly to evoke the parasympathetic nervous response. Specific massage applications using the nervous system to facilitate muscular changes are discussed in the therapeutic techniques chapter. Many conditions can affect the nervous system and its components. If the client is experiencing burning, tingling, paresthesia (pins and needles), radiating numbness or a similar sensation, nerves may be involved. You will likely encounter endangerment sites, sciatica, headaches, and thoracic outlet syndrome in your massage practice.

ENDANGERMENT SITES

Endangerment sites are places on the body where nerves and blood vessels are not well protected by muscles or bones. These sites are not pathological conditions, but you should be aware of their locations because continuous, direct, or heavy pressure or pounding on any of these sites may cause damage and are contraindicated. Massage techniques applied at these sites should include light pressure or should be avoided altogether (see Fig. 3-6).

SCIATICA

Sciatica (sahy-AT-ik-uh) is inflammation of the sciatic nerve. It is characterized by aching or cramping sensations and/or shooting or burning pain in the buttocks and down the leg into the foot. Sometimes the discomfort is accompanied by tingling, reduced sensation or numbness, paresthesia (pins and needles

sensation), and even loss of function. True sciatica involves irritation to the sciatic nerve near its root at the spinal cord, which may be caused by more serious pathology. Spinal cord or nerve root impingement should be examined and diagnosed by a healthcare professional. The nervous system is not within the massage therapy scope of practice, and treating a nerve root is inappropriate.

> *Massage is locally contraindicated for true sciatica that stems from the spinal cord or nerve root.*

The symptoms of sciatica can also be caused by irritation or inflammation of the sciatic nerve because of muscular impingement by a tight piriformis muscle, one of the deep hip rotator muscles near the ischium.

> ⚠ *Massage is indicated for sciatic nerve irritation if there is a muscular cause, because it can relax the problematic muscle tissue and relieve the pressure on the nerve.*

Many clients come in with self-diagnosed sciatica, but without a professional diagnosis, you cannot determine where the nerve is being affected. As mentioned above, massage is locally contraindicated for true sciatica, but that does not rule out massage of the deep hip rotator muscles. So you can attempt massage on the deep hip rotators to see if it relieves the discomfort at all. If massage does not decrease the symptoms, the client may have nerve root or spinal cord irritation, and you should refer such clients to their healthcare professional for further evaluation. Treatment for sciatica may include muscle relaxants, pain medication, physical therapy, traction, cortisone injections to reduce inflammation, chiropractic or osteopathic adjustment, or surgery in more severe cases.

HEADACHES

A headache is pain in the head and neck region that can be classified as muscular (tension), vascular (congestion), or traction–inflammatory (pathological). Headaches can have a sudden or gradual onset, and the pain can be on one or both sides of the head and neck. It is not within the massage therapy scope of practice to diagnose or prescribe, so all treatments mentioned, other than massage, are typically self-administered or prescribed by a healthcare professional who can prescribe treatments within their scope of practice. These treatments are mentioned because clients may already be using them when they come for a massage. You should always ask if the client has any health issues or is using treatments that may be affected by massage.

Tension Headaches

Tension headaches are the most common type of headache, caused by muscular tension, or hypertonic muscles. Some of the muscles often involved with tension headaches include the sternocleidomastoid, suboccipitals, masseter (jaw muscle), and neck extensors (splenius cervicis and splenius capitis). Tension and trigger points in these muscles refer pain into the head and contribute to tension headaches. The pain typically occurs bilaterally (both sides) in the head and neck region.

 Massage is indicated for tension headaches at all stages.

There are numerous self-treatments for tension headaches, but doctors may prescribe ice to reduce pain and muscular spasm, pain and/or antiinflammatory medication, muscle relaxants, or nutritional supplements such as magnesium and feverfew.

Vascular Headaches

Vascular headaches, also known as congestion headaches, are related to increased blood flow within the vessels in the cranium. Vasodilation can put pressure on the nerves, and pressure on nerves causes pain and discomfort. They are often associated with unilateral (one-sided) throbbing or stabbing pain, but the symptoms can also occur bilaterally.

 Massage is indicated in the subacute stage of vascular headaches.

This type of headache may require diagnostic testing such as magnetic resonance imagery (MRI) or computed tomography (CT) scan to rule out underlying pathology. Once pathology has been ruled out, professionally prescribed drug treatments may include pain medication, antiinflammatory medication, muscle relaxants, serotonin reuptake inhibitors, or tricyclic antidepressants. Other than drug therapy, doctors sometimes identify the client's nutritional sensitivities and use stress management techniques such as acupuncture, biofeedback, and exercise. All treatments other than massage should only be prescribed by the appropriate healthcare professional.

Pathological Headaches

As a massage therapist, you will not likely see a client with a pathological headache because they are caused by serious underlying conditions such as tumors, aneurysm, or CNS infection and are diagnosed and treated by a healthcare professional. These headaches are very severe and often last for days.

 Massage is systemically contraindicated for pathological headaches.

Treatment for pathological headaches is always determined and supervised by the client's healthcare professional and may require surgery and/or hospitalization.

THORACIC OUTLET SYNDROME

Thoracic outlet syndrome is impingement of the brachial plexus nerve bundle and the blood vessels going to and from the arm. As mentioned with fibromyalgia, a syndrome is a collection of specific symptoms that is not a true pathological condition. Tight muscles, cervical or rib misalignment, atrophied muscles, a herniated intervertebral disk, or spondylosis (a bone spur at the nerve root) are some of the causes of this condition. Thoracic outlet syndrome is characterized by paresthesia (pins and needles), tingling, shooting pain, weakness, numbness, feeling of fullness and possible discoloration due to diminished circulation.

Massage is indicated for thoracic outlet syndrome if the impingement is caused by muscle tightness or spasm. If it is related to any other cause, massage will be locally contraindicated at the problematic area.

If the symptoms do not diminish with massage, impingement may be due to another cause, and such clients should be referred to their healthcare professional to get a diagnosis and treatment plan. Professionally prescribed treatments for thoracic outlet syndrome that clients may be using will vary, depending on the cause that has been professionally diagnosed.

Circulatory System Conditions

One of the major benefits of massage therapy is the mechanical effect of increased circulation. It increases the delivery of oxygen and the removal of waste and lymph to and from the cells and tissues. Without oxygen, cells do not thrive and eventually die. Once the cell dies, it is destroyed, and its remains eliminated. The ends of the capillaries are very small structures and allow only small molecules to pass through. Larger particles may get caught in the very fine branches, essentially causing capillary congestion. As fragments of dead cells block the ends of the capillaries, they become less effective as transport membranes. Oxygen, other gases, and nutrients cannot get through the obstructed capillaries easily. This condition only compounds itself: the congested capillaries do not allow oxygen to pass through, the lack of oxygen causes cells to die, those cells add to the congestion, and so on. Eventually, this situation causes pain. Medically, this condition is called ischemia. Because massage mechanically enhances the circulatory system, it can alleviate ischemia by relaxing the muscles and creating more space between the muscle cells, which restores blood flow and provides better oxygen delivery and waste removal, which leads to better healing.

Increased circulation is a key to healing. Since massage techniques can mechanically enhance blood flow, they also enhance the body's healing mechanism. The healing mechanism begins when tissues are damaged:

1. Vasodilation is automatically activated to flood the injured tissues with oxygenated blood, creating additional heat and redness.
2. As the area becomes enlarged with increased blood flow, inflammation occurs.
3. The capillary walls then become thinner, allowing water to seep from the plasma, through the capillary walls, and into surrounding tissues.
4. The resultant edema, or swelling, puts extra pressure on the nerves, causing pain.
5. Once the swelling occurs, blood flow slows down and leukocytes pass through the capillaries to the injured tissues. They clean up the area, send out chemical signals to attract more leukocytes, and kill bacteria that may have entered the tissue.
6. After inflammation subsides, other healing mechanisms take place. Sometimes tissues are regenerated or scar tissue is formed to replace tissue that cannot be regenerated.

The speed of healing varies with age, health, nutrition, emotional and environmental stressors, and self-care.

> ⚠ *Generally, massage in the acute stage (24 to 72 hours) should be avoided while the tissue healing process is beginning. Massage in the subacute stage and beyond can increase tissue health via increased capillary transport of nutrition and may reduce emotional stress and be an effective element of self-care.*

Circulatory system conditions can be local or systemic. All treatments other than massage are typically prescribed by healthcare professionals who can do so within their scope of practice. Again, it is not in the massage therapist's scope of practice to diagnose or prescribe. Bruises, varicose veins, high blood pressure, edema, and fever are just a few conditions that a massage therapist may encounter.

BRUISE

A bruise (contusion) is a broken capillary or multiple capillaries in a localized area from which red blood cells seep out into the tissue, resulting from an injury such as a bump or fall. Bruises begin with, and can be recognized by, the black and bluish color that develops from deoxygenated hemoglobin molecules that cannot be resupplied with oxygen. Eventually, this hemoglobin degrades, and byproducts of the breakdown give the bruise a green and yellowish color. Generally, the healing mechanism works well and should not be disturbed.

> ⚠ *A bruise is a local contraindication for massage therapy because the injured tissue is already in the process of being repaired by the body.*

VARICOSE VEINS

Varicose veins are damaged and distended veins with internal valve damage. Without the valves to prevent backflow of blood, the deoxygenated blood pools at the last valve that is functional. Varicose veins are often found in the legs, where the blood is moving against gravity most of the time, and are recognized by their bluish, ropey, and elevated appearance.

> ⚠ *Massage should be avoided over varicose veins, but systemic massage is indicated. It is safe to massage red spider veins.*

Doctors sometimes treat varicose veins with support hose, elastic bandages, elevation of the legs, injections of chemicals into the affected vein to shut it down, or surgical removal.

HIGH BLOOD PRESSURE

High blood pressure, or hypertension, is a condition in which the blood inside the blood vessels is pushing harder than average on the walls of the blood vessels.

Typically, the presence and severity of hypertension is diagnosed by a medical doctor, and the client may be taking some type of medication for this condition.

> *For mild cases of high blood pressure, massage is indicated to reduce physical stress and encourage the parasympathetic response within the body. In severe cases, massage is systemically contraindicated until such clients get their healthcare professional's approval to receive massage treatment.*

When clients come to you for massage therapy, their doctors may have prescribed blood pressure medications or dietary changes such as reduction of salt or fat intake.

EDEMA

Edema is a lymphatic condition that occurs when excess fluid is retained between the cells. It is characterized by puffy and swollen tissue in any body area where fluid is retained.

> *When edema is related to immobility, inactivity, or musculoskeletal injury, massage is indicated.*

It can help return the lymphatic fluid to the heart by increasing the client's circulation.

> *Massage is systemically contraindicated for edema when a doctor has diagnosed a specific pathological condition, because massage can potentially make the condition and the resulting edema worse.*

Medical prescriptions for edema with an underlying pathological cause include diuretic medications that reduce the blood volume in the body by excreting more water via urine.

FEVER

Fever is the body's immune system response that raises the body's core temperature above the normal 98.6°F. Usually the result of a bacterial or viral infection, the body elevates its core temperature (brings on fever) to help destroy the invading bacteria or virus. Increased body temperature stimulates leukocyte production, prevents bacterial and viral growth by limiting the liver's release of iron, stimulates antiviral agent (interferon) production, increases the heart rate to circulate more leukocytes, and speeds

up chemical reactions and cell wall permeability. The disadvantage of fever is the accompanying discomfort. In the case of high fever involving temperatures over 104°F, complications may arise. Blood chemistry falls out of balance, and dehydration and brain damage are possible.

> *During fever, massage is strictly contraindicated because the body is going through an acute healing process.*

Respiratory System Conditions

The common cold is a viral infection of the upper respiratory tract. It may be characterized by mild fever, headache, sore throat, postnasal drip, congestion, and coughing.

> *Massage is contraindicated in the acute stage (24 to 72 hours) of a cold or if fever is present. Massage is indicated for a cold in the subacute stage (after 72 hours).*

All treatments other than massage are typically prescribed by the client's healthcare professional but many people self-prescribe for the common cold. Treatments for a cold may include rest, increased fluid intake, over-the-counter antihistamine medications, decongestants, and cough suppressants.

Digestive System Conditions

Ulcers are open sores in the digestive tract that have not healed properly. They are accompanied by burning pain in the stomach.

> *Massage is locally contraindicated for ulcers in the abdominal region.*

This condition is diagnosed by a healthcare professional who may prescribe antibiotic medication.

Urinary System Conditions

Urinary tract infection (UTI) is, by definition, an infection of the urinary tract. It is recognized by pain and burning sensations during urination as well as an increase in the frequency and urgency of urination. The urine may be cloudy or tinged with blood, and fever may or may not be present.

> **!** *Massage is systemically contraindicated in the acute stage of a UTI. In the subacute stage, massage is locally contraindicated in the abdominal region for UTI, but whole-body massage is indicated.*

Clients with professionally diagnosed UTI will typically be using prescription antibiotics and will be drinking extra water and cranberry juice. With the symptoms of UTI and because of their increased fluid intake, you will need to be aware of their need to use the bathroom during a massage session.

Reproductive System Conditions

Massage mechanically increases circulation to help maintain the health of reproductive organs. Massage can provide some relief from symptoms by reducing the stress level and by increasing circulation. Since relaxation massage induces a parasympathetic nervous response, all of the parasympathetic effects can occur, including penile erection.

BREAST CANCER

Breast cancer is malignant tumor growth in the breast tissue that may spread to the skin, muscles, lymph nodes, and the rest of the body. Although men are also diagnosed with breast cancer, most cases occur in women. Breast cancer is characterized by a small, often painless lump or thickening of the breast tissue and can be detected by mammogram.

Massage for cancer patients is a controversial subject. The treating physician should be included in the decision to include massage as part of the client's healthcare regimen, and many physicians will advise against massage.

> **!** *If you massage a client with cancer, local contraindications include any areas that are affected by edema, surgery, soreness, or numbness. With breast cancer patients, the lymph nodes, especially in the axillary area, should be avoided.*

Clients who have lost their hair because of chemotherapy treatment may especially enjoy having their scalps massaged. Medical treatment for breast cancer may include surgery, radiation treatment or chemotherapy to reduce the growth of the tumor/s, and hormone therapy.

PROSTATE CANCER

Prostate cancer occurs when malignant tumor cells are found in the prostate gland, and diagnosis is officially made by a medical doctor.

> **!** *Massage may be indicated for prostate cancer, but only if approved by the client's healthcare professional.*

Treatments prescribed by the doctor may include radiation or chemotherapy, which may reduce the growth of the tumor, or hormone therapy.

PREGNANCY

Pregnancy is not a dysfunction or pathological condition. It is, however, a special condition of the reproductive system that massage therapists must understand. During pregnancy, a woman's body undergoes many hormonal, chemical, and physical changes that require special attention during a massage. Pregnant women often suffer nausea and vomiting during the early stages of pregnancy. As the body constantly changes shape and balance, the proprioceptors constantly provide different information regarding muscle tension and position. The pregnant woman cannot "get used to" a balanced posture and can feel clumsy or uncoordinated. To make matters worse, ligaments are hormonally triggered to loosen up toward the end of pregnancy, destabilizing the pelvis. The fetus can put pressure on circulatory structures, causing complications, and the size and weight of the baby can make almost any position uncomfortable.

> **!** *In an uncomplicated pregnancy, massage is indicated with specific considerations for each trimester.*

More specific information regarding pregnancy is covered in the Special Populations chapter.

Chapter Summary

Knowing the structures and functions of the body and knowing how massage can affect these structures can help you deliver safe and effective treatment.

Massage affects the basic unit of life and, ultimately, the organism. It also gives you an opportunity to educate clients about how anatomical and physiological changes affect their health and well-being.

The main function of the skeletal muscles is to create movement, and restoration of the most functional movement is often the goal of massage therapy. Understanding the attachment points and actions of the muscles in this chapter is especially important because it means you know the structures you are manipulating, both to create benefit and avoid damage. Although massage focuses on the muscular system, massage therapy deals with all of the body systems. All of the body systems must cooperate for a person to function normally, and the interrelationships between the body systems are a critical part of the big picture of health.

You may want to supplement this text with a book that is dedicated to anatomy and physiology for more thorough information. Countless anatomy and physiology texts are available in libraries and stores, some of which are listed in the suggested reading section at the end of the chapter.

SPECIAL MUSCLE SECTION

Action/ Movement	Muscle	Origin	Insertion (bone that is moved is CAPITALIZED)	Nerve (spinal segment nerve numbers)	Plates
Shoulder					
Elevation	Levator scapula	Transverse processes of C1-C4	Medial border of SCAPULA	Cervical & dorsal scapular (C3,4,5)	Pl. 4-1
	Rhomboid major	C7, T1-T5	Medial border of SCAPULA	Dorsal scapular (C4,5)	Pl. 4-1
	Trapezius (upper)	Occiput, ligamentum nuchae	Lateral end of clavicle, lateral spine of SCAPULA	Accessory (C2,3,4)	Pl. 4-1
Depression	Serratus anterior	Outer surfaces of ribs 8-10	Anterior surface of medial border of SCAPULA	Long thoracic (C5,6,7)	Pl. 4-2
	Subclavius	Junction of first rib and costal cartilage	Inferior surface of CLAVICLE	Branch of brachial plexus (C5,6)	Pl. 4-3
	Trapezius (lower)	T4-12	Root of spine of SCAPULA	Accessory (C3,4)	Pl. 4-1
Protraction	Serratus anterior	Outer surfaces of ribs 8–10	Anterior surface of medial border of SCAPULA	Long thoracic (C5,6,7)	Pl. 4-2
Retraction	Rhomboid major	C7, T1-5	Medial border of SCAPULA	Dorsal scapular (C4,5)	Pl. 4-1
	Trapezius (middle)	Ligamentum nuchae, C7-T4	Spine of SCAPULA	Accessory (C3,4)	Pl. 4-1
Upward rotation	Serratus anterior	Outer surfaces of ribs 8-10	Anterior surface of medial border of SCAPULA	Long thoracic (C5,6,7)	Pl. 4-2
	Trapezius (lower)	T4-12	Root of spine of SCAPULA	Accessory (C3,4)	Pl. 4-1
	Trapezius (upper)	Occiput, ligamentum nuchae	Lateral end of clavicle, lateral spine of SCAPULA	Accessory (C2,3,4)	Pl. 4-1
Downward rotation	Levator scapula	Transverse processes of C1-C4	Medial border of SCAPULA	Cervical & dorsal scapular (C3,4,5)	Pl. 4-1
	Pectoralis minor	Anterior surface of ribs 3,4,5	Coracoid process of SCAPULA	Lateral pectoral (C5,6,7)	Pl. 4-3
	Rhomboid major	C7, T1-5	Medial border of SCAPULA	Dorsal scapular (C4,5)	Pl. 4-1
Forward rotation	Pectoralis minor	Anterior surface of ribs 3,4,5	Coracoid process of SCAPULA	Lateral pectoral (C5,6,7)	Pl. 4-3
Flexion	Coracobrachialis	Coracoid process of scapula	Medial side of middle of HUMERUS	Musculocutaneous (C5,6,7)	Pl. 4-4
	Deltoid (anterior)	Lateral third of clavicle	Deltoid tuberosity of HUMERUS	Axillary (C5,6)	Pl. 4-3
	Pectoralis major	Medial clavicle, sternum, costal cartilages of ribs 2–6	Greater tubercle of HUMERUS	Lateral and medial pectoral (C7,C8,T1)	Pl. 4-3

(continued)

SPECIAL MUSCLE SECTION *(Continued)*

Action/ Movement	Muscle	Origin	Insertion (bone that is moved is CAPITALIZED)	Nerve (spinal segment nerve numbers)	Plates
Shoulder *(continued)*					
Accessory muscles/assist flexion	Biceps brachii	Long head: supraglenoid tubercle of scapula; short head: coracoid process of scapula	Tuberosity of RADIUS	Musculocutaneous (C5,6)	Pl. 4-4
	Subscapularis	Subscapular fossa on anterior scapula	Lesser tubercle of HUMERUS	Subscapular (C5,6,7)	Pl. 4-3
Extension	Deltoid (posterior)	Spine of scapula	Deltoid tuberosity of HUMERUS	Axillary (C5,6)	Pl. 4-3
	Latissimus dorsi	Thoracolumbar fascia, iliac crest, inferior angle of scapula, spinous processes of T7-S3)	Bicipital groove of HUMERUS	Thoracodorsal, brachial plexus (C6,7,8)	Pl. 4-1
	Teres major	Lower third of scapula	Bicipital groove of HUMERUS	Upper and lower scapular (C5,6)	Pl. 4-1
Accessory muscles/assist flexion	Triceps brachii	Long head: infraglenoid tubercle of scapula; lateral head: upper third of posterior humerus; medial head: distal half of humerus	Olecranon process of ULNA	Radial (C6,7,8)	Pl. 4-4
Abduction	Deltoid	Anterior: lateral third of clavicle; middle: lateral acromion; posterior: spine of scapula	Deltoid tuberosity of HUMERUS	Axillary (C5,6)	Pl. 4-3
	Supraspinatus	Supraspinous fossa of scapula	Greater tubercle of HUMERUS	Suprascapular (C5,6)	Pl. 4-5
Accessory muscles/assist abduction	Biceps brachii (long head)	Supraglenoid tubercle of scapula	Tuberosity of RADIUS	Musculocutaneous (C5,6)	Pl. 4-4
	Infraspinatus	Infraspinous fossa of scapula	Greater tubercle of HUMERUS	Suprascapular (C5,6)	Pl. 4-5
Adduction	Latissimus dorsi	Thoracolumbar fascia, iliac crest, inferior angle of scapula, spinous processes of T7-S3	Bicipital groove of HUMERUS	Thoracodorsal, brachial plexus (C6,7,8)	Pl. 4-1
	Pectoralis major	Medial clavicle, sternum, costal cartilages of ribs 2-6	Greater tubercle of HUMERUS	Lateral and medial pectoral (C7,C8,T1)	Pl. 4-3
	Teres major	Lower third of scapula	Bicipital groove of HUMERUS	Upper and lower scapular (C5,6)	Pl. 4-1
Accessory muscles/assist adduction	Biceps brachii (short head)	Coracoid process of scapula	Tuberosity of RADIUS	Musculocutaneous (C5,6)	Pl. 4-4
	Coracobrachialis	Coracoid process of scapula	Middle of medial HUMERUS	Musculocutaneous (C5,6,7)	Pl. 4-4
	Teres minor	Upper axillary border of scapula	Greater tubercle of HUMERUS	Axillary (C5,6)	Pl. 4-5
Lateral rotation	Deltoid (posterior)	Spine of scapula	Deltoid tuberosity of HUMERUS	Axillary (C5,6)	Pl. 4-3
	Infraspinatus	Infraspinous fossa of scapula	Greater tubercle of HUMERUS	Suprascapular (C5,6)	Pl. 4-5

(continued)

SPECIAL MUSCLE SECTION *(Continued)*

Action/Movement	Muscle	Origin	Insertion (bone that is moved is CAPITALIZED)	Nerve (spinal segment nerve numbers)	Plates
Shoulder (continued)					
Lateral rotation *(continued)*	Teres minor	Upper axillary border of scapula	Greater tubercle of HUMERUS	Axillary (C5,6)	Pl. 4-5
Medial rotation	Anterior deltoid	Lateral third of clavicle	Deltoid tuberosity of HUMERUS	Axillary (C5,6)	Pl. 4-3
	Latissimus dorsi	Thoracolumbar fascia, iliac crest, inferior angle of scapula, spinous processes of T7-S3)	Bicipital groove of HUMERUS	Thoracodorsal, brachial plexus (C6,7,8)	Pl. 4-1
	Pectoralis major	Medial clavicle, sternum, costal cartilages of ribs 2–6	Greater tubercle of HUMERUS	Lateral and medial pectoral (C7,C8,T1)	Pl. 4-3
	Subscapularis	Subscapular fossa (anterior surface of scapula)	Lesser tubercle of HUMERUS	Subscapular (C5,6,7)	Pl. 4-5
	Teres major	Lower third of scapula	Bicipital groove of HUMERUS	Upper and lower scapular (C5,6)	Pl. 4-1
Elbow					
Flexion	Biceps brachii	Long head: supraglenoid tubercle of scapula; short head: coracoid process of scapula	Tuberosity of RADIUS	Musculocutaneous (C5,6)	Pl. 4-6
	Brachialis	Distal half of anterior humerus	Proximal tuberosity of ULNA	Musculocutaneous (C5,6,7)	Pl. 4-7
	Brachioradialis	Lateral, distal humerus	Styloid process, distal end of RADIUS	Radial (C5,6)	Pl. 4-7
Extension	Triceps brachii	Long head: infraglenoid tubercle of scapula; lateral head: upper third of posterior humerus; medial head: distal half of humerus	Olecranon process of ULNA	Radial (C6,7,8)	Pl. 4-8
Assist extension/accessory muscles	Anconeus	Lateral epicondyle of humerus	Olecranon process of ULNA	Radial (C7,8)	Pl. 4-7
Pronation	Pronator quadratus	Anterior, distal ulna	Anterior, distal RADIUS	Median (C6,7)	Pl. 4-6
	Pronator teres	Medial epicondyle of humerus, coronoid process of ulna	Middle of lateral RADIUS	Median (C6,7)	Pl. 4-6
Assist pronation/accessory muscles	Anconeus	Lateral epicondyle of humerus	Olecranon process of ULNA	Radial (C7,8)	Pl. 4-7
	Brachioradialis	Lateral, distal humerus	Styloid process, distal end of RADIUS	Radial (C5,6)	Pl. 4-7
Supination	Biceps brachii	Long head: supraglenoid tubercle of scapula; short head: coracoid process of scapula	Tuberosity of RADIUS	Musculocutaneous (C5,6)	Pl. 4-6
	Supinator	Lateral epicondyle of humerus; proximal, posterior end of ulna	Anterior, proximal third of RADIUS	Radial (C6)	Pl. 4-6

(continued)

SPECIAL MUSCLE SECTION *(Continued)*

Action/ Movement	Muscle	Origin	Insertion (bone that is moved is CAPITALIZED)	Nerve (spinal segment nerve numbers)	Plates
Wrist					
Flexion	Flexor carpi radialis	Medial epicondyle of humerus	Bases of 2nd and 3rd METACARPALS	Median (C6,7)	Pl. 4-6
	Flexor carpi ulnaris	Lateral epicondyle of humerus	Base of 5th METACARPAL	Ulnar (C7,8)	Pl. 4-6
	Palmaris longus	Medial epicondyle of humerus	Palmar aponeurosis, anterior flexor retinaculum at PALM	Median (C7,8)	Pl. 4-6
Extension	Extensor carpi radialis brevis	Lateral epicondyle of humerus	Base of 3rd METACARPAL	Radial (C7,8)	Pl. 4-9
	Extensor carpi radialis longus	Lateral supracondylar ride of humerus	Dorsal 2nd METACARPAL	Radial (C7,8)	Pl. 4-9
	Extensor carpi ulnaris	Lateral epicondyle of humerus, posterior border of ulna	Base of 5th METACARPAL	Radial (C7,8)	Pl. 4-9
Abduction	Extensor carpi radialis brevis	Lateral epicondyle of humerus	Base of 3rd METACARPAL	Radial (C7,8)	Pl. 4-9
	Extensor carpi radialis longus	Lateral supracondylar ride of humerus	Dorsal 2nd METACARPAL	Radial (C7,8)	Pl. 4-9
	Flexor carpi radialis	Medial epicondyle of humerus	Bases of 2nd and 3rd METACARPALS	Median (C6,7)	Pl. 4-6
Adduction	Extensor carpi ulnaris	Lateral epicondyle of humerus, posterior border of ulna	Base of 5th METACARPAL	Radial (C7,8)	Pl. 4-9
	Flexor carpi ulnaris	Lateral epicondyle of humerus	Base of 5th METACARPAL	Ulnar (C7,8)	Pl. 4-6
Fingers					
Flexion	Flexor digitorum profundus				Pl. 4-6
	Flexor digitorum superficialis				Pl. 4-6
Extension	Extensor digiti minimi				Pl. 4-10
	Extensor digitorum				Pl. 4-10
	Extensor indices				Pl. 4-9
Abduction	Abductor digiti minimi				Pl. 4-11
	Abductor pollicis longus				Pl. 4-10
	Flexor digiti minimi				Pl. 4-11
	Interossei				Pl. 4-12
	Lumbricals				Pl. 4-12
	Opponens digiti minimi				Not pictured
Adduction	Dorsal interossei				Pl. 4-12
	Palmar interossei				Pl. 4-12

(continued)

SPECIAL MUSCLE SECTION *(Continued)*

Action/ Movement	Muscle	Origin	Insertion (bone that is moved is CAPITALIZED)	Nerve (spinal segment nerve numbers)	Plates
Thumb					
Adduction	Adductor pollicis				Pl. 4-12
Flexion	Flexor pollicis brevis				Pl. 4-11
	Flexor pollicis longus				Pl. 4-12
Extension	Extensor pollicis brevis				Pl. 4-10
	Extensor pollicis longus				Pl. 4-9
Opposition	Opponens pollicis				Pl. 4-11
Abduction	Abductor pollicis brevis				Pl. 4-11
Hip					
Flexion	Gluteus medius	External iliac fossa	Lateral, greater trochanter of FEMUR	Superior gluteal (L5,S1)	Pl. 4-13
	Gluteus minimus	External iliac fossa (anterior to gluteus medius)	Greater trochanter of FEMUR	Superior gluteal (L5,S1)	Pl. 4-13
	Gracilis	Inferior pubis	Medial, upper TIBIA	Obturator (L2,3,4)	Pl. 4-15, 16
	Iliacus	Iliac fossa, lateral sacrum	Greater psoas tendon, lesser trochanter of FEMUR	Femoral (L2,3)	Pl. 4-14
	Pectineus	Lateral pubis	Lesser trochanter and posterior FEMUR	Obturator/sacral plexus (L2,3,4)	Pl. 4-15, 16
	Psoas major	T12, L1-4	Lesser trochanter of FEMUR	Lumbar plexus (L1,2,3)	Pl. 4-14
	Rectus femoris	Anterior, inferior iliac spine	Patellar tendon into tuberosity of TIBIA	Femoral (L2,3,4)	Pl. 4-15
	Sartorius	ASIS	Superior medial TIBIA	Femoral (L2,3,4)	Pl. 4-15, 16
	Tensor fascia latae	Iliac crest, ASIS	Iliotibial band into TIBIA and FIBULA	Superior gluteal (L4,5,S1)	Pl. 4-15, 17
Extension	Adductor magnus	Ramus of pubis, ramus of ischium, ischial tuberosity	Linea aspera and adductor tubercle of FEMUR	Sacral plexus (L4,5,S1,2,3)	Pl. 4-15, 16
	Biceps femoris	Ischial tuberosity, posterior femoral shaft	Head of FIBULA	Peroneal and sciatic (L4,5,S1,2)	Pl. 4-17
	Gluteus maximus	Upper outer ilium, sacrum, coccyx	Iliotibial band, posterior FEMUR	Inferior gluteal (L5,S1,2)	Pl. 4-13
	Gluteus minimus	External iliac fossa (anterior to gluteus medius)	Greater trochanter of FEMUR	Superior gluteal (L5,S1)	Pl. 4-13
	Semimembranosus	Lateral ischial tuberosity	Medial condyle of TIBIA	Sciatic (L4,5,S1,2,3)	Pl. 4-17
	Semitendinosus	Ischial tuberosity	Upper, medial TIBIA near tibial tuberosity	Sciatic (L4,5,S1,2,3)	Pl. 4-17

(continued)

SPECIAL MUSCLE SECTION *(Continued)*

Action/ Movement	Muscle	Origin	Insertion (bone that is moved is CAPITALIZED)	Nerve (spinal segment nerve numbers)	Plates
Hip *(continued)*					
Abduction	Gemellus inferior	Upper ischial tuberosity	Medial greater trochanter of FEMUR	Sacral plexus (L4,5,S1,2,3)	Pl. 4-13
	Gemellus superior	Spine of ischium	Medial greater trochanter of FEMUR	Sacral plexus (L4,5,S1,2,3)	Pl. 4-13
	Gluteus maximus	Upper outer ilium, sacrum, coccyx	Iliotibial band, posterior FEMUR	Inferior gluteal (L5,S1,2)	Pl. 4-13
	Gluteus medius	External iliac fossa	Lateral, greater trochanter of FEMUR	Superior gluteal (L5,S1)	Pl. 4-13
	Gluteus minimus	External iliac fossa (anterior to gluteus medius)	Greater trochanter of FEMUR	Superior gluteal (L5,S1)	Pl. 4-13
	Obturator externus	External margin of obturator foramen, obturator membrane	Medial greater trochanter of FEMUR	Sacral plexus (L4,5,S1,2,3)	Pl. 4-13
	Obturator internus	Internal margin of obturator foramen, obturator membrane	Medial greater trochanter of FEMUR	Sacral plexus (L4,5,S1,2,3)	Pl. 4-17
	Piriformis	Anterior sacrum, ilium near posterior iliac spine	Greater trochanter of FEMUR	Sacral plexus (L4,5,S1,2,3)	Pl. 4-13, 17
	Sartorius	ASIS	Superior medial TIBIA	Femoral (L2,3,4)	Pl. 4-15, 16
	Tensor fascia latae	Iliac crest, ASIS	Iliotibial band into TIBIA and FIBULA	Superior gluteal (L4,5,S1)	Pl. 4-15, 17
Adduction	Adductor brevis	Medial ramus of pubis	Linea aspera of FEMUR	Sacral plexus (L4,5,S1,2,3)	Pl. 4-15, 16
	Adductor longus	Anterior pubis	Linea aspera of FEMUR	Sacral plexus (L4,5,S1,2,3)	Pl. 4-15, 16
	Adductor magnus	Ramus of pubis, ramus of ischium, ischial tuberosity	Linea aspera and adductor tubercle of FEMUR	Sacral plexus (L4,5,S1,2,3)	Pl. 4-15, 16
	Biceps femoris	Ischial tuberosity, posterior femoral shaft	Head of FIBULA	Peroneal and sciatic (L4,5,S1,2)	Pl. 4-17
	Gluteus maximus	Upper outer ilium, sacrum, coccyx	Iliotibial band, posterior FEMUR	Inferior gluteal (L5,S1,2)	Pl. 4-13
	Gracilis	Inferior pubis	Medial, upper TIBIA	Obturator (L2,3,4)	Pl. 4-15, 16
	Iliacus	Iliac fossa, lateral sacrum	Greater psoas tendon, lesser trochanter of FEMUR	Femoral (L2,3)	Pl. 4-14
	Pectineus	Lateral pubis	Lesser trochanter and posterior FEMUR	Obturator/sacral plexus (L2,3,4)	Pl. 4-15, 16
	Psoas major	T12, L1-4	Lesser trochanter of FEMUR	Lumbar plexus (L1,2,3)	Pl. 4-14
Medial rotation	Gluteus medius	External iliac fossa	Lateral, greater trochanter of FEMUR	Superior gluteal (L5,S1)	Pl. 4-13
	Gluteus minimus	External iliac fossa (anterior to gluteus medius)	Greater trochanter of FEMUR	Superior gluteal (L5,S1)	Pl. 4-13
	Tensor fascia latae	Iliac crest, ASIS	Iliotibial band into TIBIA and FIBULA	Superior gluteal (L4,5,S1)	Pl. 4-15, 17

(continued)

SPECIAL MUSCLE SECTION *(Continued)*

Action/ Movement	Muscle	Origin	Insertion (bone that is moved is CAPITALIZED)	Nerve (spinal segment nerve numbers)	Plates
Hip *(continued)*					
Lateral rotation	Adductor brevis	Medial ramus of pubis	Linea aspera of FEMUR	Sacral plexus (L4,5,S1,2,3)	Pl. 4-15, 16
	Adductor longus	Anterior pubis	Linea aspera of FEMUR	Sacral plexus (L4,5,S1,2,3)	Pl. 4-15, 16
	Adductor magnus	Ramus of pubis, ramus of ischium, ischial tuberosity	Linea aspera and adductor tubercle of FEMUR	Sacral plexus (L4,5,S1,2,3)	Pl. 4-15, 16
	Biceps femoris	Ischial tuberosity, posterior femoral shaft	Head of FIBULA	Peroneal and sciatic (L4,5,S1,2)	Pl. 4-17
	Gemellus inferior	Upper ischial tuberosity	Medial greater trochanter of FEMUR	Sacral plexus (L4,5,S1,2,3)	Pl. 4-13
	Gemellus superior	Spine of ischium	Medial greater trochanter of FEMUR	Sacral plexus (L4,5,S1,2,3)	Pl. 4-13
	Gluteus maximus	Upper outer ilium, sacrum, coccyx	Iliotibial band, posterior FEMUR	Inferior gluteal (L5,S1,2)	Pl. 4-13
	Obturator externus	External margin of obturator foramen, obturator membrane	Medial greater trochanter of FEMUR	Sacral plexus (L4,5,S1,2,3)	Pl. 4-13
	Obturator internus	Internal margin of obturator foramen, obturator membrane	Medial greater trochanter of FEMUR	Sacral plexus (L4,5,S1,2,3)	Pl. 4-17
	Piriformis	Anterior sacrum, ilium near posterior iliac spine	Greater trochanter of FEMUR	Sacral plexus (L4,5,S1,2,3)	Pl. 4-13, 17
	Quadratus femoris	Upper, lateral ischial tuberosity	Posterior greater trochanter of FEMUR	Sacral plexus (L4,5,S1,2,3)	Pl. 4-13
Knee					
Flexion	Biceps femoris	Ischial tuberosity, posterior femoral shaft	Head of FIBULA	Peroneal and sciatic (L4,5,S1,2)	Pl. 4-17
	Gastrocnemius	Femoral condyles	Achilles tendon into CALCANEUS	Tibial (S1,2)	Pl. 4-20
	Gracilis	Inferior pubis	Medial, upper TIBIA	Obturator (L2,3,4)	Pl. 4-15, 16
	Popliteus	Lateral femoral condyle	Posterior, medial shaft of TIBIA	Tibial (S1,2)	Pl. 4-20
	Sartorius	ASIS	Superior medial TIBIA	Femoral (L2,3,4)	Pl. 4-15, 16
	Semimembranosus	Lateral ischial tuberosity	Medial condyle of TIBIA	Sciatic (L4,5,S1,2,3)	Pl. 4-17
	Semitendinosus	Ischial tuberosity	Upper, medial TIBIA near tibial tuberosity	Sciatic (L4,5,S1,2,3)	Pl. 4-17
Extension	Rectus femoris	Anterior, inferior iliac spine	Patellar tendon into tuberosity of TIBIA	Femoral (L2,3,4)	Pl. 4-15
	Tensor fascia latae	Iliac crest, ASIS	Iliotibial band into TIBIA and FIBULA	Superior gluteal (L4,5,S1)	Pl. 4-15, 17
	Vastus intermedius	Anterior, upper 2/3 of femur	Patellar tendon into TIBIA	Femoral (L2,3,4)	Pl. 4-15
	Vastus lateralis	Lateral, upper femur	Patellar tendon into TIBIA	Femoral (L2,3,4)	Pl. 4-15
	Vastus medialis	Medial femur	Patellar tendon into TIBIA	Femoral (L2,3,4)	Pl. 4-15

(continued)

SPECIAL MUSCLE SECTION *(Continued)*

Action/ Movement	Muscle	Origin	Insertion (bone that is moved is CAPITALIZED)	Nerve (spinal segment nerve numbers)	Plates
Knee (continued)					
Medial rotation	Gracilis	Inferior pubis	Medial, upper TIBIA	Obturator (L2,3,4)	Pl. 4-15, 16
	Popliteus	Lateral femoral condyle	Posterior, medial shaft of TIBIA	Tibial (S1,2)	Pl. 4-20
	Sartorius	ASIS	Superior medial TIBIA	Femoral (L2,3,4)	Pl. 4-15, 16
	Semimembranosus	Lateral ischial tuberosity	Medial condyle of TIBIA	Sciatic (L4,5,S1,2,3)	Pl. 4-17
	Semitendinosus	Ischial tuberosity	Upper, medial TIBIA near tibial tuberosity	Sciatic (L4,5,S1,2,3)	Pl. 4-17
Lateral rotation	Biceps femoris	Ischial tuberosity, posterior femoral shaft	Head of FIBULA	Peroneal and sciatic (L4,5,S1,2)	Pl. 4-17
	Gluteus maximus	Upper outer ilium, sacrum, coccyx	Iliotibial band, posterior FEMUR	Inferior gluteal (L5,S1,2)	Pl. 4-13
	Tensor fascia latae	Iliac crest, ASIS	Iliotibial band into TIBIA and FIBULA	Superior gluteal (L4,5,S1)	Pl. 4-15, 17
Ankle/foot					
Dorsiflexion	Extensor digitorum longus	Medial, upper 3/4 of fibula and lateral condyle of tibia	Dorsal aponeurosis of middle and distal PHALANGES	Deep peroneal (L5,S1)	Pl. 4-19
	Extensor hallucis longus	Middle of fibula	Dorsal distal PHALANX of big toe	Deep peroneal (L5,S1)	Pl. 4-18
	Peroneus tertius	Inferior fibula	METATARSAL V	Peroneal (L4,5,S1,2)	Pl. 4-19
	Tibialis anterior	Lateral condyle and shaft of tibia	Base of METATARSAL I	Deep peroneal (L4,5)	Pl. 4-18
Plantarflexion	Flexor digitorum longus	Posterior, middle half of tibia	Distal PHALANGES II-V	Tibial (S2,3)	Pl. 4-19, 20
	Flexor hallucis longus	Lower, posterior 2/3 of fibula	Bottom of distal PHALANX I	Tibial (S2,3)	Pl. 4-19, 20
	Gastrocnemius	Femoral condyles	Achilles tendon into CALCANEUS	Tibial (S1,2)	Pl. 4-20
	Peroneus brevis	Inferior, lateral fibula	Base of METATARSAL V	Peroneal (L4,5,S1,2)	Pl. 4-21
	Peroneus longus	Lateral head of fibula	Base of METATARSAL I	Peroneal (L4,5,S1,2)	Pl. 4-21
	Soleus	Proximal tibia and fibula	Achilles tendon into CALCANEUS	Peroneal (L4,5,S1,2,3)	Pl. 4-20
	Tibialis posterior	Tibia and fibula	TARSALS and METATARSALS	Tibial (L4,5,S1,2,3)	Pl. 4-20
Eversion (pronation/ abduction)	Extensor digitorum longus	Medial, upper 3/4 of fibula and lateral condyle of tibia	Dorsal aponeurosis of middle and distal PHALANGES	Deep peroneal (L5,S1)	Pl. 4-19
	Peroneus brevis	Inferior, lateral fibula	Base of METATARSAL V	Peroneal (L4,5,S1,2)	Pl. 4-21
	Peroneus longus	Lateral head of fibula	Base of METATARSAL I	Peroneal (L4,5,S1,2)	Pl. 4-21
	Peroneus tertius	Inferior fibula	METATARSAL V	Peroneal (L4,5,S1,2)	Pl. 4-21
Inversion (supination/ adduction)	Extensor hallucis longus	Middle of fibula	Dorsal distal PHALANX of big toe	Deep peroneal (L5,S1)	Pl. 4-18
	Flexor digitorum longus	Posterior, middle half of tibia	Distal PHALANGES II-V	Tibial (S2,3)	Pl. 4-19
	Flexor hallucis longus	Lower, posterior 2/3 of fibula	Bottom of distal PHALANX I	Tibial (S2,3)	Pl. 4-19
	Gastrocnemius	Femoral condyles	Achilles tendon into CALCANEUS	Tibial (S1,2)	Pl. 4-20

(continued)

SPECIAL MUSCLE SECTION *(Continued)*

Action/ Movement	Muscle	Origin	Insertion (bone that is moved is CAPITALIZED)	Nerve (spinal segment nerve numbers)	Plates
Ankle/foot (continued)					
Inversion (supination/ adduction) *(continued)*	Soleus	Proximal tibia and fibula	Achilles tendon into CALCANEUS	Peroneal (L4,5,S1,2,3)	Pl. 4-20
	Tibialis anterior	Lateral condyle and shaft of tibia	Base of METATARSAL I	Deep peroneal (L4,5)	Pl. 4-18
	Tibialis posterior	Tibia and fibula	TARSALS and METATARSALS	Tibial (L4,5,S1,2,3)	Pl. 4-20
	Foot muscles, dorsal view				Pl. 4-22
	Foot muscles, plantar view				Pl. 4-23
Spine/thorax					
Flexion	External obliques	Inferior ribs 5-12	Anterior ILIAC crest, linea alba	Intercostal (T7-12, L1)	Pl. 4-24, 25
	Internal obliques	Anterior iliac crest	Inferior RIBS 10-12, linea alba, PUBIS	Intercostal (T7-12, L1)	Pl. 4-24, 25
	Rectus abdominis	Pubic crest and pubic symphysis	Costal cartilages (RIBS), xiphoid process of STERNUM	Intercostal (T5-12)	Pl. 4-24, 25
Extension	Erector spinae group (ilio- costalis, longis- simus, spinalis)	Large group, multiple origins, from thora- columbar aponeuro- sis, ribs, spinous processes of verte- brae	Insertions are superior to the origins, ranging from the posterior RIBS to the mastoid process of the TEMPORAL bone and OCCIPUT	Spinal nerves (T1-12, L1-5, S1-3)	Pl. 4-27
	Multifidi	Articular processes C4-C7, transverse processes T1-12, posterior sacrum, posterior iliac spine	Spine of VERTEBRA supe- rior to origin, from one to three vertebrae higher	All spinal nerves (C1-S4)	Pl. 4-27
	Rotatores	Transverse processes C1-L5	Lamina of VERTEBRA di- rectly superior to origin	Spinal nerves (C1-S4)	Pl. 4-27
Lateral flexion/ hip elevation	External obliques	Inferior ribs 5–12	Anterior ILIAC crest, linea alba	Intercostal (T7-12, L1)	Pl. 4-24, 25
	Internal obliques	Anterior iliac crest	Inferior RIBS 10-12, linea alba, PUBIS	Intercostal (T7-12, L1)	Pl. 4-24, 25
	Quadratus lum- borum	Thoracolumbar aponeurosis, iliac crest	12th RIB, VERTEBRAE L1-4	Lumbar plexus (T12,L1,2,3)	Pl. 4-24, 25
Rotation	External obliques	Inferior ribs 5-12	Anterior ILIAC crest, linea alba	Intercostal (T7-12, L1)	Pl. 4-24, 25
	Internal obliques	Anterior iliac crest	Inferior RIBS 10-12, linea alba, PUBIS	Intercostal (T7-12, L1)	Pl. 4-24, 25
	Multifidi	Articular processes C4-C7, transverse processes T1-12, posterior sacrum, posterior iliac spine	Spine of VERTEBRA supe- rior to origin, from one to three vertebrae higher	All spinal nerves (C1-S4)	Pl. 4-27
	Rotatores	Transverse processes C1-L5	Lamina of VERTEBRA di- rectly superior to origin	Spinal nerves (C1-S4)	Pl. 4-27
Muscles of respiration					
Exhalation	External obliques	Inferior ribs 5–12	Anterior ILIAC crest, linea alba	Intercostal (T7-12, L1)	Pl. 4-24, 25

(continued)

SPECIAL MUSCLE SECTION *(Continued)*

Action/ Movement	Muscle	Origin	Insertion (bone that is moved is CAPITALIZED)	Nerve (spinal segment nerve numbers)	Plates
Muscles of respiration *(continued)*					
Exhalation *(continued)*	Internal intercostals (posterior)	Lower border of ribs, costal cartilage	Upper border of RIB and costal cartilage just inferior to origin	Intercostal (T1-12)	Pl. 4-26
	Internal obliques	Anterior iliac crest	Inferior RIBS 10-12, linea alba, PUBIS	Intercostal (T7-12, L1)	Pl. 4-24, 25
	Rectus abdominis	Pubic crest and pubic symphysis	Costal cartilages (RIBS), xiphoid process of STERNUM	Intercostal (T5-12)	Pl. 4-24, 25
	Transversus abdominis	Thoracolumbar aponeurosis, iliac crest	Abdominal aponeurosis, pubis, linea alba	Intercostal (T7-12,L1)	Pl. 4-24, 25
Inhalation	Diaphragm	Ribs 7–12, costal cartilages, xiphoid process, L1-3	Central tendon of DIAPHRAGM	Phrenic (C3,4,5)	Pl. 4-26
	External intercostals	Lower border of ribs	Upper border of RIB just inferior to origin	Intercostal (T1-12)	Pl. 4-26
	Internal intercostals (anterior)	Lower border of ribs, costal cartilage	Upper border of RIB and costal cartilage just inferior to origin	Intercostal (T1-12)	Pl. 4-26
	Scalenus anterior	Transverse processes C2-5	First RIB	Cervical plexus (C1-7, T1)	Pl. 4-28
	Scalenus medius	Transverse processes of C1-6	First RIB	Cervical plexus (C1-7,T1)	Pl. 4-28
	Scalenus posterior	Transverse processes of C4-6	Second RIB	Cervical plexus (C1-7,T1)	Pl. 4-28
Neck					
Extension	Erector spinae group (iliocostalis, longissimus, spinalis)	Large group, multiple origins, from thoracolumbar aponeurosis, ribs, spinous processes of vertebrae	Insertions are superior to the origins, ranging from the posterior RIBS to the mastoid process of the TEMPORAL bone and OCCIPUT	Spinal nerves (T1-12, L1-5, S1-3)	Pl. 4-27
	Levator scapulae	Transverse processes C1-4	Vertebral border of superior SCAPULA	Scapular (C4,5)	Pl. 4-34
	Multifidi	Articular processes C4-C7, transverse processes T1-12, posterior sacrum, posterior iliac spine	Spine of VERTEBRA superior to origin, from one to three vertebrae higher	All spinal nerves (C1-S4)	Pl. 4-34
	Rotatores	Transverse processes C1-L5	Lamina of VERTEBRA directly superior to origin	Spinal nerves (C1-S4)	Pl. 4-34
	Semispinalis	Transverse processes C4-T6	OCCIPUT, spinous processes VERTEBRAE C2-6	Cervical, thoracic (C4,5,6)	Pl. 4-33
	Splenius capitis	Spinous processes of C7-T3	Mastoid process of TEMPORAL bone	Cervical (C3-5)	Pl. 4-33
	Splenius cervicis	Spinous processes T3-6	Transverse processes of VERTEBRAE C2-4	Cervical (C4-6)	Pl. 4-33
	Trapezius (upper)	Occiput, ligamentum nuchae	Lateral end of clavicle, lateral spine of SCAPULA	Accessory (C2,3,4)	Pl. 4-33
Flexion	Scalenes	Transverse processes C2-7	First and second RIBS	Cervical plexus (C1-7, T1)	Pl. 4-28
	Sternocleidomastoid	Sternal head, medial clavicle	Mastoid process of TEMOPORAL bone, OCCIPUT	Accessory (C2,3)	Pl. 4-30, 31

(continued)

SPECIAL MUSCLE SECTION *(Continued)*

Action/ Movement	Muscle	Origin	Insertion (bone that is moved is CAPITALIZED)	Nerve (spinal segment nerve numbers)	Plates
Neck *(continued)*					
Lateral flexion	Levator scapulae	Transverse processes C1-4	Vertebral border of superior SCAPULA	Scapular (C4,5)	Pl. 4-34
	Sternocleidomastoid	Sternal head, medial clavicle	Mastoid process of TEMOPORAL bone, OCCIPUT	Accessory (C2,3)	Pl. 4-30, 31
	Trapezius (upper)	Occiput, ligamentum nuchae	Lateral end of clavicle, lateral spine of SCAPULA	Accessory (C2,3,4)	Pl. 4-33
Rotation	Levator scapulae	Transverse processes C1-4	Vertebral border of superior SCAPULA	Scapular (C4,5)	Pl. 4-34
	Multifidi	Articular processes C4-C7, transverse processes T1-12, posterior sacrum, posterior iliac spine	Spine of VERTEBRA superior to origin, from one to three vertebrae higher	All spinal nerves (C1-S4)	Pl. 4-34
	Rotatores	Transverse processes C1-L5	Lamina of VERTEBRA directly superior to origin	Spinal nerves (C1-S4)	Pl. 4-34
	Sternocleidomastoid	Sternal head, medial clavicle	Mastoid process of TEMOPORAL bone, OCCIPUT	Accessory (C2,3)	Pl. 4-30, 31
	Trapezius (upper)	Occiput, ligamentum nuchae	Lateral end of clavicle, lateral spine of SCAPULA	Accessory (C2,3,4)	Pl. 4-33
	Deep neck muscles				Pl. 4-32
Temporomandibular joint					
Elevation (closes the jaw)	Temporalis	Lateral temporal bone	Coronoid process and anterior ramus of MANDIBLE	Trigeminal (cranial V)	Pl. 4-29
	Masseter	Zygomatic arch	Angle and lateral surface of MANDIBLE	Trigeminal (cranial V)	Pl. 4-29
	Medial pterygoid	Medial pterygoid Pl.	TMJ capsule, condyle of MANDIBLE	Trigeminal (cranial V)	Pl. 4-29
Depression (opens the jaw)	Platysma	Fascia of superior thorax	Lower border of MANDIBLE, fascia around chin	Facial (cranial VII)	Pl. 4-31
	Lateral pterygoid	Lateral pterygoid Pl.	Angle of MANDIBLE	Trigeminal (cranial V)	Pl. 4-29
Accessory muscles/assist depression	Suprahyoids (digastric, geniohyoid, mylohyoid, stylohyoid)	Inferior mandible, mastoid process, styloid process of temporal bone	HYOID bone	Facial (cranial VII)	Pl. 4-35
Protraction	Lateral pterygoid	Lateral pterygoid Pl.	Angle of MANDIBLE	Trigeminal (cranial V)	Pl. 4-29
	Medial pterygoid	Medial pterygoid Pl.	TMJ capsule, condyle of MANDIBLE	Trigeminal (cranial V)	Pl. 4-29
	Masseter	Zygomatic arch	Angle and lateral surface of MANDIBLE	Trigeminal (cranial V)	Pl. 4-29
Retraction	Temporalis	Lateral temporal bone	Coronoid process and anterior ramus of MANDIBLE	Trigeminal (cranial V)	Pl. 4-29
Lateral deviation	Masseter	Zygomatic arch	Angle and lateral surface of MANDIBLE	Trigeminal (cranial V)	Pl. 4-29
	Lateral pterygoid	Lateral pterygoid Pl.	Angle of MANDIBLE	Trigeminal (cranial V)	Pl. 4-29

All plates referenced in the table above are reprinted from Clay JH, Pounds DM. Basic Clinical Massage Therapy: Integrating Anatomy and Treatment. Baltimore: Lippincott Williams & Wilkins, 2003.

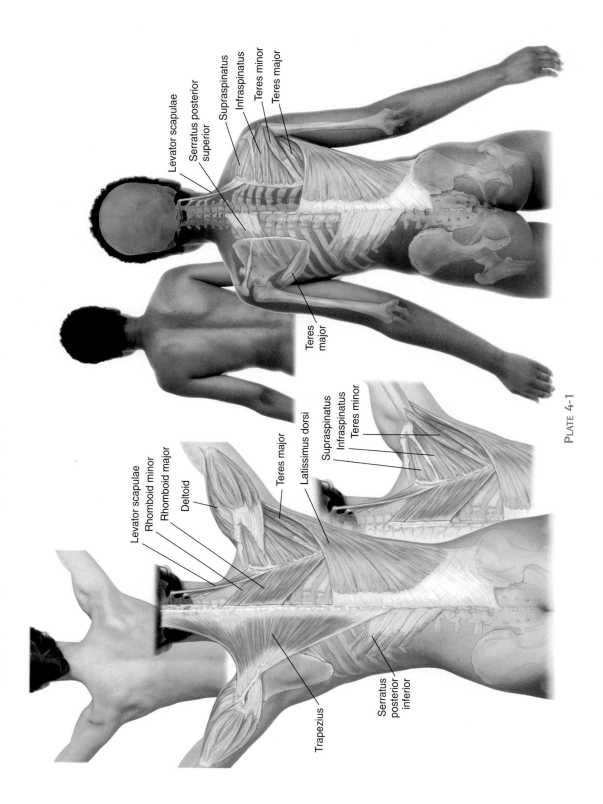

Levator scapulae
Serratus posterior superior
Supraspinatus
Infraspinatus
Teres minor
Teres major
Teres major

Levator scapulae
Rhomboid minor
Rhomboid major
Deltoid
Teres major
Latissimus dorsi
Supraspinatus
Infraspinatus
Teres minor
Trapezius
Serratus posterior inferior

PLATE 4-1

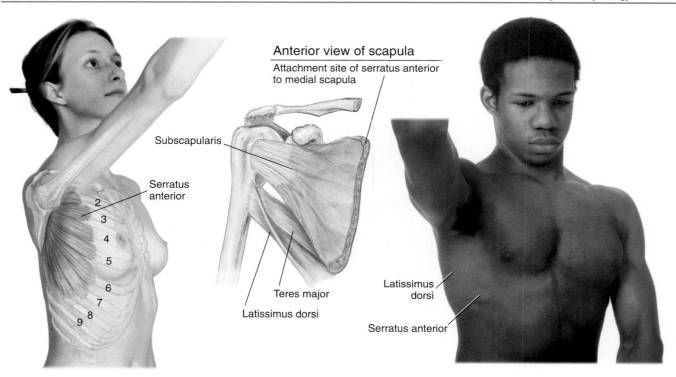

Serratus anterior

2
3
4
5
6
7
8
9

Anterior view of scapula

Attachment site of serratus anterior to medial scapula

Subscapularis

Teres major

Latissimus dorsi

Latissimus dorsi

Serratus anterior

PLATE 4-2

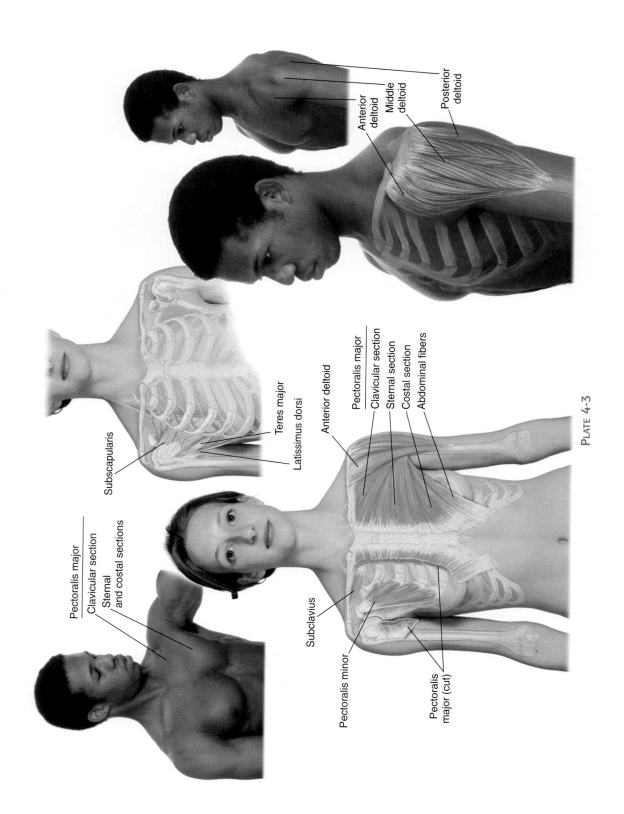

Subscapularis

Teres major

Latissimus dorsi

Anterior deltoid

Anterior deltoid

Middle deltoid

Posterior deltoid

Pectoralis major
Clavicular section
Sternal section
Costal section
Abdominal fibers

Pectoralis major
Clavicular section
Sternal
and costal sections

Subclavius

Pectoralis minor

Pectoralis
major (cut)

PLATE 4-3

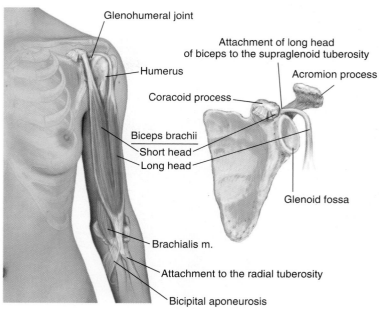

Glenohumeral joint

Attachment of long head of biceps to the supraglenoid tuberosity

Humerus

Acromion process

Coracoid process

Biceps brachii
Short head
Long head

Glenoid fossa

Brachialis m.

Attachment to the radial tuberosity

Bicipital aponeurosis

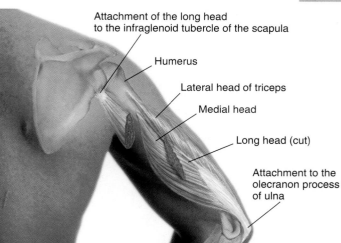

Attachment of the long head to the infraglenoid tubercle of the scapula

Humerus

Lateral head of triceps

Medial head

Long head (cut)

Attachment to the olecranon process of ulna

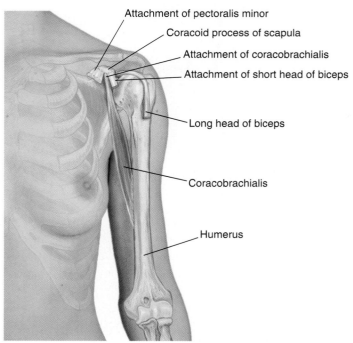

Attachment of pectoralis minor

Coracoid process of scapula

Attachment of coracobrachialis

Attachment of short head of biceps

Long head of biceps

Coracobrachialis

Humerus

PLATE 4-4

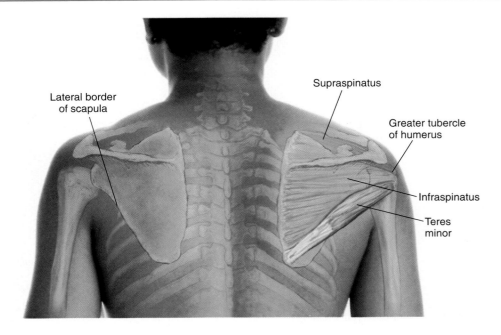

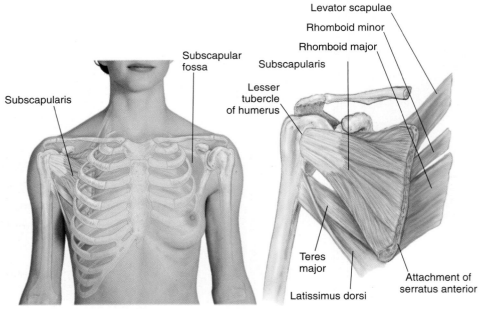

PLATE 4-5

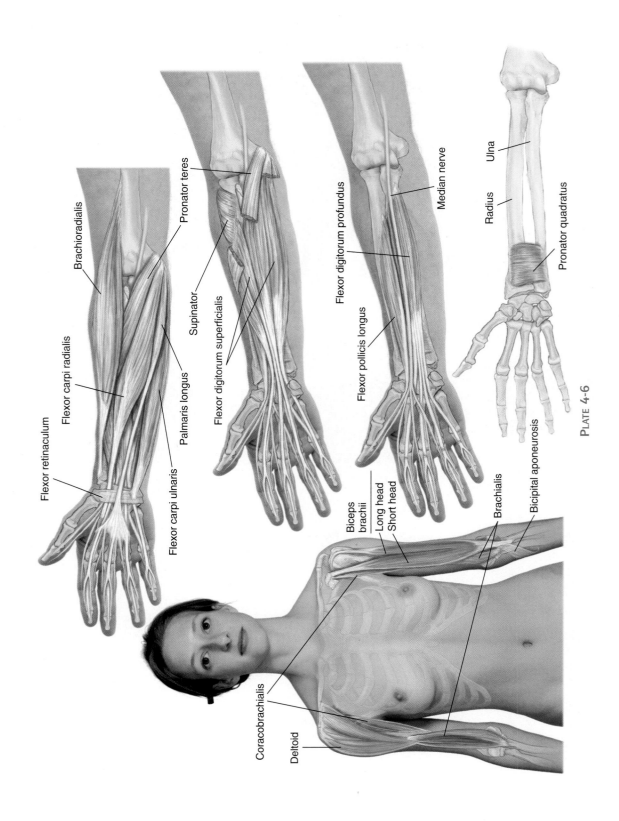

Brachioradialis

Flexor carpi radialis

Flexor retinaculum

Palmaris longus

Flexor carpi ulnaris

Pronator teres

Supinator

Flexor digitorum superficialis

Flexor digitorum profundus

Median nerve

Flexor pollicis longus

Radius

Ulna

Pronator quadratus

Biceps brachii — Long head / Short head

Brachialis

Bicipital aponeurosis

Coracobrachialis

Deltoid

PLATE 4-6

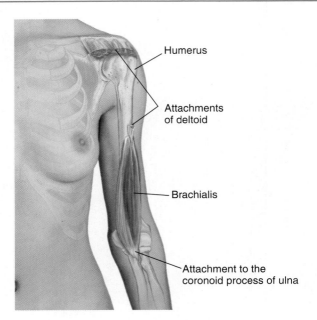

Humerus

Attachments
of deltoid

Brachialis

Attachment to the
coronoid process of ulna

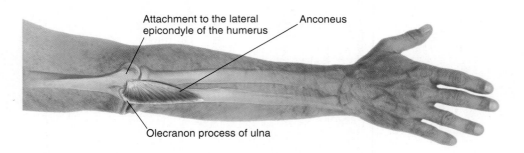

Attachment to the lateral
epicondyle of the humerus

Anconeus

Olecranon process of ulna

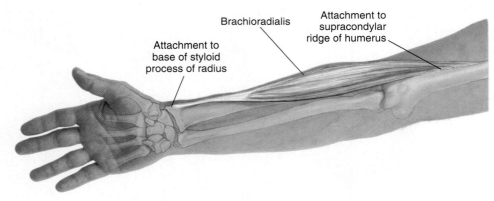

Brachioradialis

Attachment to
supracondylar
ridge of humerus

Attachment to
base of styloid
process of radius

PLATE 4-7

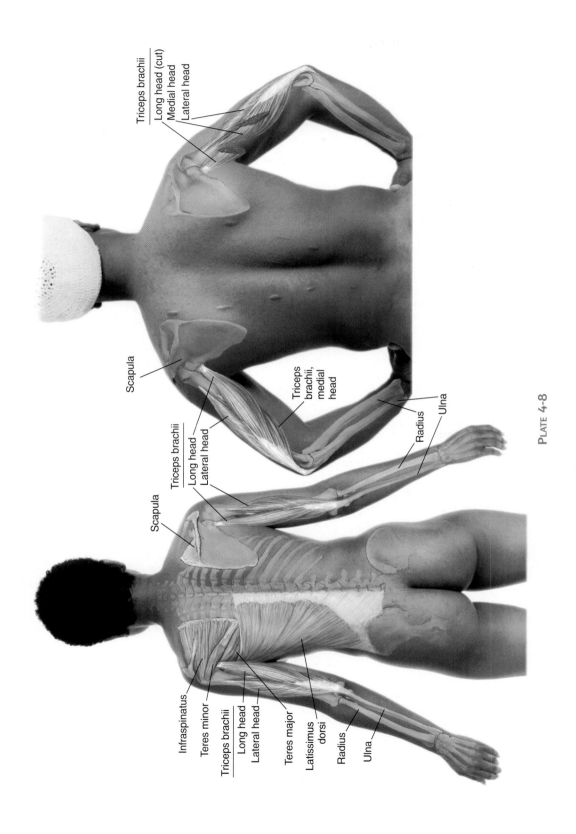

Triceps brachii
Long head (cut)
Medial head
Lateral head

Scapula

Triceps brachii, medial head

Radius

Ulna

Triceps brachii
Long head
Lateral head

Scapula

Infraspinatus

Teres minor

Triceps brachii
Long head
Lateral head

Teres major

Latissimus dorsi

Radius

Ulna

PLATE 4-8

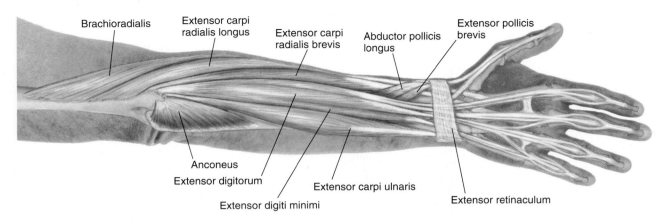

Brachioradialis

Extensor carpi
radialis longus

Extensor carpi
radialis brevis

Abductor pollicis
longus

Extensor pollicis
brevis

Anconeus

Extensor digitorum

Extensor digiti minimi

Extensor carpi ulnaris

Extensor retinaculum

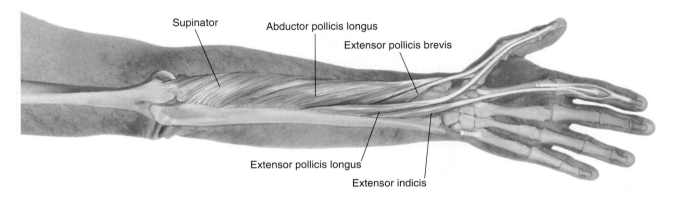

Supinator

Abductor pollicis longus

Extensor pollicis brevis

Extensor pollicis longus

Extensor indicis

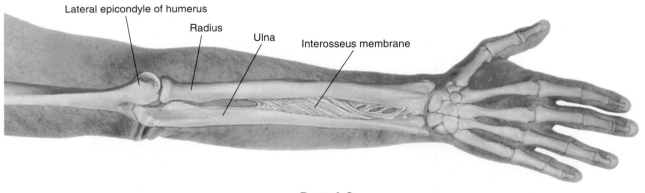

Lateral epicondyle of humerus

Radius

Ulna

Interosseus membrane

PLATE 4-9

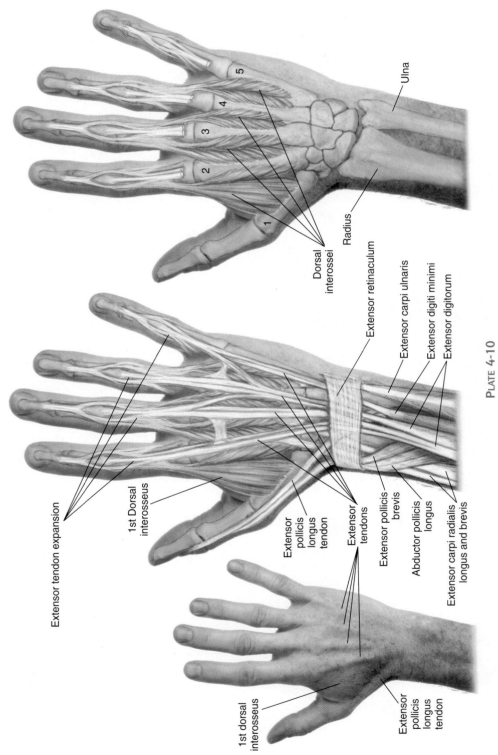

Ulna

Radius

Dorsal interossei

Extensor retinaculum

Extensor carpi ulnaris

Extensor digiti minimi

Extensor digitorum

Extensor tendon expansion

1st Dorsal interosseus

Extensor pollicis longus tendon

Extensor tendons

Extensor pollicis brevis

Abductor pollicis longus

Extensor carpi radialis longus and brevis

1st dorsal interosseus

Extensor pollicis longus tendon

PLATE 4-10

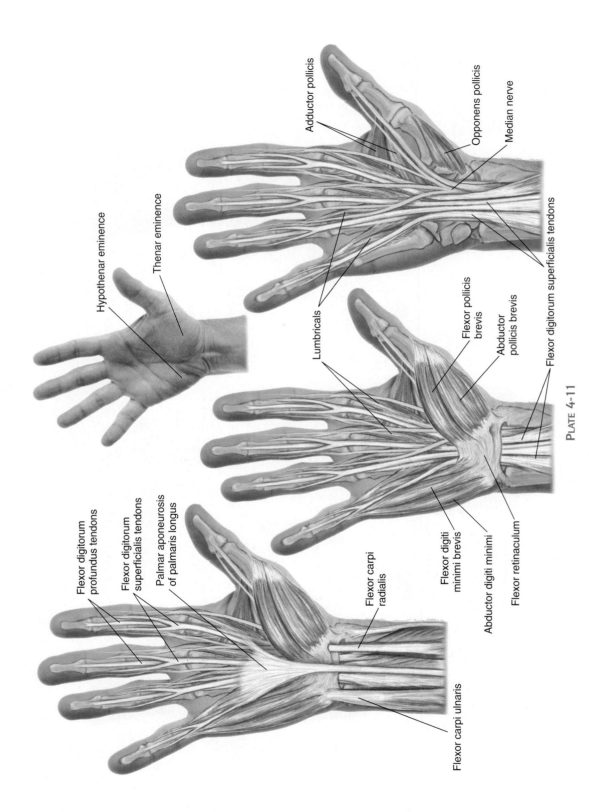

PLATE 4-11

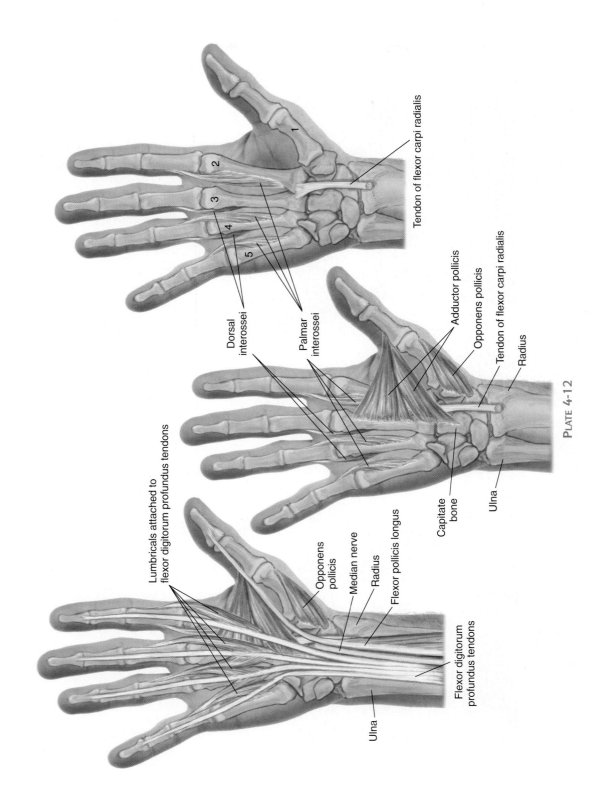

Tendon of flexor carpi radialis

1
2
3
4
5

Dorsal interossei

Palmar interossei

Adductor pollicis

Opponens pollicis

Tendon of flexor carpi radialis

Radius

Capitate bone

Ulna

PLATE 4-12

Lumbricals attached to flexor digitorum profundus tendons

Opponens pollicis

Median nerve

Radius

Flexor pollicis longus

Flexor digitorum profundus tendons

Ulna

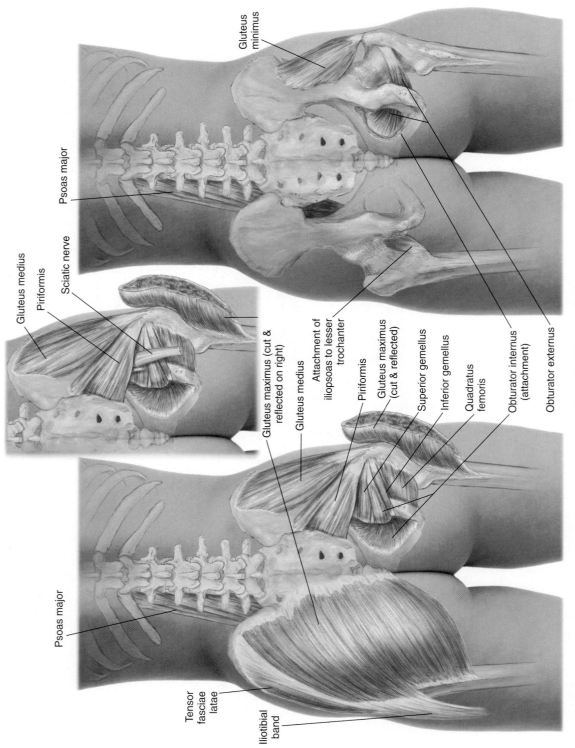

Gluteus minimus

Psoas major

Gluteus medius

Piriformis

Sciatic nerve

Gluteus maximus (cut & reflected on right)

Gluteus medius

Attachment of iliopsoas to lesser trochanter

Piriformis

Gluteus maximus (cut & reflected)

Superior gemellus

Inferior gemellus

Quadratus femoris

Obturator internus (attachment)

Obturator externus

Psoas major

Tensor fasciae latae

Iliotibial band

PLATE 4-13

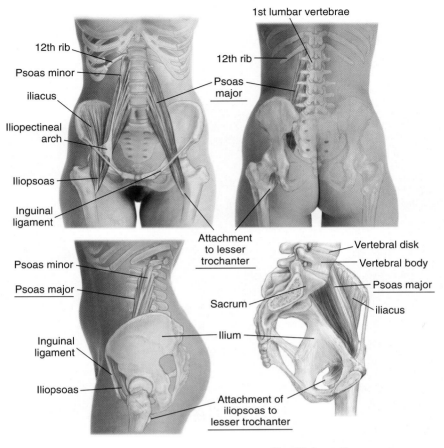

Sagittal section

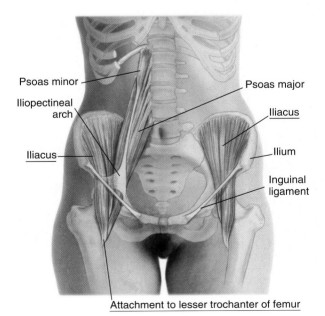

PLATE 4-14

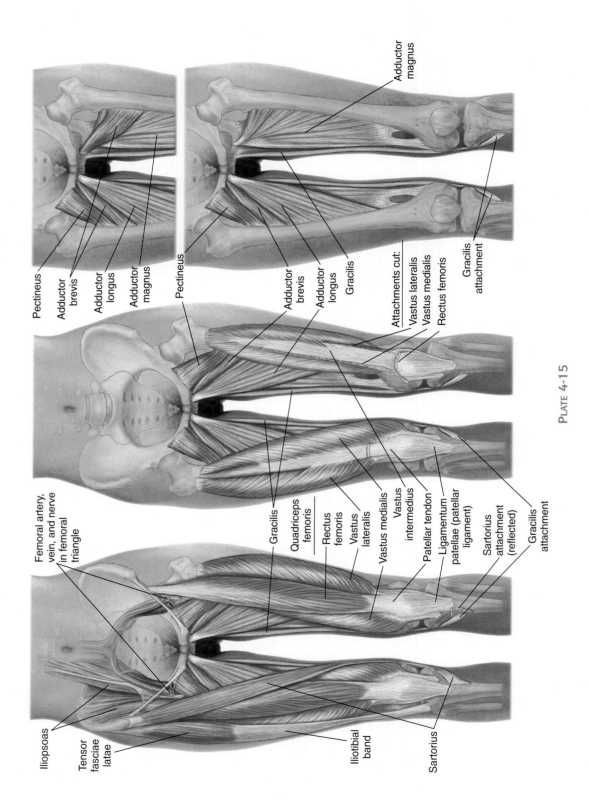

Pectineus

Adductor brevis

Adductor longus

Adductor magnus

Pectineus

Adductor brevis

Adductor longus

Gracilis

Adductor magnus

Attachments cut:
Vastus lateralis
Vastus medialis
Rectus femoris

Gracilis attachment

Femoral artery, vein, and nerve in femoral triangle

Gracilis

Quadriceps femoris

Rectus femoris

Vastus lateralis

Vastus medialis

Vastus intermedius

Patellar tendon

Ligamentum patellae (patellar ligament)

Sartorius attachment (reflected)

Gracilis attachment

Iliopsoas

Tensor fasciae latae

Iliotibial band

Sartorius

PLATE 4-15

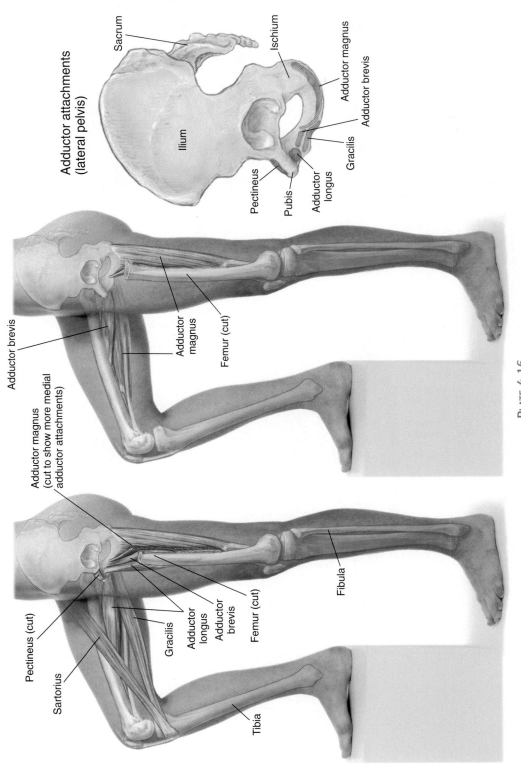

Adductor attachments (lateral pelvis)

Sacrum

Ischium

Adductor magnus

Adductor brevis

Adductor longus

Gracilis

Pubis

Pectineus

Ilium

Adductor brevis

Adductor magnus

Femur (cut)

Adductor magnus (cut to show more medial adductor attachments)

Pectineus (cut)

Sartorius

Gracilis

Adductor longus

Adductor brevis

Femur (cut)

Fibula

Tibia

PLATE 4-16

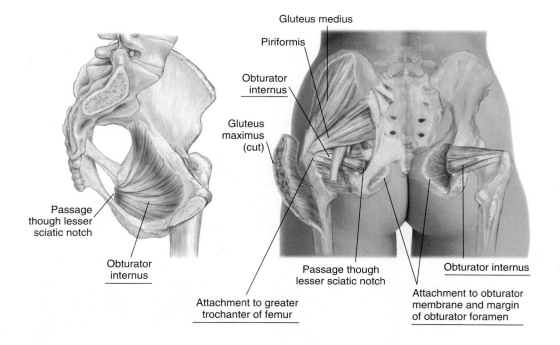

Gluteus medius

Piriformis

Obturator internus

Gluteus maximus (cut)

Passage though lesser sciatic notch

Obturator internus

Attachment to greater trochanter of femur

Passage though lesser sciatic notch

Obturator internus

Attachment to obturator membrane and margin of obturator foramen

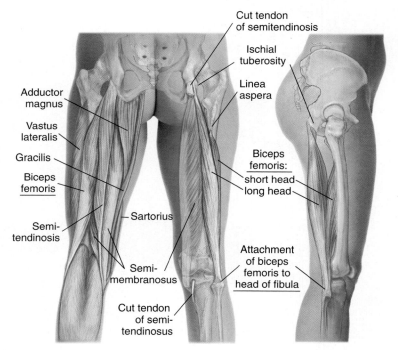

Cut tendon of semitendinosis

Ischial tuberosity

Linea aspera

Adductor magnus

Vastus lateralis

Gracilis

Biceps femoris

Semi-tendinosis

Sartorius

Semi-membranosus

Cut tendon of semi-tendinosus

Biceps femoris: short head long head

Attachment of biceps femoris to head of fibula

PLATE 4-17

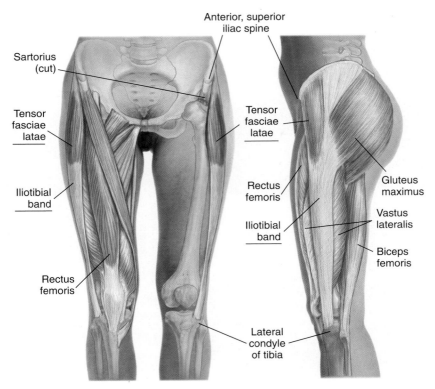

PLATE 4-17 *(continued)*

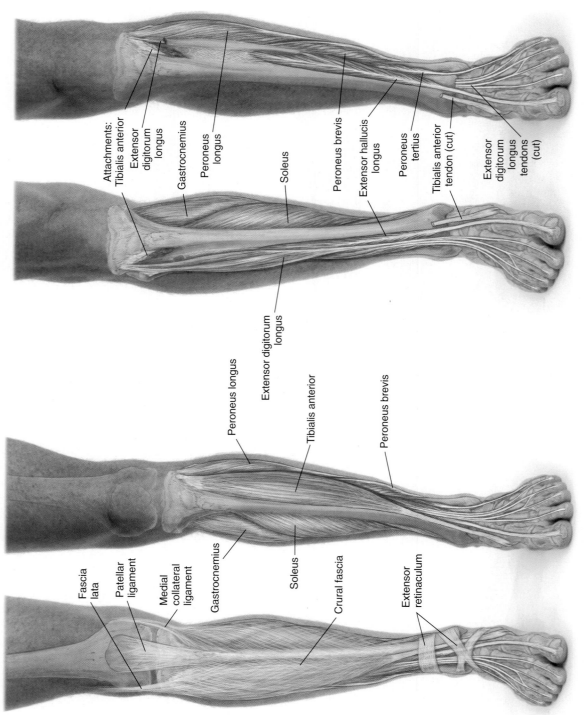

Attachments:
Tibialis anterior

Extensor digitorum longus

Gastrocnemius

Peroneus longus

Soleus

Peroneus brevis

Extensor hallucis longus

Peroneus tertius

Tibialis anterior tendon (cut)

Extensor digitorum longus tendons (cut)

Peroneus longus

Extensor digitorum longus

Tibialis anterior

Peroneus brevis

Fascia lata

Patellar ligament

Medial collateral ligament

Gastrocnemius

Soleus

Crural fascia

Extensor retinaculum

PLATE 4-18

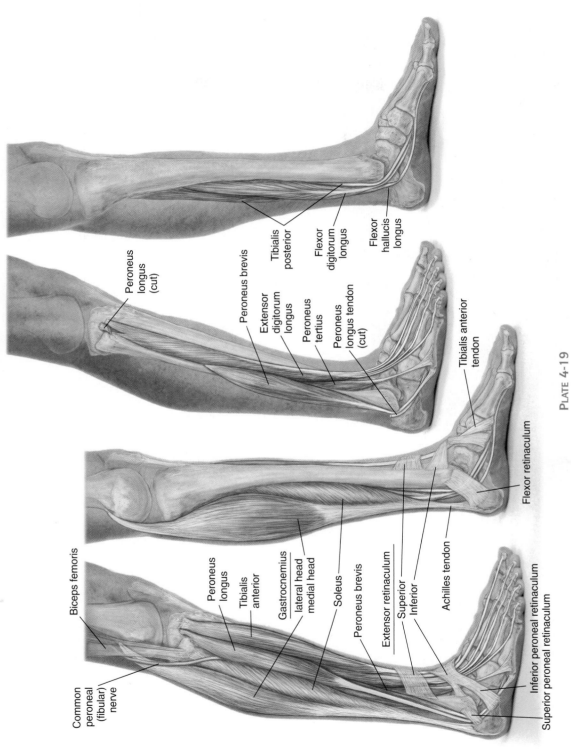

Peroneus longus (cut)

Peroneus brevis

Tibialis posterior

Flexor digitorum longus

Flexor hallucis longus

Extensor digitorum longus

Peroneus tertius

Peroneus longus tendon (cut)

Tibialis anterior tendon

Flexor retinaculum

Biceps femoris

Common peroneal (fibular) nerve

Peroneus longus

Tibialis anterior

Gastrocnemius
lateral head
medial head

Soleus

Peroneus brevis

Extensor retinaculum
Superior
Inferior

Achilles tendon

Inferior peroneal retinaculum

Superior peroneal retinaculum

PLATE 4-19

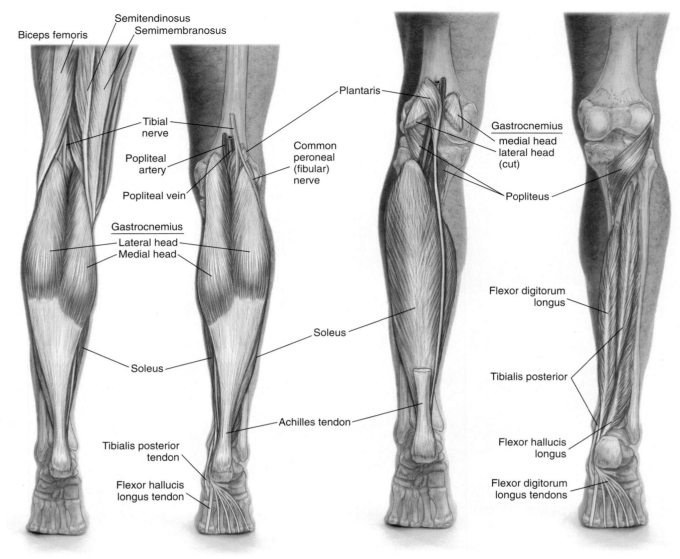

Biceps femoris

Semitendinosus
Semimembranosus

Tibial
nerve

Popliteal
artery

Popliteal vein

Gastrocnemius
Lateral head
Medial head

Soleus

Tibialis posterior
tendon

Flexor hallucis
longus tendon

Plantaris

Common
peroneal
(fibular)
nerve

Soleus

Achilles tendon

Gastrocnemius
medial head
lateral head
(cut)

Popliteus

Flexor digitorum
longus

Tibialis posterior

Flexor hallucis
longus

Flexor digitorum
longus tendons

PLATE 4-20

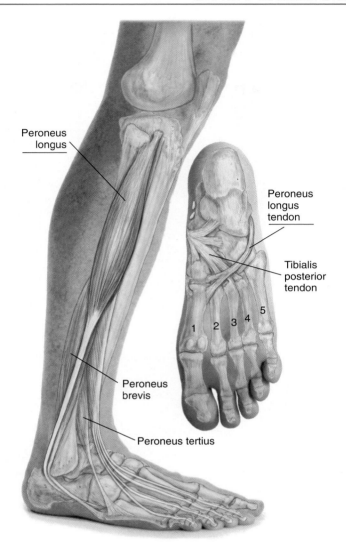

Peroneus
longus

Peroneus
longus
tendon

Tibialis
posterior
tendon

1 2 3 4 5

Peroneus
brevis

Peroneus tertius

PLATE 4-21

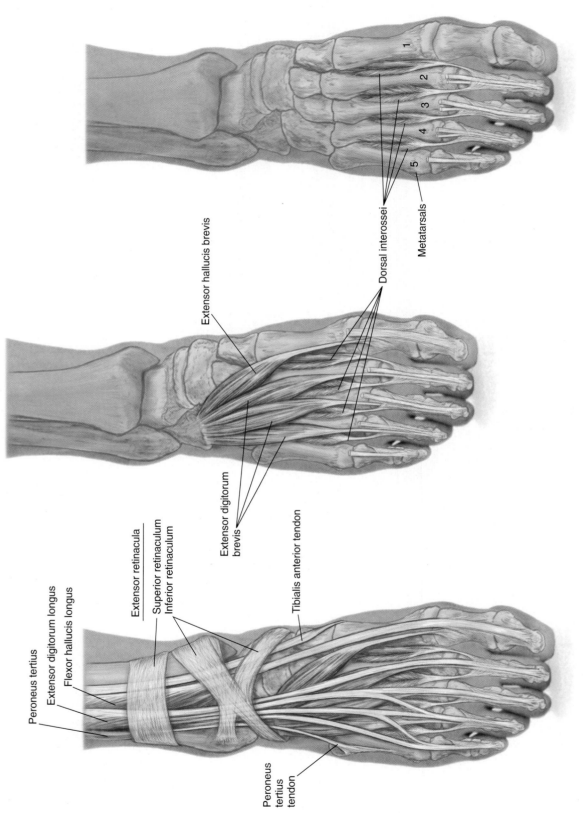

Extensor hallucis brevis

Dorsal interossei

Metatarsals

Extensor digitorum brevis

Tibialis anterior tendon

Peroneus tertius

Extensor digitorum longus

Flexor hallucis longus

Extensor retinacula

Superior retinaculum

Inferior retinaculum

Peroneus tertius tendon

PLATE 4-22

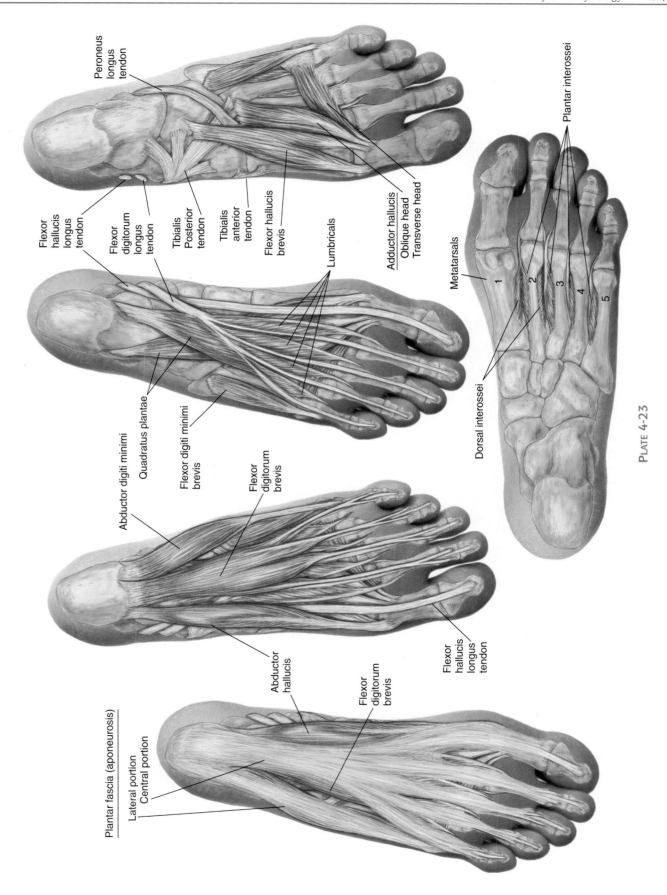

Peroneus longus tendon

Flexor hallucis longus tendon

Flexor digitorum longus tendon

Tibialis Posterior tendon

Tibialis anterior tendon

Flexor hallucis brevis

Lumbricals

Adductor hallucis
Oblique head
Transverse head

Plantar interossei

Metatarsals

Dorsal interossei

Abductor digiti minimi

Quadratus plantae

Flexor digiti minimi brevis

Flexor digitorum brevis

Abductor hallucis

Flexor digitorum brevis

Flexor hallucis longus tendon

Plantar fascia (aponeurosis)
Lateral portion
Central portion

PLATE 4-23

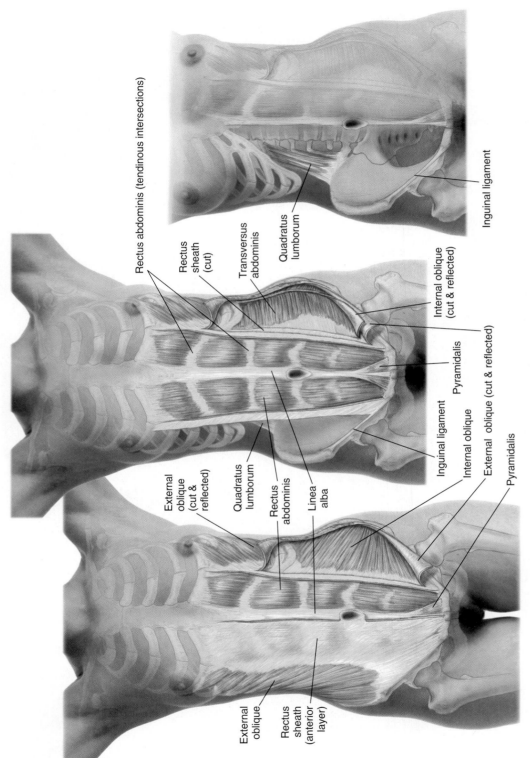

Rectus abdominis (tendinous intersections)

Rectus sheath (cut)

Transversus abdominis

Quadratus lumborum

Inguinal ligament

Internal oblique (cut & reflected)

Internal oblique

Inguinal ligament

External oblique (cut & reflected)

Pyramidalis

Pyramidalis

External oblique (cut & reflected)

Quadratus lumborum

Rectus abdominis

Linea alba

External oblique

Rectus sheath (anterior layer)

PLATE 4-24

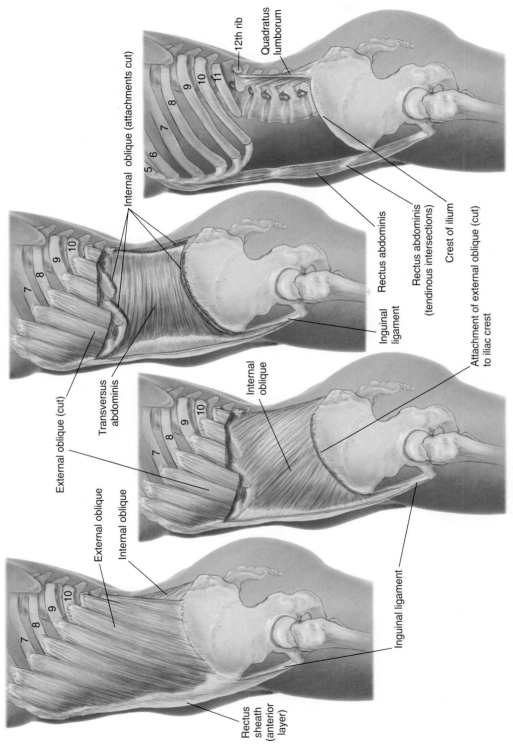

Internal oblique (attachments cut)

12th rib

Quadratus lumborum

Rectus abdominis

Rectus abdominis (tendinous intersections)

Crest of ilium

Attachment of external oblique (cut) to iliac crest

Inguinal ligament

Internal oblique

External oblique (cut)

Transversus abdominis

External oblique

Internal oblique

Rectus sheath (anterior layer)

Inguinal ligament

PLATE 4-25

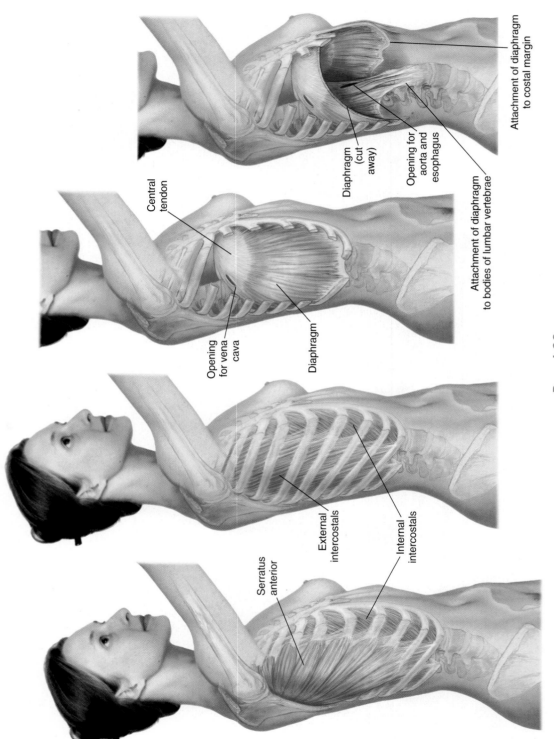

Attachment of diaphragm to costal margin

Diaphragm (cut away)

Opening for aorta and esophagus

Attachment of diaphragm to bodies of lumbar vertebrae

Central tendon

Opening for vena cava

Diaphragm

External intercostals

Internal intercostals

Serratus anterior

PLATE 4-26

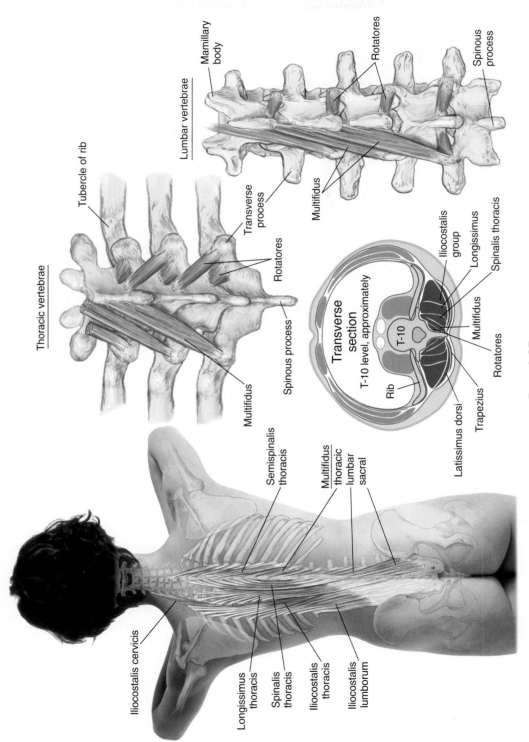

Lumbar vertebrae

Mamillary body

Rotatores

Spinous process

Transverse process

Multifidus

Thoracic vertebrae

Tubercle of rib

Rotatores

Multifidus

Spinous process

Transverse section
T-10 level, approximately

Iliocostalis group

Longissimus

Spinalis thoracis

Multifidus

Rotatores

T-10

Rib

Latissimus dorsi

Trapezius

Iliocostalis cervicis

Semispinalis thoracis

Multifidus
thoracic
lumbar
sacral

Longissimus thoracis

Spinalis thoracis

Iliocostalis thoracis

Iliocostalis lumborum

PLATE 4-27

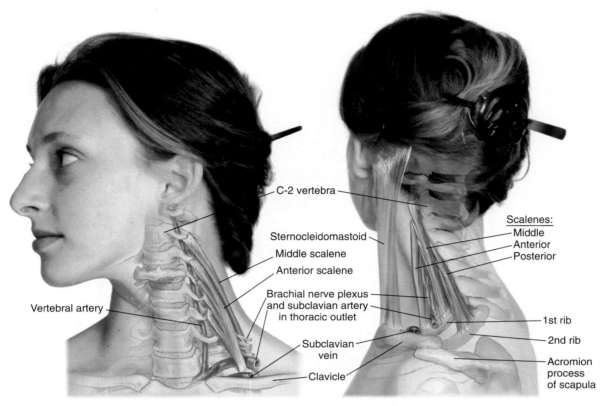

C-2 vertebra

Sternocleidomastoid

Middle scalene

Anterior scalene

Brachial nerve plexus
and subclavian artery
in thoracic outlet

Vertebral artery

Subclavian
vein

Clavicle

Scalenes:
Middle
Anterior
Posterior

1st rib

2nd rib

Acromion
process
of scapula

PLATE 4-28

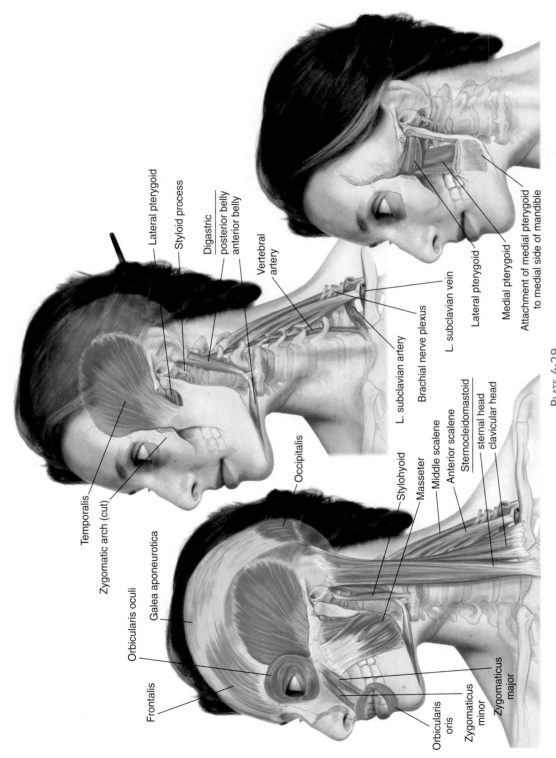

Lateral pterygoid
Styloid process
Digastric
posterior belly
anterior belly
Vertebral artery
L. subclavian vein
Lateral pterygoid
Medial pterygoid
Attachment of medial pterygoid to medial side of mandible
L. subclavian artery
Brachial nerve plexus
Temporalis
Zygomatic arch (cut)
Orbicularis oculi
Galea aponeurotica
Occipitalis
Stylohyoid
Masseter
Middle scalene
Anterior scalene
Sternocleidomastoid
sternal head
clavicular head
Frontalis
Orbicularis oris
Zygomaticus minor
Zygomaticus major

PLATE 4-29

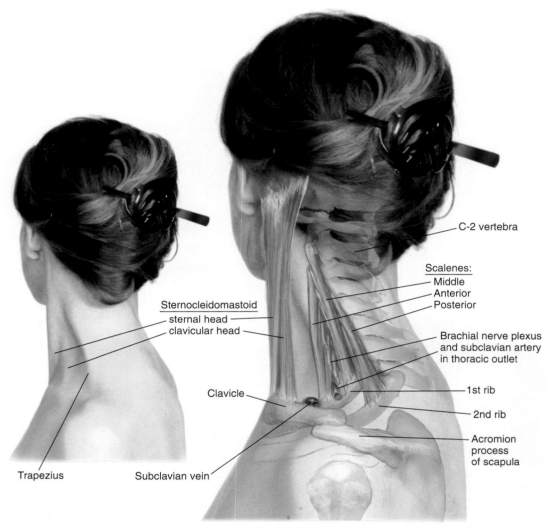

C-2 vertebra

Scalenes:
Middle
Anterior
Posterior

Sternocleidomastoid
sternal head
clavicular head

Brachial nerve plexus
and subclavian artery
in thoracic outlet

Clavicle

1st rib

2nd rib

Acromion
process
of scapula

Trapezius

Subclavian vein

PLATE 4-30

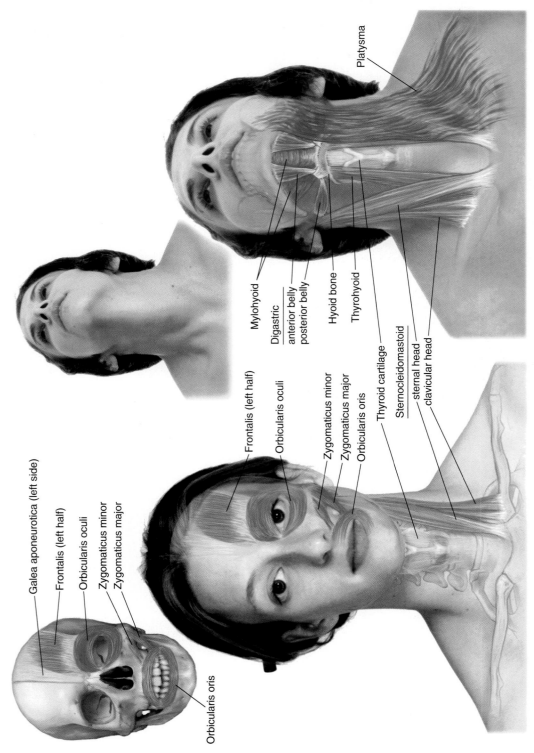

Galea aponeurotica (left side)
Frontalis (left half)
Orbicularis oculi
Zygomaticus minor
Zygomaticus major

Orbicularis oris

Frontalis (left half)
Orbicularis oculi

Zygomaticus minor
Zygomaticus major
Orbicularis oris

Thyroid cartilage
Sternocleidomastoid
sternal head
clavicular head

Mylohyoid
Digastric
anterior belly
posterior belly

Hyoid bone
Thyrohyoid

Platysma

PLATE 4-31

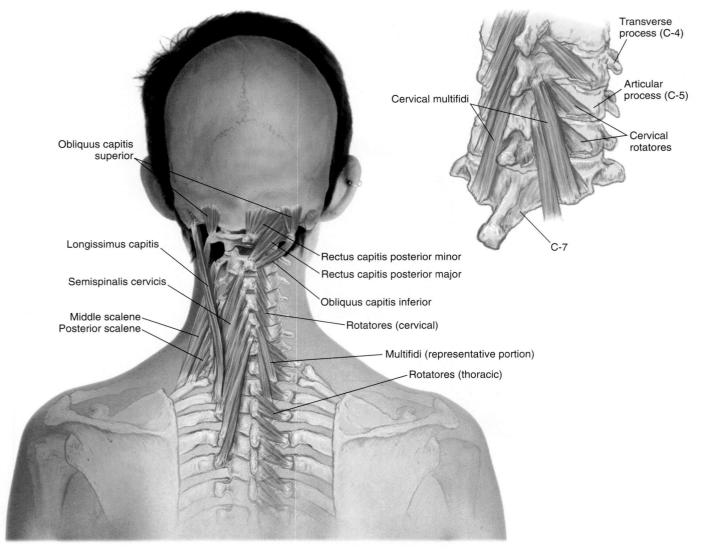

Obliquus capitis superior

Longissimus capitis

Semispinalis cervicis

Middle scalene
Posterior scalene

Rectus capitis posterior minor
Rectus capitis posterior major

Obliquus capitis inferior

Rotatores (cervical)

Multifidi (representative portion)

Rotatores (thoracic)

Transverse process (C-4)

Articular process (C-5)

Cervical rotatores

Cervical multifidi

C-7

PLATE 4-32

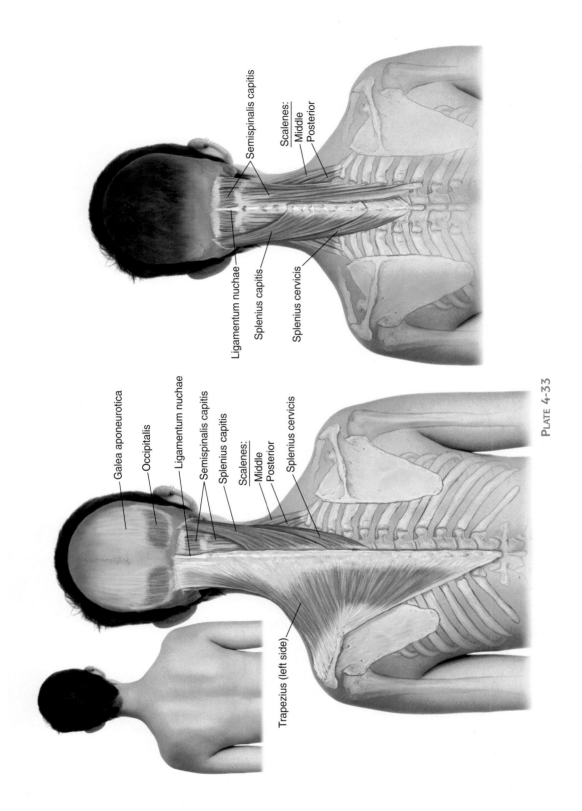

Semispinalis capitis

Scalenes:
Middle
Posterior

Ligamentum nuchae

Splenius capitis

Splenius cervicis

Galea aponeurotica

Occipitalis

Ligamentum nuchae

Semispinalis capitis

Splenius capitis

Scalenes:
Middle
Posterior

Splenius cervicis

Trapezius (left side)

PLATE 4-33

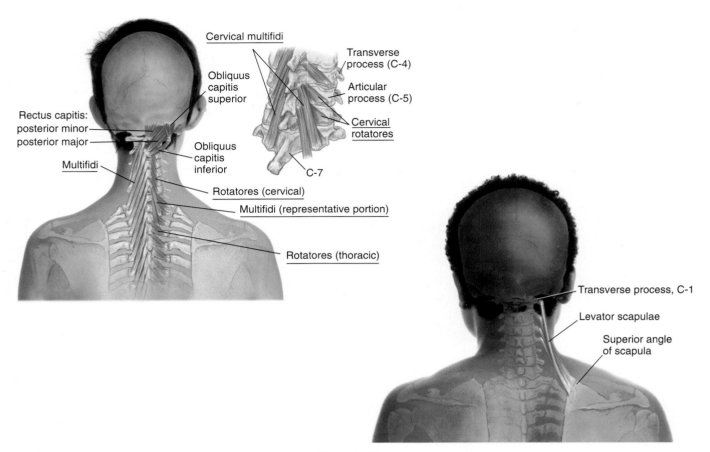

Cervical multifidi

Transverse process (C-4)

Articular process (C-5)

Obliquus capitis superior

Rectus capitis: posterior minor posterior major

Cervical rotatores

C-7

Obliquus capitis inferior

Multifidi

Rotatores (cervical)

Multifidi (representative portion)

Rotatores (thoracic)

Transverse process, C-1

Levator scapulae

Superior angle of scapula

PLATE 4-34

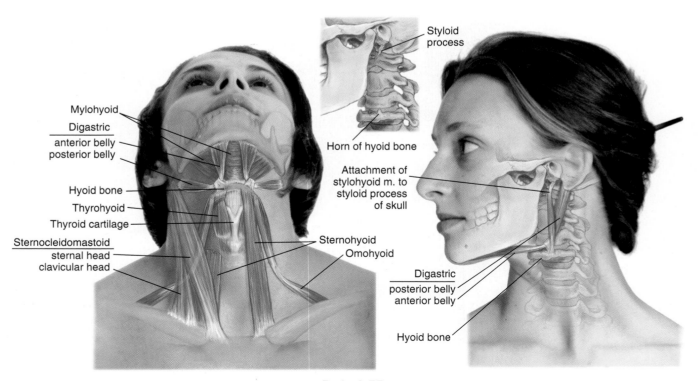

Styloid process

Mylohyoid

Digastric
anterior belly
posterior belly

Hyoid bone

Thyrohyoid

Thyroid cartilage

Sternocleidomastoid
sternal head
clavicular head

Horn of hyoid bone

Attachment of stylohyoid m. to styloid process of skull

Sternohyoid

Omohyoid

Digastric
posterior belly
anterior belly

Hyoid bone

PLATE 4-35

CHAPTER EXERCISES

1. List the six kinds of synovial joints and give at least one example of each. Then, on yourself or a partner, demonstrate the movements allowed at each joint.

2. Define the following:

   Homeostasis
   Peristalsis
   Reflex arc
   Motor unit
   Diffusion
   Osmosis
   Facilitated diffusion
   Filtration
   Exocytosis
   Endocytosis
   Neuron
   Nerve
   Muscle cell
   Muscle

3. Explain the effects of fascial restriction and describe a situation or experience that may have been the result of a fascial restriction.

4. Identify at least 10 bony landmarks on yourself or a partner.

5. Name the five functions of the muscular system.

6. List the structures of a whole skeletal muscle.

7. Demonstrate the antagonistic movement to each of the following:

   Extension
   Dorsiflexion
   Medial rotation
   Elevation
   Retraction
   Abduction
   Inhalation
   Pronation
   Lateral deviation

8. Compare and contrast the organization and bundled arrangements of the structures of a muscle, bone, and nerve.

9. Describe the similarities between the venous system and the lymphatic system.

10. Identify the prime mover, synergist, antagonist, and fixator for elbow flexion. Then identify the prime mover, synergist, antagonist, and fixator for elbow extension. Notice the relationship between prime mover and antagonist in these antagonistic movements.

11. Name at least five different kinds of sensory receptors.

12. Identify the sensory neurons involved in each of the following: stretch reflex, tendon reflex, flexor reflex.

13. Name at least five indications for massage.

14. Give five examples of local contraindications and two examples of systemic contraindications.

15. Describe the difference between sprain and strain.

SUGGESTED READINGS

Balch PA, Balch JF. Prescription for Nutritional Healing. New York: Avery, 2000.

Benjamin B, Borden G. Listen to your Pain, The Active Person's Guide to Understanding and Identifying and Treating Pain and Injury. New York: Penguin Books, 1984.

Biel A. Trail Guide to the Body. Boulder, CO: Books of Discovery, 1997.

Buchholz D. Heal Your Headache: The 1•2•3 Program for Taking Charge of your Pain. New York: Workman Publishing, 2002.

Calais-Germain B. Anatomy of Movement. Seattle, WA: Eastland Press, 1993.

Chaitow L. Fibromyalgia and Muscle Pain: Your Self-Treatment Guide. London: Thorsons, 2001.

Chaitow L. Fibromyalgia Syndrome: A Practitioner's Guide to Treatment. London: Churchill Livingstone, 2000.

Chaitow L, Bradley D, Gilbert C. Multidisciplinary Approaches to Breathing Pattern Disorders. London: Churchill Livingstone, 2002.

Clemente C. Gray's Anatomy. 30th ed. Philadelphia: Lippincott Williams & Wilkins, 1985.

Cohen BJ, Wood DL. Memmler's Structure and Function of the Human Body. 7th ed. Philadelphia: Lippincott Williams & Wilkins, 2000.

Cohen BJ, Wood DL. Memmler's Structure and Function of the Human Body. 9th ed. Philadelphia: Lippincott Williams & Wilkins, 2000.

Crowley LV, Abrams C. Physiology. Springhouse, PA: Springhouse Corporation, 1993.

Major Systems of the Body, World Almanac Library. Milwaukee, WI: Jacques Fortin, 2002.

Gray H, Lewis WH. Anatomy of the Human Body. 23rd ed. Philadelphia: Lea & Febiger, 1936.

Guinness AE, ed. ABC's of the Human Body, A Family Answer Book. Pleasantville, NY: Readers Digest Association, 1987.

Hendrickson T. Massage for Orthopedic Conditions. Philadelphia: Lippincott Williams & Wilkins, 2003.

Johnston CA. Anatomy. Springhouse, PA: Springhouse Corporation, 1993.

Kendall FP, McCreary EK, Provance PG. Muscle Testing and Function. 4th ed. Baltimore: Williams & Wilkins, 1993.

Lowe WW. Functional Assessment in Massage Therapy. 2nd ed. Corvallis, OR: Pacific Orthopedic Massage, 1995.

Marieb EN. Essentials of Human Anatomy and Physiology. 5th ed. Benjamin/Cummings Menlo Park, CA: Benjamin/Cummings, 1997.

Mauskop A, Fox B. What your Doctor May Not Tell You About Migraines: The Breakthrough Program that Can Help End Your Pain. New York: Warner Books, 2001.

Melloni JL, Dox I, Melloni HP, Melloni BJ. Melloni's Illustrated Review of Human Anatomy. Philadelphia: JB Lippincott, 1988.

Northrup C. Women's Bodies, Women's Wisdom. New York: Bantam Books, 1998.

Paulino J, Griffith CJ. The Headache Sourcebook. New York: Contemporary Books/McGraw Hill, 2001.

Physician's Desk Reference, Pocket Guide to Prescription Drugs. 5th ed. New York: Pocket Books, 2002.

Persad RS. Massage Therapy and Medications General Treatment Principles. Toronto: Curties-Overzet, 2001.

Rattray F, Ludwig L. Clinical Massage Therapy: Understanding, Assessing and Treating over 70 Conditions. Toronto: Talus, 2000.

Scanlon VC, Sanders T. Essentials of Anatomy and Physiology. 2nd ed. Philadelphia: FA Davis, 1991.

Sieg KW, Adams SP. Illustrated Essentials of Musculoskeletal Anatomy. 2nd ed. Gainesville, FL: Megabooks, 1985.

Sloane E. Anatomy and Physiology: An Easy Learner. Boston: Jones and Bartlett, 1994.

Starlanyl D, Copeland ME. Fibromyalgia and Chronic Myofascial Pain: A Survival Manual. 2nd ed. New York: New Harbinger Publications, 2001.

Takahashi T (editorial supervisor). Atlas of the Human Body. New York: HarperCollins, 1994.

Theodosakis MD, Adderly B, Fox B. The Arthritis Cure, New York: St. Martin's Press, 1997.

Travell JG, Simons DG. Myofascial Pain and Dysfunction: The Trigger Point Manual, vol I. Philadelphia: Lippincott Williams & Wilkins, 1983.

Travell JG, Simons DG. Myofascial Pain and Dysfunction: The Trigger Point Manual, vol II. Philadelphia: Lippincott Williams & Wilkins, 1992.

Utting School of Massage Lecture Notes. Seattle, WA: 1994.

Watkins J. Structure and Function of the Musculoskeletal System, Champaign, IL: Human Kinetics, 1999.

Werner R. A Massage Therapist's Guide to Pathology. Lippincott Williams and Wilkins. Baltimore: Lippincott Williams & Wilkins, 1998.

Willis MC. Medical Terminology The Language of Healthcare. Baltimore: Lippincott Williams & Wilkins, 1996.

http://aolsvc.health.webmd.aol.com/NR/internal.asp?GUID={33761E43-DAC3-44F6-B9DB-2D4A8557A6A1}, accessed 7.19.03.

http://cal.nbc.upenn.edu/saortho/chapter_03/03mast.htm, accessed June 15, 2002.

http://gened.emc.maricopa.edu/bio/bio181/BIOBK/BioBookIMMUN.html, accessed June 24, 2002.

http://infoplease.lycos.com/ce6/sci/A0804321.html, accessed June 24, 2002.

http://nk1000.nutrifit.com/, accessed June 25, 2002.

http://www.bartleby.com/107/pages/page502.html, accessed June 22, 2002.

http://www.cdc.gov/

http://www.cdc.gov/mmwr/

http://www.cell-biology.com, accessed May 15, 2002.

http://www.dermnet.org.nz/index.html

http://www.e-histology.net, accessed May 15, 2002.

http://www.factmonster.com/ce6/sci/A0843878.html, accessed June 5, 2002.

http://www.go-symmetry.com/vitamin-d.htm, accessed June 28, 2002.

http://www.hhp.ufl.edu/ess/at/AbdomenWeb/web%20page%20info/Types_of_Shock.htm, accessed June 24, 2002.

http://www.infoplease.com/ce6/sci/A0818305.html, accessed June 5, 2002.

http://www.intelihealth.com/IH/ihtIH

http://www.mayoclinic.com/invoke.cfm?objectid=43CB5F79-2B33-4F96-B7D06EC696826071, accessed June 28, 2002.

http://www.me.unm.edu/~bgreen/QEM98/ANAYAR/R6.HTM, accessed June 14, 2002.

http://www.medic-planet.com/MP_article/internal_reference/capillaries, accessed June 24, 2002.

http://www.medic-planet.com/MP_article/internal_reference/veins, accessed June 24, 2002.

http://www.mic.ki.se/Diseases/

http://www.nci.nih.gov/

http://www.nih.gov/icd/

http://www.nlm.nih.gov/medlineplus/ency/article/002338.htm, accessed June 28, 2002.

http://www.nlm.nih.gov/medlineplus/sweat.html, accessed June 28, 2002.

http://www.physsportsmed.com/index.html

http://www.unomaha.edu/~swick/2740connectivetissue.html#ret, accessed June 19, 2003.

http://www.webmd.com, accessed July 24, 2002.

http://www.Weighttrainer.virtualave.net, accessed May 21, 2002.

http://www.ahealthyme.com, accessed June 16, 2002.

http://www.webmd.com, accessed June 16, 2002.

Communication and Documentation

UPON COMPLETION OF THIS CHAPTER, THE STUDENT WILL BE ABLE TO:

- Describe at least four factors of effective communication and interviewing skills
- Define reflective listening
- List at least five specific examples of nonverbal communication
- Give at least five reasons why a massage therapist should document every massage session
- Describe the information recorded in each section of a SOAP note
- List at least 15 questions to ask when taking a client history
- Tell why it is important to educate clients about the cumulative effects of stress
- Describe the difference between short- and long-term goals
- List at least 10 abbreviations commonly used in massage treatment records.

KEY TERMS

Activity and analysis information: the massage activity and an analysis of the treatment session documented on the SOAP note

Confidentiality: information that is to be kept private unless the client expressly permits you to share it

Functional limitation: a normal activity of daily life that is limited by muscular or connective tissue conditions

Intake form: a form that documents a client's contact information, health history, or informed consent for care

Leading question: a question that focuses the client's attention to clarify or specify information and to recall missing or forgotten details

Massage treatment record: the document containing input from clients, your objective assessments of the clients' condition, the massage techniques you use, results of the treatment session, and plans for future massage treatment

Objective information: your visual, palpation, range-of-motion, and gait assessments of the client's body and soft tissues documented on the SOAP note

Open-ended question: a question that requires a descriptive answer instead of a one-word answer

Plan information: the section of the SOAP note including plans for future treatment and self-care recommendations

Rapport: mutual trust in a relationship

Reflective listening: a method with which you reiterate the client's words to convey your comprehension or to clarify a misunderstanding

SOAP: an acronym for Subjective, Objective, Activity and analysis, and Plan that refers to a format for documentation

Subjective information: verbal and written information clients share with you regarding their health documented in the SOAP note

Treatment goal: a specific goal that is determined after therapeutic massage treatment to clarify progress toward restoring functional limitations

E ffective communication, interviewing skills, and documentation are vital to the therapeutic process for both the massage therapist and the client. While the massage therapy profession evolves as part of complementary medicine, documentation contributes to the professional quality of your work.

Good documentation also helps you assess the client's condition to determine the appropriateness and type of treatment, improvements, setbacks, treatment goals, and clinical reasoning. More than just a written record, documentation provides clues regarding the client's health history as well as a "road map" to effective initial and session-to-session treatment.

Effective Communication and Interviewing Skills

Effective communication with clients is essential for obtaining accurate and pertinent data for the initial and subsequent massage treatment sessions. Before meeting with a client, focus your attention on the present and do your best to leave any personal distractions out of the treatment room. Be fully aware of your clients and their needs. Engaging the client in a good conversation helps you gather the necessary information to provide safe and effective treatment. A genuine interest in the client helps the client feel heard and understood, leading to a more trusting relationship. This is important for assisting the client throughout the healing process and helps clients cultivate a broader understanding of health. Always keep clients and their needs at the center of the treatment process to establish and support a safe, trusting, effective relationship.

You must consider several factors involved in effective communication skills and the interview process. These include establishing **rapport** (rah-POR), or mutual trust, through communication, making certain assumptions about the client, using reflective listening skills, asking open-ended and leading questions, and looking beyond the client's verbal report for nonverbal information.

The saying goes, "You never get a second chance to make a first impression." First impressions are lasting ones. It is important to present and maintain a professional atmosphere from the beginning of the therapist–client relationship. The first meeting with a client is critically important, as it provides the foundation for the professional relationship, so the following concepts should always be incorporated:

- Formal introductions that include names, a handshake, eye contact, and a statement that clearly identifies the therapist
- Verbal communication that gives the client control over the treatment. For example, a therapist may indicate when a change to a deeper or more invasive technique will occur. You should offer a

safety mechanism that allows clients to inform you if they are uncomfortable in any way, which gives them permission to request that a particular technique be altered or stopped.
- Disclosure of some of the effects of the session that could develop in the next few days, especially if the client was not familiar with the techniques used.

Establishing rapport is perhaps the single most important skill a massage therapist must have for the interviewing process. The first step to establishing rapport with a client is to offer a confident, caring handshake and a greeting using the person's first name. You must know the correct pronunciation and spelling of the client's name, and nickname, if used. One of the keys to establishing rapport is maintaining eye contact. Look clients in the eye while discussing the details of their condition and history to communicate your interest in their explanation. This also increases the client's feelings of validation and positive attention. Another technique for creating rapport is to establish and continue to build trust by acknowledging the client's input and maintaining confidentiality. Phrases such as "I hear you," or "I understand," show that you have heard what the client said, again validating the client's words.

Another step in creating and building trust and rapport in the therapist client relationship is **confidentiality.** Any information the client provides should remain confidential, meaning that the information is to be kept private and not shared with anyone else unless the client expressly permits it. There are special situations when information in clients' files is shared. The client may choose to use you as part of a healthcare team, which could require you to share session information with the other healthcare practitioners. Insurance companies sometimes request session information to reimburse you or your clients. Client information may be released to an attorney or judge upon court order as part of litigation, as in auto accident cases. To release the client's records, the client must authorize and sign a release form (Fig. 5-1). There are a number of occupations, including licensed massage therapy, that legally require reporting abusive situations and threats of deadly harm to the appropriate authorities, such as the police or other governmental agency that protects children and families. You can inform clients of this possibility when you get informed consent for care.

Clients who sense their importance to you are more likely to trust you and, as a result, provide more pertinent information. Another factor in establishing rapport is to explain to clients exactly what they can expect to have happen in the therapy session. Know-

CLIENT RECORDS RELEASE FORM

My signature below authorizes the release of my records including history forms, chart notes, reports, and billing statements to my healthcare provider, attorney and/or insurance company.

Additionally, I authorize my manual therapist to consult with any of the above regarding my health and treatment.

Name: (please print): _____

Signature: _____   Date: _____

FIGURE 5-1   Client records release form.

ing what to expect takes the mystery out of the process and makes clients more comfortable.

Certain assumptions about clients support the communication process by making sure you use a humanistic view of your clients instead of a clinical, unfeeling approach:

- Each client is unique: The extent to which you consider the individual story of each client directly affects the client's chances for improvement.
- Each client has skills: Communicating your recognition of the client's skills and using those skills as a personal strength enhances information gathering.
- Each client interacts with the environment: Recognizing that clients are significantly affected by their lives outside the massage therapy treatment area and gathering more information about their lives leads to more pertinent communication.
- Clients are like us: Considering clients as equal human beings, with similar reactions and difficulties, and maintaining equal footing with clients instead of creating a dependent relationship, facilitates the healing process.
- Clients are honest: Typically, clients give the best information they can, but it is up to you to ask the right questions to help them recall that information.
- Each client sincerely desires success: Clients do their best to achieve their treatment goals. Sometimes environmental factors prevent complete cooperation, and you must recognize these factors.
- Each client shares responsibility with you during the interview: Although you are likely more experienced with interviewing, clients also have a responsibility to help the interview be successful.

- Each client desires interaction and negotiation: Most clients attempt to understand your intent and evaluate your skills and knowledge by asking questions or negotiating instructions.
- Each client knows what the problem is: Clients are typically aware of factors contributing to their difficulties, and the therapist can learn these factors by listening carefully.
- Each client knows when success has occurred: Because clients are often the best judges of whether treatment has been successful, you should recognize that their concepts of success might be different from yours.

Though these assumptions are generalizations, they will help you maintain a client-centered focus and will support your work toward successfully reaching treatment goals.

REFLECTIVE LISTENING

Good listening skills help you to further establish rapport and ensure that the information from the client is documented accurately and completely. Maintaining a client-centered focus throughout the interview process often requires the skill of reflective listening. **Reflective listening** is a method with which you repeat or reiterate the client's words to convey your comprehension or to clarify a misunderstanding. For example, a client may say, "The pain in my shoulder gets worse after I sleep on my side all night." You may then respond to the client, "So when you sleep on one side through the entire night, the pain in your right shoulder has increased by the time you wake up?" This question determines if you have heard the client correctly and gives the client an opportunity to clarify a misunderstanding. Additionally, it helps you document the correct information. As you gain more practice with the interviewing process and use the fundamental skill of reflective listening, you will become a more effective interviewer.

Open-Ended Questions

Using your own style with reflective listening will help you formulate questions to elicit as much information from clients as possible regarding their present condition and cumulative stressors that have affected it. The best method of gathering information uses **open-ended questions.** Open-ended questions are those that require a descriptive answer instead of a one- word answer. They encourage and broaden the conversation, often helping clients remember any details they might have forgotten. For example, the closed question, "Does your shoulder hurt today?" is likely to lead to a short answer such as yes or no. In contrast, the open-ended question, "What makes your shoulder pain better or worse?" may elicit a more thoughtful, thorough response that provides more information about which soft tissues might be involved.

Leading Questions

After exploring open-ended questions, you might use leading questions to refocus the conversation to the chief complaint. **Leading questions** focus the client's attention to clarify or to give more specific types of information and to recall missing or forgotten details. For example, if a client's chief complaint is right-sided neck pain, your reflective listening skills and open-ended questions might evoke a story about a typical workday and a number of events that happened at work last week that brought the client in for a massage. You can ask leading questions regarding the neck pain to help you understand which soft tissues might be involved. "Is there any activity that you typically do with your right side, such as carry your child or talk a lot on the phone with the phone on your right side?" or "Is there an activity where you turn your head mostly to one side during a typical day?" or "What position do you sleep in?" or "Can you show me the movements that hurt the most?" These questions will help refocus the discussion to determine the plan for the upcoming massage treatment.

NONVERBAL COMMUNICATION

Gathering information from clients involves more than just collecting verbal data. Look beyond the client's words written on the history form and the client's answers from the interview to gather the whole picture, paying attention to nonverbal communication. These nonverbal cues help you better understand clients' actual perception of their conditions.

You can evaluate clients' perceptions of their condition by noticing their tone of voice, breathing patterns, and body language, including facial expression, eye contact, areas of muscular tension, and body positioning. A normal tone of voice is recognized as steady instead of shaky, not too loud or soft, not too rushed or hesitant, and not excessively emotional. Body language can be especially helpful to massage therapists because people tend to accompany the verbal description of the condition of their soft tissues with clues for massage treatment. You will notice that as clients describe pain or areas of restricted movement, they may rub the affected tissues a certain way, poke at themselves, hold their hand over affected areas, or stretch restricted soft tissues. These nonverbal messages can tell you which areas to include in the session and which techniques to use. Body language is not the only thing that indicates the techniques you should use or that only certain techniques will work, nor does it necessarily indicate the specific areas that are causing the pain or restricted function, but it does suggest that these techniques will be well-received by the client and that those tissues are most likely involved in the pain or restriction.

Sometimes the nonverbal communication reinforces the spoken words, but many times, the nonverbal cues contradict the client's words, and you have to recognize the discrepancy to sort through the input and determine the most effective approach to treatment. Consider a client who comes in and briefly requests a massage just to relax and denies any areas of pain or discomfort at the time. However, the client's words are quiet and shaky, there is no eye contact, and the client is slumped in the chair and breathing shallowly. While filling out the intake form, the client rubs his or her temples, squeezes the eyes shut from time to time, sits up straight a couple of times to hyperextend and laterally flex, and rubs the posterior aspect of the neck. The nonverbal body language suggests pain and some muscular tension in the head or neck. It also suggests that the client might respond well to massaging the posterior and lateral soft tissues of the neck and lateral flexion stretches to the neck.

Clients' nonverbal and emotional cues can also offer information about their stress levels and healing or recovery time. Generally, the higher the client's stress level, the more symptoms they may have, and the longer the recovery time will be. Conversely, lower levels of stress may be associated with fewer symptoms and shorter recovery times.

While it is beyond the therapist's scope of practice to counsel clients, you may take note of their emotions and emotional reactions to their conditions. For example, you have a client who starts crying when describing the effect of back pain on his or her life and the worthless feelings it causes. Without diagnosing any specific medical or psychological condition, you could note that the client is very distressed as a result of the back pain. This notation may offer you and other healthcare providers insight into the client's condition and response to healing.

 Be extremely careful to stay within your role as a massage therapist; your scope of practice does not include diagnosing or counseling.

It is much better to offer genuine caring and concern about the client's condition than to offer inappropriate advice.

Good documentation depends on good communication as you engage clients in effective interviews. Establishing rapport through communication, making certain assumptions about the client, using reflective listening skills, asking open-ended and leading questions, and paying attention to nonverbal messages all help you gather accurate, complete information for documentation.

Documentation

Within the healthcare community, documentation is used to create and maintain a patient's record and develop initial and session-to-session treatment plans as well as for communication between healthcare professionals. Documentation is a guideline for safe and effective treatment and proof of the client's progress. Currently, in the massage field, documentation is becoming more common. As massage continues to develop as a healthcare profession and governmental licensure becomes prevalent, the need to learn documentation becomes more critical because licensed healthcare practitioners are legally required to document patient progress. Many insurance companies require professional documentation for reimbursement. There are therapists who do not keep accurate records of client progress because they consider it unnecessary at the time, think it takes too much time, or do not want to bother clients with paperwork and interviews. Realistically, most clients are not interested in filling out forms or sitting through an interview. Most of them just want to get on the massage table, receive treatment, and go home.

REASONS FOR DOCUMENTATION

Despite the impatience of clients who "just want to get a massage," maintaining a client-centered and successful practice requires documentation of both wellness and therapeutic massage for many reasons:

- You must understand the clients' health history to ensure that there are no contraindications for massage.
- You can treat repeat clients more efficiently when you know which techniques were effective.
- You can encourage client participation by inquiring about their self-care activities.
- You have written proof to illustrate progress toward the clients' goals.
- You promote professional massage therapy as a legitimate, aboveboard healthcare practice.
- You convey and breed trust by conducting a professional interview that ensures that your treatment will be purely professional.
- You convey the importance of health history and progress by writing it down instead of trying to remember it.
- You can show clients that their goals were reached with money well spent.
- You have written records to share with insurance companies, both to get reimbursed and for accident and injury settlements.
- You have written records to share with the clients' other healthcare practitioners to ensure that treatments are cooperative rather than contradictory.
- You have written records to share with healthcare practitioners who refer clients to you, thus closing the communication loop and marketing and presenting yourself as a professional.
- You have written records to protect you in the rare case of a malpractice suit.

As you can see, keeping written records in an organized file system is a worthwhile investment for the safety of your clients, the education of your clients, the financial success of your practice, and the professional image of your practice. Client files must represent accurate information that is pertinent to treatment. The file should include client contact information, the client's signed informed consent for care (discussed in the Ethics and Professionalism chapter), and basic treatment information, whether in a SOAP note or in another format. It should include any referrals made and any self-care recommended.

 The file should not include your subjective or judgmental statements, suspected diagnoses, or behavioral inconsistencies.

The files can be used to keep track of the techniques you use, techniques clients like or do not like, techniques that work especially well for a particular

---

SOAP NOTE

Name: _____ **Date:** _____

Current illness, injury, medication: _____

_____

Primary reason for visit: _____

SUBJECTIVE

The clients' chief complaint or concern (the reason they came for massage)
- what clients say about their condition
- their perception of the condition since the last massage treatment

Information from the health history that is pertinent to the chief complaint

OBJECTIVE (Obvious differences you notice before, during, and after the massage)

Postural assessments
- levelness and evenness of bilateral landmarks, rotational deviations, landmarks that are anterior or posterior to their normal position, feet

Gait assessments
- quantity, quality, fluidity of steps and arm swing (bilateral similarities, evenness, smoothness), upright alignment (head over spine, shoulders not hunched, etc.), feet (medial or lateral deviation), knee flexion (slight flexion for shock absorption resembles a bounce in the step)

Range of motion assessments
- active range of motion, passive range of motion

Your visual observations of the clients' bodies and their soft tissues
- color, fullness, bilateral symmetry

Your palpation observations of the clients' bodies and their soft tissues
- temperature abnormalities, differences in texture and movement of skin and soft tissues, areas of abnormal fullness or swelling, body rhythms

ACTIVITY AND ANALYSIS

Massage activity
- specify where and which techniques you applied

Massage session analysis
- results of the current massage session
- prioritized functional limitations
- long and short term goals

PLAN

Plan for future massage treatment
- techniques to use or avoid, duration and frequency of future sessions
- self-care recommendations
- referrals to other healthcare practitioners

Therapist's Signature: _____ Date: _____

FIGURE 5-2 SOAP note with pertinent information.

client, and the condition of soft tissues from session to session. Documentation is not only a tool for you; it is also an important method of communication with other massage therapists or healthcare practitioners. You may work in a situation, perhaps a spa or massage clinic, where other therapists may see the same clients. Good documentation will help the treating therapist gain an understanding of the client's history and progress and learn what techniques work well with a particular client. Additionally, the uniqueness of individuals makes it impossible for any one treatment to work for every person, so clients may choose to use one or several healthcare practitioners as a collective team. The team approach can be especially beneficial, as long as the participants share pertinent and valid information. You need to keep records that a primary care physician or other healthcare practitioner can understand and, with the client's signed release of records form, share any records with referring practitioners as a professional courtesy.

DOCUMENTATION FORMS

There are different forms and formats you can use to document client assessment and massage treatment. You can choose or create the appropriate forms based on the information you will document. Essentially, you need to include contact information for your clients, health history information, informed consent for care, subjective ideas from your clients about how they feel and what they want to accomplish, your objective evaluations of clients' bodies and the condition of their soft tissues, massage activity and analysis of treatments, and future massage treatment plans.

The contact information, health history, and informed consent for care can be consolidated onto one form. Sometimes called **intake forms,** these are only filled out by clients at their first appointment, and the forms are kept in your client files. (Fig. 5-6 shows an example of an intake form.)

The **massage treatment record** contains the rest of the information you need to document: input from clients, your objective assessments, the massage techniques you use, results of the treatment session, and plans for future massage treatment. All of the information can be recorded on a printed form or just written down on a blank document, as long as the appropriate information is included.

SOAP

A common format for documenting massage sessions is SOAP. **SOAP** is an acronym for Subjective, Objective, Activity and analysis, and Plan information. Fig-

ure 5-2 is an example of a printed SOAP chart, also called a SOAP note, and indicates the pertinent information to document in each section.

Subjective Information

Generally, **subjective** data includes any information the client shares with you in both written and verbal communication. In addition to the health history information that clients share on the intake form, they may tell you what hurts, what they want to accomplish from the session, the physiological or psychosocial factors that are affecting their health, and activities they think are affected by muscular tension or pain. Use effective communication skills to obtain as much pertinent information as you can from the client to determine any potential contraindications and to create the best treatment plan. This chapter focuses on communication skills and the "S" portion of the SOAP note.

CLIENT HISTORY

To know where to begin treatment, you must first know where clients have been—know their history. The history is the first step in evaluating the client's condition, and this information is documented as subjective data on the SOAP note. Information from the client history form provides many clues about the condition of a client's structures and soft tissues even before your formal assessment. The history form should include the following client data: personal identification and contact information; current health information, health concerns, and goals for health; goals for treatment; history of injuries, illnesses, and surgeries; and consent to exchange health information with other healthcare providers as well as consent for care. Finally, clients should sign and date the form as acknowledgment and proof that they had the opportunity to discuss anything on the form with you and give their consent for massage treatment. (Examples of health history forms are shown in Figs. 5-6 and Figure 5-9.)

Some intake forms include body diagrams, which can be a helpful tool for clients, because verbalizing their symptoms and physical sensations of discomfort may be difficult. Additionally, when the client is given the opportunity to draw on the body diagram before the interview, it can simplify and expedite the interview process. Figure 5-3 is a sample health report form indicating a client's current symptoms.

Know that clients almost always have more information than they initially write down. More often than not, peo-

Provider Name _Sagamore Therapy_

Patient Name _Craig Sherman_

Date of Injury _N/A_   Insurance ID# _6012306_

HEALTH REPORT

Date _Aug. 5, 2003_

A. Draw today's symptoms on the figures.

1. Identify CURRENT symptomatic areas in your body by marking letters on the figures below. Use the letters provided in the key to identify the symptoms you are feeling today.
2. Circle the area around each letter, representing the size and shape of each symptom location.

Key

P = pain or tenderness

S = joint or muscle stiffness

N = numbness or tingling

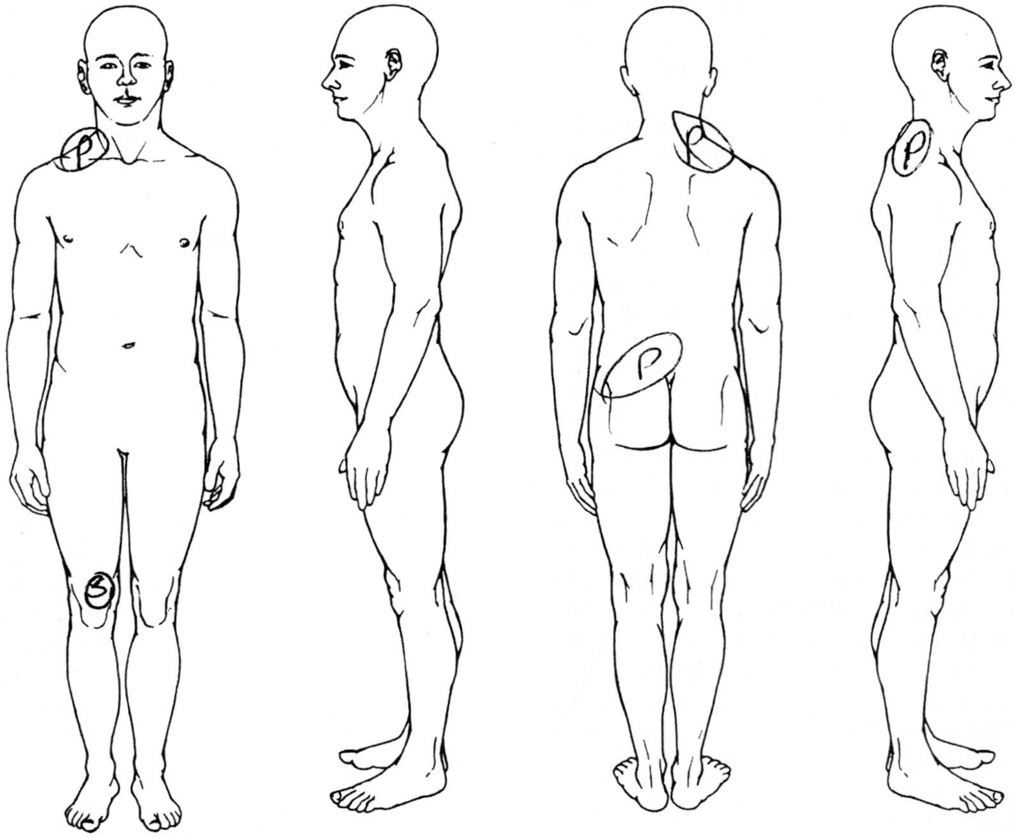

B. Identify the intensity of your symptoms.

1. Pain Scale: Mark a line on the scale to show the amount of pain you are experiencing today.

No Pain |————————X————————————————| Unbearable Pain

2. Activities Scale: Mark a line on the scale to show the limitations you are experiencing today in your daily activities.

Can Do Anything I Want |—X————————————————————| Cannot Do Anything

C. Comments

Stiff Knee from basketball

Signature _Craig Sherman_   Date _Aug. 5, 2003_

FIGURE 5-3 Health report, filled out. (Modified from Thompson DL. Hands Heal: Communication, Documentation, and Insurance Billing for Manual Therapists. 2nd ed. Baltimore: Lippincott Williams & Wilkins, 2002.)

ple forget past accidents and injuries. The muscular and nervous systems, however, do not forget. In fact, the clients' soft tissue condition and postural compensations directly reflect their cumulative stresses. Any one accident, injury, condition, hobby, or activity may not seem stressful for the body, but cumulatively or unresolved, individual stressors will manifest in the body as postural compensation patterns and physical symptoms in soft tissues.

INTERVIEW

After the client has filled out the history form and indicated symptoms on the body diagram, you begin sorting through the information. Leading questions help clarify the client's input, allowing you to identify contraindications, set appropriate session goals, and develop an effective treatment plan. Daily activities, hobbies, and environmental factors such as climbing stairs or long commutes to and from work are often the culprit of muscular tension and pain. Some categories that are commonly covered when interviewing massage clients[1]:

- General: allergies, fatigue, fever, function, illness, pain, stress
- Circulatory: cold extremities, cramps, edema, inflammation, swollen lymph nodes, varicose veins
- Musculoskeletal: aches, joint pain, muscle pain, stiffness, swelling, tension, weakness
- Neurological: numbness, radiating pain, tingling, localized weakness
- Psychosocial: lifestyle, important experiences, personal life, social life, work situation

The history is your first and perhaps most important assessment tool to understand the condition of the client and whether massage is the safest and most effective treatment.

FUNCTIONAL STRESS ASSESSMENT

Stress can be anything that takes a person out of homeostasis or balance or it can be defined as a state of bodily or mental tension resulting from factors that hinder the body from maintaining homeostasis. Stress is not necessarily a bad thing and, in fact, small doses of stress can encourage the body to become stronger. Antigens that are incompatible with our own tissues are a form of stress because they jeopardize homeostasis, but the only way our bodies can develop the appropriate antibodies is by being exposed to those antigens. The resulting antibodies effectively strengthen the immune system. Bones remodel and become stronger in response to mechanical forces, or forms of stress that push, pull, twist, or compress them.

Stress may cause problems when it is prolonged or when many individual stress factors accumulate and the body is challenged to maintain homeostasis. For example, people who work extra long hours and have to stay intense and alert for weeks on end overwork their sympathetic nervous systems. Without enough rest, the activities of the sympathetic and parasympathetic nervous systems become imbalanced, creating internal stress that threatens the ability to maintain homeostasis. Mechanical forms of stress can be caused by overusing one set of muscles on one side of the body without using the antagonists or the same set of muscles on the other side of the body as much. To maintain balance and homeostasis, the body adopts an abnormal posture that compensates for the imbalance. Another form of mechanical stress is pain, which may force the body to accommodate for the pain with an abnormal posture and compensation patterns.

Massage therapists consider the effects of stress from a functional perspective, evaluating the extent to which a client is out of balance and how the imbalance affects the client's soft tissue and postural compensation patterns as well as everyday activities. When assessing a client, you must consider specific sources of stress, such as dysfunctions or pathology, previous accidents or surgeries, activities, and nutritional habits and the overall effect of the accumulated stress factors. Several types of stress may affect the client in many areas of life, and you must recognize how each source of stress affects soft tissues and postural compensation patterns so you can develop the most effective treatment plan for each client. You should evaluate, using leading questions, if necessary, the following stress factors:

Health Conditions

1. What current soft tissue or pathological conditions is the client experiencing?
2. Are the client's conditions acute or chronic? (This provides information about the condition of soft tissues.)
3. Are the conditions genetic?
4. Has the client seen any other healthcare practitioner or had other forms of treatment for the condition? If so, what did the other healthcare practitioner conclude? What kind of treatment is currently being given?

Accidents and Surgeries

1. How many and what kinds of accidents or surgeries has the client had?
2. What kind of treatment, if any, has the client had for the accidents?
3. What are the residual soft tissue injuries or compensations?

4. How many and what kinds of surgeries has the client had? Does the client have residual scarring in the area?

Age Considerations

1. Tissue changes at different ages
2. The effects of gravity over time on postural compensation patterns

Lifestyle

1. Are there any activities the client does daily that use repetitive movements or positions that are held for extended periods of time? What postures or positions is the client in and for how many hours a day?
2. What exercise activities does the client participate in? What muscles are used most in those particular activities?

Postural Factors

1. Are there any daily postures or positions that the client holds for extended periods of time?
2. How many hours does the client work per day?

3. What position does the client sleep in?
4. How many hours does the client sleep per night?

Nutrition and Medication (nutrition is discussed in detail in the treatment plan chapter, and medication is discussed in the medical terminology and anatomy and physiology chapters)

1. What are the client's nutritional habits?
2. How much water does the client drink per day?
3. How much caffeine does the client consume per day?
4. What vitamins or nutritional supplements does the client take?
5. Does the client take any medication, prescription or over-the-counter? If so, what does the client take it for?

Emotional and Psychological Factors

As stated above, treating emotional and psychological factors is *not* within the MT's scope of practice, but any increase in stress level because of these factors

---

PROCEDURE BOX 5-1
Client Interview

1. Greet first-time clients with good eye contact and a friendly, confident handshake.
2. Explain your policies and intake form(s) and offer reasons for documentation.
3. Ask clients to fill out forms. Meanwhile, start filling out their SOAP note.
4. Interview clients:
   a. Clarify their purpose for coming to you for a massage.
      i. Is there any area in particular they want you to address or avoid?
      ii. Are there any techniques they prefer or dislike?
   b. Clarify their chief complaint, if there is one. This helps you better understand the client's current condition to know if any progress was made when you perform the posttreatment assessment.
      i. Is there anything that makes the pain worse or better?
      ii. Do they notice the discomfort all of the time, only during certain activities, or only after certain activities?
      iii. How long have they had this condition?
      iv. Ask them to try to rate the discomfort, using a scale of 1 to 10 or on a scale of mild to severe.
      v. Ask them to try to describe the discomfort (sharp, achy, numb, tingling, heavy, throbbing, etc.).
   c. Question any conditions on the history form that might present contraindications—injuries, illness, surgeries, bruises, circulatory problems.

   d. Inquire about daily activities, hobbies, and environmental factors, looking for repetitive movements or sustained positions to try to identify the soft tissues that might be involved.
      i. Do they drive/sit/stand/type/carry an infant a lot during a typical workday?
      ii. Do they garden/knit/ride horses/drive a race car most of the weekend?
      iii. Do they hold an instrument/walk a lot of stairs/breathe smoke-filled air/shift a manual transmission/look up at a screen high on the wall repeatedly?
   e. Discuss the general, circulatory, musculoskeletal, neurological, and psychosocial aspects of their health to find out if there is anything that might influence the treatment you give or the results of the treatment.
5. Evaluate their functional stress:
   a. Health conditions
   b. Accidents and surgeries
   c. Nutrition and medication
   d. Age, lifestyle, postural factors, emotional and psychological factors
6. Explain that the uniqueness of individuals, especially their stress factors, can affect the length of time it takes to restore function or create a noticeable change.

can weaken the body's ability to maintain homeostasis or balance. In turn, this can affect the client's soft tissues or postural compensation patterns. Although specific psychological conditions should not be documented, you can make notes regarding general emotions to consider when creating a treatment plan. Generally, the higher the client's stress level, the longer it will take to return to balance or homeostasis.

CUMULATIVE EFFECTS OF STRESS

After discussing the client's history, you then educate the client about how the stress has accumulated and describe your plan for the current massage session as well as future sessions. The client may be seeking treatment for relief of present stressors and the resulting pain or discomfort. You must address the current needs of the client, but you must also consider past and potential stressors. All past, present, and potential or perceived future stressors can affect the client's condition. Explain to the client that if it took years to develop a muscular or soft tissue condition, it could take numerous sessions to reduce the severity of the condition. Again, the number and accumulation of stressors influence the length of time it will take soft tissues and postural compensation patterns to return to balance or homeostasis. While there are general principles regarding soft tissue rehabilitation and recovery time, each client is affected by a unique set of accumulated stressors. Some clients may think that one massage will miraculously cure them of their aches and pains. Unless they understand how the cumulative effects of stress relate to the development of a chronic condition, clients may be quickly discouraged or decide that massage is not helpful after only one session. (See Procedure Box 5-1, Client Interview.)

Objective Information

Objective data include your assessments of a client's body and the condition of the soft tissues. Any observations and evaluations you make before, during, or after the actual massage treatment are documented in this section of the SOAP note. Visual observations to record might include areas of swelling or inflammation, unevenness of bilateral bony landmarks or muscles, postural abnormalities, compensation patterns, gait (walking) assessments, and localized areas of abnormal skin coloration, especially redness. Palpation observations are noticed when you touch the client's body and feel the soft tissues. Some pertinent palpation observations to record include hypertonic muscles, atrophied muscles, and abnormal skin temperatures, either localized or over the entire body.

You may also evaluate the client's range of motion (ROM) at one or more joints, especially if he or she complains of restricted movement, normal activities that cannot be performed, or "tightness." A goniometer (GOH-nee-AH-meh-ter) is a specific device that measures the ROM in degrees. With specific training, some massage therapists use this device; however, most massage therapists evaluate range of motion as a relative difference. Usually clients explain that they have difficulty moving a specific joint or difficulty performing an activity that they normally do without any trouble. You can easily compare the ROM of the affected joint to the ROM of the same joint on the opposite side of the body. Likewise, you can consider the ROM of the joints involved in the activities that they cannot perform or have difficulty performing and compare the client's normal ROM to the now limited function and its associated limited ROM. With additional training, you can use functional assessment tests such as manual resisted (manual muscle) and special orthopedic tests to help determine any potential contraindications or the need for referral to another healthcare practitioner. The information you need to document in the "O" section of the SOAP note is covered in detail in the next chapter, on assessments.

Activity and Analysis Information

Activity and analysis data cover the massage activity and an analysis of the session. The "A" portion of the SOAP note includes information about which techniques were used, where they were applied, and what happened as a result. The activity includes any techniques clients prefer or dislike, effective or ineffective techniques, and any changes you made to the massage or flow of the massage. Massage strokes, the flow of the massage, therapeutic techniques, and special techniques are covered later in Chapters 10–13.

The analysis of the session requires that you perform a posttreatment assessment to determine if there are any changes following the massage, including increased or reduced pain levels, ROMs, stress levels, muscular tension, and progress toward the client's goals. These assessment tools are detailed in Chapter 6.

The next two steps of the analysis of the session, prioritizing functional limitations and setting treatment goals, apply to both therapeutic and wellness massage sessions. Even though wellness massage does not address any specific soft tissue conditions or limitations, you should document these components of the analysis. You should not define clients as wellness massage clients or therapeutic massage clients because in actuality, any one client can receive both wellness and therapeutic massages. A number of people go to spas for wellness massage on a regular basis, but occasionally injure soft tissues. When that happens, a massage therapist can perform a therapeutic massage and establish the necessary treatment goals on the basis of the prioritized functional limitations.

PRIORITIZING FUNCTIONAL LIMITATIONS

After you have performed the posttreatment assessment, you can review all of the subjective, objective, and activity and analysis information to help clients prioritize their **functional limitations,** which are normal daily activities that are limited by muscular or connective tissue conditions. Using the information gathered from the intake forms, interview, and general assessments, you can guide clients to prioritize their functional limitations, deciding which activity is most important to restore. Consider a client who has trouble flexing his left hip. Functional limitations may include a struggle to get in and out of his car without severe pain, an inability to go running, and difficulty getting in and out of his bed. His main concern might be getting in and out of the car because his job, which requires a lot of driving, is significantly affected. The secondary concerns might be running and climbing in and out of bed. You may have some information about the client's past and present involvement with these limited activities: how much the client ran before the limitation or how the lack of running has affected him. All of this information will help you devise the treatment goals and treatment plan.

SETTING TREATMENT GOALS

When clients come to you for massage treatment, they typically want to relax, reduce pain, reduce stress, reduce muscular tension, and/or increase movement. These pretreatment requests, sometimes considered goals, are subjective input that can be documented in the "S" portion of the SOAP note. After the massage and posttreatment assessment, however, you and your client will integrate the client's goals with the analysis of the session to determine short- and long-term treatment goals. These **treatment goals** are functional goals that clarify a client's progress toward restoring functional limitations. Although not necessary, client participation in goal setting is helpful because it facilitates their participation in their healing and treatment process. When establishing goals, the following components must be included:

- Identify a specific activity
- Include results that can be easily recognized or are quantifiable
- Include measurable tasks that can be accomplished by the client
- Include a functional limitation that is pertinent to the client's lifestyle
- Set a limited amount of time in which to accomplish the goal

The most important quality of these goals is that you and your clients can recognize when the goals are met and the outcome has been achieved. Specifying measurable quantities and identifiable qualities makes it easy for clients to see that the goal has been accomplished. You should also make sure that the goals are reasonable and attainable. Otherwise, clients might feel too discouraged to participate in their healthcare or could be disappointed when the goals are not quickly reached. If the client is not convinced that a goal will lead to lifestyle improvements, and there is no distinguishable way to know if the goal is achievable or when it has been achieved, then that goal is useless for the therapeutic process. Creating effective and useful goals takes some practice but is important for the therapeutic process. **When clients have a solid goal before them that is attainable and easily recognized, they are usually more motivated to participate in their healthcare.**

Long- and Short-Term Goals

Long-term goals (LTGs) are set up for clients to achieve within 1 to 2 months and are based upon their primary areas of concern. This time frame varies with functional stress, chronic conditions that require to time to heal, and a client's desire to return to the most functional state of health over time. Any longer than 2 months, and clients can easily lose sight of the goal and may discontinue treatment. A long-term goal for the above client with hip problems might be being able to run 3 miles, three times a week without pain after 2 months of treatment.

To keep clients from becoming discouraged with slow progress or from doubting progress altogether, you assign short-term goals (STGs). STGs are those that can be accomplished in 1–2 weeks. They are a good source of motivation for clients to continue treatment and continue working toward restoring functional limitations. They focus on the client's primary area of concern, restoring functional limitations that are top priority, or getting clients out of an acute phase of an injury. Each STG should support the LTG, and they are typically designed to be progressive so the client is aware of the progress. For instance, consider a dog groomer who experiences shoulder pain when lifting dogs onto the grooming table. You and the client can decide on the LTG of being able to lift a 20-pound dog onto the grooming table, four times a day, 5 days a week without pain. A series of STGs to support this LTG might be

1. Within 10 days, be able to lift a dog of less than 5 pounds onto the grooming table, twice a day, 3 days a week without pain
2. Within 10 days, be able to lift a dog of between 5 and 10 pounds onto the grooming table, twice a day, 5 days a week without pain
3. Within 10 days, be able to lift a 10-pound dog onto the grooming table, four times a day, 5 days a week without pain

Following are some effective STGs to support LTGs:

- STG: Climb in and out of a car three times a day with mild pain within 2 weeks
- LTG: Run 3 miles, three times a week without pain after 2 months
- STG: Drive the car for 10 minutes, 3 days in a row, without pain within 1 week
- LTG: Drive the car for the 1-hour commute to work, 5 days a week without pain within 2 months
- STG: Sleep for 3 hours in a row, without back pain upon waking, 3 days during a week within 2 weeks
- LTG: Sleep for 6 hours in a row and wake up without back pain, 3 days a week within 2 months
- STG: Talk on the phone for 15 minutes without getting a headache, 3 days in a row, within 12 days
- LTG: Talk on the phone for 30 minutes, five times a day, 5 days a week without getting a headache, within 6 weeks
- STG: Carry the baby for 10 minutes at a time, once a day without neck and shoulder pain, 3 days in a row, within 1 week
- LTG: Carry the baby for 15 minutes at a time, five times a day without neck and shoulder pain, 7 days a week within 2 months

Recall the effects of cumulative stress. Healing time and the length of time improvements will last depend on the accumulated stress and stress factors, the amount of self-care a client performs, and the client's physical activity. You must explain to clients that accomplishing their treatment goals depends on a number of factors. The uniqueness of the individual plays a large part in restoring normal function, and although the treatment goals are reasonable and attainable, client participation with self-care activities will be helpful.

Examples of the activity and analysis of massage sessions are shown in Box 5-1.

Plan Information

The **plan** section of the SOAP note includes a plan for future treatment and recommendations for self-care. This future treatment refers to the frequency of future treatments, duration of those treatments, techniques to try, and techniques to avoid. If you refer clients to any other healthcare practitioners, you can document it in this section.

The plan section identifies the specific self-care activities that you assign and how often clients are supposed to do the activities. You can check the SOAP note from the client's previous session to know what kind of self-care the client might have used between sessions and ask whether it was used. Many clients are only interested in receiving massage to feel better and are not interested in participating in their own healthcare, so try to not get frustrated with clients who do not use the self-care activities you recommend. You can gently remind clients that self-care activities will help reduce the time it takes to accomplish goals and will increase the length of time the benefits of the massage last. One form of self-care is to redirect clients' focus from illness and pain to health and absence of pain. When clients start paying attention to how much better they feel, they better appreciate the benefits of massage and may be more likely to participate in their own healthcare. Treatment goals that focus on the absence of pain or discomfort support this redirected pattern of thinking. The treatment plan is further discussed in Chapter 7.

Putting the SOAP Together

The massage treatment record you use does not have to be the SOAP format included in this text; however, because it is commonly used in many healthcare fields, it can be helpful for sharing information with other healthcare practitioners. There are several guidelines for documenting in your practice to ensure validity and dependability of the records:

- Information should be pertinent to the client's chief complaint/s or massage treatment.
- Information should be clear but brief.
- Abbreviations used should be generally accepted industry standards.
- Use a pen.

Box 5-1

Examples of Activity and Analysis of a Therapeutic Massage Session

Andy

Andy begins the session by wanting to minimize his right-sided neck tension and pain. He has difficulty looking over his shoulder to check his blind spot when he drives, and he states that he drives in city traffic all day long for his job. Aspirin seems to reduce the pain temporarily, and as the day wears on, he can move his neck more. You observe limited ROM of the neck upon rotation and lateral flexion, especially to the left.

During the session, you notice that the muscles for neck rotation and lateral flexion are hypertonic, and you find some trigger points that radiate pain in his levator scapula muscles. You apply some light friction and trigger point release along with general massage techniques.

The posttreatment assessment shows several improvements. Andy reports reduced pain and expresses relief and gratitude. With palpation and retesting, you notice that the tension in the neck has decreased and the ROM has increased when tested for lateral flexion. Andy says that his only concern is to be able to check his blind spot without wincing in pain, which becomes his top priority functional limitation. Together you determine his long-term goal to be to be able to check his blind spot throughout the entire day, 5 days a week without pain. Some short-term goals you set from session to session might be to

1. Check his blind spot for the first hour of driving without pain at least 3 days a week, within the next week.
2. Check his blind spot all morning without pain at least 3 days a week, within 10 days.
3. Check his blind spot all day without pain at least 3 days a week, within 10 days.

Sara

Sara comes to you for massage. She says she is having trouble lifting her baby in and out of the crib, car, swing, and highchair. She complains that her neck and shoulders hurt all the time, but these particular movements create so much pain in her shoulders that she is afraid she will drop the baby. She says she suffers the same pain when doing laundry and trying to wash her hair. Before the massage, your general assessments reveal bilateral limited shoulder flexion and bilateral shoulder abduction, although worse on the right side.

During the massage, you detect hypertonic areas anterior to her glenohumeral joints, hypertonic upper trapezius muscles, and hypertonic levator scapula muscles. Adding therapeutic techniques to your typical relaxation massage flow, you feel the hypertonic tissues soften with massage.

Following the massage, Sara admits that the pain that she felt all the time is gone. You reevaluate the affected ROMs and find that she can flex and abduct both shoulders much farther than before treatment and barely notices the pain at the end of the ROM. Verbally summarizing the subjective, objective, activity and analysis information, you can then review Sara's functional limitations: lifting the baby in and out of different things, doing laundry, and washing her hair. She states that it is most important that she be able to lift the baby in and out of the crib confidently, because people are usually around to help her with the other things, such as getting the baby out of the car and doing the laundry.

Together, you determine her long-term goal to be to lift the baby in and out of the crib 3 times a day for a week without pain. Over a series of sessions, you establish the following short-term goals:

1. Within a week, be able to place four dishes on the top shelf of the kitchen cabinet daily, one at a time, without pain
2. Within a week, be able to place eight dishes on the top shelf of the kitchen cabinet daily, two at a time, without pain
3. Within 2 weeks, be able to lift the baby out of the highchair twice a day, every day, without pain
4. Within 2 weeks, be able to lift the baby out of the crib once a day, every day, without pain

---

- Only correct a mistake by drawing a single line through it and writing your initials and date near or over the line. Never use an eraser or correction fluid.
- Writing should be neat and legible.
- Records should be kept in a safe place and away from public access.

When you first start writing **SOAP** notes, you may find it challenging to write all the necessary information in a limited space and within the limited time for every massage session. There are times when you might have 15 minutes between clients to clean the table, wash your hands, put new sheets on the table for the next client, and document the session you just finished. Although it is tempting to skip the documentation for some sessions, it is important to your clients, your financial success, and the profession that each session is recorded. Brief statements, body diagrams, abbreviations, and symbols can speed up the documentation process and make **SOAP** notes easier to interpret. SOAP notes can be preprinted forms or blank documents that you fill out.

Some preprinted massage treatment records include a body diagram to indicate where on the body the client feels symptoms. (See Fig. 5-4 for an example **SOAP** note for a client from Box 5-1.) Often, symbols are used on these diagrams, and a key to the symbols is typically at the bottom of the page. These diagrams can be useful for noting changes next to the area where the change occurred, and they eliminate the need to use words to describe an area on the body.

Many abbreviations and symbols are used for efficient and effective documentation. (Table 5-1 lists

Provider Name __AMERICAN COMMUNITY MASSAGE__ **SOAP CHART-M**

Patient Name __ANDY JAMES__   Date __5-10-03__

Date of Injury __5-07-03__ Insurance ID# __N/A__   Current Meds __none__

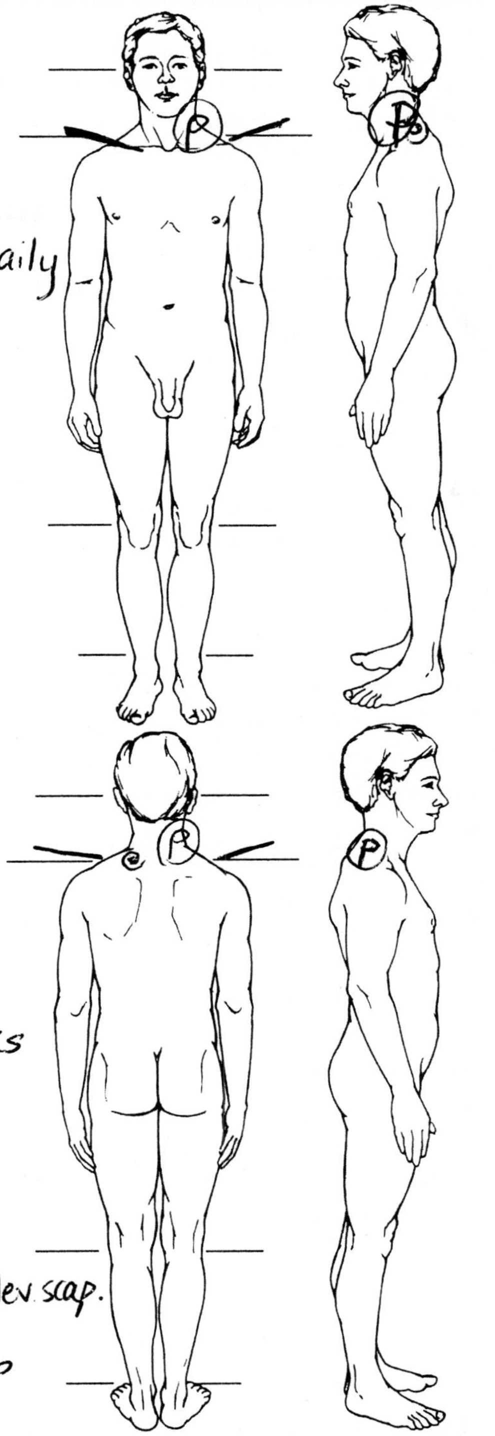

S   Focus for Today

Symptoms: Location/Intensity/Frequency/Duration/Onset

Ⓟ+ ↓ROM neck, ⒷⓁ   DOI: 3 days ago

Activities of Daily Living: Aggravating/Relieving

Can't check blind spot safely, drives daily
Aspirin ↓Ⓟ; w/o meds. Ⓟ ≈ 8 of 10 scale
ROM ↑ through the day.

O   Findings: Visual/Palpable/Test Results

Ⓛ rot, lat flex neck < Ⓡ
ⒷⓁ shoulder elev.
TP Ⓛ lev. scap.
Hypertonic ⒷⓁ lev scap, up trap, SCM

A   Modalities: Applications/Locations

FBRM, Fx ⒷⓁ lev scap, TP release Ⓛ lev scap.

Response to Treatment (see △)

↓Ⓟ (8→3), ROM ↑ ⒷⓁ neck rot, lat flex

Prioritize Functional Limitations

#1 Check blind spot!

Goals: Long-term/Short-term

LTG: Check blind spot 8 hrs/day,
5 days/wk, without Ⓟ – within 6 weeks
STG#1: Check blind spot 1 hr. w/o Ⓟ,
3 days/wk – within 7 days

P   Future Treatment/Frequency

1 hr. Ⓜ, once/5 days for 15 days,
then once every 10 days. FBRM, try PNF to ⒷⓁ lev. scap.

Homework/Self-care

Focus on ↓Ⓟ, ↑ROM, when sitting at stop
light, drop shoulders slowly & hold.

Provider Signature __Barb L. Massage__   Date __May 10, 2003__

Legend: ⒸTP   •TeP   ○ Ⓟ   ✳Infl   ≡HT   ≈SP

     ✕Adh   ≋Numb   ⌒rot   ╱elev   ⊶Short   ↔Long

FIGURE 5-4   SOAP with body diagram filled out for sample client in Box 5-1. (Modified from Thompson DL. Hands Heal: Communication, Documentation, and Insurance Billing for Manual Therapists. 2nd ed. Baltimore: Lippincott Williams & Wilkins, 2002.)

TABLE 5-1

Abbreviations and Symbols for Massage Therapy (common ones in **bold**)

Term	Symbols	Term	Symbols
Massage Terms, Modalities, Findings		hypertonic, tension	≡
client	**Cl**	**leading to, resulting**	→
connective tissue	**CT**	less than	<
contraindication	**CI**	longer than normal	↔
craniosacral therapy	**CST**	male	♂
cross fiber friction	**XFF**	numbness, tingling	≳
deep tissue	**DT**	**pain**	**P, ⓟ**
direct manipulation	**DM**	rotation	↻, ↺, ↻
direct pressure	DP	shorter than normal	⊢⊣
effleurage	**eff**	spasm	≈
energy work	**EW**	swelling, inflammation	✳
friction	**Fx**	tender point	•
ice, compression, elevation, support	ICES	trigger point	⊚
manual lymphatic drainage	**MLD**	**times, repetitions**	**X**
massage	**Ⓜ**	**up, increase**	↑
massage therapist	**MT**	**with**	**w/, c̄**
muscle energy technique	**MET**	**without**	**w/o**
myofascial release	**MFR**	*Anatomy*	
neuromuscular therapy	**NMT**	**abdominals**	**abs**
not applicable	N/A	**anterior, superior iliac spine**	**ASIS**
palpation	**palp**	biceps brachii	bi
petrissage	**pet**	**cervical, cervical vertebrae**	**C, C1-7**
physical therapy	PT	**connective tissue**	**CT**
positional release	**PR**	cranium	Cr
proprioceptive neuromuscular facilitation	**PNF**	**deltoid**	**delt**
reciprocal inhibition	**RI**	diaphragm	dia
reflexology	reflex	energy	E
somatoemotional release	SER	erector spinae	ES
tense and relax	**T&R**	**gastrocnemius**	**gastroc**
tension	tens	**gluteal muscles**	**gluts**
treatment	Tx	**hamstrings**	**hams**
adhesion	χ	head and neck	H&N
after	p, post	**iliotibial band**	**ITB, IT band**
and	&, +	**latissimus dorsi**	**lats**
approximate	≈, ~	**levator scapulae**	**lev scap**
at	@	**low back**	**LB**
before	ā, pre	**lumbar, lumbar vertebrae**	**L, L1-5**
change	Δ	**muscles**	**mm**
down, decrease	↓	occiput	occ
elevation	∕	**pectoralis muscles**	**pecs**
equals	=	**posterior, superior iliac spine**	**PSIS**
female	♀	**quadratus lumborum**	**QL**
greater than	>	**quadriceps femoris**	**quads**

TABLE 5-1

Abbreviations and Symbols for Massage Therapy (common ones in **bold**) *(continued)*

Term	Symbols	Term	Symbols
rhomboid muscles	**rhomb**	*Directional, Descriptive Terms*	
scalene muscles	**scal**	**anterior**	**ant**
sternocleidomastoid	**SCM**	**bilateral, both**	**Ⓑ🄻, Ⓑ**
sacroiliac	**SI**	constant	const
soft tissue	**ST**	excessive	xs
thoracic, thoracic vertebrae	**T, T1-12**	**external**	**ext**
tensor fascia latae	**TFL**	**internal**	**int**
temporomandibular joint	**TMJ**	**lateral**	**lat**
trapezius muscles	**traps**	**left**	**Ⓛ**
triceps brachii	tri	light, low, mild	L
Medical Record Terminology, Measurements		**medial**	**med**
as needed	prn	**moderate**	**mod**
beats per minute	bpm	normal	N
complains of	**c/o**	**posterior**	**post**
continue same	CSTx	prone	pr
could not test	CNT	**proximal**	**prox**
date of injury	**DOI**	**right**	**Ⓡ**
did not test	DNT	**severe**	**sev**
full body	**FB**	sidelying	SL
full body relaxation massage	**FBRM**	superior, supine	sup
history	**Hx**	within normal limits	WNL
long term goal	**LTG**	*Actions, Planes*	
medications	**meds**	**abduction**	**abd**
next visit	nv	**adduction**	**add**
prescriptions	**Rx**	**circumduction**	**circ**
recommendation	**rec**	depression	dep
same as	S/A	dorsiflexion	DF
same treatment	SATx	elevation	ele
treatment	**Tx**	eversion	ever
Symptoms, Maladies		**extension**	**ext**
adhesion	**adh**	**flexion**	**flex**
backache	BA	inversion	inv
chronic fatigue syndrome	CFS	**lateral flexion**	**lat flex**
diagnosis	Dx	opposition	opp
edema	ed	plantarflexion	PF
fibromyalgia syndrome	FM, FMS	pronation	pro
fibrous tissue	FT	**range of motion**	**ROM**
headache	**HA**	**active range of motion**	**AROM**
pain	**P, Ⓟ**	active assisted range of motion	AAROM
sleep disturbance	SD	**passive range of motion**	**PROM**
symptoms	Sx	**resisted range** of motion	RROM
tender point	**TeP**	**rotation**	**rot**
tension	**tens**	sidebending	SB
trigger point	**TP, TrP**	supination	sup

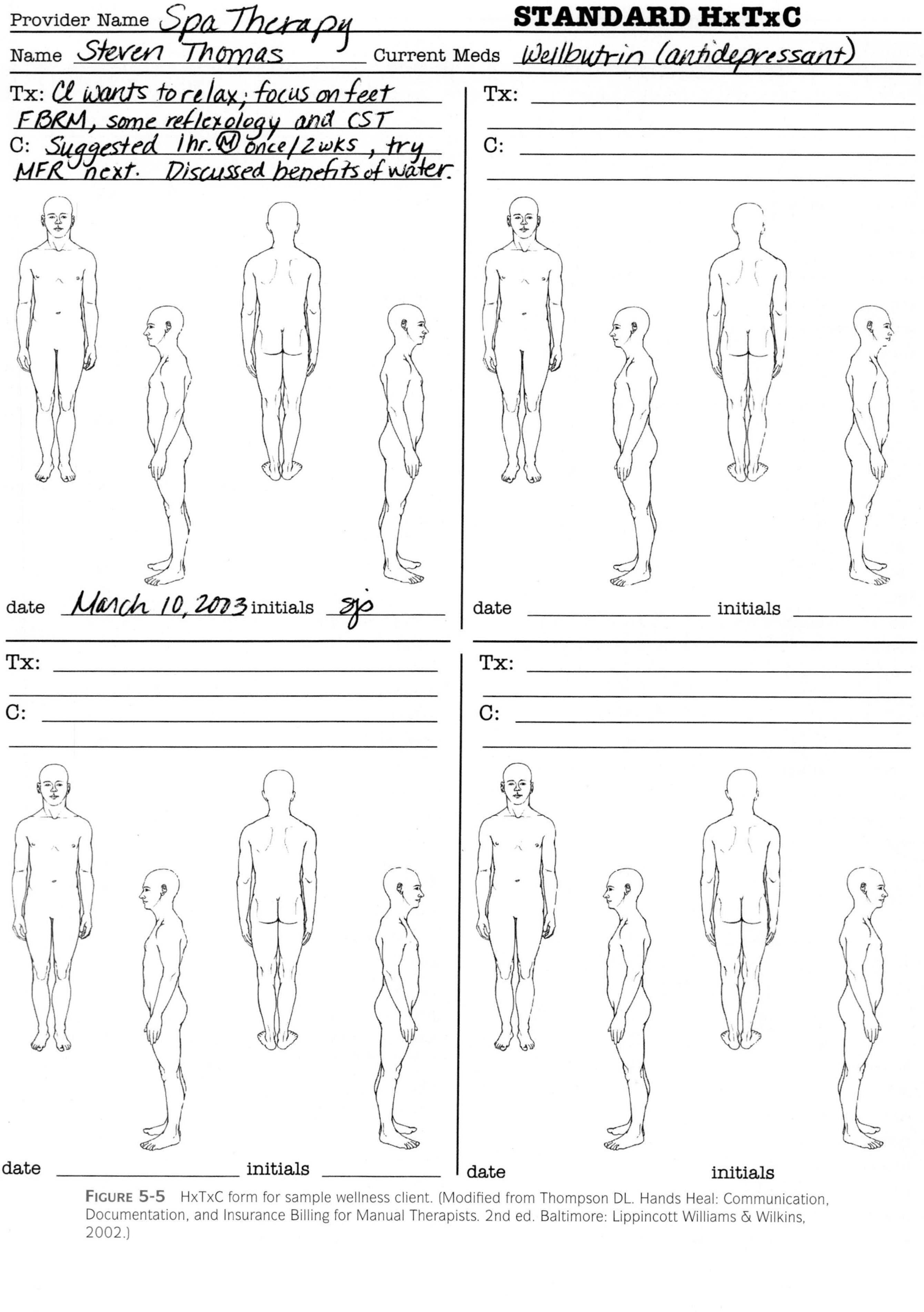

Provider Name *Spa Therapy*   **STANDARD HxTxC**

Name *Steven Thomas*   Current Meds *Wellbutrin (antidepressant)*

Tx: *Cl wants to relax; focus on feet*
FBRM, some reflexology and CST
C: *Suggested 1hr. Ⓜ once/2wks, try*
MFR next. Discussed benefits of water.

Tx: _____
_____
C: _____
_____

date *March 10, 2003* initials *sjp*   date _____ initials _____

Tx: _____   Tx: _____
_____   _____
C: _____   C: _____
_____   _____

date _____ initials _____   date _____ initials _____

FIGURE 5-5 HxTxC form for sample wellness client. (Modified from Thompson DL. Hands Heal: Communication, Documentation, and Insurance Billing for Manual Therapists. 2nd ed. Baltimore: Lippincott Williams & Wilkins, 2002.)

abbreviations and symbols for massage treatment records, identifying the more common ones.) Some of the more helpful symbols you may use include delta (Δ), the standard symbol for change, or an arrow (→) to indicate posttreatment assessment findings. The changes you indicate will typically be positive changes due to treatment, but if symptoms worsen, you can still use these symbols. For instance:

- Full body relaxation massage resulted in reduced pain and increased left lateral flexion of the neck.
  FBRM → ↓P + ↑(L)lat flex neck
- The client complains of moderate pain in the right shoulder.
  Cl c/o mod P (R)shoulder
- The left anterior, superior iliac spine was higher than the right before the massage, but they were even after the massage.
  (L)ASIS↑ Δ (L)ASIS=(R)ASIS

Typically, not much time is available to fill out a SOAP note, so you may be inclined to wait until the end of the day to document all the SOAP notes. Unfortunately, the longer you wait to fill out the SOAP, the less accurate your documentation will be, especially if you have to fill out numerous SOAP notes at one time. After several different clients have come and gone, it is often difficult to remember details specific to each client. Information is more accurate when you document immediately after the session. Since these documents are used as the basis for future treatments and may also be used by other healthcare professionals as well as attorneys and insurance companies, your accuracy is critical. Using appropriate abbreviations can speed up the process of documentation, allowing you to fill out the SOAP note immediately after each massage session.

SOAP NOTE VARIATIONS

All of the previous examples of SOAP notes are full-page forms that provide space for recording the pertinent details for therapeutic massage sessions. There are a number of variations available. A shortened form can be used when a client is treated for general concerns or given a wellness massage. One of the shortened forms is called the HxTxC (Fig. 5-5). Hx refers to history, including current and most recent injuries, health and soft tissue conditions, and medications taken on the treatment day. Tx refers to treatment, and you document general information on

treatment and results. C refers to comments, including brief recommendations for another treatment and self-care. The form shown here includes a body diagram for you to note specific data.

INTRODUCING . . . THE CASE STUDIES

Three different case studies are presented throughout this text. The participants are introduced in this chapter with brief biographies followed by the documentation forms used to record their information: health history and SOAP notes. The SOAP note highlights the subjective information, which was detailed in this chapter. In the following chapters, you will see the same SOAP note highlighting sections that are appropriate for those chapters. Here, we introduce Rob Blackwell, Timothy Roberts, and Kirsten Van Marter.

PROGRESSIVE CASE STUDY 1

Rob Blackwell

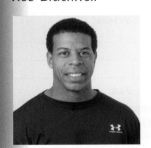

Rob Blackwell is a 42-year-old man who is trying massage for the first time and hopes to restore his sleep and reduce pain in his neck, shoulder, back, and knees so he can lift weights and golf as he used to. Rob says his shoulder pain interferes with his activities the most. He complains that his sleep is affected by his pain, and his health history reveals osteoarthritis and tendinitis in his knees, multiple sprains in his ankles, sinus trouble, and multiple head injuries. Your interview determines that the osteoarthritis diagnosis was made more than 10 years ago. On a pain scale of 1 to 10, with 10 being the worst pain, Rob says all of his areas of concern are about 4. He soaks in the hot tub, which helps the pain, and he occasionally takes ibuprofen, which could affect his pain perception during massage. All of the information Rob tells you is subjective information, and you record anything that is pertinent to his chief complaints (See Figs. 5-6 and 5-7).

The massage for Rob is designed to reduce pain and tension and find fascial adhesions, but you focus on the condition of the soft tissues in his shoulders. You use your standard massage flow, with the addition of some therapeutic techniques. After the massage, you perform the posttreatment assessment, prioritize Rob's functional limitations, and determine short- and long-term treatment goals. You make treatment plan recommendations regarding future treatment, self-care, and referrals to other healthcare practitioners.

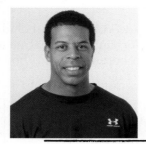

Therapeutic Massage Works

HEALTH INFORMATION

Patient Name Rob Blackwell
Date 4.2.02

Date of Injury _____ **Insurance ID#** N/A

A. Patient Information

Address 120 Main St.
City Indianapolis **State** IN **Zip** 46220
Phone: Home 317-555-2345
Work same **Cell/Pgr** 317-555-3333
Date of Birth 10/29/60
Employer self-employed
Occupation Personal Trainer
Emergency Contact Wife (Stephanie)
Phone: Home same as above
Work (317)5552346 **Cell/Pgr** N/A

Primary Health Care Provider
Name None
Address _____
City/State/Zip _____
Phone: _____ **Fax** _____

I give my manual therapist permission to consult with my referring health care provider regarding my health and treatment.

Comments _____
Initials _____ **Date** _____

B. Current Health Information

List Health/Concerns Check all that apply
Primary neck/shoulder
☒ mild ☐ moderate ☐ disabling
☒ constant ☐ intermittant
☒ symptoms ↑ w/activity ☐ ↓ w/activity
☐ getting worse ☐ getting better ☒ no change
treatment received none
Secondary back
☒ mild ☐ moderate ☐ disabling
☒ constant ☐ intermittant
☒ symptoms ↑ w/activity ☐ ↓ w/activity
☐ getting worse ☐ getting better ☒ no change
treatment received none
Additional knee
☐ mild ☒ moderate ☐ disabling
☐ constant ☒ intermittant
☐ symptoms ↑ w/activity ☒ ↓ w/activity
☐ getting worse ☐ getting better ☒ no change
treatment received none

Have you ever received Manual Therapy before? ☐ Y ☒ N Frequency? _____

List all conditions currently monitored by a Health Care Provider N/A
_____

List the medications you took today (include pain relievers and herbal remedies)
N/A
_____

List all other medications taken in the last 3 months Ibuprofen

List Daily Activities
Work training 8+ hours/day

Home/Family _____

Social/Recreational Workout: lift weights, bicycling; Basketball 3x/mo, golf
Circle the activities affected by your condition,
☒ all of the above
Check other activities affected: ☒ sleep
☐ washing ☐ dressing ☒ fitness
How do you reduce stress? Workout

Pain? Ibuprofen

What are your goals for receiving Manual Therapy? restore sleep, reduce pain, restore ability to lift weights at prior level, be able to play golf again

C. Health History
List and Explain. Include dates and treatment received.
Surgeries appendix 9/78

Accidents _____

Major Illnesses N/A

Check All Current and Previous Conditions Please Explain **HEALTH INFORMATION** page 2

General

current	past		comments
☐	☐	headaches	___
☒	☐	pain	___
☒	☐	sleep disturbances	___
☒	☐	fatigue	___
☐	☐	infectious	___
☐	☐	fever	___
☐	☒	sinus	___
☐	☐	other	___

Skin Conditions

current	past		comments
☐	☐	rashes	___
☐	☒	athlete's foot, warts	___
☐	☐	other	___

Allergies

current	past		comments
☐	☐	scents, oils, lotions	___
☐	☐	detergents	___
☐	☐	other	___

Muscles and Joints

current	past		comments
☐	☐	rheumatoid arthritis	___
☒	☐	osteoarthritis	*Knees*
☐	☐	osteoporosis	___
☐	☐	scoliosis	___
☐	☐	broken bones	___
☐	☐	spinal problems	___
☐	☐	disk problems	___
☐	☐	lupus	___
☐	☐	TMJ, jaw pain	___
☐	☐	spasms, cramps	___
☐	☒	sprains, strains	___
☐	☒	tendonitis, bursitis	*Knees*
☒	☐	stiff or painful joints	___
☐	☐	weak or sore muscles	___
☒	☐	(neck)(shoulder) arm pain	___
☐	☐	low back, hip, leg pain	___
☐	☐	other	___

Nervous System

current	past		comments
☐	☒	head injuries, concussions	*1980, 1981, 1982*
☐	☐	dizziness, ringing in the ears	___
☐	☐	loss of memory, confusion	___
☒	☐	numbness, tingling	___
☐	☐	sciatica, shooting pain	___
☐	☐	chronic pain	___
☐	☐	depression	___
☐	☐	other	___

Respiratory, Cardiovascular

current	past		comments
☐	☐	heart disease	___
☐	☐	blood clots	___
☐	☐	stroke	___
☐	☐	lymphadema	___
☐	☐	high, low blood pressure	___
☐	☐	irregular heart beat	___
☐	☐	poor circulation	___
☐	☐	swollen ankles	___
☐	☐	varicose veins	___
☐	☐	chest pain, shortness of breath	___
☐	☐	asthma	___

Digestive/Elimination System

current	past		comments
☐	☐	bowel dysfunction	___
☐	☐	gas, bloating	___
☐	☐	bladder/kidney dysfunction	___
☐	☐	abdominal pain	___
☐	☐	other	___

Endocrine System

current	past		comments
☐	☐	thyroid dysfunction	___
☐	☐	diabetes	___

Reproductive System

current	past		comments
☐	☐	pregnancy	___
☐	☐	painful, emotional menses	___
☐	☐	fibrotic cysts	___

Cancer/Tumors

current	past		comments
☐	☐	benign	___
☐	☐	malignant	___

Habits

current	past		comments
☐	☐	tobacco	___
☐	☐	alcohol	___
☐	☐	drugs	___
☐	☐	coffee, soda	___

Contract for Care

I promise to participate fully as a member of my health care team. I will make sound choices regarding my treatment plan based on the information provided by my manual therapist and other members of my health care team, and my experience of those suggestions. I agree to participate in the self care program we select. I promise to inform my practitioner any time I feel my well-being is threatened or compromised. I expect my manual therapist to provide safe and effective treatment.

Consent for Care

It is my choice to receive manual therapy, and I give my consent to receive treatment. I have reported all health conditions that I am aware of and will inform my practitioner of any changes in my health.

Signature _RobBlackwell_   Date _4·2·02_

Signature of parent or guardian ___   Date ___
(If patient is a minor)

FIGURE 5-6 *(continued)* Health information form for Rob Blackwell.

Provider Name _Therapeutic Massage Works_

SOAP CHART-M

Patient Name _Rob Blackwell_   **Date** _4.2.02_

Date of Injury _N/A_   **Insurance ID#** _N/A_   **Current Meds** _ibuprofen prn_

S   Focus for Today

Symptoms: Location/Intensity/Frequency/Duration/Onset

Cl c/o neck, shoulder and back Ⓟ, Ⓟ is mild and constant; Sx ↑ c̄ activity; also c/o knee Ⓟ, mod c̄ intermittant Sx ↓ c̄ activity

Activities of Daily Living: Aggravating/Relieving

workout and basketball are affected by Sx & Ⓟ; sleep is also affected

O   Findings: Visual/Palpable/Test Results

Client standing; anterior view

① ≡, X, @ᴾ SCM, pec major & minor; ≡ & @ suboccipitals, traps -Ⓑ Ⓛ; ≡ Ⓡ scalenes & pec minor, mod Ⓟ upon digital pressure to Ⓡ SCM ② ≡ & X to Ⓑ Ⓛ quads; I.t. band & T.f.l.

A   Modalities: Applications/Locations

XFF & DF to affected mm c̄ X, mfr c̄ P.R. to Ⓡ SCM & scalenes & suboccipitals.

Response to Treatment (see Δ)

Prioritize Functional Limitations

① ↓ neck, shoulder and back Ⓟ

② ↓ knee Ⓟ

Goals: Long-term/Short-term

LTG: ↓ Ⓟ to functional level

STG: workout and play basketball c̄ minimal Ⓟ & Sx

P   Future Treatment/Frequency

Tx 1x/wk for 4 weeks; then reevaluate

Homework/Self-care

ice to affected areas, stretching for SCM, scalenes & pecs; ↑ H₂O intake

Provider Signature _Ms Therapist_   **Date** _4.2.02_

Legend:

℮ TP	• TeP	○ Ⓟ	✳ Infl	≡ HT	≈ SP
✕ Adh	≋ Numb	◯ rot	╱ elev	⊱⊰ Short	↔ Long

FIGURE 5-7 SOAP note for Rob Blackwell, subjective information highlighted. (Modified from Thompson DL. Hands Heal: Communication, Documentation, and Insurance Billing for Manual Therapists. 2nd ed. Baltimore: Lippincott Williams & Wilkins, 2002.)

PROGRESSIVE CASE STUDY 2

Timothy Roberts

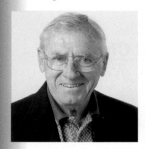

Timothy Roberts is an elderly gentleman who is primarily interested in relaxation. A person his age is considered part of the senior (geriatric) population, but treatment should be based upon the condition of the soft tissues and general state of health. He indicates no specific areas of concern or chief complaints, but you notice that he takes blood pressure medication and has a history of skin cancers (See Fig. 5-8).

The main focus of Timothy's massage will be relaxation and circulatory enhancement. During the massage, you find fascial restrictions and reduced PROM in his left ankle. Following the massage, you briefly discuss plans for future massage treatment and self-help activities.

PROGRESSIVE CASE STUDY 3

Kirsten Van Marter

Kirsten Van Marter is a 38-year-old woman in her third trimester of pregnancy. She has received monthly massage treatments in the past but is a first-time client for you. Her primary complaint is mild but constant back pain. Her secondary concern is mild pain in her hips, pelvis, neck, and shoulders. She is looking for pain reduction in her areas of concern, restored sleep, and restored normal fitness level, and she wants to be able to pick up her child without pain. She says that she worries that she will drop her daughter because of the pain. She is physically active and in good health, except for anemia and gestational diabetes during this pregnancy. You record any information Kirsten shares with you that is pertinent to her areas of concern as subjective information (See Figs. 5-9 and 5-10).

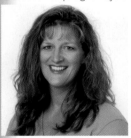

There are a number of techniques and areas to avoid for prenatal massage and special considerations to make. You keep Kirsten in the side-lying position for most of the massage and provide a relaxation massage with some therapeutic techniques. After the massage, you perform a posttreatment assessment, prioritize her functional limitations, and determine short- and long-term treatment goals. You make specific recommendations for future treatment and self-care.

Chapter Summary

Based on the events in the history of massage and the concepts of ethics and professionalism, you can see why effective communication and documentation are important. Without effective communication, you cannot gather appropriate and important information or accurately document activity that occurred. Inaccurate records provide an undependable history, they can lead to misunderstanding, and they can compromise your integrity and professionalism. Ethics and professionalism are cornerstones for a successful practice. Your understanding of medical terminology, anatomy, and physiology help you read and write useful massage treatment records that contain helpful information for you and the other members of your clients' healthcare team.

Gathering information through effective communication with clients is vital to good documentation. Establishing rapport and mutual trust and validating the client's condition and perceptions are necessary for creating a client-centered focus for safe and effective massage treatment. Effective communication, reflective listening skills, asking useful questions, and considering nonverbal communication all help make the interview more effective and lead to the most thorough picture of a client's current condition. This information is recorded on a SOAP chart or other documentation format. Documentation is essential for the safe and effective treatment of clients as well as for communication with other healthcare providers.

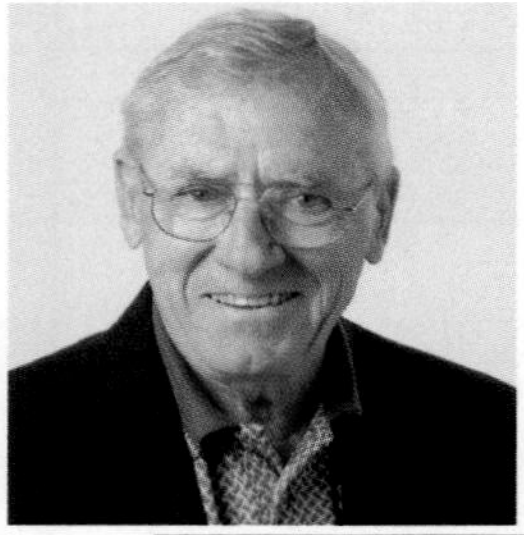

Therapeutic Massage Works STANDARD HxTxC Chart-M

Name ___Timothy Roberts_____ Date _9/10/03_

Phone __317-555-1234___ Address __110 Main St, Indianapolis, IN 46220_

1. What are your goals for health, and how may I assist you in achieving your goals? _____
   _relaxation_____.

2. Are you currently experiencing any of the following? If yes, please explain.

pain, tenderness	☑ No	☐ Yes: _____	stiffness	☑ No	☐ Yes: _____
numbness or tingling	☑ No	☐ Yes: _____	swelling	☑ No	☐ Yes: _____
allergies	☑ No	☐ Yes: _____			

3. List all illnesses, injuries, and health concerns you have now or have had in the past 3 years.
   (Examples: arthritis, diabetes, car accident, pregnancy) _moderate blood pressure,_
   skin cancer, broken (L) ankle

4. List medications and pain relievers taken today. _Blood pressure medication_
   _____

5. I have provided all my known medical information. I acknowledge that manual therapy is not
   a substitute for medical diagnosis and treatment. I give my consent to receive treatment.

   Signature _Timothy Roberts_____ Date _2/21/02_

   Tx: _FBRM c̄ circulatory enhancement focus; during_
   (m) _noticed ↓ ROM & X in (L) ankle –_
   C: _Cl has no complaints today_
   next session XFF to (L) ankle

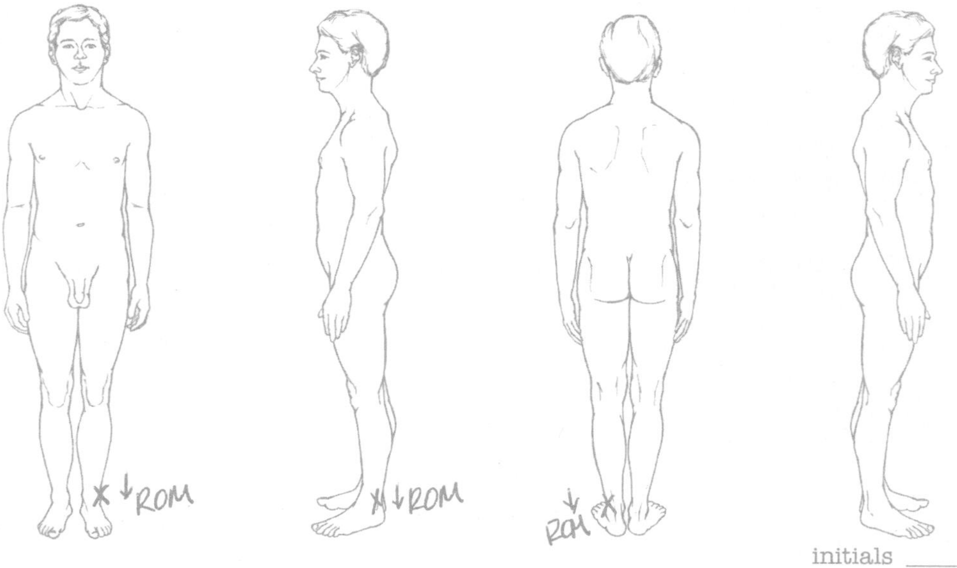

FIGURE 5-8 Standard HxTxC chart for Timothy Roberts. (Modified from Thompson DL. Hands Heal: Communication, Documentation, and Insurance Billing for Manual Therapists. 2nd ed. Baltimore: Lippincott Williams & Wilkins, 2002.)

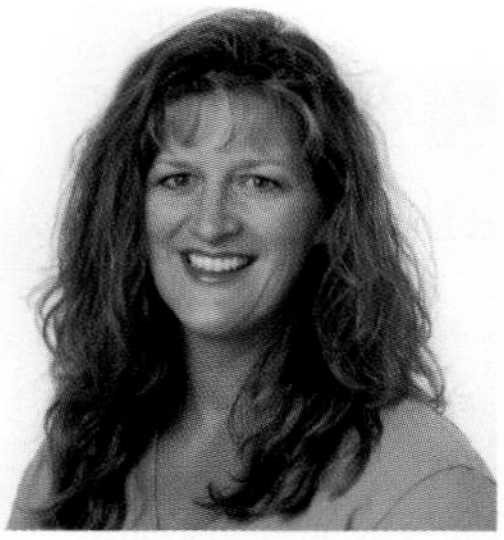

Therapeutic Massage Works   **HEALTH INFORMATION**

Patient Name ___Kirsten Van Marter___   Date ___4.9.02___

Date of Injury ___N/A___   Insurance ID# ___N/A___

A. Patient Information

Address ___130 Main St___
City ___Indianapolis___ State ___IN___ Zip ___46220___
Phone: Home ___317-555-3456___
    Work ___317-555-456___ Cell/Pgr ___317-555-4114___
Date of Birth ___6-17-63___
Employer ___ABC Hospital___
Occupation ___Health Program Coordinator___
Emergency Contact ___husband (Tom)___
Phone: Home ___Same___
    Work ___317-555-6789___ Cell/Pgr ___N/A___

Primary Health Care Provider

Name ___Dr. Daniels___
Address ___555 N. America___
City/State/Zip ___Indianapolis, IN 46220___
Phone: ___317 555 5555___ Fax ___317 555 5556___

I give my manual therapist permission to
consult with my referring health care provider
regarding my health and treatment.

Comments _____
Initials ___KVC___   Date ___4.9.02___

B. Current Health Information

List Health/Concerns Check all that apply
Primary ___Back Pain___
☒ mild ☐ moderate ☐ disabling
☐ constant ☒ intermittant
☒ symptoms ↑ w/activity   ☐ ↓ w/activity
☐ getting worse ☐ getting better ☒ no change
treatment received ___massage___
Secondary ___Hip Pain___
☒ mild ☐ moderate ☐ disabling
☐ constant ☒ intermittant
☒ symptoms ↑ w/activity   ☐ ↓ w/activity
☐ getting worse ☐ getting better ☒ no change
treatment received ___massage___
Additional ___neck & shoulder___
☒ mild ☐ moderate ☐ disabling
☐ constant ☒ intermittant
☒ symptoms ↑ w/activity   ☐ ↓ w/activity
☐ getting worse ☐ getting better ☒ no change
treatment received ___massage___

Have you ever received Manual Therapy
before? ☒ Y ☐ N Frequency? ___1x/mo___
List all conditions currently monitored by a
Health Care Provider ___pregnancy___
_____

List the medications you took today
(include pain relievers and herbal remedies)
___prenatal vitamin, iron supplement___
_____

List all other medications taken in the last
3 months ___tylenol, antibiotic___
_____

List Daily Activities

Work ___computer entry, fitness instructor 3x/wk___

Home/Family ___cleaning, laundry, care
for 2½ year old___
Social/Recreational ___walk 1-2x/wk,
strength train 1x/wk___
Circle the activities affected by your condition,
☒ all of the above
Check other activities affected: ☒ sleep
☐ washing ☐ dressing ☒ fitness
How do you reduce stress? ___exrcise,
massage___
Pain? ___stretching, pain relief meds___

What are your goals for receiving Manual
Therapy? ___reduce back & hip pain, neck/shoulder
pain, restore normal sleep, restore normal
fitness level, pick up 2½ year old daughter___

C. Health History

List and Explain. Include dates and treatment
received.
Surgeries ___1979 - (R) knee - cartilage removed,
1999 - C-section___
Accidents ___N/A___

Major Illnesses ___Hepatitis A - Aug 2000___
_____

FIGURE 5-9   Health information form for Kirsten Van Marter.

Check All Current and Previous Conditions   Please Explain   **HEALTH INFORMATION** page 2

General

current	past		comments
☒	☐	headaches	pregnancy
☒	☐	pain	"
☒	☐	sleep disturbances	"
☒	☐	fatigue	"
☐	☒	infectious	
☐	☒	fever	
☐	☒	sinus	
☐	☐	other	

Skin Conditions

current	past		comments
☐	☐	rashes	
☐	☒	athlete's foot (warts)	
☐	☐	other	

Allergies

current	past		comments
☐	☐	scents, oils, lotions	
☐	☐	detergents	
☒	☐	other	sulfa drugs

Muscles and Joints

current	past		comments
☐	☐	rheumatoid arthritis	
☐	☐	osteoarthritis	
☐	☐	osteoporosis	
☐	☐	scoliosis	
☐	☐	broken bones	
☐	☐	spinal problems	
☐	☐	disk problems	
☐	☐	lupus	
☐	☐	TMJ, jaw pain	
☐	☐	spasms, cramps	
☐	☒	sprains, strains (L) ankle	
☐	☐	tendonitis, bursitis	
☐	☐	stiff or painful joints	
☐	☐	weak or sore muscles	
☒	☐	neck, shoulder, arm pain	
☒	☐	low back, hip, leg pain	
☐	☐	other	

Nervous System

current	past		comments
☐	☒	head injuries, (concussions)	7yrs old
☐	☐	dizziness, ringing in the ears	
☐	☐	loss of memory, confusion	
☐	☐	numbness, tingling	
☐	☐	sciatica, shooting pain	
☐	☐	chronic pain	
☐	☐	depression	
☒	☐	other anemia – due to pregnancy	

Respiratory, Cardiovascular

current	past		comments
☐	☐	heart disease	
☐	☐	blood clots	
☐	☐	stroke	
☐	☐	lymphadema	
☐	☐	high, low blood pressure	
☐	☐	irregular heart beat	
☐	☐	poor circulation	
☐	☐	swollen ankles	
☐	☐	varicose veins	
☐	☐	chest pain, shortness of breath	
☐	☐	asthma	

Digestive/Elimination System

current	past		comments
☐	☐	bowel dysfunction	
☐	☐	gas, bloating	
☐	☐	bladder/kidney dysfunction	
☐	☐	abdominal pain	
☐	☐	other	

Endocrine System

current	past		comments
☐	☐	thyroid dysfunction	
☐	☒	diabetes	gestational

Reproductive System

current	past		comments
☐	☐	pregnancy	
☐	☐	painful, emotional menses	
☐	☐	fibrotic cysts	

Cancer/Tumors

current	past		comments
☐	☐	benign	
☐	☐	malignant	

Habits

current	past		comments
☐	☐	tobacco	
☐	☐	alcohol	
☐	☐	drugs	
☒	☐	coffee, soda	tea

Contract for Care

I promise to participate fully as a member of my health care team. I will make sound choices regarding my treatment plan based on the information provided by my manual therapist and other members of my health care team, and my experience of those suggestions. I agree to participate in the self care program we select. I promise to inform my practitioner any time I feel my well-being is threatened or compromised. I expect my manual therapist to provide safe and effective treatment.

Consent for Care

It is my choice to receive manual therapy, and I give my consent to receive treatment. I have reported all health conditions that I am aware of and will inform my practitioner of any changes in my health.

Signature _Kirsten Van Marter_   Date 4.9.02

Signature of parent or guardian _____   Date _____
(If patient is a minor)

FIGURE 5-9   *(continued)* Health information form for Kirsten Van Marter.

Provider Name: Therapeutic Massage Works

SOAP CHART-F

Patient Name: Kirsten Van Marter   Date: 4.9.02

Date of Injury: N/A   Insurance ID#: N/A   Current Meds: N/A

S Focus for Today

Symptoms: Location/Intensity/Frequency/Duration/Onset

Cl c/o mild & intermittant @ lower & upper back ⓟ; also c/o mild and intermittant hip ⓟ, Ⓑⓛ; mostly ® exacerbated by pregnancy; cl states she is in last trimester

Activities of Daily Living: Aggravating/Relieving

aggravating ADL: teaching fitness class, computer entry, household activities, child care, workouts

relieving ADL: massage, stretching, exercise and pain meds prn

O Findings: Visual/Palpable/Test Results

Client standing, anterior view

① Ⓑⓛ ≡ pec major & minor, subscap, rhomboids, traps. Ⓑⓛ X in erector spinae; TeP in Ⓑⓛ traps & rhomboids @ in Ⓑⓛ pec.

② Ⓑⓛ ≡ QL, esp Ⓛ, ≡ hams; Ⓛ ≡ gastroc, peroneals, quad, t.fl., itband

A Modalities: Applications/Locations

light mfr to neck, back and hips; Light XFF to erector spinae

Response to Treatment (see Δ)

Prioritize Functional Limitations

① ↓ ⓟ in work and household activities

② ↓ ⓟ while working out

Goals: Long-term/Short-term

LTG: ↓ ⓟ in ADL

STG: ↓ ⓟ in affected areas

P Future Treatment/Frequency

massage 1x/wk for 1 month

Homework/Self-care

↑ H₂O intake; stretches for neck and back

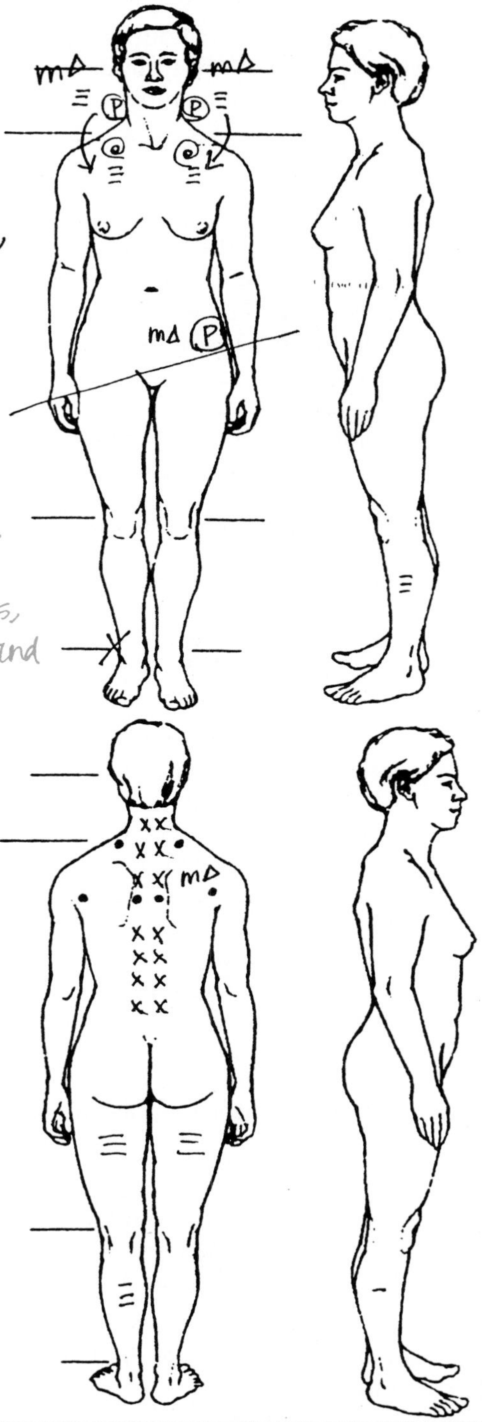

Provider Signature: TMS Therapist   Date: 4.9.02

Legend: ⓒ TP   • TeP   ○ ⓟ   ✳ Infl   ≡ HT   ≈ SP
          X Adh   ≋ Numb   ⌒ rot   ╱ elev   ⊁ Short   ↔ Long

FIGURE 5-10 SOAP note for Kirsten Van Marter.

CHAPTER EXERCISES

1. Using the procedure outlined in this chapter, perform at least five different client intake interviews with friends or family members.

2. Using the procedure outlined in this chapter, take at least five different client histories from friends or family members.

3. Identify the stress factors for yourself and five other people.

4. Identify the appropriate section of the SOAP note (subjective, objective, activity and analysis, plan) for documenting the following information:
   a. Within the next week, the client should be able to lift 10 pounds at a time, three times a day, for 5 days with no shoulder pain.
   _____
   b. Applied a full-body relaxation massage using therapeutic techniques on the left quadriceps femoris muscles. _____
   c. Client complains of low back pain.
   _____
   d. Client was referred to Dr. Bob Smith for skin abnormality. _____
   e. Upon posttreatment assessment, the client's lateral neck flexion and neck rotation to the right increased. _____
   f. Next session, try to address the right biceps femoris muscle with therapeutic techniques.
   _____
   g. The client's skin was red and hot around the left scapula. _____
   h. The client barely swings her left arm when walking. _____
   i. After the massage, the client says he has to be able to lift 50 pounds at a time, repeatedly throughout the day, for his job.
   _____
   j. The client responded well to vibration over the levator scapula muscles.
   _____

5. List the signs and symptoms of the following categories that you should ask about during a client interview: General, Circulatory, Musculoskeletal, Neurological, Psychosocial.

6. List at least seven assumptions that help maintain a humanistic view of clients in the communication process.

7. Identify the five components of an effective goal.

8. Write down at least five different functional limitations you have experienced in your life and describe how they were restored.

9. Use abbreviations and symbols from Table 5-1 to shorten the following sentences:
   a. The client complains of pain in the right levator scapula muscle.
   b. Lateral flexion of the neck increased with massage.
   c. I applied a full-body relaxation massage with a lot of effleurage bilaterally over the quadratus lumborum muscles.
   d. The client has decreased range of motion at the left ankle, and no dorsiflexion is possible.
   e. The client came in with a headache and a fever, which is a contraindication, so I explained that he could return for a safe massage treatment when his fever has subsided.

10. Design your own client intake form by following the steps below:
    a. What client contact information do you want to record?
    b. Do you want clients' insurance information?
    c. What questions do you want to include regarding the current condition of the clients' soft tissues?
    d. What health history information do you want to know about?
    e. Do you want to know about daily activities?
    f. Do you want to include a body diagram for the client to use?
    g. Do you want to include the informed consent for care on your intake form?

SUGGESTED READINGS

Ford RD, ed. Health Assessment Handbook. Springhouse, PA: Springhouse Corporation, 1985.

Loeb S (executive editorial director). Mastering Documentation. Springhouse, PA: Springhouse Corporation, 1995.

Newell R. Interviewing Skills for Nurses and Other Health Care Professionals: A Structured Approach. New York: Routledge, 1994.

Rattray F, Ludwig L. Clinical Massage Therapy: Understanding, Assessing and Treating over 70 Conditions. Toronto: Talus Incorporated, 2000.

Thompson DL. Hands Heal: Documentation for Massage Therapy, A Guide to SOAP Charting. 1st ed. Seattle, WA: Diana L. Thompson, 1993.

Thompson DL. Hands Heal: Communication, Documentation and Insurance Billing for Manual Therapists. 2nd ed. Baltimore: Lippincott Williams & Wilkins, 2002.

Werner R. A Massage Therapist's Guide to Pathology. Philadelphia: Lippincott Williams & Wilkins, 1998.

Willis MC. Medical Terminology The Language of Healthcare. Philadelphia: Lippincott Williams & Wilkins, 1996.

Assessment

UPON COMPLETION OF THIS CHAPTER, THE STUDENT WILL BE ABLE TO:

- List the five kinds of observations included in general assessments
- Describe why massage therapists should understand fascial adhesions
- Define compensation pattern
- Identify at least three characteristics to evaluate during postural assessment
- Name the six aspects of gait assessment
- Name the two different kinds of range-of-motion evaluations
- Define end feel
- Name the three characteristics to assess with palpation
- Describe the purpose of functional assessments

KEY TERMS

Active range of motion (AROM): joint movement that requires clients to actively use their own energy to demonstrate how much of the full range can be completed comfortably and without restriction

Assessment: the process of evaluating a client's condition

Compensation pattern: a postural offset that is the body's attempt to correct an imbalance or protect a primary dysfunction or injury

Direction of ease: the direction in which tissues move with least resistance

End feel: a unique feel when a joint reaches the end of its passive range of motion (PROM) determined by specific structures that stop the movement

Fascial adhesion (fascial restriction): an area where the fascia has adhered to nearby tissues or has been crumpled or kinked

Gait: a walking pattern

Palpation: the skillful art of client evaluation that uses touch to locate and assess the quality of different structures

Passive range of motion (PROM): joint movement that requires the therapist to move the relaxed client through a range of motion to determine how much of the full range can be completed comfortably and without restriction

Range of motion (ROM): the end-to-end distance of a specific joint movement that is structurally possible

Well-trained massage therapists are soft tissue experts with a solid understanding of muscular system anatomy and physiology. **Assessment** is the process of evaluating a client's condition to determine which muscles and soft tissues of the client's body to work on and which massage techniques to use. Good assessment skills go hand in hand with skilled and effective treatments. They help you evaluate the condition of the client's soft tissues to

- Determine which techniques to use to reach the client's treatment goals
- Identify compensation patterns
- Determine whether massage therapy is indicated or the client needs to be referred to a healthcare professional for further evaluation

The physical condition of clients, in addition to their treatment goals, will guide your approach to treatment. Using techniques that are too aggressive or too subtle can be inappropriate or ineffective, as can massage sessions that are too short or too long and techniques that are too slow or too fast.

Although assessment skills help you determine the condition of the client's tissues for massage and discover contraindications, you do not use them to diagnose any specific medical conditions or prescribe treatments. Medical diagnosis and prescription are out of the massage therapy scope of practice and should not be performed by massage therapists under any circumstance.

Many assessment tools can be used to evaluate the condition of soft tissues. The massage therapist's first assessment tool is the client's health history. The initial interview process gives you a general idea of the condition of the soft tissues and the past and present stress factors that influence the healing process. Clients often come to you with specific areas of concern and functional limitations that serve as a starting point for your assessment. Some common areas of concern are neck tension, low back pain, and shoulder stiffness. The accompanying functional limitations can include the inability to turn the neck to check blind spots while driving, the inability to sit for long periods of time, and difficulty brushing and washing hair.

Along with the health history that provides information about the client's condition, there are general assessments and functional assessments. General assessments include postural, gait, range-of-motion (ROM), visual, and palpation (tactile) observations. More advanced, functional assessments can help you determine whether a specific pain or injury condition warrants massage or whether massage may be contraindicated. Functional assessments include manual muscle testing, manual resistive testing, and orthopedic tests. They require additional training because to elicit accurate and useful information, you need careful technique and supervised practice. Referring clients for further evaluation to rule out contraindications conveys the message that you know your limits and that the client's health and well-being is at the center of care. Understand that massage is not necessarily the appropriate treatment for all soft tissue conditions. Often when medical conditions that present contraindications have been ruled out, massage is one of the best treatments for soft tissue conditions.

General Assessments

The general assessments you perform prior to all wellness and therapeutic massage sessions include postural, gait, ROM, visual, and palpation (tactile) observations. For clients seeking nonspecific relaxation massage for wellness, the general assessment process does not need to be extensive or time-consuming, but it still needs to be done. Without an initial assessment, it is more difficult for you and your clients to recognize the results of the massage treatment, and it is also more difficult to write an effective treatment plan. The assessments pertinent to the areas of concern are documented on your massage treatment records. When clients have concerns about health conditions beyond the massage scope of practice (soft connective tissues), you should refer them to the appropriate healthcare professionals who can perform the necessary examinations to determine whether there are any contraindications for massage.

WELLNESS VERSUS THERAPEUTIC MASSAGE ASSESSMENTS

The general assessment process for wellness and relaxation massage is usually completed in less than 2–3 minutes. You can use the following guidelines for a short but complete assessment:

1. Ask a series of two or three questions to elicit the client's goal(s) for the treatment session.
2. Ask a couple of questions to determine if there are any functional limitations, areas to concentrate on, or areas to avoid.
3. Look for obvious visible differences in the evenness or levelness of the body, especially in the client's area of concern or area of functional limitation.
4. Before or during the massage, evaluate one or two movements that relate to the functional limitation or area of previous injury.
5. During the massage session, pay attention to the general texture and movement of soft tissues.

Many clients who initially come to you for relaxation massage on a regular basis can benefit from therapeutic massage if their pain pattern becomes worse or if they sustain an injury. When these clients look for more than a relaxation massage, your general assessments can last 5 minutes or longer because you need more information to determine safe and effective treatment. The assessment process for therapeutic massage can include the following:

1. Determine the client's goal(s) for the session.
2. Ask a series of leading questions to understand the condition of the client's soft tissues.
3. Ask a series of leading questions to determine the client's functional limitations and how they affect the client's lifestyle.
4. Before the massage, perform the general assessments shown in Procedure Box 6-1 to evaluate posture, gait, and ROMs.
   Evaluate each movement of the joint(s) involved in the functional limitations.

PROCEDURE BOX 6-1
General Assessments for Therapeutic Massage

Standing Postural Assessment

(You can use the body diagram on the general assessment form)

1. With the client fully clothed, shoes off, ask the client to stand comfortably with heels about 3 inches apart, arms hanging in a relaxed position.

   You can use a door frame as a vertical reference line by asking the client to stand in front of it so that the vertical part of the frame can be seen centered between the client's feet.

2. View the client's anterior aspect to look for obvious differences in the height of bilateral surface or bony landmarks or obvious deviations off the midsagittal plane (off to one side).
   a. Head (nose, chin, ears)
   b. Shoulders (acromion process)
   c. Sternum
   d. Navel
   e. Pelvis (ASIS and iliac crest)
   f. Hands (fingertips, wrists)
   g. Knees (patella)
   h. Feet—flat, normal, or high arches, lateral deviation (toes point out) or medial deviation (toes point in), how client wears out soles of shoes

3. Ask the client to turn around and face the door frame in the same relaxed position.

4. View the client's posterior aspect to look for obvious differences in height of bilateral surface or bony structures, or obvious deviations off the midsagittal plane.
   a. Head (ears)
   b. Shoulders (acromion process)
   c. Spine
   d. Pelvis (iliac crest or PSIS)
   e. Hands (fingertips, wrists)

5. Ask the client to turn so the door frame is behind the ankle and stand in the same relaxed position.

6. View the client's lateral aspect to look for obvious deviations toward the anterior or posterior.
   a. Head (ear just anterior to midsagittal line)
   b. Shoulders (center of glenohumeral joint on midsagittal line)
   c. Hands (palms directed medially)
   d. Pelvis (greater trochanters on midsagittal line)
   e. Knees (center of joint on midsagittal line)

7. Ask the client to turn and face the other direction, in the same relaxed position, with the door frame behind the ankle.

8. View the second side to confirm the anterior or posterior deviations observed on the first side or to show differences from right to left, suggesting rotation.
   a. Head (left ear is anterior to the right ear, or vice versa)
   b. Shoulder girdle (left acromion process is anterior to right, or vice versa)
   c. Pelvis (right ASIS is anterior to the left, or vice versa)

9. Document any obvious differences or deviations on the general assessment form and in the objective portion of the SOAP chart.

Gait Assessment

1. Ask the client to walk across the floor.
2. Observe how the client walks, paying attention to the quantity, quality, and fluidity of steps (bilateral symmetry, evenness of steps, smoothness).
3. Observe the alignment of the head over the spine and the position of the shoulders.
4. Observe the arm swing for bilateral symmetry and smooth movement.
5. Observe the medial or lateral deviation of the feet (indicating rotation of the hip).
6. Observe the knee flexion upon a step and the bounce in the step or lack thereof.
7. Document any deviation from the normal gait pattern on the general assessment form and in the SOAP note's Objective section.

Active Range of Motion Assessment

1. Determine the possible movements of the joint.
2. Starting and ending in the anatomical position, demonstrate the ROM to clients, moving slowly and steadily, keeping the body very still to isolate the joint movement.
3. Explain that there are no successful results or failures possible because it is not a test. Ask clients to tell you if there is any sensation of discomfort or pain.
4. Ask clients to demonstrate the ROM slowly and steadily, starting with the joint on the side that is unaffected or least affected, and ending when there is any sensation of restriction, tightness, or discomfort.
5. Evaluate clients' movement.
   a. Glitches or hesitations
   b. Facial expressions
   c. Changes in breathing patterns
   d. Variations in speed or fluidity
   e. Recruitment of other muscles to complete the range
   f. Completeness or limitations to the ROM
6. Ask clients to repeat the ROM using the affected joint, with a slow, steady movement while holding the body still.
7. Evaluate clients' movement of the affected side as in step 5.
8. Document any findings from your evaluations of AROM on the general assessment form and in the SOAP note's Objective section.

Passive Range of Motion Assessment

1. Identify the movements possible at the particular joint and the muscles and passive structures involved with the joint movement.
2. Explain that clients relax their bodies while you slowly and gently move them through a ROM and to let you do the work. Reassure clients with your confidence and sufficient stabilization, holding them securely and using a gentle but knowledgeable tone of voice.
3. Explain that there are no successful results or failures possible because it is not a test. Ask clients to tell you if there is any sensation of discomfort or pain.

(continued)

4. Ask clients to sit or lie comfortably while you start with the joint on the uninvolved or less involved side.
5. Holding the client's body securely, slowly, steadily, and gently move through the ROM of the joint.
6. Evaluate the movement.
   a. Glitches or hesitations
   b. Resistance
   c. Changes in breathing patterns
   d. Variations in fluidity of movement
7. Move to the affected side, telling the client to remain relaxed while you repeat the process on the other side.
8. Holding the client's body securely, slowly, steadily, and gently move the affected joint through the ROM.
9. Evaluate the movement for the same factors as in step 6.
10. Document any findings from your evaluations of PROM on the general assessment form and in the SOAP note's Objective section.

Appearance of Tissues

1. Before and during the massage, visually evaluate clients.
   a. Differences in color (areas of redness or paleness)
   b. Differences in fullness or thickness of soft tissues
   c. Bilateral symmetry of soft tissues
   d. Marks, bruises, moles, wounds, scars
2. Document any visual findings on the general assessment form and Objective portion of the SOAP note.

Palpation Assessments

1. During the massage, take note of what you feel.
   a. Differences in temperatures (cold areas or hot areas)
   b. Textural differences in skin and soft tissues
   c. Movement of skin and soft tissues
   d. Areas of fullness or swelling
   e. Body rhythms
2. Document any palpation findings on the general assessment form and the Objective portion of the SOAP note.

5. During the massage session, pay attention to the textures and movement of soft tissues throughout the body.

The general assessments give you a better idea of whether or not a client presents any contraindications for massage, which soft tissues you should address, and how you should address them.

There are also occasions when therapeutic massage clients reach a point at which relaxation massage is indicated and a brief assessment is sufficient. Either way, you need to have a thorough understanding of the assessment process to determine how much assessment is necessary to ensure the most appropriate massage treatment.

FASCIA

When assessing the soft tissue, remember the widespread nature of fascia. As described in the anatomy and physiology chapter, fascia is very pervasive, wrapping around and running between all the organs, muscles, and layers of tissue. Its tough, pliable, plastic structure provides support and protection and forms a sort of spider web throughout the body. The protein fibers in fascia can get crumpled, kinked, or stuck together, making it difficult for muscle fibers to slide back and forth for smooth contraction and movement. These **fascial adhesions,** also called **fascial restrictions,** are disruptions in the smooth fascia that can result from

- Insufficient hydration
- Injury
- Accumulated scar tissue
- Tissue dehydration
- Repetitive motions

- Sustained positions
- Postural deviations

In addition to the local restrictions and tightness, fascial adhesions have far-reaching effects on other soft tissues because of the intertwined, three-dimensionality of fascia.

For massage, fascial adhesions are particularly important to understand because fascia's involvement with muscle tissues can cause the location of your clients' pain to differ from where the pain originates. Fascia is much like a sheet of plastic wrap. When a sheet of plastic wrap is pulled on at one corner, the tension creates deformities that extend across the plastic in lines. When a section in the middle of a sheet of plastic is crumpled, it creates several lines of tension that radiate out from the crumpled area. If there is a local restriction in the muscle and soft tissues, there will be similar lines of tension, called fascial lines, that extend out to other areas of the body. (Fig. 6-1 illustrates lines of tension that reach out from a restriction to other areas, similar to the way a

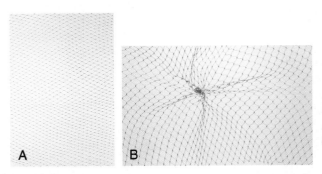

FIGURE 6-1 Fascia photo showing fascial lines. **A.** Representation of unrestricted fascia. **B.** Representation of fascial restriction; notice the fascial lines created by the fascial restriction.

fascial adhesion can pull on structures far away.) Restricted movement, compensation patterns, reduced circulation, muscular tension, and pain in seemingly unrelated areas can all result from fascial tension. Generally, the longer the restriction exists, the more the fascia will be deformed and the longer it will take for the client's tissues to return to normal. For example, right shoulder pain can be caused by structures in and immediately around the glenohumeral joint, but it can also be caused by fascial tension that originates in the abdomen or near the spine. The length of time the pain and restriction have existed, in addition to stress factors and client participation, will determine the best treatment techniques and the amount of time it could take to "unwind" the restriction.

COMPENSATION PATTERNS

The body's objective is to have all the muscles in balance to remain upright, in ideal posture and moving efficiently. When the body deviates from this balanced state, muscles become shortened or overstretched to compensate for the imbalance. **Compensation patterns** are postural offsets that attempt to protect a primary dysfunction or injury or correct an imbalance. Some examples of injury compensation patterns are a limp for a sore ankle, the excessive use of one arm because the other is in a cast, and turning the entire thorax to look over your shoulder because neck rotation is limited and painful.

Sustained postures and repetitive motions can also cause compensation patterns. When muscles continually hold the body in place or are continually used to perform the same movement, they are actively contracted on a regular basis without being lengthened regularly by their antagonists. As a result, the muscles that repeatedly contract or hold contractions for extended periods of time adopt a shorter resting length (they are posturally shortened), and their antagonists develop longer resting lengths (they are overstretched). The body must make up for the imbalance between the antagonistic muscles by adjusting the posture in other areas with functional compensation patterns. Sitting at a computer all day using a mouse requires your body to hold a single position for an extended period of time. Cashiers repetitively turn to their left and sweep products from right to left. Musicians are especially prone to functional compensation patterns because they have to hold their bodies in asymmetric positions for extended periods while they perform repetitive motions with their hands and fingers. All of these activities result in functional compensation patterns that show up as postural asymmetries or deviations. (See Procedure Box 6-2 for the steps to determine compensation patterns.)

✓ PROCEDURE BOX 6-2
Compensation Patterns

1. Identify the client's primary area(s) of complaint.
2. Identify the client's postural deviations as noted on the general assessment form and/or the objective portion of the SOAP chart.
3. Consider relationships between the postural deviations, the area(s) of concern, and pain patterns.
4. Determine the original imbalance or primary dysfunction or injury that caused the postural offsets:
   a. Ask if there is an area that has been painful longer than the others.
   b. Ask if there was an event (such as an injury, trauma, fall, twisted joint, prolonged period in one position, extended period of repetitive motion) that started the pain pattern.
5. Identify the joint(s) involved in the original imbalance or primary dysfunction.
6. Evaluate AROM and PROM of the movements of those joints, looking for restrictions or limitations, and for pain upon PROM, suggesting problems with the passive structures that require a medical referral.
7. Evaluate AROM and PROM of the movements of nearby joints, looking for restrictions that may have resulted from the original imbalance.
   > For example, an injury to the right foot could be compensated by a limp to relieve pressure on the right foot. The limp could require extra work from the hamstring muscles to flex the knee, the rectus femoris muscle to flex the right hip, the right quadratus lumborum to elevate the right side of the pelvis, and the left levator scapula and upper trapezius to elevate the left shoulder. The muscles that are overworked will likely be posturally shortened and will restrict ROM of the joints they move.
8. Document compensation patterns in the Objective section of the SOAP chart.
9. Document any medical referrals in the Plan section of the SOAP chart.

Compensation patterns begin when the imbalance or injury occurs, and ideally, as balance is restored or the injury heals, the compensation patterns work themselves out. Unfortunately, a lot of compensation patterns do not go away completely and can develop areas of chronic hypertonic muscles and restricted fascia. A sprained ankle ligament that occurred a week ago will have an associated compensation pattern that could dissipate over several months, as long as the ligament healed well and the ROMs were restored safely and completely. On the other hand, a 40-year-old man who has had flat feet all his life and has never been medically treated for them will have developed and reinforced a compensation pattern over several decades. Restoring the shortened and

Client Name: _____

Standing Postural Assessment (Evaluate level and position of the following)

Cranium (ears)

Shoulder girdle (acromion process)

Pelvic girdle (ASIS, iliac crest, PSIS)

Hands and fingers

Knees (patella)

Feet : flat, normal, high arch
       lateral or medial deviation
       wear pattern on soles of shoes

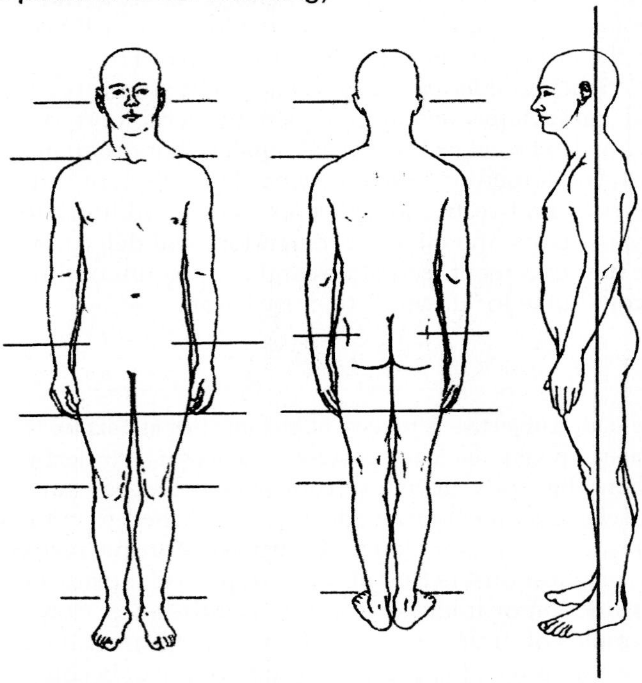

Gait Analysis (quantity, quality, fluidity, alignment, arm swing, foot deviation, knee flexion):

Range of Motion Evaluation:
    Joint: _____ Movement: _____ Normal or reduced
    Pain or discomfort with AROM? ___ PROM? ____

    Joint: _____ Movement: _____ Normal or reduced
    Pain or discomfort with AROM? ___ PROM? ____

    Joint: _____ Movement: _____ Normal or reduced
    Pain or discomfort with AROM? ___ PROM? ____

    Joint: _____ Movement: _____ Normal or reduced
    Pain or discomfort with AROM? ___ PROM? ____

Appearance of Tissues (color, fullness, bilateral symmetry):

Palpation Findings (temperature, texture, movement, fullness, rhythms):

Therapist's signature: _____ Date: _____

FIGURE 6-2 Blank general assessment form. (Modified from Thompson DL. Hands Heal: Communication, Documentation and Insurance Billing for Manual Therapists. 2nd ed. Baltimore: Lippincott Williams & Wilkins, 2002.)

overstretched muscles to their normal resting lengths and breaking up the fascial adhesions that have settled into the tissues could take years, especially if the man continued to go without medical corrective treatment and continued to reinforce the source of the imbalance.

The body's compensation is registered not only in the muscles, but also in the nervous system via nerve tracks, which are discussed in the nervous system section of the anatomy and physiology chapter. The longer a compensation pattern has existed, the more the compensated body positions and the functionally shortened and overstretched muscles are locked into these figurative grooves in the nervous system. Imagine drawing a circle in the sand with a stick. The more circles you draw, the deeper the groove becomes. Over time, compensations are reinforced and become more difficult to change.

Implications for Massage

Once you discover compensation patterns in your postural assessment, you can determine which muscles are functionally shortened or overstretched. Postural deviations, imbalances, or restrictions in movement can be documented with symbols and abbreviations on body diagrams or in the text of your massage treatment records.

Your findings can determine the type of techniques to use and the length of time it may take to restore the most functional balance for the client. Several factors affect massage treatment and the time it will take for healing and restoration of balance and functional movement to occur:

- Lifestyle
- General health
- Length of time the client has been compensating
- Number of planes involved in the compensation
- The client's continuation to repeat any activity that reinforces the imbalance or compensation pattern
- Reinjuring the affected muscles

ASSESSMENT DOCUMENTATION

Your initial observations of postural symmetry, gait, ROM, soft tissue appearance, and soft tissue textures can be recorded as objective information in the SOAP note or on specific forms that only include general assessment data. (See Fig. 6-2 for an example of a general assessment form.) If you use a general assessment form for the client's initial visit, you can record general assessments made in subsequent massage sessions in the Objective portion of the SOAP chart.

Postural Assessment

Posture is the position of the upright, relaxed body. Although many people pay little attention to posture, it can significantly affect a person's health and well-being. The efficiency of the entire organism, or person, depends on cooperation of all the separate anatomical structures working efficiently, with little friction and minimal energy. Any interference can create muscular and soft tissue strain, extra energy requirements, and reduced efficiency in movement. These interferences can result in stress, exhaustion, and health problems that affect the circulatory and digestive systems, spleen, liver, and kidneys. Correct posture provides the best conditions for the bones, joints, muscles, and organs. Incorrect posture can lead to discomfort, pain, organ dysfunction, and disability.

You can evaluate posture to see how "straight" clients stand by looking at how surface landmarks and bony landmarks are positioned, relative to vertical and horizontal reference lines. Your vertical reference can be a plumb line, a line that hangs perfectly vertically as the result of gravity. It can be fashioned with a small weight at the end of a string that hangs from a level higher than the client's head. The client's stance is positioned such that the line falls exactly between the feet. (Fig. 6-3 shows a plumb line and its position relative to the client.) As simple as it is to hang a plumb line, most massage therapists do not have one in their office. Instead, you can use a door frame as a vertical reference, which is readily available in every massage treatment room. Some door frames are not perfectly vertical, but they still give you a reference line to work with.

IDEAL POSTURE

Ideal posture minimizes stress and strain while maximizing efficiency. To evaluate posture for massage, you will look at the anterior, posterior and lateral aspects of your clients and check the alignment and position of surface landmarks. Figure 6-3 illustrates anterior, posterior, and lateral views of ideal posture.

Looking at the anterior aspect of ideal posture, there are a number of surface and bony landmarks that fall on the midsagittal line, which runs vertically down the center of the body: nose, chin, sternum, spine, and navel.

Looking at the anterior or posterior view of ideal posture, there are a number of bilateral landmarks that are both at the same horizontal level: ears, shoulders (acromion process), pelvis (ASIS, PSIS, and iliac crest), hands (fingertips), and knees (patella).

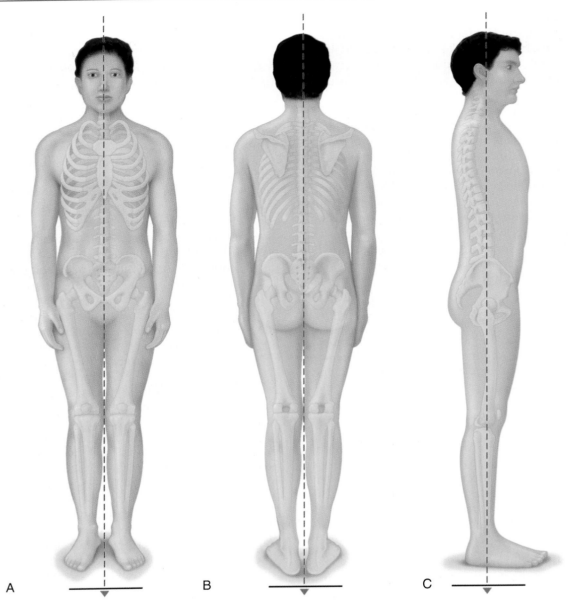

FIGURE 6-3   Ideal posture. **A.** Anterior view. **B.** Posterior view. **C.** Lateral view.

When you evaluate the lateral aspect of your clients, your reference is a vertical line that runs just anterior to the lateral malleolus (ankle). In ideal posture, the vertical line will run through the center of the ear, through the center of the glenohumeral joint, through the bodies of the lumbar vertebrae, through the center of the greater trochanter of the femur, and through the center of the knee joint.

ANTERIOR POSTURAL ASSESSMENT

To view the client's anterior postural alignment, ask clients to stand comfortably, shoes off, arms hanging at the sides, and heels about 3 inches apart. Make sure that your vertical reference line falls midway between the heels and that the client's body does not touch the line. Using the position of bony landmarks in ideal posture as a comparison, evaluate the position of the client's

- Ears (both ears at the same level)
- Nose (on the midsagittal line)
- Chin (on the midsagittal line)
- Shoulders (both acromion processes at the same level and the same distance from the midsagittal line)
- Sternum (on the midsagittal line)
- Navel (on the midsagittal line)
- Pelvis (ASIS or iliac crests at the same level)

- Hands (fingertips at the same level, same amount of space between the body and each hand)
- Knees (patellae at the same level)

If bilateral landmarks are higher on one side than on the other (i.e., horizontal level is different), the landmarks are said to be located off the transverse plane (the chapter Medical Terminology describes planes of division). For example, a right shoulder that is noticeably higher than the left shoulder exhibits a deviation off the transverse plane. Another way to recognize bilateral landmarks at different levels is to use the term elevation. Using the previous example, the right shoulder is elevated. This can be documented on the SOAP note or general assessment form with a diagonal line on the body diagram at the shoulders that is higher on the right. (Figs. 6-10, 6-11, 6-13, and 6-14 below show the documentation of elevation)

If left and right landmarks are at the same horizontal level but farther to the left or the right, they are said to deviate off the sagittal plane. Some examples of deviations off the sagittal plane include a body part that is abducted or adducted more on one side than the other or a body that leans to one side. These can be recorded on the body diagram with an arrow at the location of the deviation, pointing in the direction of the deviation.

When evaluating the anterior view of your client's standing posture, you consider symmetry. Determine whether the client's landmarks are in similar positions on both sides, as described above, but also look for side-to-side differences in fullness, space, and body surface curves. There are sometimes differences in the fullness of tissues from side to side. For instance, one arm might be noticeably larger than the other. The space between the arms and body should also be about equal, but occasionally one arm will hang much closer to the body than the other. You might notice symmetrical differences in the curves, such as the curve at the waist, or the creases of the body such as at the axilla (armpit). (Fig. 6-6, illustrating scoliosis, shows these differences in symmetry.) These observations can be noted on the general assessment form and the Objective portion of the SOAP note.

POSTERIOR POSTURAL ASSESSMENT

To evaluate the client's postural alignment in the posterior view, clients should stand in the same, relaxed position and not touch the line, but instead of facing you, their back is to you. Using the ideal posture in Figure 6-3 for comparison, evaluate the position of the client's

- Cranium (ears at the same level)
- Shoulders (acromion processes at the same level)

- Spine (along the midsagittal line)
- Pelvis (PSIS or iliac crest at the same level)
- Hands (fingertips at the same level, same amount of space between the body and each hand)

You check for bilateral symmetries when evaluating the posterior view of your client's standing posture, just as you did with the anterior view: positions of landmarks, fullness, space, and body curves. The differences can be recorded on the general assessment form and the Objective portion of the SOAP note.

LATERAL POSTURAL ASSESSMENT

When you evaluate the side view, the client's feet maintain the same kind of positioning, but the vertical reference line should run just anterior to the lateral malleolus. You can use Figure 6-3C, lateral view of ideal posture, as a comparative standard when evaluating your clients for

- Cranium (ear just anterior to the line)
- Shoulder (center of the glenohumeral joint should be on the line)
- Hands (palms should be directed medially)
- Pelvis (greater trochanter should be on the line)
- Knee (center of the knee joint should be on the line)

If a landmark is found more toward the anterior or posterior of the client's body, the deviation is off the frontal plane. A client whose head and shoulders are anterior appears to stand slightly bent forward in what is sometimes called a forward posture. The deviation can be documented on a body diagram with an arrow located at the area that is noticeably deviated, with the arrow pointing in the direction of the deviation. (See Figs. 6-10 and 6-11 below, which show documentation of deviation off the frontal plane.) Clients who wear shoes with a heel are shifted forward, off the frontal plane, and their bodies have to compensate by pulling the head and shoulders posteriorly. In fact, the higher the heel, the farther the forward shift and the more the body has to compensate.

POSTURAL DEVIATIONS

Sometimes posture contributes to, or is the source of, soft tissue dysfunction. Seemingly minor postural deviations can cause major problems in some clients, yet significant postural deviations may not be accompanied by any symptoms. Generally, however, incorrect posture is learned and reinforced from soft tissue imbalances that occur over time and lead to discomfort, pain, and compensation patterns. A deviated an-

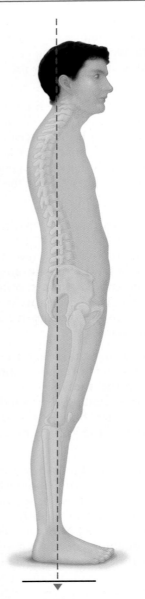

FIGURE 6-4 Sway posture.

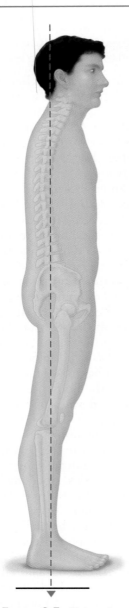

FIGURE 6-5 Flat posture.

gle of the sacrum can distort the symmetry and balance of the body, causing rounded shoulders, spinal curve deviations, and abdominal deformations, which can affect internal organs. In animals that walk on four legs, the ventral wall of the abdomen supports the organs. In people, however, the ligaments and mesentery suspend the organs, which rest on each other. Abnormal positioning of the organs can interfere with the circulatory and digestive systems. Because all body systems are functionally interrelated, even the spleen, liver, and kidneys can be affected. Massage therapists may relax the soft tissue surrounding the postural deviation, and although that may not cure symptoms, it allows the body to use its energetic resources where they are best needed, rather than to fight against posture-created strain.

Abnormal Spinal Curvature

There are a number of postural deviations your clients may have, often accompanied by excessive spinal curvature:

- Sway-back posture—easiest to see from the lateral view: excessive kyphosis, head is anterior, shoulder is slightly anterior, palms of hands are directed posteriorly, pelvis is anterior, knees are often hyperextended (Fig. 6-4)
- Flat-back posture—easiest to see from the lateral view: reduced lordotic curve, head is anterior, pelvis is anterior, knees are posterior and often hyperextended (Fig. 6-5)
- Scoliosis (lateral curvature of spine)—easiest to see from the posterior view: ears may not be at

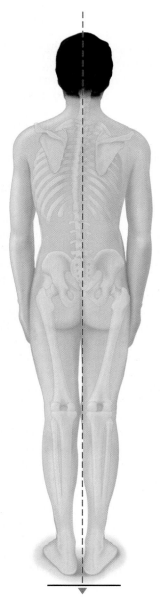

FIGURE 6-6 Scoliosis.

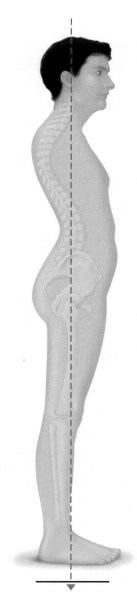

FIGURE 6-7 Kyphosis–lordosis.

the same level, shoulders may not be at the same level, spine is not directly along midsagittal line, iliac crests are not at the same level, PSIS are not at the same level, space between hands and body differs from side to side (Fig. 6-6)

■ Kyphosis-lordosis (excessive lordosis and kyphosis)—easiest to see from the lateral view: head anterior, shoulder posterior, pelvis anterior, knees posterior and slightly hyperextended (Fig. 6-7). In this case the musculature will compensate for the abnormal curvature with shortened neck extensors and hip flexors, as well as elongated, weakened neck flexors, upper sections of the erector spinae group, and external obliques.

Many clients have a forward posture, with the head anterior to the spine. Their scalenes, sternocleidomastoid, and other neck flexor muscles might be hypertonic, or excessively tight. As a result, the antagonistic neck extensor muscles are overstretched, creating tension on the musculotendinous juncture or the tenoperiosteal juncture. This tension often causes pain because the overstretched muscles are continually attempting to bring the head back into balance, over the spine. Clients commonly feel pain in their upper back because of overstretched neck extensors resulting from chronically tight neck flexor muscles associated with their forward posture.

The massage therapy scope of practice includes manipulation of soft tissue but not bony structures.

In other words, we do not attempt to realign the skeleton. Sometimes, in our attempt to normalize the soft tissues of the body to restore function, the client's posture and skeletal alignment improve.

 Do not make it your intent to manipulate skeletal structures.

Chiropractors and osteopathic physicians perform spinal manipulations (adjustments) to realign the spine and bony structures of the body. Their work is very complementary to massage because the skeletal structures and soft tissue structures are so interactive in maintaining posture and creating movement.

Rotation

Rotation, or torque, occurs around the vertical or longitudinal axis. This is an imaginary axis that runs straight up and down through the center of the body or through the center of a long bone. For example, when clients stand face forward with their feet parallel, and their shoulders appear to be turning to face another direction, they exhibit rotation of the thorax. The left and right acromion processes are both on the same horizontal level, but one is anterior to the frontal plane and one is posterior. A laterally rotated femur may be present, for example, when a client's patella is directed more laterally than anteriorly. Rotation is a significant factor in soft tissue compensation, although it is unfortunately often ignored. Document your initial observations on the general assessment form as well as in the Objective section of the SOAP chart.

A complex movement at the glenohumeral joint that rolls the structures of the shoulder joint forward and down is sometimes called shoulder rotation, but it is not a true rotation. A more appropriate description is an anterior roll, which is recorded as "shoulders rolled forward." You can document a shoulder roll by drawing a curved line in the direction of the roll on the body diagram. (Figs. 6-10, 6-11, 6-13, and 6-14 below show documentation for rolled shoulders.)

FEET

As the foundation for our balance, the feet are important to healthy posture. If you have ever stepped on something sharp or injured a toe, you are familiar with the compensation your body makes to keep you from putting any pressure on the injury. **Imbalances of the feet can result in the development of multiple compensation patterns because our structure balances on top of** our feet. When the compensation patterns are not relieved (rebalanced) within a month or two, muscles develop shorter resting lengths and fascial restrictions are established.

Postural assessment is performed with shoes off, giving you an opportunity to take a look at your clients' feet. You can check the height of their arches, see if the feet are deviated medially (toes point in) or laterally (toes point out), and observe the wear pattern on the soles of their shoes. The arch affects how people stand on their feet, as does the wear pattern on the soles of the shoes, and the deviation can indicate rotation of the femur.

Arches and wear patterns can provide information about their stance. Pronation causes wear on the medial edge of the sole, and supination wears the lateral edge of the sole. If the client's feet pronate, the peroneus muscles will develop a shorter resting length, and the antagonistic muscles will be overstretched. As a result of this imbalance starting at the feet, compensation patterns can develop all the way up the body as we try to maintain balance. If you judge that supination or pronation may be causing compensation patterns throughout the body, you may refer the client to a podiatrist (poh-DAHY-ah-trist), chiropractor, or other healthcare professional. There are some medical devices and treatments that can rectify pronation and supination. Massage therapy can provide temporary relief for these compensation patterns, but unless the client can walk and stand in a new, balanced state, the compensation patterns will be perpetuated. Wearing old, worn out shoes is one of the worst things a client suffering from foot imbalances can do, because those shoes reinforce the imbalance and can potentially make the situation worse. Proper stance and muscle balance, on the other hand, facilitate good health. This information can be used to educate clients and is a source of good self-care. Once you make observations of the feet, record your findings on the general assessment form and in the Objective portion of the SOAP note. For example, supination of both feet can be recorded as (BL) foot sup.

Gait Assessment

Observing the body in motion is another assessment tool you can use. Evaluating **gait,** or the walking pattern, is a process of observing how the client walks, in which you pay attention to the following aspects:

- Quantity, quality, fluidity, and evenness of steps
- Alignment of the head over the spine
- Position of the shoulders

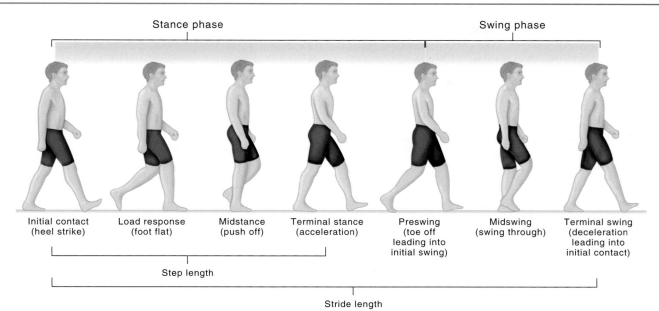

Stance phase   Swing phase

Initial contact (heel strike) — Load response (foot flat) — Midstance (push off) — Terminal stance (acceleration) — Preswing (toe off leading into initial swing) — Midswing (swing through) — Terminal swing (deceleration leading into initial contact)

Step length

Stride length

Figure 6-8 Gait pattern.

- Arm swing is equal from side to side
- Medial or lateral deviation of the feet
- Extent of knee flexion upon a step and the amount of bounce in the step

The proper, normal gait pattern is shown in Figure 6-8. Some clients will swing one arm less than the other, some will walk with their head anterior to the spine, and others will use their toes to absorb the shock of a step instead of their knees. Document any deviations from the normal gait pattern on the general assessment form and in the SOAP note's Objective section.

Range of Motion Assessment

Evaluating ROM is another way of assessing the body in motion. When your clients tell you what their primary area of concern is, you use that information to determine which joint movements are affected, how they are affected, and which soft tissues might be involved. The first joint you check is the one closest to the client's area of concern. Assess each movement of that joint for limitations and the quality of movement and use the information for your analysis of the massage session.

Each joint can move in specific directions to varying extents. The **range of motion** (ROM) is the end-to-end distance of a specific joint movement that is structurally possible. It can be measured in degrees by a device called a goniometer (GOH-nee-AH-meh-

ter), but massage therapists generally evaluate the quality and restriction of a client's joint movement instead of specifically measuring degrees of movement.

There are two kinds of ROM, active and passive. **Active range of motion (AROM)** is joint movement that requires clients to actively use their own energy to demonstrate how much of the full range can be completed comfortably and without restriction. It provides information regarding condition of the active structures of movement, such as the muscles and tendons. **Passive range of motion (PROM)** is joint movement that requires the therapist to move the relaxed client through a ROM to determine how much of the full range can be completed comfortably and without restriction. PROM evaluations can help determine the likelihood that there is a dysfunction in anatomical structures that are passively involved in movement, such as ligaments and joints. **AROM assesses active structures and PROM assesses passive structures.**

Massage therapists work with muscles and soft tissues, not bones and structures of the joints. Pain and discomfort caused by PROM can suggest problems with the ligaments and joint structures, which are outside the massage scope of practice. If you suspect that a client's area of concern could be a contraindication for massage, you can use ROM evaluations to help you make the determination and refer to the appropriate healthcare professional. Medical, osteopathic, and chiropractic doctors can diagnose medical conditions and prescribe treatment for injuries to bones and joint structures.

ACTIVE RANGE OF MOTION

AROM assesses the muscles and tendons actively involved in the joint movement. The following factors are critical to evaluating AROM and gathering useful information:

- Movement should be slow.
- Movement should be performed at a steady speed.
- Movement must be isolated, and the rest of the body must be still.
- Movement should continue through the normal range until the client feels restriction, tightness, or discomfort. When the movement is not slow and steady, you will not easily notice hesitations, glitches, facial expressions, changes in breathing patterns, variations in speed or fluidity, recruitment of other muscles to complete the range, or limitations to the ROM. Isolating the movement is a finer point of the evaluation. Clients often recruit other muscles to perform AROM, partly because of their natural compensation patterns and sometimes because of a desire to successfully "pass the test." For example, neck rotation is easily and commonly altered with lateral flexion of the neck, and shoulder flexion is often accompanied by shoulder elevation. Keeping the body still, except for the movement of the joint being evaluated, helps reveal any recruitment of other muscles to accomplish the whole range of joint movement (Fig. 6-9A).

To evaluate AROM, there are a series of steps to follow (see Procedure Box 6-1). You should always demonstrate the movement before asking your client to perform the movement. During your demonstration you can point out the slow, steady speed and the stillness of your body that helps isolate the joint movement. Let clients know that if there is any restriction, pain, or discomfort, they should tell you. Clients then slowly move one joint through the specified range and back to anatomical position, minimizing any other body movement during the evaluation, while you look for compensation and recruitment activities. Then they demonstrate AROM for the joint on other side and you compare the quality and quantity of the two sides.

When AROM is evaluated to rule out the possibility of a condition that would contraindicate massage, the uninvolved or unaffected side should be observed first to determine the client's normal ROM. Explain this concept to clients, emphasizing that you are only comparing their left and right sides. Sometimes this helps clients realize that AROM is not a test or a competition. After the evaluation has been made on the unaffected side, you can evaluate the involved side, looking for any limitations, hesitation, fluidity, compensation, recruitment, and facial expressions.

Always ask clients to let you know if there is any restriction, discomfort, or pain during AROM. Clients perceive pain at different levels or may have a diminished awareness of pain. They may not use the word "pain" or "weakness" to describe a restriction of movement, instead thinking of it as "pressure," "tension," or a feeling of being "stuck." Be sensitive to this terminology and watch for any abnormal movement, unusual facial expressions, or movement-created sensations. Any findings can be recorded as a positive test result on the general assessment form or in the Objective section of the SOAP note. For a client who complains of pain in the right shoulder when demonstrating active range of motion, you can record: Cl c/o (P) in ® shoulder w/ AROM.

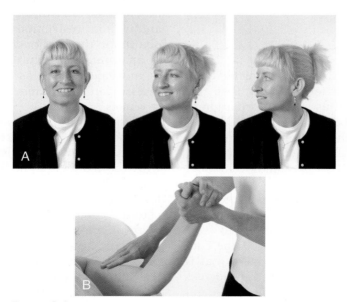

FIGURE 6-9   **A.** Active range of motion. **B.** Passive range of motion.

PASSIVE RANGE OF MOTION

PROM evaluates passive tissues including ligaments, joints, and joint capsules. Using PROM can give you a better idea of whether the client's area of concern can benefit from massage or whether the client should be referred out for further evaluation. Clients relax during PROM while you do the work. You hold and support their body parts, slowly and gently moving their body through the individual joint ranges of motion. If they feel that you might drop their arm or leg, they will "help" you by holding up their own body part to prevent it from being dropped. When clients "help" you hold their body, they introduce muscular tension that interferes with the PROM evaluation. By holding clients securely and using a gentle and knowledgeable tone of voice, clients are more likely to relax their body (Fig. 6-9B illustrates the gentle but secure way to hold a client during PROM). PROM requires a certain amount of trust from your client and must be performed carefully to avoid injuring your clients.

Before evaluating PROM, clients should demonstrate AROM for the same joint movement because it gives you a good idea of the limits of the range. With AROM, the actively contracted muscles can impede movement, but with PROM, those muscles are relaxed and can be compressed to allow a greater ROM.

Evaluating PROM follows a series of steps similar to the AROM procedure (see general assessment Procedure Box 6-1 for PROM). Starting with the client's area of concern, you determine the joint that may be affected, determine the movements of that joint, and observe the client's AROM of the joint to get a general idea of the limits to the ROM. Explain the PROM process to your clients, demonstrating passive elbow flexion on your own arm if they need clarification. Express the importance of being relaxed, encourage clients to tell you if there is any pain or discomfort, and provide sufficient stabilization.

Gently and slowly guide the client's joint through its range, watching and feeling for glitches or hesitations in movement, resistance, changes in breathing patterns, and variations in fluidity of movement. Test the uninvolved side first to determine the client's normal PROM for the joint and then test the affected side. Record any differences you notice from side to side and note any pain or discomfort as a positive test result on the general assessment form and in the Objective portion of the SOAP chart.

> **!** *If passive ROM elicits pain or discomfort, the client may have a condition outside the scope of massage therapy.*

Massage therapists do not treat joint or joint capsule injury, and clients with those conditions should be referred to the appropriate healthcare professional. If PROM results are negative, meaning that there is no pain or discomfort with passive movement, massage therapy is indicated.

End Feels

When moving any joint through a ROM, you need to know when to stop pushing or pulling. It is possible to injure a client with PROM if the joint is moved past its safe stopping point. It requires practice to be able to feel the limitation of a joint's ROM. An **end feel** is resistance sensation as a joint reaches the end of its PROM and the client's body resists further movement. Specific structures that stop the ROM have a unique end feel. Normal end feels are created by normal anatomical structures that stop the movements and determine the full ROM. Normal end feels are classified as hard, soft, or firm. Abnormal end feels are the result of abnormal anatomical conditions or some kind of problem in or around the joint. Abnormal end feels are classified as hard, soft, firm, springy block, empty, or spasm. More important than learning the difference between the abnormal end feels, which takes a lot of practice, is being able to recognize an end feel as normal or abnormal. Table 6-1 describes the normal and abnormal end feels and gives examples of each. You should learn the normal end feels and get comfortable with determining a firm end feel. The firm end feel is caused by muscular or fascial tension, which is within the scope of practice for massage therapy. When PROM is limited by a firm end feel, massage is indicated to relieve the muscular tension and soft tissue restrictions. You must learn and practice these end feels with a qualified instructor to avoid injuring a client.

When a joint is put through passive ROM, the position at the end of the range passively contracts the muscle that is responsible for that movement. In other words, a muscle in passive contraction is in a shortened position, but is not actively contracting. Passive contraction brings the muscle's origin and insertion closer together and puts the muscle in a relaxed, soft position that is especially helpful for massaging deep tissues.

Direction of Ease

There are a lot of clients who want to "help," but verbally encouraging these clients to relax is not always effective. The **direction of ease** concept can be a good tool to use in these situations. This concept uses the direction in which the tissues move with least resistance. You let clients position themselves the way they want to (in the direction that "eases" their pain or discomfort), and you can even encourage them to display that

TABLE 6-1

End Feels

NORMAL (PHYSIOLOGICAL) END FEELS

End Feel	Description	For Example
Hard (bony)	When movement comes to an abrupt, hard stop and bone contacts bone	Passive elbow extension: the olecranon process contacts the olecranon fossa
Soft (Soft tissue apposition)	When two exterior body surfaces come together and a soft compression of tissue is felt	Passive knee flexion: the posterior aspects of the calf and thigh come together
Firm (Soft tissue stretch)	When muscles are stretched and elicit a firm or springy sensation that has some give	Passive ankle dorsiflexion with the knee in extension: tension from the gastrocnemius muscle
(Capsular stretch)	When joint capsule or ligaments are stretched and provide a hard arrest with some give	Passive external rotation of humerus

ABNORMAL (PATHOLOGICAL) END FEELS

End Feel	Description	For Example
Hard	When bone contacts bone or there is a grating sensation like rough articular surfaces moving past each other, there will be an abrupt, hard stop to movement	A joint with loose components, degenerative joint disease or bone fracture
Soft	When movement is stopped with a squishy or yielding sensation	Presence of synovitis or soft tissue edema
Firm	When there is a springy sensation or hard stop with a little give	Muscular, capsular, or ligamentous shortening
Springy block	When the client jumps or withdraws with discomfort (a rebound) to the end feel	Torn meniscus of the knee
Empty	When the therapist cannot reach the end feel because the client experiences considerable pain and requests to stop ROM	Acute bursitis, joint inflammation, or a fracture
Spasm	When PROM comes to a hard, sudden stop and the client often suffers pain	Acute or subacute arthritis or a fracture

position, and then slowly but gently ease them into the position or activity you desire. Clients who continue to tense their muscles despite your polite requests and suggestions to relax during PROM may respond to your attempts to use the direction of ease concept. You can firmly hold their body in a fixed position and ask them to gently push or pull against your resistance, which gives them the opportunity to activate their muscles, which is what their body wants to do. After 5 seconds or so, you can ask them to relax slowly and gently, which again gives them control over their body. The muscles will likely be more relaxed than before they pushed against you, and you can attempt the PROM evaluation again.

Appearance of Tissues

Once clients are on your massage table, visual assessments provide information regarding the condition of their soft tissues. Look for variations of skin coloration, differences in bilateral symmetry of tissues, and any kind of marks or wounds on the skin.

Areas of redness often indicate a localized area of increased circulation. Areas that appear paler than the rest of the skin can result from ischemia, which is a localized area of reduced blood supply. Either condition indicates some kind of dysfunction that may affect the condition of the client's soft tissues.

Sometimes you notice differences in the fullness or thickness of soft tissues or bilateral asymmetry of soft tissues. If your client's left gastrocnemius is smaller than the right one, your client likely that has some compensation patterns to maintain balance. Differences in the size and fullness of soft tissues can be caused by hypertonicity, a difference in muscle mass, or edema (swelling caused by accumulated interstitial tissue fluids that are not drained by the lymph system). Checking the fullness of muscles and comparing the left to right can point out hypertonic muscles or compensation patterns, which gives you more information on where you might focus your massage techniques.

Visual assessments should also include open wounds, rashes, bruises, moles, varicose veins. and scars. You may notice changes on a client's skin before he or she does. Remember that any open skin wounds, bruises, or varicose veins are local contraindications for massage. Visible scars are important because the skin and underlying tissues are usually pulled toward the scar in the healing process. and they can even lead to compensation patterns. All of these visual findings are recorded on the general assessment form and the Objective portion of the SOAP note. For a client with a bruise on the right gastrocnemius, you could record bruise on ® gastroc.

Palpation Assessment

Palpation is the skillful art of touching and exploring the body, locating different structures, and assessing the quality of structural characteristics. It requires a thorough knowledge of the functional anatomy of the body and continually improves with practical experience. With practice, you will learn to use all of your senses with increased awareness and become more sensitive to what is underneath your hands. Good palpation skills are critical for massage therapy. Massage therapists with good palpation skills become soft tissue experts. Working with relaxed hands will help you gain even the subtlest sensory information about the client's soft tissues. **There are more nerve endings in the skin than any other body part—600,000 overall in an adult; 50,000 per square inch in the fingertips. A single touch receptor in a fingertip can detect pressure of less than 1/1400 of an ounce, or the weight of an average housefly.**

The saying, "Less is more" applies to palpation and treatment of soft tissues. People tolerate being poked, prodded, and invaded, but nobody is particularly comfortable or pleased with such intrusions. Moving too fast and too deep can activate the body's protective response to push the intrusion back out by contracting muscles. You can test this phenomenon by slowly poking yourself in a relaxed muscle such as the masseter, which is located in the lower cheek. Notice how your finger sinks into the relaxed muscle tissue. Now, actively contract the muscle by clenching your teeth and feel the contraction of the muscle push your finger out. This protective mechanism is activated subconsciously by the sympathetic nervous system in situations of potential and perceived danger. When you quickly jab a finger into someone's arm, they can respond with surprise, pain, discomfort, and recoil. If you very slowly push your finger into their relaxed arm, your finger can penetrate deeper and you might be able to feel the muscle relax and soften. This approach is less intrusive and less painful for clients and gives you a better feel for the condition of the soft tissues.

Your palpation assessment evaluates and notices different temperatures, textures, and movements of soft tissues:

- Temperature—localized areas of heat or cold, or a noticeably elevated body temperature
- Textures—hypertonic muscles, scar tissue, restricted fascia, trigger points, and tissue edema (swelling)
- Movements—fascial adhesions and restrictions, which can be localized or cover large areas of the body, sometimes feel stuck, sticky, or resist movement; hypertonic muscles limit ROM
- Rhythms—breathing, pulse, craniosacral

ASSESSMENT OF SKIN TEMPERATURE

Temperature can be an indicator of circulation. Excessive heat can be caused by a fever or by the increased circulation of an inflammatory process that is the body's response to an injury. Fever is a systemic contraindication for massage, meaning you should not massage clients who have a fever. If the inflammatory process is causing the elevated temperature, you need to know how long the pain and discomfort have been present. An acute injury that has existed less than 72 hours is a local contraindication for massage, but general massage will help the rest of the body relax and may decrease the likelihood of the formation of compensation patterns.

Cold skin temperatures can indicate decreased circulation. Ischemia is a condition of reduced blood supply that is sometimes caused by fascial adhesions and hypertonic muscles. These conditions restrict circulation and prevent adequate blood supply. Massage is especially beneficial for ischemia caused by restricted soft tissues because it can relax and create more space in them or normalize them and restore their blood supply.

TEXTURES AND MOVEMENT OF SOFT TISSUES

As you gain experience with palpation and massage, you will easily notice the different textures associated with soft tissues. Scar tissue and restricted fascia can feel as if the tissues are bound down and stuck together, and sometimes they have a grainy texture. Hypertonic muscles feel tight and resistant when they are in a relaxed position or are passively contracted. Trigger points feel like little knots within a muscle, and they elicit pain or discomfort upon palpation, which radiates to another part of the body. Without the radiating pain, these localized areas of hypertonic muscle tissue are considered tender points. Tissue edema (swelling) can feel spongy or full and squishy.

Textures and Movement of Muscles

Normal, healthy muscles feel warm and pliable; they open up to receive additional pressure, they slip smoothly past neighboring tissues, and they are not painful. When muscles lack nutrition, are injured, or are chronically contracted or overstretched, they will not feel like healthy muscle tissue. Tissues suffering from poor nutrition feel deteriorated and nonsubstantial, as if they are falling away or dissolving under the palpation pressure. Tissue that seems to dissolve under pressure feels different from tissue that opens up to receive additional pressure. The difference is subtle at first, but with experience, you can easily differentiate between the two.

Injured muscle tissue that develops fascial adhesions and scars has a ropelike feel that may elicit pain or discomfort with applied pressure and force. When your massage stroke travels across fascial restrictions, your hand or forearm may slow down or bounce over the tissue with a skidding or jumpy movement.

Muscles used for repetitive motions and muscles that are posturally shortened can become hypertonic, or excessively tight. Hypertonic muscles can create trigger points, areas of pain and hypersensitivity, and fascial adhesions. They feel tight upon palpation, even in a passive contraction, and can feel resistant, tough, inelastic, and sticky.

RHYTHMS

There are different body rhythms you can learn to distinguish and evaluate. These rhythms can provide you with more information about your client's overall condition. Once you recognize the normal range of the different rhythms, you can recognize aberrations. The repeated inhalation and exhalation of breathing produces a rhythm that you can feel. The regular contractions of the heart ventricles that create the cardiac pulse can be detected along the arteries. The craniosacral rhythm is a subtle ebb and flow of cerebrospinal fluid that, with practice, can be felt in different parts of the body, but most easily on the cranium.

Breathing Rhythm

By placing your hands lightly on the back of a prone client or on the shoulders of a supine or seated client,

you can relax your hands and use a light touch to detect the breathing rhythm. The movement of the rib cage may feel easy and fluid, freely movable, restricted, hesitant, or difficult. The more freely the rib cage moves, the more deeply and effectively the client can breathe. Slow, deep breathing usually indicates relaxation and parasympathetic nervous system activity. Shallow, fast breathing generally indicates stress or sympathetic nervous system activity, and it usually involves upper chest breathing. You may feel shallow breathers' shoulders move up and down as they breathe because they are using their scalenes, the accessory muscles that raise the rib cage, instead of the diaphragm muscle to pull air into the lungs. Upper chest breathing overworks the scalene and anterior neck muscles and can lead to neck and shoulder tension and headaches. The muscular involvement in breathing is a good topic for client education and self-care because getting oxygen into the body not only helps the soft tissue, but also overall health and well-being. (Remember that without oxygen, cells will eventually die.) A number of resources are available to explain breathing techniques, which you may suggest to clients.

Cardiac Pulse

Your palpation observations can include assessment of the client's heartbeat, or cardiac pulse. The pulse is the rhythmic throbbing felt along the arteries, and it indicates the rate at which the heart is pumping oxygenated blood through the arterial system. More common places to detect and evaluate the pulse are the radial artery (at the distal end of the anterior radius), carotid artery (anterolateral aspect of the neck), and temporal artery (anterior aspect of the temporal bone). Use your middle and index fingers to firmly compress the artery and then relieve the pressure gradually to feel the pulse. The average pulse rate is about 75 beats per minute, but for massage, you will be checking more for differences in the strength of the pulse from side to side. Hypertonic muscles and fascial adhesions can restrict the blood vessels and thus reduce the blood flow to an area. For example, if you detect a stronger radial pulse on the right than on the left, you could use ROM evaluations to see if some soft tissue restrictions near the shoulder might be constricting blood flow through the brachial artery.

Craniosacral Rhythm

You may notice the extraordinarily subtle craniosacral (KRAY-nee-oh-SAY-krahl) rhythm while you perform massage, which is an ebb and flow of cerebrospinal fluid (CSF). The CSF surrounds the brain and spinal cord, acting as a source of protection and nourishment. It is produced in the brain, is contained within the dural tube as it bathes the spinal cord, and is reabsorbed in the brain. The CSF is released and reabsorbed in a slow rhythm, and the flow creates a wavelike pulsation that is almost imperceptible, but the rhythm can be palpated on the body.

The rhythm may be easiest to detect at the cranium by positioning your relaxed fingertips so that they touch different bones of the cranium. For example, you could touch the occipital, parietal, and temporal bones. With a very light touch, you might feel those bones move outward very slightly (1–2 mm) over a period of about 4 seconds, which feels like the entire cranium is expanding ever so slightly, and then a short pause that is followed by all the bones moving inward a similar distance and at a similar rate. Feeling the craniosacral rhythm depends on a delicate, refined technique that can be learned with advanced training in the field of craniosacral therapy. This rhythm can be evaluated for quality, quantity, and fluidity. The parasympathetic nervous system arises from the cranial and sacral sections of the spinal cord and is sometimes referred to as the craniosacral system. Restricted CSF flow, which can be caused by soft tissue restrictions, may hinder the parasympathetic nervous system response. Massage can relieve soft tissue restrictions and restore the parasympathetic response, which involves the activities of resting and digesting, relaxing, and restoring energy. Without these activities, a body cannot resolve stress effectively.

Functional Assessments

For the entry-level student, using massage techniques to reduce pain and tension and restore muscle balance can help minimize or eliminate functional limitations over time. The general assessments you use before the initial and subsequent massage sessions help you determine the soft tissues that might be involved with your clients' areas of concern, the techniques you should use or avoid, and a treatment plan that is focused on achieving treatment goals. Functional assessment (FA) tests specifically evaluate the client's area of concern to discover the likelihood of specific dysfunctions and conditions that require medical diagnosis. These tests, which include manual muscle tests, manual resistive tests, and special orthopedic tests, are more definitive than general assessments. Some resources refer to active and passive ROM evaluations as functional assessment.

Manual muscle tests require clients to perform isometric muscle contractions against your counterforce. The test results help you determine whether muscles are functioning abnormally because they are shortened, overstretched, or weak. Manual resistive tests are similar, involving active isometric muscle contractions, but they help you determine whether there may be problems with a muscle or a tendon, a breakdown in the neuromuscular communication, or a more severe neurological condition. There are orthopedic tests that are designed to discover the likelihood of specific medical conditions related to fascia, ligaments, nerves, and joints. For instance, there are orthopedic tests that examine symptoms of carpal tunnel syndrome, tendinitis, ankle sprain, and sciatica to indicate whether or not these conditions are likely.

The concepts of these functional assessments are introduced so you know that they are available as assessment tools. Once you have an established a practice and find that many of your clients come to you with health conditions that may need further evaluation, or if you want to work specifically with clients who have injuries, you might want to take additional training on FA techniques so you can deliver safe and effective massage treatments and continue to keep the client's health and well-being at the center of your care. Performing good FA tests requires good technique and supervised practice to elicit valid test results that can be incorporated into your treatment plan.

Posttreatment Assessment

Following the massage treatment, you need to analyze progress with posttreatment assessments, or reassessment observations. These assessments are the same ones you used before the treatment, but they help you analyze the massage. For a client who begins the session complaining of a tight left shoulder, your initial assessment may discover bilateral hypertonicity in the upper trapezius and levator scapula muscles, left shoulder elevation, and reduced AROM and PROM upon left shoulder flexion and abduction. Posttreatment assessment would reevaluate your original findings to look for any changes in the hypertonic muscles, shoulder elevation, or ROMs. Tightness can be assessed during the massage after you apply techniques to this area. Assess the shoulder elevation and ROMS after the client is off the table and dressed. Document these changes in the Activity and Analysis portion of the SOAP note. For this sample client, you could record

- A moderate change that reduced hypertonicity in the bilateral upper trapezius and levator scapula muscles: mod. $\Delta\downarrow \equiv$ (BL) up trap + lev scap

■ After a full body relaxation massage, the left shoulder elevation was reduced: FBRM → ↓ (L) shoulder elev

(See SOAP notes with posttreatment assessment findings noted in Figs. 6-11 and 6-14)

Box 6-1

Rob Blackwell's Compensation Pattern

1. Primary areas of concern are neck, back, and knees.
2. Rob's right shoulder is elevated and rotated (rolled) forward.
3. The right shoulder elevation and roll could cause the neck and back pain, but the knees do not fit into the local pain pattern.
4. Rob indicates that his bilateral knee pain has been with him the longest, for about 10 years. He was diagnosed with osteoarthritis in both knees over 10 years ago but remembers badly twisting his left knee playing basketball before then.
5. Assume that the knee is the joint originally involved in the imbalance.
6. Evaluate AROM and PROM for flexion and extension of the left knee.
   a. You find reduced AROM with discomfort.
   b. PROM is reduced and painful, indicating that passive structures are involved in addition to active structures. Treating passive structures is outside our scope of practice!
7. Evaluate AROM and PROM for all movements of the left and right hips, spine, and shoulders.
   a You find reduced AROM and PROM of left hip flexion, extension, and abduction.
   b. You find greater AROM for lateral flexion of the spine to the left than to the right.
   c. AROM for neck rotation is reduced to both sides.
   d. You find reduced AROM upon bilateral shoulder abduction.
      His right shoulder elevation and roll could be com-pensation for the original left knee injury.
8. Document your general assessment findings, including the compensation pattern, in the Objective portion of the SOAP note, and/or on the general assessment form.
   a. ® shoulder elev + roll, ↓ROM + (P) w/ (L) knee flex + ext, ↓ROM (L) hip flex + ext + abduct, AROM lat flex spine (L) > ®, ↓ AROM (BL) neck rot + shoulder abduct
   b. ® shoulder compensation for (L) knee?
9. Because there was pain upon PROM of left knee, refer Rob to a medical doctor for a more current diagnosis to make sure massage is not contraindicated. Document your referral in the Plan section of the SOAP note.

Case Studies

This chapter highlights the documentation of objective information.

PROGRESSIVE CASE STUDY 1

Rob Blackwell

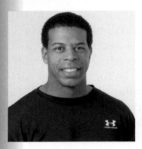

Rob Blackwell's health history form and intake interview provide the starting point for your assessment process. His goals are to restore sleep, reduce pain, restore his previous abilities to lift weights and play golf. You ask questions to determine that he especially likes golf and is frustrated because his shoulder pain has significantly affected his game.

The anterior postural assessment shows some extra wrinkles in his shirt at the right axilla and elevation of the right shoulder. From the posterior aspect, you confirm right shoulder elevation. The lateral view of Rob's posture indicates that his right shoulder is rolled forward and his head is forward.

His gait pattern is smooth and symmetrical with no noticeable abnormalities.

To sort through the different areas of pain, you determine Rob's compensation patterns. (See Box 6-1). Both active and passive ROM for flexion of the left knee are reduced and painful. You find reduced active and passive ROM upon left hip flexion, extension, and abduction. AROM shows lateral flexion of the spine is greater to the left than to the right. AROM is reduced for bilateral shoulder abduction and neck rotation to the left and right.

During the massage, you do not notice any visual differences. You feel a number of hypertonic muscles on the right: sternocleidomastoid, pectoralis major, levator scapula, and rhomboids. The upper trapezius, deltoids, and tensor fascia lata muscles are hypertonic bilaterally. Quadratus lumborum is hypertonic on the left. You feel fascial adhesions around the right levator scapula, right rhomboids, and bilateral iliotibial bands. All of these general assessments are recorded in the Objective section of the SOAP note. You also use a general assessment form, as shown in Figure 6-10).

You perform the appropriate massage, analyze the results, prioritize functional limitations, and determine treatment goals. You determine a treatment plan, including recommendations for future treatment and self-care activities to help him maintain the progress made during the first massage (Fig. 6-11).

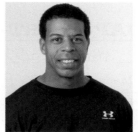

General Assessment Form

Client Name: _Rob Blackwell_

Standing Postural Assessment (Evaluate level and position of the following)

Cranium (ears) _forward_

Shoulder girdle (acromion process)
Ⓡ elevated, rolled forward

Space between body & arm Ⓛ > Ⓡ

Pelvic girdle (ASIS, iliac crest, PSIS)

Hands and fingers
Ⓡ higher than Ⓛ
Ⓡ palm directed posteriorly
Knees (patella)

Feet : flat, ⟨normal⟩, high arch
⟨lateral⟩ or medial deviation
wear pattern on soles of shoes _-even_

Gait Analysis (quantity, quality, fluidity, alignment, arm swing, foot deviation, knee flexion):
smooth, symmetrical

Range of Motion Evaluation:
Joint: _Ⓛ Knee_ Movement: _flexion + exten_. Normal or ⟨reduced⟩
Pain or discomfort with AROM? _✓_ PROM? _✓_

Joint: _ⒷⓁ shoulder_ Movement: _abduction_ Normal or ⟨reduced⟩
Pain or discomfort with AROM? ___ PROM? ___

Joint: _neck_ Movement: _rotation_ Normal or ⟨reduced⟩ _both sides_
Pain or discomfort with AROM? ___ PROM? ___

Joint: _Spine_ Movement: _lat flex_ Normal or reduced ⟨Ⓛ⟩ > Ⓡ
Pain or discomfort with AROM? ___ PROM? ___

Appearance of Tissues (color, fullness, bilateral symmetry):
∅

Palpation Findings (temperature, texture, movement, fullness, rhythms):
Hypertonic - Ⓡ SCM / pecs / lev.scap / rhomb, Ⓛ QL, ⒷⓁ up trap / delt / TFL
Adhesions - Ⓡ rhomb, ⒷⓁ IT band, Ⓡ lev scap

Therapist's signature: _Anne Therapist_ Date: _4-2-02_

FIGURE 6-10 General assessment form for Rob.

Provider Name Therapeutic Massage Works **SOAP CHART-M**

Patient Name Robert (Rob) Blackwell Date 4-2-02

Date of Injury N/A Insurance ID# N/A Current Meds ibuprofen prn

S Focus for Today ↑sleep, ↓Ⓟ

Symptoms: Location/Intensity/Frequency/Duration/Onset
c/o neck, shoulder, back Ⓟ constant 4 on 10 scale
Knee Ⓟ 4 on 10 scale, 10 yrs +, intermittent

Activities of Daily Living: Aggravating/Relieving
Aggravate: weights, bball, golf
Relief: ibuprofen, hot tub

O Findings: Visual/Palpable/Test Results
↓A/PROM Ⓛ Knee flex PROM w/ Ⓟ
↓A/PROM Ⓛ hip flex, ext, abd
Lat flex Ⓛ > Ⓡ
↓AROM BL shoulder abd., neck rot.
≡ Ⓡ SCM, pecs, lev scap. rhomb, Ⓛ QL, BL up trap, delts, TFL
X Ⓡ rhomb, lev scap, BL IT bands

A Modalities: Applications/Locations
XFF BL IT bands, MFR Ⓡ pec area, Ⓡ scap, Ⓛ QL
PNF Ⓡ up trap, Ⓡ pecs

Response to Treatment (see Δ)
↑AROM shoulder abd, neck rot, Ⓟ 4 → 1

Prioritize Functional Limitations
1. Swing golf club
2. lift weights
} both due to shoulder Ⓟ

Goals: Long-term/Short-term
LTG: Within 6 wks, lift 30 lb. w/ shoulder abd, 3 sets of 10, 5 days/wk
STG: Within 1 wk, lift 10 lb. w/ shoulder abd, 1 set of 10, 3 days/wk

P Future Treatment/Frequency
1 hr. Ⓜ, 1X/wk for 6 wks. Try vibration at Ⓡ pecs
Refer to Dr. Christian for knee eval to rule out CI

Homework/Self-care
rec: ice Ⓡ up trap 20 min 1X/day everyday
rec: door jamb pec stretch & passive SCM stretch 1X/day 5 days/wk as demo'd
rec: 100 oz. H_2O/day

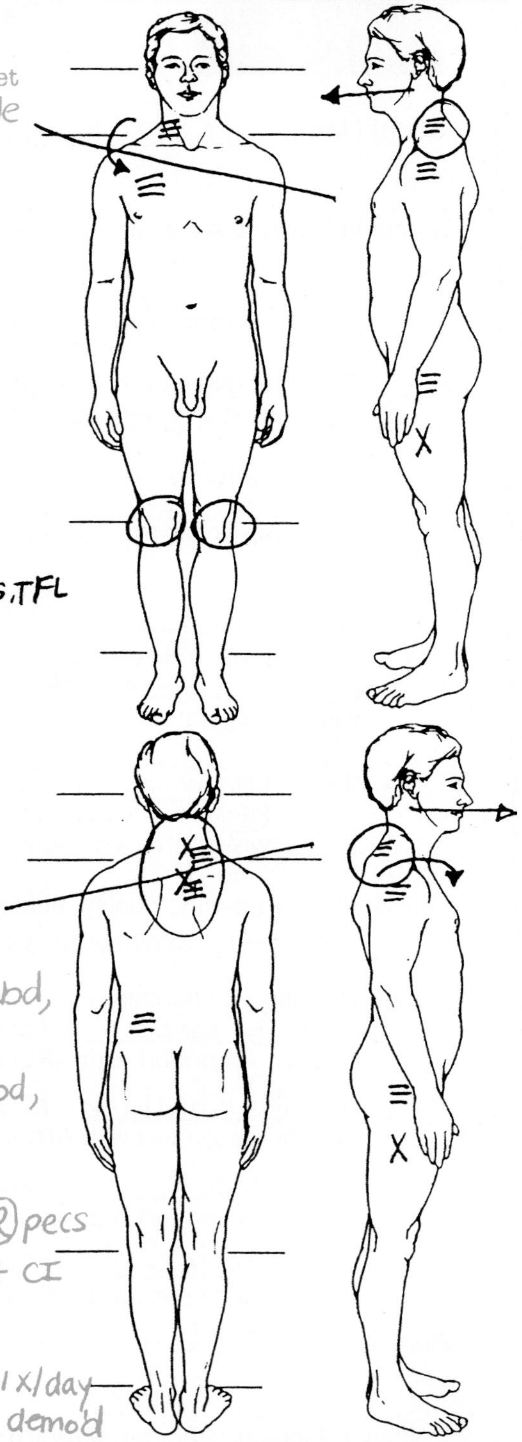

Provider Signature Jane Therapist Date 4.2.02

Legend: @ TP • TeP ○ Ⓡ ⋇ Infl ≡ HT ≈ SP
X Adh ≷ Numb ◯ rot / elev ≻≺ Short ⟷ Long

FIGURE 6-11 SOAP note for Rob, highlighting O. (Modified from Thompson DL. Hands Heal: Communication, Documentation and Insurance Billing for Manual Therapists. 2nd ed. Baltimore: Lippincott Williams & Wilkins, 2002.)

PROGRESSIVE CASE STUDY 2

Timothy Roberts

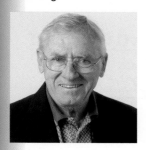

Timothy has made a first-time appointment for relaxation massage. To assess the general condition of his health and soft tissues, you look over the HxTxC form he filled out, looking for any specific complaints to confirm that he does not want therapeutic treatment. He states impatiently that he just wants a massage and asks if all the paperwork is really necessary. To strike a balance between gaining his trust and remaining professional, your assessments are brief. You quickly ask if there are any specific areas he wants you to work on, or if there are any areas he wants you to avoid. He quickly says no and starts taking off his shoes. As he is sitting in front of you and starts to stand up, you look for any obvious postural deviations. While he is getting onto the table, you use your office references to determine that the combination of relaxation massage and blood pressure medication could lower blood pressure further. You know to be especially careful when he gets off the table.

During the massage, you notice some fascial adhesions around his left ankle and that PROM is limited for that ankle. Like many seniors, Timothy may have hypertonic areas where ROM is reduced without associated pain.

Following the massage, you make recommendations for future treatment and self-care. Your assessments and recommendations are recorded on the HxTxC form (Fig. 6-12).

PROGRESSIVE CASE STUDY 3

Kirsten Van Marter

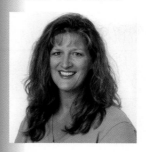

Kirsten's information from the history and intake interview provides the basis for your assessment process. She wants to reduce her back, hip, neck, and shoulder pain; restore sleep; restore her previous fitness level; and lift her child. She has been receiving massage regularly for years, and she knows that massage cannot deliver all of these benefits at once. She says that she is especially concerned that she cannot lift her child without pain and is afraid it will only get worse as the pregnancy progresses.

Postural assessments show that both shoulders are rolled forward and her left hip is elevated. When you evaluate her gait, you notice that she is starting to compensate for the growing fetus by widening her stance and pulling her shoulders back. AROM is limited with pain upon bilateral shoulder flexion, but PROM is not painful.

During the massage, you notice hypertonicity in a number of areas: bilateral pectoralis major and minor, rhomboids, and upper trapezius muscles and left quadratus lumborum and left tensor fascia latae muscles. You feel adhesions in the superior erector spinae muscles and bilateral iliotibial bands. She has trigger points in her bilateral pectoralis minor muscles and many tender points in her trapezius and rhomboid muscles. You do not notice any visual differences in tissue color, but you do notice some swelling around her ankles. All of your observations are recorded as objective information on the SOAP note or on a general assessment form (Fig. 6-13).

Following the massage, you and she prioritize her functional limitations, determine treatment goals, and come up with a treatment plan that is feasible for her (Fig. 6-14).

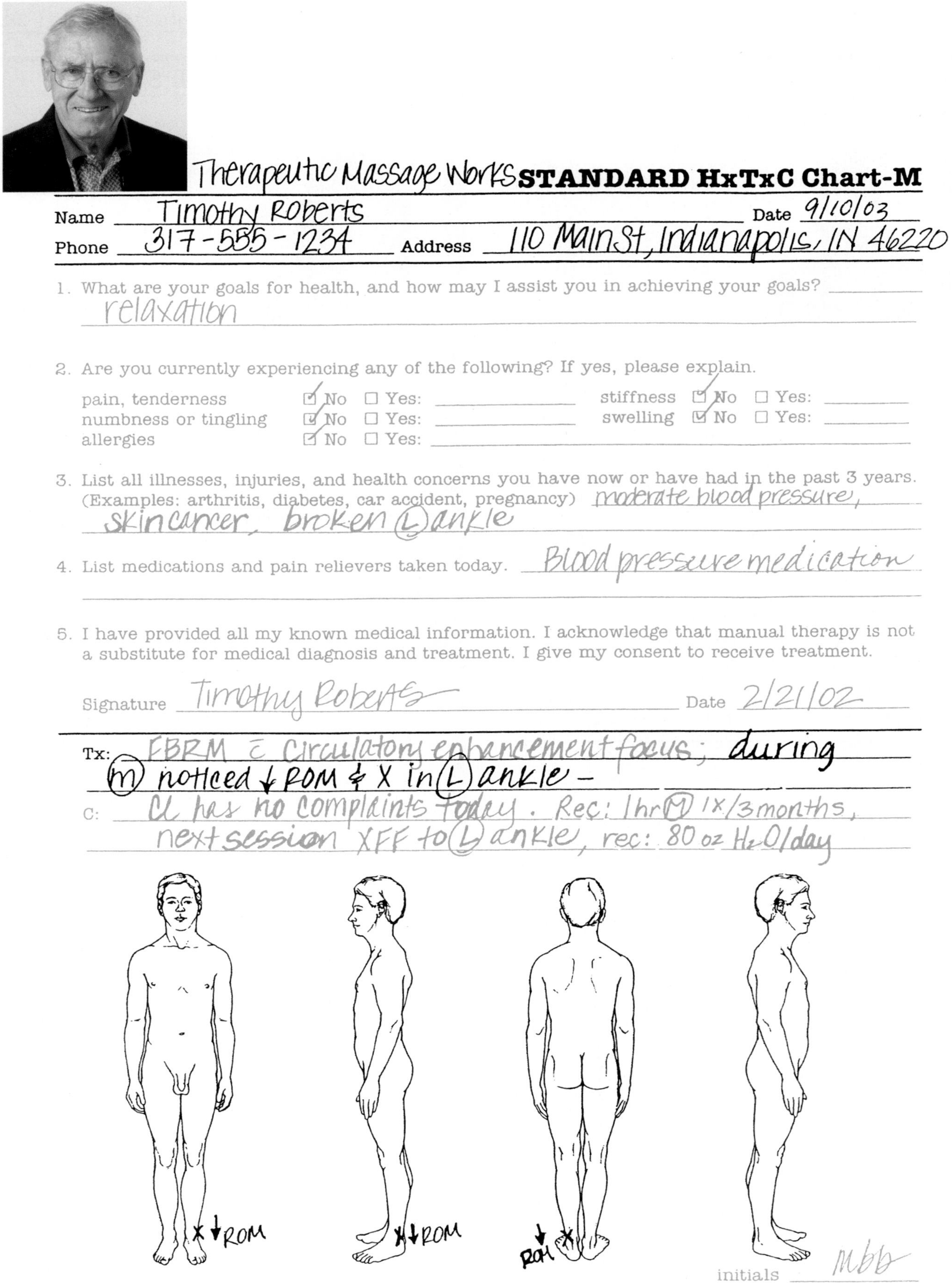

Therapeutic Massage Works STANDARD HxTxC Chart-M

Name __Timothy Roberts__   Date __9/10/03__

Phone __317-555-1234__   Address __110 Main St, Indianapolis, IN 46220__

1. What are your goals for health, and how may I assist you in achieving your goals? _____
   __relaxation__

2. Are you currently experiencing any of the following? If yes, please explain.

   pain, tenderness   ☑ No   ☐ Yes: _____   stiffness   ☑ No   ☐ Yes: _____
   numbness or tingling   ☑ No   ☐ Yes: _____   swelling   ☑ No   ☐ Yes: _____
   allergies   ☑ No   ☐ Yes: _____

3. List all illnesses, injuries, and health concerns you have now or have had in the past 3 years.
   (Examples: arthritis, diabetes, car accident, pregnancy) __moderate blood pressure,__
   __skin cancer, broken (L) ankle__

4. List medications and pain relievers taken today. __Blood pressure medication__
   _____

5. I have provided all my known medical information. I acknowledge that manual therapy is not
   a substitute for medical diagnosis and treatment. I give my consent to receive treatment.

   Signature __Timothy Roberts__   Date __2/21/02__

   Tx: __FBRM c̄ circulatory enhancement focus; during__
   __(M) noticed ↓ ROM & X in (L) ankle —__

   C: __Cl has no complaints today. Rec: 1hr (M) 1X/3months,__
   __next session XFF to (L) ankle, rec: 80 oz H₂O/day__

x ↓ ROM   X↓ROM   ↓ ROM X

initials __Mbb__

FIGURE 6-12 Client health report for Timothy, highlighting O. (Modified from Thompson DL. Hands Heal: Communication, Documentation and Insurance Billing for Manual Therapists. 2nd ed. Baltimore: Lippincott Williams & Wilkins, 2002.)

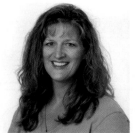

General Assessment Form

Client Name: _Kirsten Van Marter_

Standing Postural Assessment (Evaluate level and position of the following)

Cranium (ears)

Shoulder girdle (acromion process)
(BL) rolled forward
Space between body & arm (R) X (L)

Pelvic girdle (ASIS, iliac crest, PSIS)
(L) elevated

Hands and fingers

Knees (patella)

Feet : flat, (normal,) high arch
(lateral) or medial deviation
wear pattern on soles of shoes N/A
(new shoes)

Gait Analysis (quantity, quality, fluidity, alignment, arm swing, foot deviation, knee flexion):
wide stance, not much knee flexion, increased arm swing

Range of Motion Evaluation:
Joint: (BL) shoulder   Movement: flexion   Normal or (reduced)
Pain or discomfort with AROM? ✓ PROM? ∅

Joint: _____ Movement: _____ Normal or reduced
Pain or discomfort with AROM? ___ PROM? ___

Joint: _____ Movement: _____ Normal or reduced
Pain or discomfort with AROM? ___ PROM? ___

Joint: _____ Movement: _____ Normal or reduced
Pain or discomfort with AROM? ___ PROM? ___

Appearance of Tissues (color, fullness, bilateral symmetry):
Inflammation (BL) ankles

Palpation Findings (temperature, texture, movement, fullness, rhythms):
Hypertonic - (BL) pecs/rhomb/up trap, (L) QL, TFL
Adhesions - (BL) sup. erector spinae, IT bands
TP - (BL) pec minor
TeP - (BL) traps/rhomb
Therapist's signature: _June Therapist_   Date: 4-9-02

FIGURE 6-13 General assessment form for Kirsten.

Provider Name **Therapeutic Massage Works**　　**SOAP CHART-F**

Patient Name __Kirsten Van Marter__　　Date __4-9-02__

Date of Injury __N/A__　　Insurance ID# __N/A__　　Current Meds __N/A__

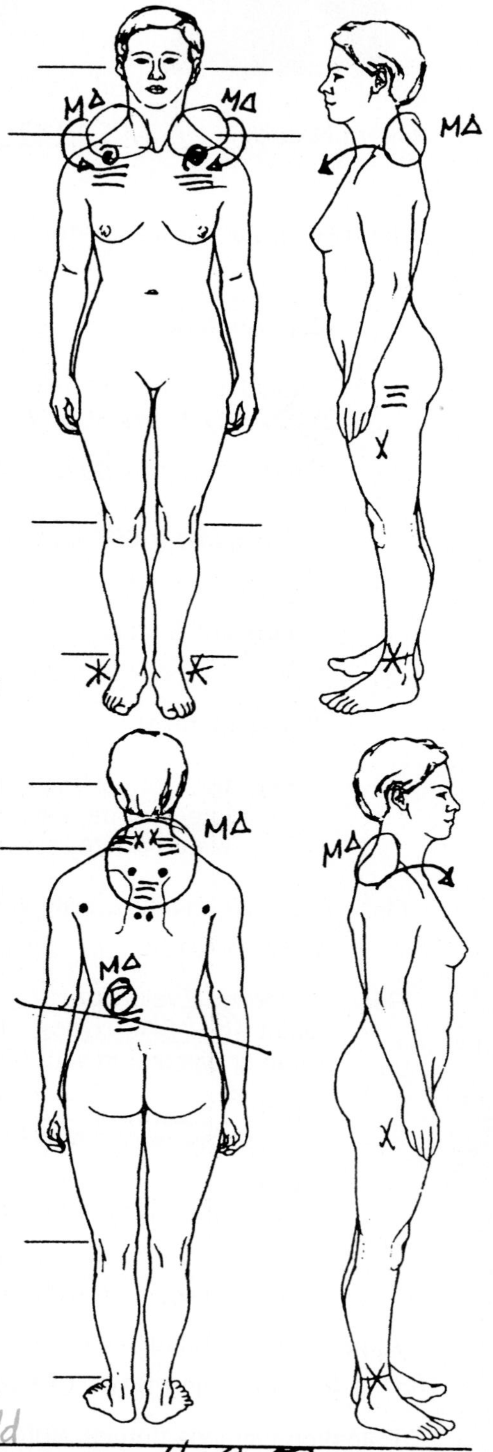

S Focus for Today ↓Ⓟ, ↑sleep, ↑fitness level

Symptoms: Location/Intensity/Frequency/Duration/Onset
c/o mild, constant back Ⓟ (5 on 10 scale)
mild hip, neck, shoulder Ⓟ (3 on 10 scale)
All Ⓟ for 3 months w/ pregnancy

Activities of Daily Living: Aggravating/Relieving
Aggravating: computer work, childcare, housework
Relieving: Ⓜ, stretches, exercise, pain meds prn.

O Findings: Visual/Palpable/Test Results
↓AROM + Ⓟ Ⓑ shoulder flex, No Ⓟ c̄ PROM
≡ Ⓑ pecs, rhomb, up trap, Ⓛ QL, TFL
✗ Ⓑ sup. erector spinae, IT bands
✳ Ⓑ ankles
TP Ⓑ pec minor, TeP Ⓑ traps, rhomb

A Modalities: Applications/Locations
Prenatal sidelying FBRM, circ. enhance, light XFF erectors
Response to Treatment (see Δ)　　PNF to TP, TeP
Ⓟ 5→2, 3→1, ↑AROM Ⓑ shoulder flex

Prioritize Functional Limitations
1. Lift daughter

Goals: Long-term/Short-term
LTG: Within 4 wks, lift child into highchair
2x/day w/o Ⓟ, 3 days/wk.
STG: with 1 wk, put dishes away into top
cabinet 1x/day w/o Ⓟ, 3 days/wk.

P Future Treatment/Frequency
1 hr Ⓜ 1x/wk, 4 wks, use more bolsters

Homework/Self-care
rec: 70 oz. H₂O/day
rec: door jamb stretches for pec. major + subscap
1x/day, every day as demo'd

Provider Signature _Anne Therapist_　　Date __4-9-02__

Legend: ℮ TP　　• TeP　　○ Ⓟ　　✳ Infl　　≡ HT　　≈ SP
✗ Adh　　≷ Numb　　◯ rot　　╱ elev　　⊢ Short　　↔ Long

FIGURE 6-14 SOAP note for Kirsten, highlighting O. (Modified from Thompson DL. Hands Heal: Communication, Documentation and Insurance Billing for Manual Therapists. 2nd ed. Baltimore: Lippincott Williams & Wilkins, 2002.)

Chapter Summary

Relaxation massage often provides temporary relief from pain and tension, but determining the underlying cause of the problem and using therapeutic techniques when they are indicated is more beneficial and offers longer-lasting results. Clients should be evaluated for their chief complaints to determine the condition of their soft tissues as well as their overall health. A new mother complaining of tight shoulders, for example, probably suffers fatigue, guilt, lack of rest, and insufficient aerobic exercise. These other factors can affect her overall health as much or more than the hypertonic shoulders and associated fascial restrictions.

Although we cannot avoid stress completely, we can learn to cope with it. Holding onto tension and stress requires a lot of energy, which then depletes the body's resources for functioning properly. Compensation patterns require a part of the body to work excessively to compensate for a dysfunction or imbalance in another part of the body, and they can increase the potential for injury. By relieving compensation patterns, we can facilitate the client's ability to relax and experience more energy and vitality. Compensation patterns should always be suspected and, when they exist, treated to restore optimal function and movement. **As a guideline, treat where it hurts, where it is compensated, and at the ends of the fascial restriction.**

The concepts of ethics and professionalism, effective communication and documentation, and assessment skills can be combined with your anatomy and physiology knowledge to develop a treatment plan with the objective of promoting overall health and well-being with a client-centered focus.

CHAPTER EXERCISES

1. Using the procedure outlined in this chapter, perform general assessments on at least five friends or family members. (Try to use the same people who filled out client histories and participated in the intake interview exercises.)

2. Watch people (on television, in a shopping mall, in the break room, at the beach, etc.) to make quick postural assessments and write a list of at least 20 observations. For example, you might notice one shoulder higher than the other, a hunched posture, uneven arm swing, or a tilted head.

3. Demonstrate AROM for each of the movements possible at the following joints, remembering to use a slow, steady speed while keeping your body very still:
   a. Glenohumeral joint
   b. Knee
   c. Elbow
   d. Temporomandibular joint
   e. Ankle
   f. Neck

4. Using flexion of the elbow
   a. Ask someone to quickly and casually show you the movement, without giving them any specific directions.
   b. Watch the movement and notice where the ROM ends.
   c. Then demonstrate slow and steady elbow flexion, isolating the joint movement.
   d. Ask your partner to perform the movement again, this time using the technique you demonstrated.
   e. Compare the range that was performed quickly to the range that was performed slowly and write down any differences you notice.

5. Practice evaluating body rhythms on at least three different people.
   a. Ask the person to lie in a prone position, on the stomach.
   b. Gently place one hand over the person's lumbar spine and the other over the thoracic spine.
   c. Relax your hands and tune in to their breathing—the rhythm, the amount of movement, the location of the movement.
   d. Try to notice other rhythms, such as the heartbeat or the craniosacral rhythm.
   e. Compare the different rhythms of different people.

6. Perform AROM for elbow flexion. Perform PROM for elbow flexion with your own arm. If they have different end feels or different limits to the range of motion, list some reasons why they might differ.

7. Considering the guideline to treat where it hurts, where it is compensated, and at the ends of the fascial restriction, describe how fascia is involved in muscle tissue and compensation patterns.

8. Position yourself in an abnormal standing posture (hips forward, shoulders forward, shoulders shrugged upward, head forward, shoulders backward, etc.).

a. Walk around with that posture for 2–3 minutes and then return to your normal, relaxed posture.

b. Describe any areas that feel hypertonic or uncomfortable.

c. Consider the long-term effects of that abnormal posture and identify some of the muscles that might become posturally shortened.

9. Use abbreviations and symbols to document the following objective assessments:

a. The client's right elbow flexion had a reduced active range of motion .

b. The client's skin was red and hot over the right quadratus lumborum muscle.

c. The client's left anterior superior iliac spine was higher than the right anterior superior iliac spine.

d. Upon active range of motion of the neck rotating to the left, the client shrugged the left shoulder and dropped the chin.

e. Passive range of motion of neck rotation to the left was greater than the active range of motion of neck rotation to the left.

10. Take several deep breaths while doing the following, and compare how the different postures affect your breathing:

a. Tighten the muscles in your pelvic floor and squeeze your abdominal muscles.

b. Hunch forward at the shoulders.

c. Slump in your chair, rolling your pelvis downward.

d. Raise your arms over your head.

e. Stand in your normal, relaxed position.

f. Sit in your normal, relaxed position.

SUGGESTED READINGS

Biel A. Trail Guide to the Body. 2nd ed. Boulder, CO: Books of Discovery, 2001.

Clarkson HM. Musculoskeletal Assessment Joint Range of Motion and Manual Muscle Strength. 2nd ed. Philadelphia: Lippincott Williams & Wilkins, 2000.

Dickson FD. Posture Its Relation to Health. Philadelphia: JB Lippincott, 1930.

Kendall FP, McCreary EK, Provance PG. Muscles Testing and Function with Posture and Pain. 4th ed. Baltimore: Williams & Wilkins, 1993.

Kendall HO, Kendall FP, Boynton DA. Posture and Pain. Baltimore: Williams & Wilkins, 1952 (reprinted by Robert E. Krieger Publishing Company, Malabar, FL, 1985).

Lowe W. Functional Assessment. Bend, OR: OMERI, 1997.

Rattray F, Ludwig L. Clinical Massage Therapy: Understanding, Assessing and Treating over 70 Conditions. Toronto: Talus, 2000.

Souriau M, transl. and ed. Souriau P. The Aesthetics of Movement. Amherst, MA: The University of Massachusetts Press, 1983.

Thompson DL. Hands Heal: Communication, Documentation and Insurance Billing for Manual Therapists. 2nd ed. Baltimore: Lippincott Williams & Wilkins, 2002.

Trager M, Hamond C. Movement as a Way to Agelessness A Guide to Trager Mentastics. Barrytown, NY: Station Hill Press, 1995.

http://www.back-pain-solved.com/trcmuscletest.html, accessed 9/8/02.

http://www.cofc.edu/~futrellm/mmtbasics.html, accessed 9/8/02.

http://www.dpdc-mbf.com/MBDFArtl.htm, accessed 9/8/02.

http://www.kinesiologycentral.com/cgi-in/gate2?~aaaMB4Aljo.o9A4aUaCoBkvj , accessed 9/8/02.

http://www.kinesiology.net/kinesiology/, accessed 9/8/02.

http://www.neurogenics.net/What%20is%20Applied%20and%20Specialized%20Kinesiology.html, accessed 9/8/02.

http://www.painreleaseclinic.com/muscletest.html, accessed 9/8/02.

http://www.systemsdc.com/ofmtest.htm, accessed 9/8/02.

http://www.uskinesiologyinstitute.com/faq.htm, accessed 9/8/02.

Treatment Plan

UPON COMPLETION OF THIS CHAPTER,
THE STUDENT WILL BE ABLE TO:

- Identify the three primary components of a treatment plan
- List the five aspects of future treatment to address in a treatment plan
- Describe why it is important for clients to participate in the therapeutic process
- Name at least five topics that are commonly used for self-care recommendations
- Describe at least three different self-care recommendations
- Write at least five specific treatment plans, using abbreviations and symbols

KEY TERMS

Ergonomics: the science that designs and coordinates people's activities with the equipment they use and the working conditions of their environment

Hydrotherapy: the use of water as a treatment

Refer: recommend that someone see a specific healthcare practitioner

Self-care (self-help): activities that clients can use between massage sessions to participate in their healing process and help them achieve their treatment goals

Treatment plan: your recommendations for future treatment, self-care activities, and referrals to other healthcare professionals

Therapists who understand how to read and write all components of the massage treatment record demonstrate a professional image and, more importantly, can make their treatments more effective. Your **treatment plan** is the intended path you recommend for clients to reach their goals, and the three primary components include your suggestions for future treatment, your suggestions for self-care, and referrals to other healthcare professionals. Future treatment refers to the frequency, duration, expected length of treatment, techniques, and reevaluation tips for future massage sessions. **Self-care** (also called **self-help**) refers to activities that clients can use between massage sessions to help maintain any progress made during the massage session and encourage the healing process. They are excellent tools for getting clients involved in their own healthcare. If you think clients should see another healthcare professional for further evaluation and diagnosis, you can **refer** them, or recommend that they see a specific healthcare practitioner. This component of the treatment plan is not always included, as it is not always necessary.

Treatment plans can be used for both wellness and therapeutic massage. Even in a spa, where the focus is typically wellness massage, clients occasionally ask for therapeutic massage because of a strained muscle or excessive muscular tension. Writing treatment plans for all clients keeps your documentation consistent, and consistency helps you keep track of your clients' progress toward their goals. Additionally, if you work in a setting where other therapists may be working on clients you have treated, they must be able to use your massage treatment records to design a massage that continues progress toward the treatment goals.

Planning Process

Treatment planning is a process of examining a client's unique information and making an educated guess at the best way to reach the treatment goals. The plan should be flexible, allowing for alterations and changes of course with each massage session because clients sometimes reprioritize the original goals or develop new soft tissue dysfunctions that change the priorities. **The plan is a guide and should be adapted to the client's condition at the time of treatment. Most importantly, the treatment plan should always reflect how to continue progressing toward the prioritized goals.** The components of a plan for client care include

- Duration of sessions
- Frequency of sessions
- Length of treatment
- Techniques or specific areas to incorporate or avoid
- Self-care recommendations
- Referrals to other healthcare practitioners

Keeping all of these components in mind, you ask a series of questions to develop the treatment plan. Ask leading questions about repetitive motions, sustained positions, and the likelihood of reinjuring the area and determine new compensation patterns. Use that information, paired with your assessment of the client's overall health, to determine the frequency, duration, and length of treatment as well as techniques, self-care activities, and referrals, if necessary, to other healthcare professionals. Before recording the treatment plan, discuss it briefly with clients to ensure that it is feasible for them and give them an opportunity to ask any questions. Then document the specifics in the Plan portion of the SOAP note.

Developing the initial treatment plan is a slightly different process from reevaluating the plan for subsequent massage sessions, since you have more information to use during subsequent sessions.

INITIAL SESSION

The first time clients come to you for massage, you have to make an educated guess at your plan for reaching treatment goals. You can engage clients in a conversation during the initial session to find out how they typically handle stress, how long it usually takes to recover from illness or injury, or how physically active they tend to be. Determining the goals and designing the treatment plan at an initial mas-

---

✔ PROCEDURE BOX 7-1
Initial Treatment Plan

1. Evaluate the internal healing environment.
   a. Health history
      i. Injuries
      ii. Length of time condition has been present
      iii. What makes condition better or worse
   b. Client interview
   c. Accumulated stress factors
   d. General assessments
   e. Lifestyle
      i. How do you typically handle stress?
      ii. How long does it typically take to recover from illness or injury?
      iii. How physically active are you?
   f. Participation
      i. Generally, do you typically take medications or use lifestyle changes as a remedy?
      ii. Are you conscientious about leading a healthy lifestyle?
2. Make an educated guess about the client's ability to heal or recover from illness or injury (the following are just generalities).
   a. Strong—minimal number of chronic conditions, few injuries, few stress factors, actively manages stress, usually heals within a week or two, daily exercise, uses lifestyle changes instead of medications for treatments, tries to eat balanced meals, drink sufficient water
   b. Weak—several chronic conditions, several injuries, many stress factors, does not dissipate stress, usually takes months to heal, eats fast food, drinks a lot of coffee, smokes cigarettes, no time or energy to lead a healthy lifestyle
3. Consider the client's treatment goals and ability to heal to suggest a treatment plan.
   a. Future treatment
   b. Frequency
   c. Duration
   d. Length of treatment
   e. Techniques or areas to include or avoid
   f. Reevaluation suggestions
   g. Self-care
   h. Specific activities
   i. Specific frequency, duration, and amounts
   j. Referrals, if appropriate
   k. Healthcare practitioner's name
4. Discuss the plan with clients to make sure it is feasible for them and to address any questions.
5. Document the treatment plan recommendations in the Plan section of the SOAP note.

sage session is often a collaborative effort in which you make suggestions for future treatment, and the clients decide whether those parameters are reasonable for them. To make initial suggestions and plan effective guidelines for reaching treatment goals, you consider your client's health history, the client interview, general assessments, lifestyle, and their willingness to participate in the process. These are the factors that affect the internal healing environment, or ability for the body to recover from illness and injury (Procedure Box 7-1).

For example, a new client comes to you who has a high-pressure job, is going through a divorce, eats fast food, drinks six cups of coffee daily, does not exercise or drink much water, and has had multiple injuries. She has a relatively poor internal healing environment, so you could set treatment goals that are easily attainable and recommend a fairly aggressive treatment plan. Long-term goal (LTG)—Within 2 months, be able to lift her toddler in and out of the highchair twice a day, three times a week, without pain. Short-term goal (STG)—Within 2 weeks, be able to put dishes into the above-counter cabinets once a day, three times a week, without pain. Given those goals, your treatment plan could recommend 60-minute massages, once a week, for 2 months. You might want to try myofascial release work, proprioceptive neuromuscular facilitation work, and vibration for the muscles involved in shoulder flexion. You could mention that if she consumed at least 60 ounces of water each day and applied ice to both shoulders for 20 minutes, at least three times a week, she might be able to reach her goals faster. All of this information is recorded in the Plan section of the SOAP note.

SUBSEQUENT SESSIONS

In each subsequent massage session, you ask questions to reevaluate the previous treatment plan and make necessary changes (Procedure Box 7-2). You review the prior session's treatment notes to know how clients responded to the last treatment and follow up on self-care activities and any referrals. Additionally, you assess their current stress level by asking them how they feel that day, how they are doing, how life is treating them, and where their body hurts. Their answers are recorded in the Subjective section of the SOAP chart because it is information that clients tell you. If there are new areas of pain or discomfort, you perform the appropriate assessments to discover new compensation patterns, which muscles might be affected, and any new contraindications. The new assessments are recorded in the Objective portion of the SOAP note.

PROCEDURE BOX 7-2
Session-to-Session Treatment Plan

1. Review the SOAP note from the previous massage session.
2. Ask clients about the self-care recommendations.
   a. Were you able to incorporate the (insert specifics here)?
   b. Did you have any trouble with any of the self-care?
   c. Did any of the self-care make noticeable changes?
3. Ask clients about any referrals.
   a. Were you able to talk with (insert practitioner's name here)?
   b. If so, did the practitioner make any diagnoses, prescribe any treatments, or make any recommendations?
4. Ask clients how they felt after the previous massage.
   a. Better, worse, or no change?
   b. How long did that last?
5. Ask about the client's current condition.
   a. How are you feeling today, in general, or, how is life treating you?
   b. Describe today's pain level or discomfort and the areas of discomfort.
   c. Are there any new medications or other new treatments?
   d. Are there any new areas of concern, cuts, or bruises?
      ■ If so, perform the appropriate assessments and record them as Objective information on today's SOAP note.
6. Consider the client's progress toward treatment goals and results of the previous treatment to determine whether you will continue with the original treatment plan or make adjustments to:
   a. Future treatment recommendations
   b. Self-care activities
   c. Referrals
7. Discuss the treatment plan with clients to make sure it is feasible for them and to address any questions.
8. Properly document the current treatment plan in the Plan section of your current SOAP note.
9. If the client had an appointment with the referred healthcare practitioner, remember to obtain copies of the medical records, either formally or informally.

If clients seem to have continued progress between massage sessions, you can use the treatment plan from the previous session as a springboard, incorporating similar techniques into the current massage. If their condition seems worse or if they express doubt, you can design a massage that is very different from the previous session. Document techniques you use and the clients' responses in the Activity and Analysis section of the SOAP note.

Consider the sample client used to illustrate the initial treatment plan. A year later, she may have delegated some of her work responsibilities, settled the divorce, received massages once a month, and started to exercise and drink at least 50 ounces of water every day. Her healing environment is much better, and she would be able to reach more aggressive treatment goals with less treatment. LTG—Within 2 months, be able to lift her toddler in and out of the crib twice a day, 5 days a week without pain. STG—Within 2 weeks, be able to lift her toddler in and out of the highchair three times a day, 3 days a week without pain. The treatment plan could recommend 60-minute massages, twice a month, for 2 months. Your recommendations for techniques could be primarily relaxation techniques with a little extra attention to the muscles involved in shoulder flexion. You could mention that warm baths at least twice a week could help her relax and that consuming at least 60 ounces of water each day would help maintain the soft tissue work that was accomplished.

Future Treatment

The treatment plan includes your recommendations for clients' future massage treatments. You should refer to the duration and frequency of future sessions, length of treatment, techniques to include or avoid, and specific suggestions for reevaluation. The amount of time a client's body requires to change the condition of soft tissue strongly affects your determination of future treatment. Document the future treatment information in the Plan section of the SOAP chart. To recommend 60-minute massage sessions once a week for 8 weeks, incorporating myofascial release at the left iliotibial band, you could write 1-hr (M) 1X/wk for 8 wks, try MFR on (L) IT band.

These notes are particularly helpful because they help you determine progress and design each massage session. Besides, it is often difficult to remember details for each client, especially when seeing many clients in your practice.

HEALING TIME

Approximated healing time, or the length of time that may be required to restore normal function, influences the treatment plan. Healing time is affected by the client's internal healing environment, which you evaluate by learning about their physical, emotional, mental, and nutritional stressors in addition to their lifestyle, illness, injuries, and the general length of their recovery or healing times. It takes longer for clients to recover from illness or injury when they lead an unhealthy lifestyle with a lot of stressors than when their life is relatively uncomplicated and they

are comfortable and content. Healing time is unique to an individual and can only be estimated as a relative amount of time for that person. You should not compare the healing time of one client to that of another. In other words, your best estimations for healing time are based on information that you accumulate over a period of months or years. A strong healing environment allows a more aggressive treatment plan, with longer or more frequent massages and more aggressive techniques. A weak healing environment is best treated with a conservative plan, including shorter or less frequent massages and less aggressive techniques.

DURATION OF FUTURE SESSIONS

How long should the next massage last? The duration of each future massage session is the first consideration when developing a treatment plan. Massage sessions can be 15, 30, 60, or 90 minutes long. Most massage sessions are 60 minutes long, so most treatment plans imply future sessions of 60 minutes. Occasionally, your clients might be better served with a shorter or longer session. A shorter session may be warranted if clients are uncomfortable during the massage, for any reason. Discomfort can outweigh the benefits of the massage, and clients who are uncomfortable throughout the massage, either physically or mentally, can actually feel worse after the massage. Your effective communication skills, especially with nonverbal cues, are critical for determining whether future sessions should be limited in duration.

If clients experience pain, uneasiness, or lack of trust in you or your practice, those feelings can last for days. Thirty-minute sessions give those clients an opportunity to develop trust with you as a professional therapist who understands that everyone has different needs. Some clients, such as elderly clients and chronic pain clients, are uncomfortable lying on your massage table for extended periods of time. Rather than subject them to hour-long sessions, you can try 30-minute sessions to see if there is less discomfort and more overall benefit. Clients who are focusing specifically on healing a soft tissue injury may benefit from shorter sessions to avoid making their condition worse, or exacerbating it. There is a delicate balance between beneficially treating and overtreating an injury.

At the other end of the spectrum, some clients may benefit from a 90-minute massage session. As long as their internal healing environment is good, you might recommend a 90-minute session for clients with multiple compensation patterns or those who need a longer period of time to feel relaxed.

FREQUENCY OF FUTURE SESSIONS

Healing input influences healing output. This concept is a factor in determining the frequency of future sessions for both wellness and therapeutic massage. Massage enhances the healing process by mechanically increasing the circulation of blood and lymph to and around the area of concern. Nutrients and oxygen are brought to the area by the arterial system, and waste products are removed by the lymphatic and venous systems. Massage is also beneficial by mechanically reducing physical tension and reflexively inducing the parasympathetic nervous response, both of which encourage relaxation.

Determining the frequency of massage sessions depends on the condition of your clients' soft tissues and their lifestyle. For clients whose soft tissues are healthy, treatments as frequent as twice a week can be beneficial for maintaining relaxation, reducing muscular tension, and relieving fascial adhesions that cause compensation patterns. On the other hand, you can get too much of a good thing, including massage. The problem with receiving massage too frequently is that it can overwhelm the body and can easily exacerbate the original condition.

There are a number of reasons, both for your clients' best interest as well as yours, to recommend no fewer than one massage every few months. Clients can benefit from a regular investment in health maintenance. Occasional massage can help minimize the stressors and reduce the accumulation of stress to improve health and the internal healing environment. Clients who regularly get an occasional massage benefit your practice. Seeing clients once every few months allows you to develop relationships, which can lead to more trust and stronger rapport. It also establishes a regular and dependable client base, which is what you depend on for a financially stable practice.

The benefits of massage are cumulative, and your recommendations are based on how much healing input clients need to restore function and reach their treatment goals. You must balance the frequency of sessions such that you can make steady progress but do not overtreat. Most likely, the frequency of treatment is somewhere between once a week and once every few months. Clients are ultimately responsible for the frequency of their massage treatments, taking into consideration their financial situation, transportation arrangements, schedules, and childcare.

LENGTH OF TREATMENT

The length of treatment you recommend should not exceed the time frame of the LTGs, which should be attainable and recognizable within 1 to 2 months. It is relatively easy for clients to commit to this kind of time frame, considering finances, transportation, schedules, and childcare.

TECHNIQUES AND AREAS TO INCLUDE OR AVOID

During the massage, you may try specific strokes or techniques that are ineffective or disliked by a client. On the other hand, you may find techniques that are especially effective on a particular client or techniques that a client enjoys. Some clients do not want to be touched in certain areas, such as their abdomen, feet, or face. For a client who does not want abdominal massage, but likes trigger point techniques and responds well to them, you could write Cl - avoid abdomen, likes TP work. Use TP next session. **It is a good idea to ask clients prior to their massage session if there is any area of their body that they prefer not to have touched.**

There are occasions when you do not have enough time during the session to use all of the techniques you want or you think of a technique that might be good to try during the next session. Sometimes the massage is almost finished when you discover an area of restricted fascia that you suspect could be the primary imbalance causing the client's compensation patterns. Rather than start therapeutic techniques on that area at the end of the massage, you can recommend that these techniques be incorporated into the next session.

REEVALUATION

Reevaluation is performed when the original treatment goal has been reached, but it is also important for determining the progress toward STGs and LTGs. You may want a particular area or joint movement reevaluated before the next massage session, especially if the self-care activities were focused on that area. For example, your plan might include a suggestion to reevaluate right shoulder flexion for hesitation upon active range of motion (AROM). While you are continually reevaluating clients during each session, you might use some of the general assessments you performed in their initial visit. Any new assessment findings are documented in the "O" portion of the SOAP note.

Self-Care Recommendations

You typically treat clients for 30 to 90 minutes at a time, which is enough time to make progress. Between massage sessions, clients can help to maintain and advance the progress by using self-care, which is similar to doing homework assignments that support the treatment goals and reduce physical tension. This is not to say that clients will not benefit from the massage treatment alone, but that the benefits usually increase and goals can be reached sooner if clients participate between sessions with self-care techniques. Self-care gives clients an opportunity to participate in the maintenance and improvement of their health. Using the concept that healing input influences healing output, you can educate your clients about participating in their healthcare and following self-care recommendations to progress toward their goals faster.

It is not in the massage therapy scope of practice to prescribe, but there are clients who assume that massage therapists have the same responsibilities and capabilities as medical professionals who are allowed to diagnose and prescribe. Emphasize to clients that self-care activities are suggestions for enhancing the effects of the massage session and improving the health of the soft tissues and *not* in any way a prescription. Clarify that you treat only soft tissue conditions via massage and emphasize that any other conditions should be diagnosed and treated by the appropriate healthcare professional. It is your responsibility to ensure that clients experience no confusion regarding diagnosis, prescription, or treatment. To avoid any misconceptions, you can offer handouts and a suggested reading list with information about self-help activities you recommend.

Self-care is recorded in the Plan section of the SOAP note. Try to be specific but brief and refer to the specific activities, frequencies, durations, and amounts you recommend. For instance, you recommend a client increase water intake to 60 ounces per day and stretch the left triceps twice a day, five times a week. You demonstrate the stretch by flexing the left shoulder and elbow and, using your right hand to slowly push upward on the distal humerus, increase flexion of the left shoulder. You could write rec: ↑ H_2O to 60 oz/day, perform (L) triceps stretch 2X/day, 5X/wk, as demonstrated.

CONSIDERATIONS FOR SELF-CARE

Consider your clients' lifestyle and time constraints when making self-care recommendations. If your recommendations do not fit within either of these, they are not likely to comply or, even worse, their confidence in the treatment process may be diminished. Clients can feel empowered to take responsibility for their health and well-being when they are comfortable with the self-care you suggest, so activities should be added gradually.

Many clients feel burdened with self-care, as if it were a dreaded homework assignment. Limit the number of activities you recommend to minimize the number of things they have to remember and the amount of time and energy they have to commit. Too much too soon can overwhelm the body and even lengthen the healing process. For example, it is beneficial for a client to receive massage treatment, increase water intake, and use one or two stretches for the connective tissue in the affected area. However, adding a vigorous exercise program, using heat and ice therapy, radically changing the diet, and adding five specific stretches on a daily basis could overwhelm the body. The combination of all these activities could add more stress, the body might not be able to distinguish or integrate so many changes, and the client's initial condition could be aggravated.

Nevertheless, massage therapists often see clients resist self-care and resist progress toward their goals. This situation can be very frustrating and you must be aware of this behavior. Many persons have suffered from chronic conditions for so long that they stop paying attention to the discomfort. Their compensation patterns, pain patterns, and coping skills become part of their everyday routine and can even become part of a person's identity. The clients' goals for moving toward a better and more balanced state of health may effectively take away a part of their identity. Life without pain and discomfort may be unknown territory for a person with a chronic condition. Most people are somewhat uncomfortable about change and unfamiliar experiences. This is exactly the situation that may occur when clients start making progress toward their goals. It may seem strange, but it will make sense as you see it occur in your practice. For example, clients who have had a chronic pain condition for years can get attention and concern from friends and family. Losing this attention may deter them from letting go of their pain and from participating in their healing process. You have a professional obligation to support clients in making progress toward their goals, but you must not judge or harbor negative feelings toward a client who is hesitant or does not want to participate in the healing process.

Making self-care recommendations is the massage therapist's responsibility, whether clients choose to participate or not. Some self-help topics include internal and external hydrotherapy, rest and sleep, nutritional awareness, specific stretches for the areas of concern, physical awareness, and ergonomics.

HYDROTHERAPY

Hydrotherapy is the use of water as a treatment. It can be used internally to support cells and organs, and it can be used externally. Water, the universal solvent, is so inexpensive and readily available that it is often overlooked as a valid therapeutic approach. Because of its simplicity and availability, water is excellent for self-care.

Internal Hydrotherapy

Water has many functions in the body: elimination of waste, delivery of nutrients and oxygen to the cells, maintenance of tissue pliability and function, cushioning of joints, and regulation of body temperature. The muscles are composed of about 75% water, and blood about 90%, and those percentages must be maintained with sufficient water intake or the health of those tissues will suffer. Muscle tissue and fascia can get stuck together and cause fascial adhesions, muscle contractions can become less efficient, blood becomes more viscous, blood volume decreases, the ability of blood to flow decreases, and thus the delivery of oxygen to cells is reduced.

One of the most common self-care recommendations is for clients to drink enough water to stay hydrated. After a massage session, adequate water intake helps flush the waste out of the body that would otherwise sit in the tissues, impeding healing and restoration of function. Hydration further enhances relaxation of the muscles and surrounding soft tissue during the massage session. Encouraging clients to drink enough water after a massage and in between sessions is an important self-care activity. Recommendations vary widely, but a general rule is to drink ½ ounce per pound of body weight. The intake should be increased with physical exercise, salty food, alcoholic beverages, exposure to sun or heat, and illness. Any time you discuss hydrotherapy, provide safe guidelines rather than simply telling clients to drink more water.

Insufficient water intake leads to diminished cellular function, which in turn reduces the body's ability to recover from injury and maintain a healthful state. It makes tissues sticky and more difficult to heal. It is harder to attain STGs when tissues are dehydrated, and it requires more time to reach the LTGs. Dehydration occurs when the body does not get enough water or loses too much fluid, which can result in diminished soft tissue function, muscle cramps, fatigue, headaches, and dizziness.

The average person is typically dehydrated because of insufficient water intake and substances that rob the body of water such as alcohol and salt. Instead of judging clients' habits and tendencies, you can teach them about the effects of alcohol and salt. Alcohol is a diuretic, meaning that it causes excess amounts of water to be eliminated from the body, and it can actually cause dehydration. As alcohol is consumed, the tissues are prone to dehydration and

may require more time to heal. Consuming excessive amounts of salt makes the body shed extra amounts of water in an effort to maintain homeostasis. The negative effects of alcohol and salt can be counteracted to some extent by additional water intake. A common misconception is that caffeine contributes to dehydration, but numerous scientific studies have shown that caffeine has no effect on dehydration. You can educate clients about hydration and health, but it is up to them to decide what they will and will not consume.

The color of urine is a simple and sometimes useful indicator of hydration. Generally, pale yellow or clear urine usually indicates adequate hydration. Although deep yellow or dark coloring can indicate concentrated urine and dehydration, it can also reflect chemicals, vitamins, and minerals that are being eliminated.

Persons who are retaining water tend to drink insufficient amounts of water. They falsely believe that the less water they consume, the less water they retain. Actually, the opposite is true. As a cactus in the desert retains all of its water because of minimal rain, the body retains its precious supply of water when insufficient water is consumed. This is one of the many homeostatic mechanisms that protect and maintain our health. Drinking more than the generally recommended amount of water makes the homeostatic mechanisms eliminate any excess water that was being retained, thus reducing water retention.

External Hydrotherapy

External hydrotherapy refers to applications of cold and heat, because those temperatures were initially only provided by water in its solid (ice), liquid (water), and gaseous (steam) states. Today, there are chemical forms of cold and heat, but the original term remains. Hydrotherapy is covered extensively in the Therapeutic Applications chapter, but self-care information for clients is summarized here.

Ice and cold applications reduce circulation and nervous system activity.

 Ice should be avoided for persons with circulatory problems.

Ice is typically used in acute conditions in which inflammation, spasms, and pain are present. Any time you use deep fiber friction techniques, you can recommend ice to prevent inflammation and promote healing. Ice, or an equally cold substitute, should be applied for a maximum of 20 minutes.

A plastic bag filled with ice works, and crushed ice conforms nicely to the body. Ice can be used directly on the skin, but a washcloth or towel helps to hold onto the melting ice, and it soaks up the resulting water. Chemical gel packs are available that also conform to the body, and many people have them in their freezers at home. They must be used cautiously because they are colder than 32°F and can damage the skin.

 Use a layer of fabric between a chemical gel pack and the skin.

Heat applications enhance circulation, which can increase healing.

 Heat should be avoided if there are signs of inflammation, heat, or redness.

Heat relaxes people and may be used for acute conditions in the muscles surrounding an injury, muscle spasms, or other forms of pain. For chronic conditions in which techniques other than friction are used, heat may be applied for up to 20 minutes to increase circulation in the affected muscles. Heat may also be used concurrently while the client is applying ice to help maintain the body's core temperature and to distract the client from the unpleasant effects of ice.

STRETCHES

Stretching the muscles and surrounding connective tissue in the clients' affected areas may be the second most common self-care recommendation. Although massage lengthens muscles and stretches tissues, the body will adapt to the mechanical changes and new positions faster when clients reinforce those changes between massage sessions with additional stretches. Remember, massage therapists do not diagnose nor prescribe treatment, so be careful to educate clients only about how stretches affect soft tissues and enhance the massage treatments. Clients must understand that stretches are not a substitute for treatment from other healthcare professionals that may be necessary. If you recommend stretches to clients for self-care, you should have books and handouts in your office that illustrate specific stretches (see Suggested Readings). To keep from overwhelming clients with "homework," suggest one or two stretches at most.

As with all self-help, thoroughly explain effective stretching to clients. They should understand how to

do the stretch properly, the possible contraindications, and the expected results. Ideally, take time to demonstrate the stretch for clients and observe them as they try it. This way you can ensure that they are stretching the correct area with a safe technique. You can describe the end feel of a stretch and make sure they are not compromising any anatomical structures or triggering the stretch reflex. Always provide specific information about the frequency and duration of stretches and techniques to use.

REST

Most people underestimate the value of rest for promoting healing and regeneration. Essentially, rest is a period when mental, physical, sensory, and emotional activity slows or ceases, allowing the body to redirect its energy to restoration. People lead very busy lives, often moving from one event to another and taking little time for rest until they fall into bed in the evening, exhausted from the day's events. Taking time for a massage is one way for people to slow down and rest; however, it is most likely not enough to completely rejuvenate the body and mind. Clients should be told that it is good to take time for massage and that adequate rest can maximize the benefits of massage.

Sleep

Sleep is a deep state of rest when tissues regenerate, repair, and prepare the body for new activity. Oftentimes, sleep positions are the cause of pain and discomfort, which may include stiff necks, aching backs, and numbness and tingling in the arms or hands. It can be difficult for people to change their sleep positions, but you can educate clients about sleep positions and leave it up to them to try to incorporate the changes. Sleep positions can cause pain and discomfort, and yet sometimes pain and discomfort cause problems with sleep.

Stomach sleepers tend to develop stiff necks because they have to turn their heads to the side to breathe. Additionally, stomach sleepers may hyperextend their lumbar spine, which may create pain. They can benefit from sleeping in a different position. Persons who sleep on their side sometimes complain of back pain, which can result from the torque and tension on the pelvis and hip when the top leg drops down to the bed. You can suggest a body pillow to support the top leg and relieve the torque on the pelvis. Sometimes side sleepers complain of numbness and tingling in their arms and hands, which can be caused by nerve impingement from compression on the shoulder they sleep on. They can be relieved by sleeping on their backs. Persons who sleep on their backs sometimes complain of back pain, which can be caused by the lordotic curve of the spine. Supporting the knees with a pillow reduces the lordotic curve sometimes relieves pain.

Sleep disruption can cause irritability, concentration difficulty, poor muscle coordination, increased sensitivity to pain, fatigue, sluggishness, a diminished sense of well-being, an inability to cope with the physical and mental challenges of life, and, in some cases, depression. Too little sleep creates "sleep debt," which is similar to being overdrawn at a bank. In time, the body will demand that the debt be repaid. Our bodies do not adapt well to getting less sleep than required, and while we may get used to a sleep-depriving schedule, our judgment, reaction time, and other functions are still impaired.

When massage clients discuss their lack of sleep, you can educate them about the importance of sleep for health and healing and offer some self-help recommendations. Sleep can be affected by a number of factors, and you can recommend that clients examine their daily habits to see if any of them are affecting their sleep patterns:

- Eating or drinking too close to bedtime
- Eating or drinking too much caffeine
- Eating or drinking too much sugar
- Smoking cigarettes with nicotine
- Medications or medication schedules
- Lack of physical activity
- Temperature of the bedroom
- Insufficient body support
- Bedtime schedules
- Amount of sleep necessary for optimal daily function
- Other individuals who might be keeping them awake

Clients who are chronically sleep deprived and cannot seem to change their sleep pattern may need to be referred to a medical doctor, who can look for a diagnosis and make a prescription. If you do refer your clients to other healthcare practitioners, you should document the referral in the Plan portion of the SOAP note and follow up by writing a letter to that practitioner.

In addition, clients can be encouraged to take "minibreaks" during the workday to stretch or walk for a few minutes once every other hour or so. Our body rhythms create a dip in brain activity in the middle of the afternoon, which creates a natural naptime. A short, 15- to 20-minute nap sometime between 1 and 4 PM can be refreshing and is least likely to affect that night's sleep.

NUTRITION

Nutritional awareness is another form of self-care a therapist may encourage in a client. Unless you are a properly trained dietitian or nutritionist, you should be very careful not to offer professional advice in this area. With this in mind, massage therapists can make nutritional recommendations from an educational standpoint as they pertain to soft tissue health. Have nutritional references on hand for clients who are interested. Vitamin C is required for tissue repair and thus is important to include in the diet. Nerve cells and muscle cells require sodium and potassium to conduct electrical charges properly, so it is generally recommended that these electrolytes be included in a balanced diet. Calcium and magnesium are critical for proper muscle contraction, making them necessary dietary elements. Nutritional recommendations generally accepted by the public are usually valid, but myths and false information are widespread. Massage therapists can demonstrate professionalism by sorting through nutritional information and guiding clients toward scientifically proven, valid facts with reasonable explanations. There are a number of herbal and "natural" remedies on the market that claim all kinds of benefits, but because many of them have not been scientifically proven, it is best to refer clients with questions about these products to a nutritional or herbal specialist. For specific dietary and nutritional recommendations, however, therapists should practice the rule "When in doubt, refer out."

BODY AWARENESS

Increasing a client's physical awareness is not only a benefit of massage; it can also be recommended to clients as a self-help activity. As mentioned above, many persons with chronic conditions do not remember what it is like to be without pain or to have unlimited function. Some get used to gauging their days by the amount of pain they experience, or they regularly describe their pain to friends and family. Sometimes the pain and discomfort become so much a part of their identity that they do not know how to let go of it. Having lived with tension or pain in an area for so long, they get used to it being there and are generally unaware of times when they do not feel pain. You may encourage clients to shift their focus to times when the tension or pain is absent, even if it is just for a few moments a day. Another approach is to get clients to periodically check for pain at mealtimes or at other regular intervals during their day. It can help them realize that being without pain is acceptable and can help them look forward to less pain and discomfort and encourage them to participate in the progress toward their goals. You could write rec: Cl record (P) every day at mealtimes.

Massage therapy can be compared to peeling layers of an onion—the layers of compensation are treated with a series of massage sessions. You must inform clients that the tension or pain may get worse as these layers are removed, that you are addressing the core of their condition, and that this is a normal part of the progress. The old adage "change is good" applies in this context. Massage treatment that increases or decreases the client's pain and ROM indicates that the body is responding to the work. If significant therapeutic work was done, the mechanical effects can be uncomfortable but not extremely painful. Discomfort resulting from massage usually decreases within 2 to 3 days as the body accommodates the mechanical changes. If it does not, it is possible that you overtreated the client, and you should adjust the massage techniques for the next session. If this is the case, you must look over your documentation notes and reevaluate

- The client's condition
- Contraindications
- Your treatment
- Possible referral to another healthcare practitioner

You have a responsibility to address your clients' responses to your treatment. A thorough general assessment may be necessary, and you may need to ask more leading questions to elicit information that might suggest contraindications that you did not identify before the previous session. The techniques you used might have been too aggressive or inappropriate for the client's condition and relative tissue health. If you cannot determine how pain resulted and why it did not go away, you may need to refer the client for further evaluation by another healthcare practitioner to maintain a client-centered practice. It is in the client's best interest to refer them for conditions that you do not understand, which makes it also in your best interest.

When no change occurs after a massage, it suggests that the massage treatments are ineffective. If no change occurs, you should also reevaluate the above factors and make adjustments to your treatment.

ERGONOMICS

Ergonomics is the science that designs and coordinates people's activities with the equipment they use and the conditions of their working environment. Ergonomics focuses on minimizing the mechanical stress placed on the body and soft tissues, which is usually accomplished by maintaining body positions that are as close to our natural and relaxed standing position as possible. For example, chairs with a flat seat and a flat back provide no support for our natural spinal curves. After sitting in that kind of chair for extended periods of time, we tend to slump, which puts mechanical stress on the spine and the nerves that exit the spine, and some persons can suffer nerve impingement as a result. Ergonomic chairs are designed to provide support for our natural spinal curves to reduce the mechanical stress on our body. There are computer keyboards that are ergonomically designed to accommodate the natural resting position of our wrists and hands to reduce compression of the carpal tunnel in the wrist. This compression is sometimes responsible for impinging the radial nerve and causing neurological symptoms of numbness and tingling in the first few phalanges.

Special equipment is not required to make ergonomic changes. Instead of looking at a computer screen that is above or below your head, which forces your neck into hyperextension or flexion, you can position the screen at eye level. Instead of carrying a purse or backpack on the same shoulder all the time, which can create chronically hypertonic muscles and fascial restrictions, you can occasionally switch the shoulder you carry the bag on. These kinds of ergonomic changes are a good source for self-care recommendations and they tie into body awareness.

Referral to Other Healthcare Professionals

With a few exceptions, massage is a good form of treatment for soft tissue dysfunction, injury recovery, and stress reduction, but it is not a cure for everything. Some conditions require the care of other healthcare professionals, and as a professional massage therapist, you have an ethical responsibility to refer clients to the appropriate healthcare practitioner. You should also be aware of professional etiquette when contacting that practitioner regarding the referral.

Whether you suspect a problem with the client's skin, nervous system, teeth, body temperature, feet, emotional instability, joints, or skeletal structure, if it is not soft tissue, massage therapists *do not* treat it. Generally, you refer clients to their primary caregiver who further evaluates or diagnoses the condition.

 Even if you feel confident of a diagnosis, it is not in your scope of practice to share that diagnosis in any form of communication, verbal or written.

Again, clients often see their massage therapist as a healthcare professional who can diagnose medical conditions. As a massage professional, you must ethically and legally educate clients that diagnosing medical conditions is in no way a part of a massage therapist's scope of practice.

By referring clients to other healthcare professionals when it is appropriate, you maintain the core principle of client-centered care. Maintaining this principle creates a ripple effect of respect and trust not only with your client, but also with other healthcare professionals. The key to the ripple effect is your ability to recognize when a condition is out of your scope of practice and needs to be addressed by another professional. This is essential for upholding the standards of practice and ethical codes of the massage therapy profession as well as preserving client-centered care. Document your recommendations for referral to other healthcare professionals in the Plan section of the SOAP chart. If you recommend that a client see his or her primary care physician (PCP) for further evaluation of the left shoulder, you could write rec: Cl see PCP for further evaluation of (L) shoulder.

FOLLOW-UP COMMUNICATION

Professional communication skills and a command of the common professional language facilitate effective communication between you and other healthcare practitioners. Correct pronunciation of anatomical and physiological words, scientific terms, and techniques is required to convey true knowledge. Proper spelling, grammar, and use of terminology are also critical for communicating a sense of understanding, especially when you are trying to develop a respectful working relationship with other healthcare professionals. Working *with* other professionals is always better than working apart from them, because clients generally feel better when everyone is working together, toward the same goal—their health and well-being.

Once a referral is made, you can ask clients to keep you in the communication loop, which makes you part of their cooperative team of healthcare professionals. You should request copies of medical reports and medical updates so you are aware of any medical diagnoses, treatments, and test results. The client-centered focus encourages determination of whether massage treatment is appropriate for the client. Without team communication, you cannot make the best decisions for soft tissue treatment, which can result in over- or undertreating the soft tissues. Conversely, if a healthcare practitioner refers a client to you, you should contact them to complete the communication loop and start creating a healthcare team.

Keeping the above in mind, there is a protocol for communication between you and other healthcare practitioners. You should keep all communication simple and to the point. Rarely, do other healthcare providers have time to sort through pages of information to ascertain what you are requesting or communicating. Essentially, you should summarize the details and state the progress of the client's condition. You should know how to make a written or verbal request for copies of medical reports and updates, how to discuss a client's condition, how the referral process with another healthcare professional works, and how to communicate with insurance companies so you can be reimbursed for massage treatments.

Requesting Copies of Medical Records

You can request copies of medical reports and updates either formally or informally. To request copies of medical information formally, your client must fill out a records release form (see Chapter 5, Fig. 5-1), and you must send a copy to the practitioner along with a cover letter stating your request. (Fig. 7-1 gives an example of a cover letter.) Informally, you can ask clients to request copies from their healthcare practitioner and bring them to you. These forms are kept in the client's file.

Discussing a Client's Condition

On occasion, you may need to discuss a client's condition with another healthcare practitioner. For example, the healthcare practitioner may need some information about your soft tissue treatment before writing a prescription. Before contacting the healthcare practitioner, you must first get written permission from the client to share the information in the massage treatment records. You can include such a statement in your client history forms rather than use a separate permission form. (See Chapter 5, Fig. 5-9 for a health information form that asks for the client's permission to consult with the referring health care provider.)

Communication for Referral and Insurance Reimbursement

Insurance laws vary from state to state, so if you are seeking insurance reimbursement, you must be aware of the insurance laws in your state and research how those laws affect reimbursement for massage. The information presented here is very general and is intended to give you a basic idea of how communication flows in this process.

Currently, clients have direct access to massage therapy, meaning they can seek treatment without a

MassageWorks!
123 North Main Street
Indianapolis, IN 46220
317.555.1234

Sam Jones, DC
Family Chiropractic
2222 Healing Way
Indianapolis, IN 46220

re: Susie Smith

28 August 2003

Dear Dr. Jones:

Hello! I am Jane Therapist and Susie Smith is currently a client in my massage therapy practice. I would like a copy of her most recent MRI report to identify any potential effects on Ms. Smith's soft tissues so that I may deliver the most appropriate treatment for her condition.

Please find enclosed a signed release form granting permission to release Ms. Smith's records.

Thank you for your assistance. Please call me should you have any questions.

Kindest regards,

Jane Therapist

Jane Therapist, CMT
Encl.

FIGURE 7-1 Cover letter.

formal referral or prescription from another healthcare practitioner. In spite of direct access, most insurance companies will not reimburse without a medical prescription or formal referral for treatment as well as treatment notes. A prescription is a written order from a medical professional who is legally allowed to prescribe, and it pertains to treatment for a specific condition. A prescription typically includes the referring healthcare practitioner's name and contact information, date, patient's name, diagnosis, diagnosis code, and the prescribed treatment with frequency and duration parameters.

Since massage therapists cannot write prescriptions, you can use a referral form to get a prescription from the physician for initial or additional mas-

sage treatment. The form should include space for your contact information and the client's name, and it should be clear that you need to have the physician write the diagnosis, precautions, body areas to treat, frequency and duration of massage treatment, and whether progress updates are requested as well as how they wish to receive them, a reevaluation date, and the physician's signature and contact information. Figure 7-2 is an example of a prescription and referral form. You can fill out your contact information and the client's (patient's) name and send the form to the client's physician. The physician can then fill in the treatment protocols and return the form to you. You then make a copy to send to the insurance company and keep a copy in the client's file. Notice

MassageWorks!
Jane Therapist, CMT
123 North Main Street
Indianapolis, IN 46220
317.555.1234

Prescription and Referral

Client name _____ Date _____
Date of Injury _____ Insurance ID# _____

Diagnosis (Include Codes)   Condition is related to
_____   ☐ Automobile Accident
_____   ☐ Work Injury
_____   ☐ Other _____
_____   _____

Cautions/Contraindications:

_____
_____
_____

Medically Necessary Treatment: Follow Plan Prescribed

Body areas to be treated: **Treatment Type:**

☐ Head _____   ☐ Discretion of the massage therapist
☐ Neck _____   ☐ Massage Therapy _____
☐ Chest _____   ☐ Hydrotherapy _____
☐ Shoulders _____   ☐ Self-Care Education _____
☐ Back _____   ☐ Other _____
☐ Lowback/Hips _____
☐ Upper Extremities _____   **Treatment Goals:**
☐ Lower Extremities _____   ☐ Decrease Pain
☐ All of the above _____   ☐ Decrease Muscle Tension/Spasm
☐ Other _____   ☐ Decrease Compensation patterns
                                                  ☐ Increase Mobility
Duration and Frequency   ☐ Increase Function
☐ Daily   ☐ Other _____
☐ _____ x per wk for _____ wks   _____
☐ _____ x per month for _____ months
Reevaluation Date: _____

Additional Instructions:

_____
_____

Referring Healthcare Provider (HCP)

Contact Information   **Progress Updates**
Provider Name _____   ☐ Send Progress Report after Initial Session
Provider No. _____   ☐ Send at end of Prescription
Address _____   ☐ Send copies of Treatment Notes at end of Prescription
_____   ☐ Mail ☐ Fax ☐ Email
Phone _____
Fax _____
Email _____
Provider Signature _____ Date _____

FIGURE 7-2 Prescription and referral form.

whether an initial treatment report and/or progress notes are requested in return. Your initial treatment report should include a note of thanks to the physician for referring the client to you for massage in addition to your initial findings and massage treatment plan. Essentially, it summarizes the SOAP notes and general assessment form information. (Fig. 7-3 contains an example of an initial treatment report.) A progress report is often requested by the referring physician, and it is basically a summary of the Subjective and Objective sections of the SOAP notes. If you are recommending further care, specify the new duration and frequency parameters. Generally, a progress report is sent to the healthcare provider every 30 days or for the length of the prescription. (Fig 7-4 contains an example of a progress report.)

MassageWorks!
Jane Therapist, CMT
123 North Main Street
Indianapolis, IN 46220
317.555.1234
email: Jane@massageworks.com

Sam Jones, DC
Family Physicians
2222 Healing Way
Indianapolis, IN 46220

28 August 2003

Re: Susie Smith

Dear Dr. Jones:

Thank you for referring Susie Smith to me for massage treatment. Ms. Smith had her first appointment on 28 August 2003.

Ms. Smith presented herself for massage treatment with bilateral neck pain and tension. Her immediate goal is to get relief from the neck pain and tension. Ms. Smith would like to able to work at her computer for 2 hours a day during her workweek without neck pain and tension. Initially, our treatment goal is to have her working at the computer for 15 minutes a day with moderate pain and tension.

Together, Ms. Smith and I will work toward the treatment goals as follows: Massage and Myofascial release 2 times a week for 1 month with specific focus on the bilateral neck muscles and surrounding soft tissue, hydrotherapy to reduce any muscle spasm and/or inflammation and self-care recommendations.

I will report back to you in 30 days with Ms. Smith's progress. Please contact me should you have any questions, remarks or concerns.

Kindest Regards,

Jane Therapist

Jane Therapist, CMT

FIGURE 7-3 Initial treatment report.

MassageWorks!
Jane Therapist, CMT
123 North Main Street
Indianapolis, IN 46220
317.555.1234
email: Jane@massageworks.com

Client name Susie Smith _____ Date _30 September 2003_
Date of Injury _15 August 2003_____ Insurance ID# _123-45-6789_

Client's Current Condition
After 8 sessions of Myofascial release, Ms. Smith has reached her initial goals of relief
from her neck pain and tension as well as working 15 minutes a day with moderate neck
pain and tension. _____

Subjective Findings:
Body areas

☐ Head _____
☒ Neck _BL neck P and ≡_____
☐ Chest _____
☐ Shoulders_____
☐ Lowback/Hips _____
☐ Upper Extremities _____
☐ Lower Extremities _____
☐ All of the above _____
☐ Other _____

Objective Findings:

☐ Muscle Spasm _____
☒ Increased mobility _____
☐ Decreased mobility _____
☐ Hypersensitivity _____
☐ Increased Tension _____
☒ Decreased Tension _△ mod_
☐ Increased Pain _____
☒ Decreased Pain   _△ mod_
☐ Other _____

Recommendations for Further Care:
Duration and Frequency
Additional Care Needed
☐ None needed
☐ Daily
☐ _____ x per wk for _____ wks
☐ _____ x per month for _____ months
☐ PRN max visits _____ per _____

Please contact me with any questions, remarks or concerns. Thank you for your referrals.

Jane Therapist _____ Jane Therapist, CMT _30Sep03_ Date

FIGURE 7-4 Progress report.

Presenting the Treatment Plan

The process of developing treatment plans may seem awkward at first, but with practice, you will become very skilled at making recommendations for treatment. In the beginning, you may find it easier to leave out the treatment plan for initial appointments and only consider a treatment plan after subsequent massage sessions. This gives you time to analyze the history and assessment findings and get a feeling for your client's internal healing environment and participation in healthcare. Presenting the plan is a way of educating clients about the information you used to determine your recommendations, essentially telling them why you are making the recommendations.

Clients are more likely to commit and comply with your recommendations if they know why they are doing it.

TREATMENT RECOMMENDATIONS

The first question clients typically ask is, "How long it will take to (stop hurting, return to "normal" function, or stay relaxed for longer than a day)?" There is no single answer, much to their disappointment. You can explain that health and healing times are affected by the physical, emotional, mental, and nutritional stress that a person has accumulated and that healing time can be reduced with the help of massage and self-care. Once you educate your clients about the "whys" of your recommendations, you can discuss the treatment plan and use their input to make adjustments to the plan. All of your recommendations for future treatment are documented in the Plan section of the SOAP note.

REFERRAL RECOMMENDATIONS

If in your assessment of the client you discover a health condition that presents a contraindication for massage or is outside the scope of practice, it is in the client's best interest to refer the client to the appropriate healthcare professional. Anything in the client's best interest is in your best interest. Sometimes clients are aware of their conditions and sometimes not. If not, you may need to have a delicate conversation to refer them to a medical professional without making a diagnosis or alarming them.

Remember to be very careful not to suggest that clients may have "XYZ" condition, because they could misinterpret your statement as a diagnosis, assume they have it, and tell their friends, family, or healthcare practitioner. For example, if you detect some inflammation at or around a musculotendinous juncture, *do not* say that it might be tendinitis or that you think it could be tendinitis. Instead, you could say, "From my assessment, I have determined that I can effectively treat your soft tissue condition with massage." Conversely, if you suspect clients may need further examination, you could say, "From my assessment, I have determined that massage might not be helpful for you, and before I do any harm, I recommend that you see your primary healthcare practitioner for further examination. Once your doctor has determined that massage is indicated, I would be happy to continue treatment." There are more complex situations, such as rotator cuff injuries, in which clients have one condition that indicates massage and another that presents a contraindication for massage. In this situation, you could say, "After my assessment, I have determined that you have a soft tissue condition that I can treat, and you also might have a condition that I do not treat. I recommend that you see your primary healthcare professional for further evaluation, and when your doctor authorizes massage treatment, I can confidently continue treatment."

Case Studies

The treatment plans for Rob Blackwell, Timothy Roberts, and Kirsten Van Marter are based upon the initial treatment plan procedure.

PROGRESSIVE CASE STUDY 1

Rob Blackwell

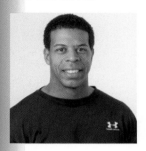

Considering Rob Blackwell's health history, interview, and assessment process, you determine that Rob's internal healing environment is good and that he is very likely to participate in his healing process. His involvement with sports and his self-employment as a personal trainer suggest that he is moderately likely to repeat the motions that created his neck and shoulder pain or reinjure the affected tissues. Rob's right shoulder is elevated and rolled forward, and there are a number of associated hypertonic muscles. Despite his good internal healing environment, the hypertonic muscles, associated fascial restrictions, and his likelihood to reinjure the tissues could increase the healing time.

Since his musculature is so developed and healthy, his body could withstand 90-minute massages without suffering overtreatment, but his financial situation cannot support them. Rob's initial treatment plan includes 60-minute massages once a week for 6 weeks, at which point the goals will be reevaluated. For the next session, you suggest vibration over the right pectoralis muscles. You mention that there are some self-care activities that he could use to help maintain progress made during the massage and reduce the length of the course of treatment. He could apply ice to his right upper trapezius for 20 minutes, at least once a day, every day. You could demonstrate some specific stretches for the pectoralis major and sternocleidomastoid muscles, explaining that he could use these stretches at least once a day, 5 days a week. He could also increase water intake to 100 ounces per day. You refer Rob to Dr. Christian for an evaluation and current diagnosis of his knees to make sure massage is not contraindicated. These recommendations are highlighted in the Plan section of Rob's SOAP chart in Figure 7-5.

PROGRESSIVE CASE STUDY 2

Timothy Roberts

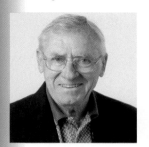

Timothy is only seeking relaxation massage, and he reports no pain, numbness, or stiffness. From the client interview and general assessment, you notice some restrictions in ROM of the left ankle, but you also detect his impatience with the assessments. To strike a balance between gaining his trust and remaining professional, your assessments are brief, primarily looking for any contraindications. For wellness clients like Timothy, you complete the initial treatment plan procedure mostly for consistency in your documentation. Should he seek more therapeutic treatment in the future, you would need to perform a more thorough intake and assessment as well as use the initial treatment plan procedure to determine a more specific plan. His initial treatment plan is simply to receive 60-minute relaxation massages at least once every 3 months, but you suggest trying cross-fiber friction on the left ankle. You can offer him a glass of water following the massage, briefly mentioning that if he were to drink at least 80 ounces of water a day, it would help his body retain the benefits of the massage. Timothy's treatment plan information is highlighted in his massage treatment record (See Fig. 7-6).

PROGRESSIVE CASE STUDY 3

Kirsten Van Marter

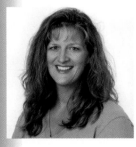

Although she is a new client to you, Kirsten's health information form indicates that she has received regular massage in the past. The information from the history and assessment process lets you know that her internal healing environment is good, but because of her hectic lifestyle of taking care of her child, being pregnant, and working two separate jobs, she may not find time to participate in her healing process. She will probably repeat the motions that created the soft tissue condition as she continues her work and household activities. Both of her shoulders are rolled forward, and her left hip is elevated. Even though she is in her third trimester of pregnancy, the distribution of her weight will continue to change, and her hip pain could get worse. Healing and restoring function may be a challenge until after the baby is born.

Kirsten's muscles and soft tissues are fairly healthy because of her regular exercise and massage. The initial treatment plan suggests 60-minute massages once a week for 4 weeks. Since she is uncomfortable with her pregnancy, it would be good to try more bolsters. You educate Kirsten about the benefits of proper hydration and offer her a glass of water following the massage, asking whether she drinks at least 70 ounces of water a day. You also demonstrate specific stretches for pectoralis major and subscapularis muscles, explaining that if she were to use those stretches at least once a day, everyday, it could help her retain the benefits of the current massage. Kirsten's SOAP note highlights the treatment plan information (See Fig. 7-7).

Provider Name **Therapeutic Massage Works**   **SOAP CHART-M**

Patient Name **Robert (Rob) Blackwell**   Date **4-2-02**

Date of Injury **N/A**   Insurance ID# **N/A**   Current Meds **ibuprofen prn**

S Focus for Today ↑sleep, ↓℗

Symptoms: Location/Intensity/Frequency/Duration/Onset
C/o neck, shoulder, back ℗ constant 4 on 10 scale
Knee ℗ 4 on 10 scale, 10 yrs +, intermittent

Activities of Daily Living: Aggravating/Relieving
Aggravate: weights, bball, golf
Relief: ibuprofen, hot tub

O Findings: Visual/Palpable/Test Results
↓A/PROM Ⓛ Knee flex PROM w/℗
↓A/PROM Ⓛ hip flex, ext, abd
Lat flex Ⓛ > Ⓡ
↓AROM ⒷⓁ shoulder abd., neck rot.
≡ Ⓡ SCM, pecs, lev scap. rhomb, Ⓛ QL, ⒷⓁ up trap, delts, TFL
X Ⓡ rhomb, lev scap, ⒷⓁ IT bands

A Modalities: Applications/Locations
XFF ⒷⓁ IT bands, MFR Ⓡ pec area, Ⓡ scap, Ⓛ QL
PNF Ⓡ up trap, Ⓡ pecs

Response to Treatment (see Δ)
↑AROM shoulder abd, neck rot, ℗ 4→1

Prioritize Functional Limitations
1. swing golf club
2. lift weights } both due to shoulder ℗

Goals: Long-term/Short-term
LTG: Within 6 wks, lift 30 lb. w/shoulder abd,
3 sets of 10, 5 days/wk

STG: Within 1 wk, lift 10 lb. w/shoulder abd,
1 set of 10, 3 days/wk

P Future Treatment/Frequency
1 hr. Ⓜ, 1x/wk for 6 wks. Try vibration at Ⓡ pecs
Refer to Dr. Christian for knee eval to rule out CI

Homework/Self-care
rec: ice Ⓡ up trap 20 min 1x/day everyday
rec: door jamb pec stretch & passive SCM stretch 1x/day
rec: 100 oz. H₂O/day   5 days/wk as demo'd

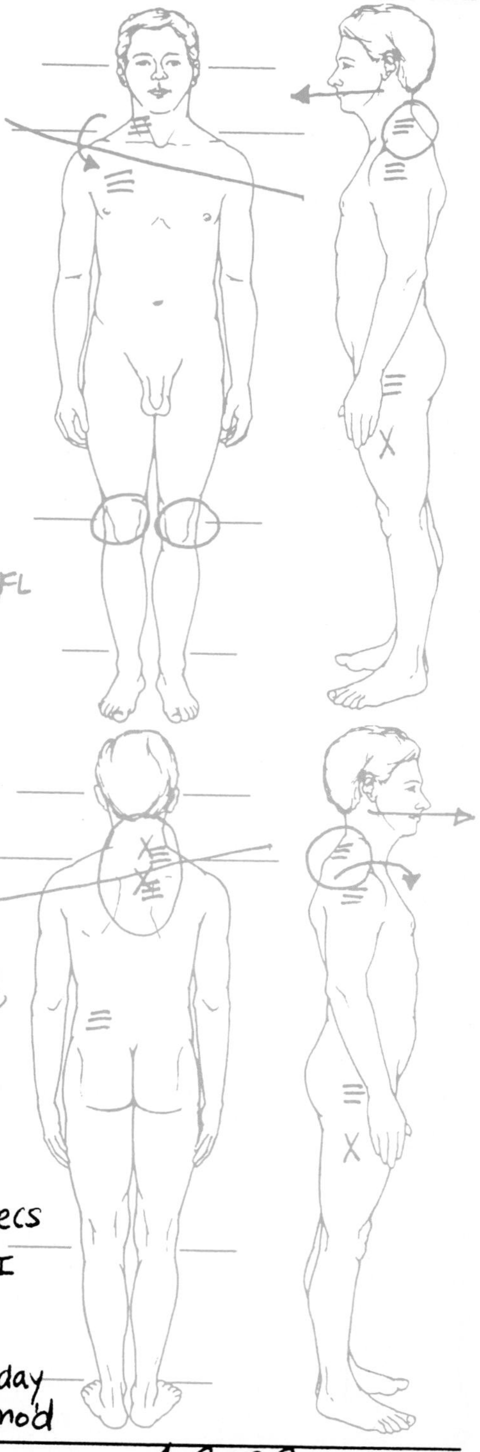

Provider Signature _Jane Therapist_   Date **4.2.02**

Legend: ⊙ TP   • TeP   ○ Ⓡ   ＊ Infl   ≡ HT   ≈ SP
X Adh   ≷ Numb   ⌒ rot   ╱ elev   ⤚ Short   ↔ Long

FIGURE 7-5 Rob's SOAP note, highlighting plan. (Modified from Thompson DL. Hands Heal: Communication, Documentation and Insurance Billing for Manual Therapists. 2nd ed. Baltimore: Lippincott Williams & Wilkins, 2002:240.)

Provider Name _Therapeutic Massage Works_ **STANDARD HxTxC Chart-M**

Name __Timothy Roberts__ Date __9/10/03__

Phone __317-555-1234__ Address __110 Main St, Indianapolis, IN 46220__

1. What are your goals for health, and how may I assist you in achieving your goals? _____
   relaxation

2. Are you currently experiencing any of the following? If yes, please explain.

   pain, tenderness   ☑ No   ☐ Yes: _____   stiffness   ☑ No   ☐ Yes: _____
   numbness or tingling   ☑ No   ☐ Yes: _____   swelling   ☑ No   ☐ Yes: _____
   allergies   ☑ No   ☐ Yes: _____

3. List all illnesses, injuries, and health concerns you have now or have had in the past 3 years.
   (Examples: arthritis, diabetes, car accident, pregnancy) _moderate blood pressure,_
   skin cancer, broken (L) ankle

4. List medications and pain relievers taken today. _Blood pressure medication_

5. I have provided all my known medical information. I acknowledge that manual therapy is not
   a substitute for medical diagnosis and treatment. I give my consent to receive treatment.

   Signature _Timothy Roberts_ Date _2/21/02_

   Tx: _FBRM c̄ circulatory enhancement focus; during_
   ⓜ _noticed ↓ ROM & X in (L) ankle –_
   C: _Cl has no complaints today. Rec: 1hr Ⓜ 1X/3 months,_
   next session XFF to (L) ankle, rec: 80 oz H₂O/day

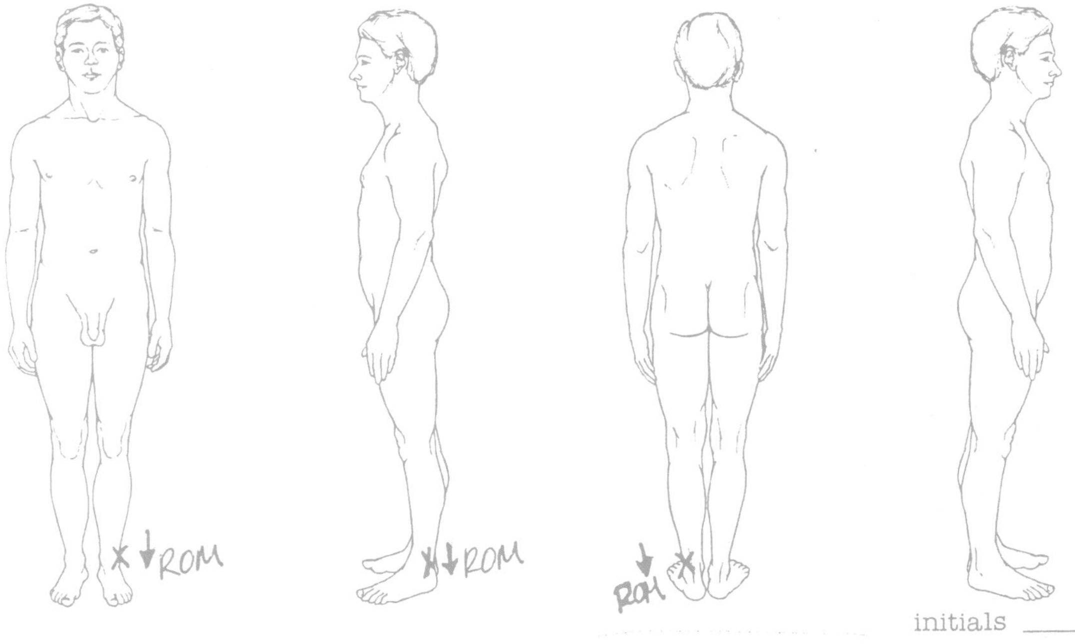

X ↓ROM   X ↓ROM   ROM X   initials _MB b_

FIGURE 7-6 Timothy's HxTxC, highlighting plan information. (Modified from Thompson DL. Hands Heal: Communication, Documentation and Insurance Billing for Manual Therapists. 2nd ed. Baltimore: Lippincott Williams & Wilkins, 2002:247.)

Provider Name __Therapeutic Massage Works__   **SOAP CHART-F**

Patient Name __Kirsten Van Marter__   Date __4-9-02__

Date of Injury __N/A__   Insurance ID# __N/A__   Current Meds __N/A__

S Focus for Today ↓ ⓟ , ↑ sleep, ↑ fitness level

Symptoms: Location/Intensity/Frequency/Duration/Onset

c/o mild, constant back ⓟ (5 on 10 scale)
  mild hip, neck, shoulder ⓟ (3 on 10 scale)
All ⓟ for 3 months w/ pregnancy

Activities of Daily Living: Aggravating/Relieving

Aggravating: computer work, childcare, housework

Relieving: Ⓜ, stretches, exercise, pain meds prn.

O Findings: Visual/Palpable/Test Results

↓ AROM + ⓟ Ⓑⓛ shoulder flex, No ⓟ c̄ PROM

≡ Ⓑⓛ pecs, rhomb, up trap, Ⓛ QL, TFL

✗ Ⓑⓛ sup. erector spinae, IT bands

✳ Ⓑⓛ ankles

TP Ⓑⓛ pec minor, TeP Ⓑⓛ traps, rhomb

A Modalities: Applications/Locations

Prenatal sidelying FBRM, circ. enhance, light XFF erectors
                                    PNF to TP, TeP

Response to Treatment (see Δ)

ⓟ 5→2, 3→1, ↑ AROM Ⓑⓛ shoulder flex

Prioritize Functional Limitations

1. Lift daughter

Goals: Long-term/Short-term

LTG: Within 4 wks, lift child into highchair
    2x/day w/o ⓟ, 3 days/wk.

STG: With 1 wk, put dishes away into top
    cabinet 1x/day w/o ⓟ, 3 days/wk.

P Future Treatment/Frequency

1 hr Ⓜ 1x/wk, 4 wks, use more bolsters

Homework/Self-care

rec: 70 oz. H₂O/day
rec: door jamb stretches for pec. major & subscap
        1x/day, everyday as demo'd

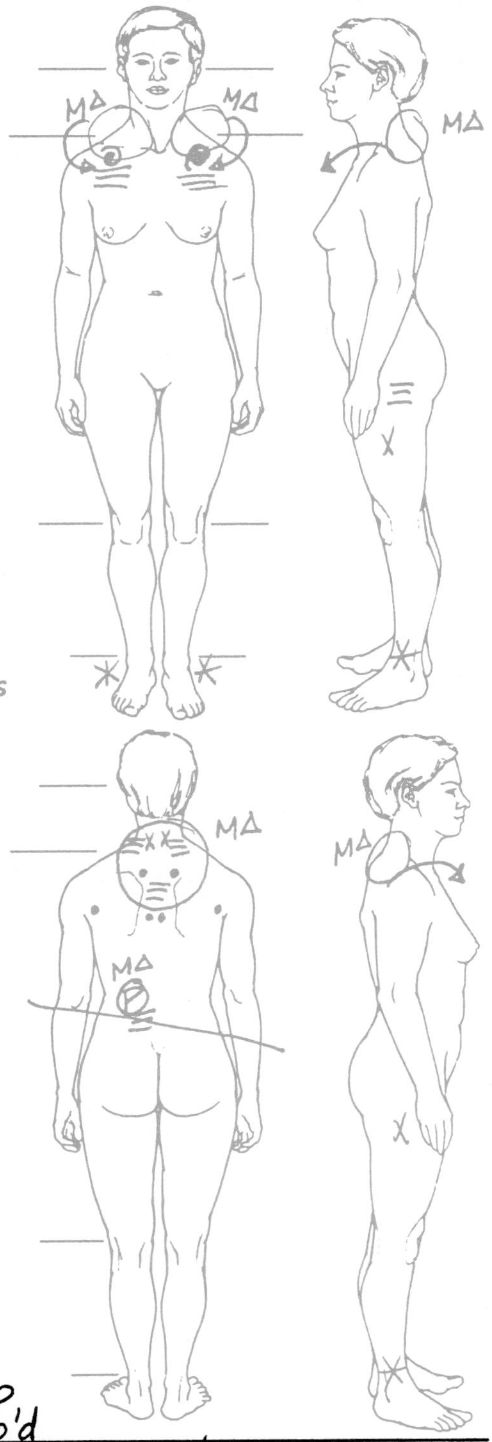

Provider Signature __June Therapist__   Date __4-9-02__

Legend: ℮ TP   • TeP   ○ ⓟ   ✳ Infl   ≡ HT   ≈ SP
          ✗ Adh   ≋ Numb   ⟲ rot   ╱ elev   ⟩—⟨ Short   ↔ Long

FIGURE 7-7 Kirsten's SOAP note, highlighting plan. (Modified from Thompson DL. Hands Heal: Communication, Documentation and Insurance Billing for Manual Therapists. 2nd ed. Baltimore: Lippincott Williams & Wilkins, 2002:239.)

Chapter Summary

Massage therapists should always maintain a client-centered focus for care. The treatment plan for client care is part of that professional focus. With space and time constraints, you can write only brief notes in your massage treatment records, but you still need to document details accurately. Another therapist should be able to read your **SOAP** note and understand what the treatment plan includes, which self-care activities were recommended between sessions, and any referrals you may have made.

Self-help techniques give you a good topic of discussion for the next session, asking about which self-help techniques clients used or which ones were more effective. Soft tissue health and healing should always be the objective of self-help techniques to clients. The effective and efficient documentation of treatment and self-care are vital aspects of a professional practice.

 CHAPTER EXERCISES

1. Use abbreviations and symbols to rewrite the following treatment plans:
   a. 60-minute massages, twice a month, for 2 months. Try vibration over the left scapula, and stay away from the client's feet. Reevaluate **AROM** of left shoulder extension to see if the triceps stretches that were demonstrated and recommended once a day, every day, were helpful.
   b. 90-minute full body relaxation massages, once a month, for 3 months. Avoid proprioceptive neuromuscular facilitation and active range of motion evaluations, because the client does not like to actively participate during the session. Referred to Dr. Park for pain upon right elbow **PROM**.
   c. 30-minute massages, once a week, for 4 weeks. Only use supine, since client is claustrophobic and does not like to be prone. Discussed use of a bolster under the knees during sleep to relieve low back pain.

2. Develop and properly document treatment plans for the following sample clients:
   a. A 20-year-old man, at least 50 pounds overweight, quietly complains of bilateral knee pain. His physical activity is limited to his walk to and from work, 5 days a week. At work, he sits at a computer all day and drinks diet soft drinks all day long. He eats fast food every day and does not like to drink water. Your general assessments discover bilateral symmetry with a forward posture, rolled shoulders, and knock-knees. He reports pain upon active and passive ROM of his knees, suggesting that some passive structures that are outside the massage scope of practice are involved.
   b. A 50-year-old man, who appears in good physical condition explains that his friend got a massage from you and convinced him to try one even though he has no areas of concern. He swims for 30 minutes, at least five times a week, and drinks at least 60 ounces of water a day. He has a wife, three kids, and two dogs and is self-employed in an established and stable business. His posture is bilaterally symmetrical, but his head is forward, and he experiences occasional neck pain and tightness. You found fascial restrictions all around the cervical area, but did not have enough time to address it. He reports that he was able to relax but not until the massage was almost over and asks if massages can be longer than 60 minutes.
   c. A 70-year-old woman has been coming to you regularly, once a month, for over a year. She is retired and enjoys her gardening club activities and worldwide travel. Every day, she drinks a glass of juice, a cup of tea, a glass of water, and a cup of coffee. Every day, she eats a lot of fruits and vegetables, very few carbohydrates, and a small amount of protein. In the past, she has always responded well to a full-body relaxation massage that includes some craniosacral work. She has not incorporated any self-help in the year you have been treating her, but she always asks about what she should do between sessions.

3. Explain the difference between an initial treatment plan and a treatment plan for the subsequent massage sessions.

4. List the six components included in the plan section of the **SOAP** note.

5. List at least five questions you can use to evaluate clients' internal healing environment to estimate their healing time and length of treatment.

6. Explain why it is not always better to recommend massage sessions that last longer and are more frequent.

7. Explain why it is not always better to recommend a lot of self-care activities.

8. Explain why we encourage clients to participate in self-care activities.

9. Name at least seven factors that can disrupt sleep.

10. Describe at least three different reasons why you need effective communication skills to follow up on your treatment plan.

SUGGESTED READING

Batmanghelidj F. You're Not Sick, You're Thirsty: Water for Health, for Healing, for Life. New York: Warner Books, 2003.

Bicknell J, Benjamin BE. The importance of water. American Massage Therapy Association's Massage Therapy Journal, 2003;Winter, pages 28–36.

Chopra D. Restful Sleep: The Complete Mind/Body Program for Overcoming Insomnia. New York: Three Rivers Press, 1994.

George M. Learn to Relax: A Practical Guide to Easing Tension & Conquering Stress. San Francisco: Chronicle Books, 1998.

Kneipp S. The Kneipp Cure: An Absolutely Verbal and Literal Translation for "Meine Wasserkur" (My Water Cure). New York: Nature Cure Publishing, 1949.

Sapolsky RM. Why Zebras Don't Get Ulcers: An Updated Guide to Stress, Stress-Related Diseases, and Coping. New York, NY: WH Freeman, 1998.

Thompson D. Hands Heal Communication, Documentation and Insurance Billing for Manual Therapists. 2nd ed. Lippincott Williams & Wilkins, Baltimore: 2002.

Tobias M, Sullivan JP. Complete Stretching: A New Exercise Program For Health and Vitality. New York: Alfred A. Knopf, 1994.

Yee R, with Zolotow N. Yoga the Poetry of the Body. New York: Thomas Dunne, 2002.

http://my.webmd.com/content/article/1674.50313, accessed 12.03.02.

http://my.webmd.com/content/article/1685.52630, accessed 12.03.02.

http://my.webmd.com/content/asset/miller_keane_30561, accessed 12.03.02.

http://my.webmd.com/encyclopedia/article/4117.732, accessed 12.03.02.

http://www.21c-online.com/2001-pickering-sleep.htm, accessed 12.03.02.

http://www.aimt-hi.com/05.html, accessed 12.03.02.

http://www.boston.com/globe/search/stories/health/how_and_why/011298.htm (The Boston Globe web site, "What Percentage of the Human Body is Water and How is This Determined?"), accessed 12/09/02.

http://www.bottledwater.org/public/hydratio.htm, accessed 12.01.02.

http://www.healthyroads.com/mylibrary/data/ash_ref/htm/art_waterrequirementshelpyourbodymaintainnormalfunction.asp, accessed 12.01.02.

http://www.jointhealing.com/pages/productpages/cryotherapy.html, accessed 12.03.02.

http://www.ninds.nih.gov/health_and_medical/pubs/understanding_sleep_brain_basic_.htm, accessed 12.03.02.

http://www.water.com, accessed 8.18.03.

Equipment and Environment

UPON COMPLETION OF THIS CHAPTER, THE STUDENT WILL BE ABLE TO:

- Properly set the height of the massage table
- Describe the difference between a stationary and a portable massage table
- List at least two reasons to use massage lubricants
- Identify at least five factors that contribute to your massage environment
- Describe at least four different massage environments created by the location of a massage practice
- Describe the purpose of standard precautions
- Demonstrate the proper hand-washing procedure

KEY TERMS

Draping: the use of sheets and towels to cover clients during the massage for warmth and modesty

Lubricants: wet and dry products that reduce friction between your skin and the client's skin and increase the comfort of the massage strokes

Outcall: a massage appointment in which you take your massage table to a client's home, hotel, or office

Pathogen (or pathogenic microorganism): a microscopic organism that can cause disease in other organisms, commonly called a germ

Standard precautions: specific procedures that maintain a hygienic and sanitary practice and reduce the risk for germ transmission

The foundation for a basic massage session includes properly assembled, dependable equipment and a comforting environment that is safe and sanitary. Most of the equipment used in a massage practice is designed to keep the client comfortable, but it also influences the massage you give by determining how much access you have to the client's body. The table, which is the primary piece of equipment, holds clients in a relaxed position during the massage, along with a variety of accessories that provide additional support and comfort. Massage chairs, massage mats, and body cushions are alternatives to the massage table that you can incorporate into your practice. Additionally, massage tools and gadgets can reduce the stress on your joints and reduce the amount of physical work required to do massage for a living. Some of the supplies you will need are so important for the comfort and safety of the client that they may be considered pieces of equipment. These include lubricants, sheets and other draping supplies (towels and blankets), a collection of massage music, a sound system, treatment room furnishings, disinfectants, and safety-related items.

Your equipment, the location of your practice, and your treatment room create the environment of your massage practice. Whether you treat clients in an office building, a spa, your home, their home, or outdoors, the location of the practice sets the initial tone for your massage and contributes significantly to the massage environment. Regardless of the kind of environment you want to establish, sanitation and safety are critical components that you must incorporate. The health and well-being of the client are the primary goals for massage therapy, so every therapist should know how to maintain a healthy, hygienic, safe practice with specific methods called standard precautions.

There are a wide variety of thoughts and opinions about which massage equipment and environment are best. This chapter covers the basics as well as guidelines to options available at the time of publication and general rules for entry-level massage therapists with regard to equipment and environment. As you gain experience and interact with other massage therapists, you will undoubtedly form your own opinions and discover what works best for you.

Equipment

The equipment and supplies you need to practice massage are available in a huge range of prices, sizes, types of construction, appearance, durability, and maintenance requirements. New equipment is readily available in specialty stores, in catalogs and magazines, and through online suppliers. A number of manufacturers specialize in massage therapy equipment and make quality products. Occasionally they sell discontinued models, discontinued colors, or demonstration models at discounted prices.

Used equipment is available and much less expensive, but you need to know its history: where it has been, how old it is, how long it was used, any substances or odors it was exposed to, if it has been damaged or repaired, and how it has been maintained. Without knowing the equipment's history, its reliability is questionable. Some sources for used and more reliable equipment are massage schools and massage therapists. Students who were unable to complete their massage education may be interested in selling their gently used equipment. Practicing therapists may know people who were unable to maintain a massage business and need to sell their used equipment.

Another alternative to purchasing new equipment is to borrow it. Recent graduates interested in helping new students may be interested in sharing their tables for a short time. Even better, some massage schools offer equipment rental to their students. Learning massage requires hands-on practice to develop good techniques, so whether you buy a new table, buy a used one, or borrow one, make sure you have one.

EQUIPMENT SPECIFICATIONS

The process of choosing your equipment can be challenging, especially because of the many options available. Once you start looking at the brochures and advertisements, you will discover the seemingly endless choices. Massage suppliers feature equipment with a range of prices, comfort levels, strength and stability specifications, and warranties. Sifting through all the numbers and tests and comparing specifications can make it difficult to know what to look for.

Price

To build a successful practice you have to give clients an experience that invites them back. Clients form impressions about you and your massage practice on the basis of many factors from your massage to your table and other accessories. With this in mind, think of the equipment you purchase as an investment in your professional image and the success of your practice. You weigh your options between saving a minimal amount of money and having the best equipment for your massage career.

Comfort

To build and sustain your practice you want to always keep your focus on client-centered care. Delivering the experience of comfort and relaxation will also encourage clients to come back. Just the right table and face rest (face cradle) padding and covering as well as quality construction will further enhance your client's experience. Minimal padding, low-quality covering, and a squeaky table provide a client with quite a different experience from that of equipment that has generous foam padding, ultrasoft covering, and solid construction. When determining which equipment to purchase, ask yourself, "Will this equipment enhance the comfort and relaxation of my client or detract from it?"

Strength and Stability

Strength and stability in a table come from quality construction in which each component reinforces the other components of the table. Your equipment holds your clients and allows them to relax, so its stability and structural integrity are very important. Underwriters Laboratories (UL) listing and static and dynamic load capacities specify the strength and stability of a table.

Underwriters Laboratories Inc. is an independent, nongovernmental, not-for-profit company that objectively tests products for safety. Products that pass their tests receive the UL listing, and products that do not pass do not get the listing. The results are vague and not necessarily helpful in deciding what to buy. Basically, massage equipment with the UL listing has been tested and determined to be safe if used properly.

Equipment companies boast static loading capacities of 3000 pounds or more and show photos of a truck, a pyramid of people, or a pile of barbell weights on a massage table. Static loading simply tests how much weight a table can withstand as long as the weight is evenly distributed and not moving. The images are impressive, to say the least, but are generally not useful when determining the working strength and stability of your table. Essentially, tables that can carry static loads of 2000 pounds or more have a strong structure that is dependable.

Dynamic loading measures the weight that can be loaded unevenly on the table. Some companies refer to this measurement as the table's working weight. It tests the amount of weight that can be set on one end of the table or on the center of a hinged table. Testing the dynamic load, or working weight, best replicates how you and your clients will use your table, making it the most helpful statistic to check. The dynamic loading capacities of good-quality massage tables will be about 450 pounds or more.

Warranty

Most reputable equipment companies offer product warranties (guarantees) that can also be a bit confusing, often with different durations and transferability. For instance, a massage table made by a respectable company may have a 5-year warranty on the padding and a 3-year warranty on the vinyl covering, all of which is transferable if the table is sold. Another table made by the same company may have a non-transferable guarantee of only 2 years on the padding and vinyl. The specifics of these guarantees are not as critical as the company's willingness to stand behind the products and replace or repair anything that they designed or made poorly. A company that guarantees its workmanship likely makes a good-quality product that should stand the test of time as long as you use it properly. All of the guarantees exclude any damage that occurs to the tables due to accident, neglect or improper use.

Tables

For most massage therapists, the primary piece of equipment is a massage table. It provides a flat surface that allows clients to lie down during the massage in a position that gives you access to their whole body. Almost all tables have a padded rectangular top with a washable covering that is supported by a stabilized wooden framework. Some massage tables are made with an aluminum framework, and although they are not as popular, they withstand exposure to water much better than wood. There are also electric-lift, stationary massage tables, whose height you can adjust by a foot pedal; however, these can be very expensive, so, it might not be an option for a beginning practitioner. Generally, massage tables are categorized as portable or stationary because the purpose and design of the two are so different. The wide variety of massage table sizes, features, and prices is mostly a function of the table top and the support structure.

TABLE TOP

The most common shape of massage table tops is a rectangle, but there are also rectangles with rounded corners, contoured shapes, ovals, and a relatively new option of a breast recess. Table widths range from 22 to 33 inches, and lengths run between 65 and 78 inches. The most common table tops are about 28 to 30 inches wide and 72 to 73 inches long. Some tables are designed for special applications such as Feldenkrais techniques, prenatal or pregnancy tables, or an easy access end panel for several different techniques (Fig. 8-1).

A wider top provides a larger and more comfortable base for your clients to lie on, increasing their comfort and security, but there are some disadvantages of a wide table to consider. Accessing the center of the clients' bodies requires a longer reach, which is especially problematic for shorter therapists. The wider the table, the heavier it is and the more awkward it is to transport.

There is a breast recess option for the table top that can help therapists perform more effective work with less effort (Fig. 8-2). Traditionally, the table top of a massage table is flat, which compresses the clients' breasts and elevates their torsos. This position rolls the shoulders forward and moves the scapulae laterally, pulling and lengthening the muscles that are medial to the scapulae. Instead of being soft and pliable, these muscles get stretched out like a tight rubber band, becoming taut and more challenging to massage. A table with breast recesses maintains a more natural position for the scapulae and can minimize the tightness that accompanies soft tissues that are pulled taut. It makes these regions more pliable and gives you deeper access to the muscles and tendons with less effort.

The table top is padded for comfort. The padding is usually made of foam or multiple layers of different kinds of foam. Padding is usually between 2 and

3 inches thick, and although thicker and firmer padding is more comfortable for clients, it tends to be heavier and bulkier. If you plan on carrying your table a lot, you may want to consider a 2-inch layer of padding instead of 3 inches (Fig. 8-3). Natural fibers such as cotton and wool are also available as padding material but usually as a separate layer that rests on top of the finished table.

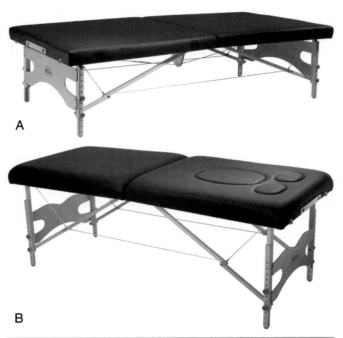

A

B

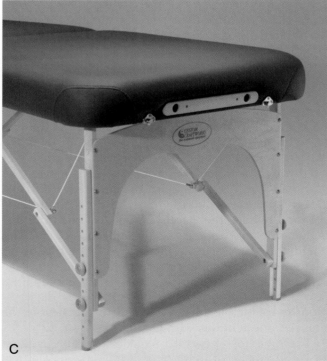

C

FIGURE 8-1   Specialty tables. **A.** Feldenkrais. **B.** Pregnancy. **C.** Easy access panel. (Photos courtesy of Customcraftworks.)

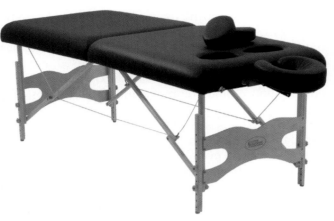

FIGURE 8-2   Breast recess table. (Photo courtesy of Customcraftworks.)

Over the foam, the entire table top is covered by a durable, leatherlike or vinyl fabric that can withstand regular cleaning with disinfectant. The covering is available in almost any color, giving you an opportunity to individualize your practice and express your personality. Dirt and stains are more noticeable on the lighter colors, but clients usually only see the sheets or towels on top of your table instead of any stains or the color of the table.

Some table coverings are buttery soft and supple to the touch. They are more expensive than the standard vinyl, implying that they are better or more comfortable. These soft coverings tend to be less durable than the standard vinyl and are more susceptible to scratches and tears. The inexpensive vinyl is a more practical option for tables that are moved around a lot or that receive a lot of use.

TABLE SUPPORT

Massage table tops are supported by four wooden or metal legs or a single metal pedestal. Tables are occasionally constructed with a fixed height, but most tables can be adjusted to different heights, providing the following benefits:

- Different therapists of different heights can use the same table.

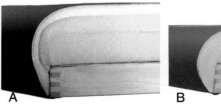

FIGURE 8-3   Foam padding. **A.** Three layer. **B.** One layer. (Photos courtesy of EarthLite.)

- Clients of different sizes and thicknesses can be positioned at the same working height.
- Variable table height accommodates multiple bodywork techniques.

Electric-lift tables can be raised and lowered with the push of a button, making height adjustment quick and easy. They are supported by a central hydraulic pedestal instead of four legs at the corners of the table. These high-end tables are typically only used in clinical settings such as doctor's offices and hospitals, because the price is prohibitive for most independent therapists (Fig. 8-4).

Manually adjustable tables are less than half the price of electric-lift tables, which is why they are the most common. The legs are constructed of two pieces of wood or metal that can be bolted together in different positions to create different lengths. As clients get on and off the table and as the table is moved or cleaned, the table experiences torque, or twisting forces, and uneven weight distribution. These mechanical forces can wiggle the bolts loose, making the table leg weak and wobbly.

 The table leg bolts must be checked for tightness on a regular basis to maintain the table's stability.

A guideline for checking leg bolts is every five to ten clients or each time the table is moved. An unstable massage table can flex, shift, and squeak during the massage. The movement and noises can distract clients into thinking the table might collapse, which obviously does not promote a feeling of comfort and safety.

The stability of the table is reinforced with bracing to keep the table from collapsing. There are usually wooden dowels and/or plastic-coated wire cables that attach the legs to the table top. Between the two legs at either end of the table, wooden panels or cross braces of different shapes and sizes provide additional stabilization.

Proper Table Height

You need to set your table at the proper height to use it efficiently. Most tables can be adjusted to heights between 24 and 34 inches, but special Shiatsu tables, mat tables, and Feldenkrais tables can be set as low as 17 inches. For general relaxation massage, if you are standing next to the table with your arms relaxed at your sides, the top of the table should be about even with the middle of your index finger or the middle of your thigh. This is a general guideline for setting your table height, but experience may lead you to a different, more comfortable setting (Fig. 8-5). When the table legs are set at different heights, as sometimes may happen when you adjust the height, the table undergoes mechanical stress that can damage it and is not safe for clients. In class, you can begin adjusting the height of the table with a partner, to help you reduce the stress on the table and prevent damage. Ideally, if you have to make height adjustments by yourself, you lay the table on its side, which eliminates the mechanical stress and maintains the integrity of your table. Realistically, you make adjustments carefully and make sure no one puts any weight on the table while you are changing the lengths of the legs.

Massage school tables are typically used by multiple students of different heights and are adjusted daily. It is likely you will have to adjust the table you use in class. Remember the number of holes above or below the bolts to help you adjust the height quickly, without wasting valuable class time. This system works best for tables made by the same company because they have the same pattern of holes, but it sometimes works for tables of different manufacturers.

 Make sure all four legs are adjusted to the same setting and the bolts are all secured before anyone gets on the table.

STATIONARY TABLES

Now that you have discovered the commonalities of massage tables, you can explore the different purposes and designs of stationary and portable tables.

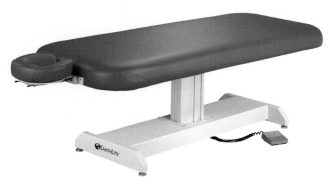

FIGURE 8-4 Electric-lift table. (Photo courtesy of EarthLite.)

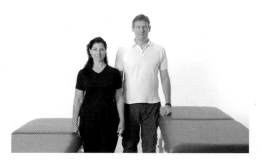

FIGURE 8-5 Proper table height.

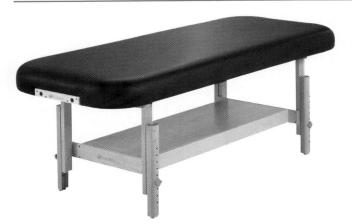

FIGURE 8-6   Stationary table. (Photo courtesy of EarthLite.)

Stationary massage tables are intended to stay in one place for long periods. They are designed and constructed as solid, stable, permanent pieces of equipment that are very sturdy and heavy (Fig. 8-6). The benefits of a stationary table are also its disadvantages, depending on the table's purpose and your needs. In a treatment room, the stationary table remains in place and everyone and everything must work around it. The permanence gives some people a sense of familiarity and comfort, but for those who need to take their table to different places, a stationary table is impractical.

PORTABLE TABLES

If you plan on taking your table to different locations such as sporting events, outcall appointments, or your home, you need a portable table. Portable massage tables are designed and built for transport with minimal trouble, so their construction is very different from the stationary ones (Fig. 8-7). They have four collapsible legs and a top that can be folded in half via a hinge that is secured to both

halves. The hinge is a structural weak spot, so a hinge that spans the width of the table provides more stability than a couple of small hinges placed along the fold. There are usually two clasps at the end of the table to keep it locked in the folded position for safe transport.

The portability of the table is relative. Even folded up, these tables are still awkward to carry around because of their size, shape, and weight. The lightest table, which is about 22 pounds, is still unwieldy. The folded table may or may not fit in the trunk or back seat of your car, so you should try to fit different-sized tables into your car before buying a table.

There are equipment accessories that make carrying your table a lot easier (Fig. 8-8). Carrying cases are available and highly recommended. They have a shoulder strap and handle that make it easier to carry the table, and their rugged fabric protects tables from bumps, scratches, and tears. Another option, which you can use with or without a carrying case, is a set of wheels. You can put your table on a luggage dolly, massage table skate, or massage table cart to roll it around instead of carrying it. Using both the carrying case and a set of wheels greatly reduces the stress and strain on your body.

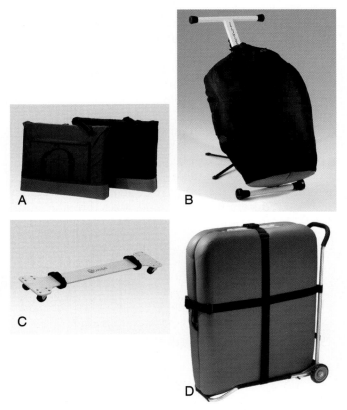

FIGURE 8-8   Massage accessories. **A.** Massage table bag. **B.** Massage chair bag. **C.** Massage table skate. **D.** Massage table cart. (Photos A–C, courtesy of EarthLite; D, courtesy of Customcraftworks.)

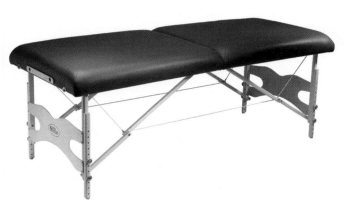

FIGURE 8-7   Portable table. (Photo courtesy of Customcraftworks.)

Setup Procedure for a Portable Massage Table

1. First, gently set the table on its edge, on the little rubber feet.
2. Unlock the clasps and open the table up slightly.
3. Flip the clasps closed to keep them from sticking out and poking someone.
4. Continue to open up the table, unfolding the legs and the top.
5. Adjust the cable system or wooden crosspieces and open the table completely while it is on its side.
6. Stand between the legs of the table, facing the center hinge.
7. Hold the handles on the side of the table (or grab the edge of the table with your hands, one hand for each half of the table top) and slowly walk backward while pulling down gently on the handles.
8. Let the legs that are closest to the ground stay in place while you tip the table to an upright position.

Portable Table Setup and Breakdown

Setting up a portable massage table is not complicated, but it does take some practice. See Procedure Box 8-1 for the portable table setup procedure. Again, if you have to stand the table up by yourself, avoid any torque or twisting motion by pulling on the handles evenly. Better yet, ask someone to help you pick up a table. Each of you can grab an end of the table with both hands, carefully rotate it until it is upright, and gently set it down.

The breakdown procedure is just the opposite of setup. Carefully place the table on its side, on the little rubber feet, fold up the legs and top, making sure the cables or dowels are stored in their appropriate places, and then lock the clasps. Check with your massage equipment manufacturer for specific directions and procedures for setting up your table, adjusting your table, and putting your table away.

Once you have practiced table setup and breakdown as well as transporting a table in and out of buildings and cars, you may find that you like it or that it is too much trouble. You may decide that you do not want a massage table of any kind or that you want to add variety to your practice with other equipment. Some equipment options include massage chairs and massage mats.

Massage Chairs

Massage chairs are designed to support fully clothed clients in a seated position, leaning forward and relaxed. They have a padded seat that tilts forward,

padded platforms for the client's shins, chest, and arms, and a padded face cradle (Fig. 8-9). Different designs and construction are available, and their weight varies accordingly. Like massage tables, the size and shape are more troublesome than the weight.

The main benefit to using a massage chair is that they can be used almost anywhere. They are portable and take up less floor space than massage tables. Since clients remain fully clothed, privacy is not an issue. As a result, you can give chair massages at public venues, health fairs, conference halls, and business offices. Chair massage is an excellent marketing and promotion tool for your business because you can demonstrate massage therapy in public, out in the open, to large numbers of people.

The primary disadvantage to massage chairs is that they limit your access to clients' bodies. You cannot use some of the basic massage strokes because clients are clothed, preventing skin-to-skin contact. Since the design of the chair holds clients in a fairly confined position, it restricts your ability to manipulate their bodies and move them around during the massage.

When clients have trouble getting into the chair, you can offer your assistance or provide an alternative. You can put a pillow or pillows on a table in front of an ordinary chair, and clients can lean forward

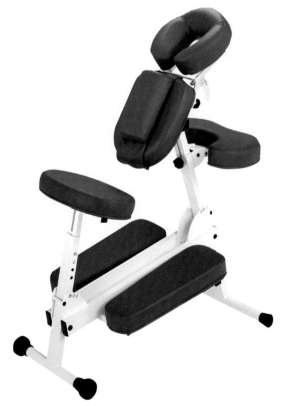

FIGURE 8-9 Massage chair. (Photo courtesy of EarthLite.)

onto the pillow and relax without being confined. This arrangement offers less support to your clients and restricts your access to their bodies even more than a massage chair, but it is an alternative you can consider if it makes your clients more comfortable.

Massage Mats

Rather than using a massage table or chair, you can also use a massage mat or shiatsu mat as your primary piece of equipment. These padded mats are placed on the floor and provide a supportive, comfortable surface for your clients to lie on. They come in a variety of prices and styles, ranging from those with organic cotton padding and coverings to those that resemble the tops of massage tables. The construction and materials of massage mats determine their ability to be rolled up or folded for storage and transport.

A variation of the massage mat is a set of specially shaped cushions called body cushions, body support systems, or body positioning cushions. By placing them on a large, flat surface such as the floor or a table, these cushion systems can be used as a lightweight alternative to massage tables that can be used in almost any home or office. They offer a less expensive alternative, but some drawbacks accompany their versatility. It may not be possible to properly disinfect the table or floor that supports the cushions, clients may find them unpleasant to lie on, and you may have difficulty accessing a client's body.

Depending on which support pieces you use, and in what combination, these cushion systems can also be used on top of a massage table for additional support and comfort. They reduce pressure on joints, tilt the pelvis forward to relax the lower back, and allow clients to keep their necks neutral (facing forward) and still breathe comfortably in the prone position.

Accessory Equipment

Accessories are available that can increase client comfort and reduce the stress and strain on your own body. Although they are not necessary, these accessories are good to have.

BOLSTERS

A bolster is a pillowlike cushion that offers additional support for client positioning. Massage equipment manufacturers sell vinyl-covered bolsters in a variety of sizes and shapes (Fig. 8-10). They are convenient because they can be easily disinfected, are durable,

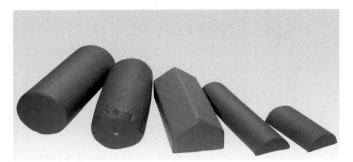

FIGURE 8-10 Bolsters. (Photo courtesy of EarthLite.)

and are slippery, making them easy to position and remove. Another option is to make your own bolsters with rolled up towels, pillows, or foam of various shapes (Fig. 8-11). Towels and pillows are more versatile, more convenient, and less expensive than retail bolsters; however, they must be laundered and disinfected after every use or have a covering that can be disinfected or removed after every use (as discussed below in this chapter).

When clients are in the side-lying position, bolsters are especially important for comfort and necessary support in the following places: under the neck and head to prevent neck strain, under the top leg that is flexed forward, under the top arm that is flexed forward, and along the client's back. Supine clients can also benefit from properly placed bolsters, including the cervical curve of the neck and the head, under the knees, and under the entire lower leg, including the knees, lower legs, and feet. In the prone position, bolsters are typically used under the ankles, under the pelvis, and under the chest, just below the sternal notch. Specific draping explanations and illustrations are included in Chapter 9, Client Positioning and Body Mechanics.

FACE CRADLES

Even though bolsters offer clients in the prone position a little extra comfort, the most awkward part of lying face down is the head placement. Generally,

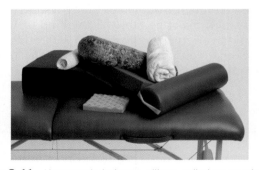

FIGURE 8-11 Homemade bolsters: pillows, rolled up towels, foam.

clients are most comfortable when the neck is in a neutral position (no neck rotation, lateral flexion, excessive extension, excessive flexion, projection, or retraction). The face cradle allows clients to keep a neutral neck and still breathe through their nose and mouth. Some clients are uncomfortable with face cradles, despite the neutral neck position. They can feel confined, have too much pressure on their sinuses, or have difficultly breathing through the hole. Most people, however, prefer using a face cradle.

Sometimes called a face rest, headrest, or head support, this horseshoe-shaped support is padded and covered like a massage table (Fig. 8-12). The covered padding is usually attached to a wooden support base with Velcro, so you can remove the padded part and use it as a neck bolster in the supine position. The Velcro also makes it possible for you to adjust the position of the padding closer to or farther from the table, essentially extending the length of your table or using it as a neck bolster, which works especially well for the side-lying position.

Fixed face cradles attach to the end of the table, and their padded surface is level with the padded table top. They eliminate neck rotation and lateral flexion, but the size or posture of your clients may force their necks into flexion, extension, projection, or retraction.

Adjustable face cradles also attach to the end of the table; however, they can be adjusted to accommodate differences in clients as well as provide greater access to the neck area. Most adjustable face cradles offer tilt adjustment that uses a pivot mechanism to raise or lower the forehead. Some adjustable face cradles also offer height adjustment that uses a telescoping mechanism to raise and lower the face cradle while keeping its surface horizontal. This is especially beneficial for persons with a large frame or a large chest. The prices vary with construction and gradually increase with additional adjustable options.

TABLE EXTENSIONS

Table extensions are not used as much as some of the other accessories, but they offer clients additional support and comfort. They are especially beneficial for clients who are tall or wide or whose arms rest in an abducted position. Table extensions such as footrests and ankle rests attach to the end of the table to increase its length. Arm shelves hang beneath the face cradle to give clients a place to rest their arms while in the prone position. Armrests attach to the sides of the table, adding extra width that allows clients to rest their arms comfortably at their sides (Fig. 8-13).

MASSAGE TOOLS

When you give several massages on a daily basis, your body will, at some point, develop aches and pains. You may want to try using some of the many tools and gadgets that can minimize the physical stress of giving a massage. These are widely available in retail stores, and many of them are marketed toward people who are not massage therapists. The professional tools are advertised in the massage trade journals and magazines and are marketed and demonstrated at various massage trade shows. The tools you might incorporate into your practice include the knoblike devices that provide localized areas of pressure.

Since standing requires more work than sitting, you can do some of your work while you sit down. Ordinary chairs are adequate, but rolling chairs or rolling stools are preferred because they let you keep

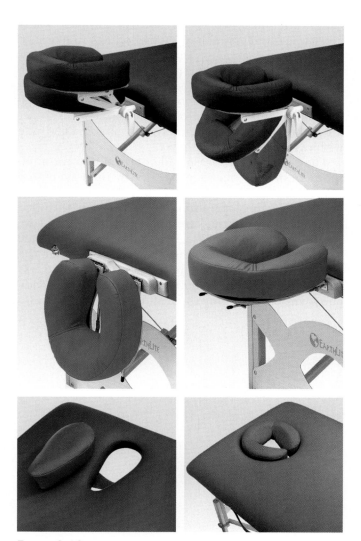

FIGURE 8-12 Face cradle assortment. (Photos courtesy of Earth-Lite.)

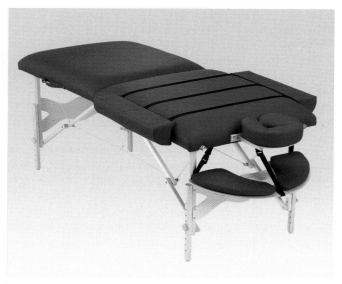

FIGURE 8-13 Table with arm shelves and arm rests. (Photo courtesy of EarthLite.)

your hands on your clients while your feet reposition the chair. Step stools are handy for clients who need help getting on and off your table (Fig. 8-14).

Instead of using your own thumb or finger to deliver the pressure, which puts undue stress on your joints, you can hold tools in the proper position in your hand and simply lean on them to deliver the pressure. There are electric massage machines that thump and vibrate, which are good for clients with very restricted tissues. Sometimes, when such clients get on the table, it can take 20 minutes or more to soften the tissues enough to work through the layers. Instead of using your own physical work to soften and warm those restricted tissues, you can use the machine to do that work. These tools can also be recommended to clients to use for self-care, as long as you remember to specify durations and frequencies for using them.

Lubricants

Lubricants are products used to reduce friction between your skin and the client's skin and increase the comfort of the massage strokes (Fig. 8-15). Most people think of lubricants as wet substances such as oils, lotions, creams, and gels; however, you can also use dry powders as massage lubricants. Experiment with a variety of products to get an idea of

- How much slip they provide
- How long they stay slippery on the skin before they dry out
- How much you need to use for the amount of slip you want
- How easily they can be dispensed during a massage
- Cost

Lubricants can be expensive, so rather than purchase different types, try to find free samples. Some lubricant suppliers market their products to massage schools and massage students by giving out trial-sized samples. These suppliers usually have online stores or phone numbers you can use to request samples. Retail stores occasionally offer samples of massage lubricants, but one of the simplest ways to get different kinds of lubricants is to share and trade with other massage therapists.

The lubricants you use will contribute to the environment of your massage practice by influencing the strokes and techniques you use. The information here is to help you familiarize yourself with lubricants. Lubricants that are slipperier deliver a very smooth and comfortable massage stroke, but they can leave the client feeling greasy or oily after the massage. On the other hand, lubricants that are less slippery allow you to manipulate the client's body parts without dropping them and use deeper pressure

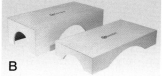

FIGURE 8-14   **A.** Rolling stool. **B.** Step stool. (Photos courtesy of EarthLite.)

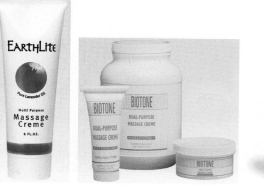
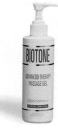

FIGURE 8-15   Lubricants. (Photos courtesy of EarthLite.)

without slipping, but clients may feel their skin getting dragged or pulled during the massage strokes. With practice, you will be able to determine just the right amount of lubricant to use with the technique you are applying.

Scented lubricants are widely available and can strongly affect the atmosphere and environment. You can create your own aromatherapy oils by adding plant and flower essences to unscented carrier oils. Guidelines to follow when using aromatherapy are discussed in more detail below in this chapter. Without being aware of it, you may be overwhelming clients with fragrances on your body, in your hair, in the air, on the carpet, in the laundry, in the bathroom, and in candles. Too many fragrances can cause the nervous system to "ignore" the sensory input and not respond to it. Basically, if you use a lot of scented products, you could actually decrease the effect of any one fragrance or essential oil by overstimulating the client's nervous system.

OILS

Oil spreads easily, and a little goes a long way. You can use oil for clients who have a lot of body hair because it is slippery and helps you slide over the body hair rather than pull it. The client is not likely to tell you when body hair is pulled during a massage, so it is up to you to use oil as your lubricant or use sufficient amounts of other lubricants. It is easy to use too much oil, and unfortunately, oil often stains sheets and clothing and is difficult to clean out of carpet.

Oils can degrade with heat, sunlight, and air, so they must be stored in a cool, dark place in an airtight container. A flip-top or pump bottle that holds just a small amount of oil is best to use in the treatment room because it allows you to store most of your oil properly and minimizes the amount of oil you can spill during a massage. Oils made from natural sources, such as fruits, vegetables, and nuts, are preferable because they are gentle on the skin and are not associated with the health risks of mineral and animal-based products. Prolonged, repeated exposure to mineral oil can irritate the skin and mucous membranes and increases the risk for cancer.[1] Additionally, lanolin is an animal-based product made with various ingredients, depending on the manufacturer. It can cause skin irritation, but more importantly, it can contain cancer-causing pesticides, making lanolin a controversial ingredient in lubricants.[2]

> *Some persons have sensitivities to nut oils, so be sure to ask the client if they have any skin allergies.*

LOTIONS, CREAMS, GELS

Lotions, creams, and gels are wet lubricants that offer an alternative to water- or oil-based products. Although laundry is not the determining factor for lubricant choice, the water-based products and water-dispersible oils are easier to wash out of sheets and clothing. Dispensing wet lubricants with pumps and flip-top bottles is an easy, one-handed operation except when you use the thicker creams. Since it is not easy to get thick lubricants out of a bottle, you can use a small disposable dish or cup that holds just enough cream for one massage. The benefit to using thick lubricants is that they cannot be spilled, which is helpful when you are learning how to do massage because you can focus on technique instead of your lubricant.

POWDERS

Dry lubricants such as cornstarch and chalk are not used very often; however, they have some benefits. Dispensing dry lubricants is tricky to do without making a cloud of dust that can irritate the client's and/or your respiratory system, but the advantages are worth considering. Powders work particularly well when you use both gliding strokes and deep compressive strokes in one massage, because they let you slide across the skin yet still apply deep pressure without slipping. Clients who need to return to work after their massage will not want to feel greasy or sticky afterward. To avoid that altogether, you can use dry lubricants.

Cornstarch is a plant product that is safe to use because it does not have any toxic effects. Chalk is available as a powder with negligible health risks, but because it is a mineral product, it can irritate the skin.[3] Talcum powder is not recommended because it is a mineral product that often contains asbestos-like structures associated with cancer risks and respiratory illness.[4]

LUBRICANT STORAGE

To protect your lubricants from contamination, there are some sanitary practices you should follow. Basically, the lubricant should be isolated so that it only comes in contact with skin when it is dispensed into your hands for immediate use on a client. Isolate your lubricant by using two different containers: a small dispenser and a larger storage container. In your treatment room, keep the lubricant in a small container that does not contact the client's skin such as a pump dispenser, flip-top bottle, or squeezable tube. The larger supply of lubricant can be kept in a big container either in or outside the treatment room, as long as it is kept at room temperature and kept out of direct sunlight. When your smaller dispenser runs low on lubricant, you can refill it from the large supply container. Oils and thin lotions can be poured directly into your dispenser with minimal risk of contamination, but you may need to transfer thicker lotions, creams, and gels with a spoon or pump mechanism. If you use a spoon or other scooplike tool, it should be disinfected before being introduced into your supply. Isolating your lubricant as much as possible minimizes the chance of it being contaminated with germs from the environment, you, or your clients. The biggest problem with contamination of your lubricant is the risk for cross-contamination, in which germs are passed from person to person via the lubricant.

APPLICATION OF LUBRICANTS

It takes practice to learn to use lubricants effectively and efficiently. First, lubricants should always be dispensed into your own hands instead of being applied directly to the client's skin. Although the recommended amount of lubricant to use varies, depending upon the type of lubricant, your school, the instructor, the area of the body receiving the lubricant, the techniques you use, and the condition of the client's skin, there are sometimes directions for use on the product label. Generally, more lubricant is used for wellness massage than for therapeutic massage because there are several therapeutic techniques that require minimal slip on the skin or require you to hold and move your client's body securely.

Since it is easier to add more lubricant than remove it, it is more practical to start out with a small amount. **Less is more when it comes to the amount of lubricant you use.** A series of steps for dispensing and applying the lubricant is outlined below. (Note: the specific directions for the left and right hands are for right-handed persons; if you are left handed, use the opposite hands as specified in the directions.)

1. Leave your left hand on the client's skin while you dispense about a penny- or nickel-sized amount of lubricant.
    a. If you are using a pump dispenser, use your right hand to push the pump once and catch the lubricant.
    b. If you are using a squirt bottle or squeezable tube, use your right hand to pick up the bottle and squirt lubricant into the palm of your left hand.
    c. If you are using an open cup or dish, use one or two fingers from your right hand to scoop out some lubricant and smear it onto your left palm.
    d. If you are using a powder, use your right hand to lift the container and carefully shake or pour a thin layer of powder into your left palm.
2. Rub your palms together to spread the lubricant evenly on both hands and warm it up a little.
3. Gently apply the lubricant to your client's skin.
4. If you feel your strokes pulling on the client's skin or body hair, you can try using more lubricant.

Lubricants are usually spread thinly and evenly in a slow, sweeping motion using both hands. The objective is to dispense enough lubricant to cover the whole area you will be immediately working on so you will not need multiple applications of lubricant to one area. The massage will flow more smoothly and you will be less distracted if you use enough lubricant on the first application.

Initial touch has a stimulating effect on the body, whereas sustained touch has a more relaxing effect. For this reason, you should minimize the number of times you break contact with the client's skin during the massage, even when you need more lubricant.

Occasionally you will find that your lubricant dispenser is out of reach when you need it. This is an awkward situation for the beginning student who wants to maintain contact but needs to retrieve the lubricant dispenser. When this happens, you have some options:

- You can break contact briefly to retrieve the dispenser.
- You can slowly "walk" your hands along the client's body to retrieve the dispenser.
- You can slowly and gently slide your contact hand along the client's body to retrieve the dispenser.

You can avoid this situation altogether by having several containers of lubricant placed in strategic places around the room or by keeping your lubricant dispenser in a holster that straps to your waist. Lubricant holsters keep you from dropping your lubricant or leaving it out of reach. Massage supply companies offer holsters for containers of different sizes and shapes. Before you buy one, try using one for a few massages, if possible. Although these holsters sound very helpful, some therapists do not like to use them.

Draping

Modesty can be defined as levels on a continuum of openness regarding personal privacy or sexual subject matter. You must protect the modesty of your clients to gain their trust and provide a comfortable, relaxing experience. Because people have different levels of modesty, all massage sessions should be performed with a professional level of modesty, as if all clients are very modest and uncomfortable about exposing their bodies. Clients can keep their clothing on during the massage, but usually they undress in private and lie on the table with a covering draped over them. **Draping** is the process of keeping clients covered with sheets, blankets, pillowcases, or towels in various combinations to keep them comfortable, warm, and secure. There are many draping techniques, but sheet draping and towel draping are most common. Both methods include a table drape, or draping that covers the table, and a face cradle cover that keeps clients from lying directly on the vinyl. With practice and working with a variety of different clients, you will develop your own techniques for draping that will coincide with the flow of your massage session.

Environment

The massage environment plays a key role in the professional presentation of the massage therapist and the comfort level of the client. As mentioned above, your equipment, lubricant, and draping are factors that contribute to the environment. Consider how your equipment influences the massage environment with its visual impact. An electric-lift table and a biohazard trash can present a clinical image suggesting a medical environment, whereas a massage mat on a carpeted floor presents a casual environment. The location of your practice will affect the environment as well. Wherever you decide to locate your practice, it must present a professional image and make the client feel comfortable and safe to receive massage. Different types of sensory input—lighting, sights, smells, sounds, draping fabrics, temperature, and décor affect the atmosphere of your practice. Sanitation and safety procedures also affect the massage environment. **Standard precautions,** which are specific procedures that maintain a hygienic and sanitary practice, reduce the risk for germ transmission. Fire codes are government regulations for fire safety at a place of business, which deal with evacuation plans, smoke detectors, fire extinguishers, and electrical cords and outlets. Clearly, your treatment room should be sanitary and safe, but so should any other space clients use: parking lot, walkway, stairs, halls, waiting area, and restroom.

Have everything ready for clients before they arrive. Adjust the table properly, have the face cradle in place or readily available, put sheets or other draping on the table, have extra towels and blankets on top of the sheets or nearby, have bolsters nearby, have your music selected and playing or make sure it is ready to be played, and gather any necessary paperwork. Being prepared for clients demonstrates your commitment to professionalism and to your clients.

LOCATION

Once you have decided to establish a business and collect income for your massage, you have to decide where you want to practice. Location is important in determining the success of any business, thus the saying "Location, location, location." The ease or difficulty with which clients can get to your place of business, in terms of distance, traffic, and parking will influence your success, as will the appearance and atmosphere of the neighborhood and surroundings. Basically, the location of your practice sets the stage for the massage environment. Consider the different scenarios of the following locations and think about how they influence the massage environment:

- Practicing in your own home
- Practicing in an office outside your home
- Traveling to your clients for outcalls
- Taking a massage chair to various public venues or corporate settings
- Working outdoors at sporting events
- Traveling with competitive teams

Setting up a practice in your own home creates an environment that is very personal and trusting. By inviting clients into your home for massage, you reveal where and how you live—our neighborhood, organization, and cleanliness. Therapists who practice massage in their own homes convey a sense of trust and openness because they allow clients into their personal space.

A massage business in someone's home feels very different from a massage practice in a hospital or at a sporting event. The atmosphere is different, and the environment affects the massage. For instance, getting a massage in a public venue will feel different from a massage you receive in your own home.

There are a number of opportunities to practice massage without an established treatment room. You can take your table to your clients at their homes, hotels, or offices for massage appointments known as **outcalls.** You can also take your massage table or chair to public venues, corporate offices, or outdoor sporting events. There are also growing opportunities to travel with competitive sports and auto racing teams and to perform veterinary massage.

TREATMENT ROOM ATMOSPHERE

Most massage therapists work in a treatment room at home or in an office building, spa, clinical setting, or fitness center. Anything clients see, hear, smell, taste, and touch influences the atmosphere of the treatment room. All of those factors, in addition to your consideration of the client's level of comfort and safety, contribute to the massage environment.

Privacy

One of the most important concerns for a treatment room should be privacy. To offer clients your focused attention, without distraction, privacy is important. Professional and ethical therapists want their clients to feel comfortable in the massage environment because comfort and relaxation can help people benefit from massage. Most importantly, clients must have privacy when they undress.

You should always step out of the treatment room when clients undress, regardless of their modesty level. Some clients start undressing while you are still in the room, but you can simply say, "I'm going to step out and wash my hands while you undress and get on the table. I'll knock before I come back in just to make sure you are situated under the covers." Usually that stops them and gives you the opportunity to leave the room, close the door behind you, and wash your hands.

If you are using a space that does not have a door, offer clients a private area where they can undress and get onto the table without being seen by others. Set up a series of fabric screens or hang some long curtains to give clients privacy. Windows in the room should have blinds or drapes that can be closed while clients are undressed and on the table. Although there are exceptions, most people do not want to be watched while they are undressing or getting a massage.

Some therapists offer clients a separate room in which to undress. This creates an awkward scenario in which clients undress in one room and need to walk, undressed, to the treatment room. You need to pay more attention to sanitation, safety, and modesty issues in this situation, but it is possible to incorporate a separate dressing room into a professional massage practice. See Procedure Box 8-2. After the massage is finished, you can use diaper draping (see Chapter 9) to cover clients modestly enough to sit up, put their socks on, and walk to the dressing room without exposing themselves.

Even though privacy is important, treatment room doors should not be locked. Not only is the locked door a fire hazard, it may threaten your client's emotional safe space. Clients should always feel empow-

PROCEDURE BOX 8-2
Instructions for Using a Separate Dressing Room

1. Show clients the treatment room, the table, and the separate dressing room.
2. Explain the draping on the table and show them how to use the draping to cover themselves after they get on the table. (See Chapter 9 for specific draping directions.)
3. Offer clients a clean robe and explain that they can go to the dressing room and
   a. Undress, leaving their socks on and removing as many undergarments as they comfortably can; usually clients remove all clothing, but there are exceptions
   b. Put on the robe
   c. Walk to the treatment room
   d. Get on the table, with the robe on, under the appropriate drape
4. After clients are back in the treatment room, knock on the door to ask if they are situated and enter the room.
5. Create a tent with the top drape by holding it up with two hands.
6. Ask clients to take the robe off while you hold the tented drape.
7. Take the robe, lower the drape, and place the robe on a nearby chair or hook.

ered to leave the treatment room of their own accord, and a locked door can take away their sense of control over the session. To keep people from walking into the treatment room during a massage, you can hang a "Please do not disturb, massage in session" sign (or something like it) from the doorknob.

Visual Input

Clients can make judgments based on anything they see, so all of the visual aspects of your practice, from the parking area to the treatment room, must be considered. The neatness, lighting, and decor of the facility all play into clients' perceptions of your practice. Your practice reflects your personality, and if clients see messy piles of papers and overflowing trash cans, they may think you are messy and question the overall cleanliness of the practice.

Ideally, the light fixtures are not directly over the massage table and the lights in your treatment room can be dimmed. During the client intake interview and during assessments, lights should be bright enough to read and fill out forms easily. During the massage, however, you want to dim the lights to help clients relax. If you cannot dim the overhead lights, use one or two lamps to provide a small amount of light. Relaxation massage and darkness cause the pupils of the eyes to dilate and let in more light. At the end of the massage, when clients are relaxed, gradually increase the amount of light in the room so as not to overwhelm the eyes with light.

Décor and furnishings create the scenery for your massage and let you express your personality. You can and should prominently display your diplomas, certifications, license (if applicable or required by law), and continuing education certificates. This helps assure the client that you are an appropriately credentialed, professional, legitimate massage therapist. Muscle and skeletal charts can be hung on the walls as sources for reference and client education. Since color can influence the atmosphere, pay attention to the colors in your treatment room: the floor, walls, your curtains or blinds, and your linens. Decorate the walls with things that you like to look at and that help you relax and focus, because you will be looking at the walls more than anyone else. Depending upon the quality, some white and very light-colored linens can be transparent, so patterns and darker solid colors may be more appropriate for draping purposes. Generally, all linens are suitable as long as they are not transparent and the client's modesty is protected.

The size of your treatment room will determine how much furniture you need. Minimally, you need a massage table and something for clients to put their clothes on, such as a chair or a hook. Better yet, you can include

- A table or desk
- A rolling stool for yourself
- A step stool to help clients on and off the table
- A clock
- A radio or sound system
- A trash can
- A box of Kleenex
- A bookshelf with some good references and self-help resource books

Since cleanliness is part of the atmosphere, make sure your décor and furniture are in good repair and are kept clean.

Auditory Input

Think about the sounds of dogs barking, babies crying, traffic, nearby conversation, a nearby television, a washing machine, clothes tumbling in the dryer, trains rushing by, kids playing, and birds singing. Depending on the person, any one of these sounds could promote relaxation or create stress, so try to minimize background noises. If some noise is unavoidable, use a small fan or white noise machine to reduce the noise. Most therapists use music in their massage sessions, which promotes relaxation and guides your timing for the session.

The physical properties of sound can be applied to human anatomy and physiology, resulting in some fascinating healing properties of music. The electrical activity of the brain can be measured objectively with an electroencephalogram (EEG) and displayed on a chart as a wave pattern. Different forms of brain activity are associated with different frequencies of electrical activity, or brain waves:

- Beta (BAY-tuh) waves, 14–20 hertz, are the highest-frequency brain waves, which occur while people are awake and thinking and when they are experiencing strong negative emotions
- Alpha (AL-fuh) waves, 8–13 hertz, occur while people are in states of calm and heightened awareness
- Theta (THAY-tuh) waves, 4–7 hertz, occur while people are very creative, are meditating, and are sleeping
- Delta (DEHL-tuh) waves, 0.5–3 hertz, are the slowest-frequency brain waves and occur during deep sleep, deep meditation, and unconsciousness

Music with a pulse, or tempo, of about 60 beats per minute can cause brain waves to shift from beta waves to alpha waves. In other words, you can use music with a tempo of 60 beats per minute to help people relax or to ease them from a distracted mindset to a calm and clear-thinking mindset. Entrainment is the process by which specific kinds of music can encourage a change in the brain wave frequencies. For example[5]:

- Shamanic drumming can encourage theta waves.
- Mozart or baroque music can shift an unfocused mood to one more aware and calmer.
- Romantic, jazz, or New Age music can help an analytical mindset be more adaptable, flexible, or emotional.
- Fast, loud music can encourage beta waves and cause someone to lose concentration and make mistakes.
- Music with a slow tempo or long, slow tones can slow down brain waves and help someone calm down.

Music and sounds can affect our brain wave activity, heartbeat, breathing rate, and blood pressure. Paying attention to your clients' verbal and nonverbal messages can help you recognize if the music is encouraging relaxation or inducing stress. You can ask clients to choose the music or bring their own, but most clients want some kind of gentle, quiet music. If possible, collect a lot of music of different kinds, including instrumental, piano, vocals, chants, synthesized, and nature sounds. The sounds of a babbling brook are usually soothing sounds of nature, but some people respond to the sound of running water with an urge to go to the bathroom; be aware whether the sounds of running water are in your massage music or from a nearby decorative fountain.

Olfactory Input

Olfactory input, or smells, can strongly affect a person's response to the environment. Smells are powerful memory triggers, and emotions can accompany those memories. Be aware of smells in or around your massage room that could offend clients: cooking smells, household chemicals, garbage odors, pet odors, cigarette smoke, cigar smoke, body odor, or breath odor. Scented products that you find pleasant may be offensive to others. Some clients may even be sensitive or allergic to your scented fabric softeners and detergents. To avoid a negative reaction to scents or odors, include a question on your intake form about sensitivities or allergies.

Practicing daily personal hygiene for your hair, teeth, and body will help you manage your body and breath odor. Before you use scented products to hide any body or breath odor, try using products that absorb or neutralize odors. Again, too many smells can overwhelm the client's nervous system and desensitize it, which could reduce the effects of any aromatherapy products you use.

True aromatherapy uses essential oils from flowers and plants to induce different physiological responses. Essential oils are frequently added to lubricants to make them more pleasant and therapeutic. Lavender and chamomile essences are especially popular and generally safe to use, but not for everyone.

 Ask clients about sensitivities and allergies before using any product.

Tactile Sensations

Tactile sensations are things you physically feel with the sensory receptors in your skin. Anything that clients physically touch and feel is a factor of the massage environment. Pay attention to all surfaces clients touch, including the feel of the sheets, your skin and fingernails, temperature and humidity of the room, and even the amount of fresh air or breeze.

The primary consideration for tactile input is the fabric of your linens because most of the client's skin touches the draping. Material components and

thread count, which are usually listed on the outside of the packaging, pertain to the quality of the sheets. All cotton sheets tend to be softer than polyester and cotton blends. Flannel and jersey sheets feel especially soft and comfortable, but they may stick together during the massage and complicate the draping process. Thread counts refer to the density of the threads in the fabric: 200 or more is usually considered a high thread count, and 180-count is considered low. High-thread-count sheets feel silkier, they help clients feel substantially covered, and they hold up to repeated laundering better than lower- thread-count sheets. The lower-thread-count sheets sometimes have a gauzelike quality that can make them transparent and feel thin and insubstantial to clients. Since draping is used to keep clients covered and comfortable and protect their modesty, you do not want see-through sheets.

Clients also feel the condition and temperature of your skin and hands. Make sure your skin and hands are soft, smooth, and clean, and that your nails are in good condition and kept short and smooth. Looking at your palm, your fingernails should be trimmed and filed so that you cannot see them extending beyond your fingertips, and there are no sharp or "pokey" edges.

Wash and dry your hands while clients are getting undressed and on the table. (Proper hand hygiene practices are discussed below in this chapter.) After you dry your hands, the residual moisture on your hands quickly evaporates and cools your hands off. Initial touch with cold hands can be uncomfortable and startling, activating the sympathetic nervous system's fight or flight response. Before you initiate touch with cold hands, let your clients know that your hands are cold and reassure them that your hands will warm up very quickly during the massage. Conscious preparation for your cold hands can reduce the shock and the sympathetic nervous response and help a client relax sooner. Although the initial touch has a stimulating effect, your sustained touch soon stops that response and allows clients to relax. Initial touch with warm hands allows much faster relaxation. You can warm your hands with friction by briskly rubbing them together just before you initiate touch.

The room should be kept between 72 and 74°F, with moderate humidity. Although the temperature may feel too warm to you, it is comfortable for most clients during a massage. During the massage, clients are typically undressed and covered by a single sheet, and as they relax, the parasympathetic nervous response reduces their heart rate, breathing rate, and blood pressure. Consequently, they can easily feel cold and uncomfortable, which hinders relaxation. Heating pads can be placed on the massage table, underneath the draping, to provide a source of warmth to keep clients comfortable. When the humidity, or the amount of water vapor in the air, is low, it can dry out mucous membranes and skin. A humidifier or decorative water fountain can add moisture to the air, but make sure to keep it clean and sanitary to avoid transmission of pathogens. Pathogen transmission is covered in detail below in this chapter. High humidity can make the air feel oppressive and difficult to breathe; a dehumidifier or air conditioner can lower the humidity. Generally, fresh air is better than stagnant, recirculated air unless there are high levels of pollution and allergens outside. Stagnant air can make a room feel stuffy and oppressive. An open window or fan can move the air around, but a breeze that feels good to you may cause clients to feel cold. If you still want to feel a breeze, make sure you have extra blankets or covers to offer clients. For the most part, you want the air in your treatment room to feel comfortable and warm.

Hygiene, Sanitation, and Safety

A successful therapist understands and practices good personal hygiene, standard precautions, sanitation procedures, and fire codes. A clean and safe practice minimizes the risk of getting sick and getting hurt, both for you and your clients. Thus, this section focuses on understanding the methods necessary for preventing disease transmission, minimizing the risks for allergic responses, and preparing for a fire emergency. Some of the massage laws and regulations (accessible through www.careeratyourfingertips.com) include guidelines for sanitation and safety, but national regulations for massage have yet to be standardized.

Your client-centered focus demands that you do everything you can to keep your clients healthy. Instead of blindly following the guidelines for sanitation and safety, you need to know about diseases and how they are transmitted before understanding how to prevent the spread of diseases.

DISEASE

Diseases are abnormal conditions of the appearance, structure, or function of an organism or its parts. They can be separated into two categories: noninfectious and infectious.

Noninfectious Disease

Noninfectious diseases are caused by internal and external factors that cannot be transmitted with any kind of contact. Noninfectious diseases can be generally separated into the following nonexclusive categories:

- Cancer—cells replicate and grow at abnormally high rates and cause symptoms (examples: breast cancer, leukemia, skin cancer)
- Degenerative—part of the organism is deteriorating and causing symptoms (examples: Alzheimer's disease, multiple sclerosis, osteoarthritis, osteoporosis, and autoimmune diseases such as AIDS and lupus erythematosus)
- Environmental—chemicals, particles and, radiation from the environment cause symptoms (examples: lead poisoning, asbestosis, allergies)
- Genetic—the genetic coding in the DNA is abnormal and causing symptoms (examples: Down syndrome, cystic fibrosis, hemophilia)
- Metabolic—the cells or tissues function abnormally and cause symptoms (examples: cardiovascular disease, diabetes, hypoglycemia)
- Neurologic–Psychiatric—a complex interaction of brain chemicals and psychological disorders cause symptoms (examples: addiction, depression, seasonal affective disorder)
- Nutritional—deficiency of nutrients acquired through the diet causes symptoms (examples: iron deficiency anemia, scurvy)

For the most part, massage therapists cannot protect clients from noninfectious diseases. However, massage therapists can help clients manage diseases, and especially the ones with environmental or nutritional causes. Take special precautions for the many people who have environmental sensitivities and allergies to chemicals, pets, pollen, and materials. Inquire about clients' allergies and sensitivities and make sure that the offending allergens or products are not present in your practice. Some allergies are life threatening, and if you know that clients are allergic to something in your practice, you have a responsibility to share that information with them and offer them a referral to another qualified therapist. Sensitivities are not as critical as allergies, but you should still make clients aware of anything in your practice that could trigger an immune reaction. Let those clients decide whether they want to continue with treatment or accept a referral to another therapist. Specific nutritional recommendations are not within your scope of practice, but you can educate clients about nutritional deficiencies and refer them to the appropriate healthcare practitioner.

Infectious Disease

Infectious diseases are more critical to understand because they can be transmitted by contact with germs. A germ is a common term for a **pathogen,** or pathogenic microorganism, which is a microscopic organism that can cause disease in other organisms. There are thousands of different kinds of microorganisms, which come in the forms of algae, bacteria, fungi, protozoa, and viruses, but only a small percentage of them are pathogens. In fact, there are normally millions of microorganisms in and on our bodies that are nonpathogenic and beneficial to us. For a pathogen to be transmitted, it must be acquired by an organism in one of three ways:

- Contact transmission
  - Direct contact—a host organism physically transfers a pathogen to another person via touching, kissing, or sexual intercourse
  - Indirect contact—a host organism leaves a pathogen on a fomite, or inanimate object such as a doorknob, table, or chair, and the pathogen is transferred to someone else who touches that fomite
  - Droplets—a host organism forcefully expels mucus by spitting, sneezing, or coughing on another person, and a pathogen in the mucus is transferred to another person
- Vehicle transmission
  - Air—pathogens are either suspended in a mist of very fine mucous droplets or have become airborne as a result of evaporation of a mucous droplet, and they are transferred to someone who contacts them in the air
  - Food—pathogens residing in food are transferred to persons who eat the contaminated food
  - Liquid—pathogens residing in water or other liquids are transferred to persons who drink the contaminated liquid
- Vector transmission
  - Mosquitoes
  - Flies
  - Rats

Healthy immune systems normally inactivate or destroy acquired pathogens, but when the immune system does not do its job, pathogens can establish themselves, multiply, and cause disease in the host organism. You cannot know how effective your clients' immune systems are or who might be carrying pathogens. **Do your best to keep everyone healthy with isolation procedures that prevent any existing pathogens from being transmitted.**

PREVENTING TRANSMISSION OF PATHOGENS

There is a good chance that you will not know if you or your clients are harboring harmful pathogens. Assume that pathogens are present and use the appro-

priate procedures to keep them from being transmitted via direct contact, indirect contact, and vehicles such as air, food, and liquids. In 1987, the Centers for Disease Control and Prevention (CDC) designed a set of universal precautions to prevent the spread of blood-borne pathogens such as human immunodeficiency virus (HIV) and hepatitis B. The CDC updated its infection control protocols in 1996 and designed a set of standard precautions to prevent the spread of pathogens that reside in *all* body secretions—blood, semen, vaginal secretions, tears, saliva, nasal secretions, urine, feces, and vomit. Standard precautions include

- Proper hand hygiene
- Barrier techniques
- Proper cleaning and sanitizing procedures
- Proper disposal techniques

In addition to the standard precautions that are intended to prevent pathogen transmission by direct contact, by indirect contact, and through the air, you will also need to use some common sense to keep your clients safe from germs. If you know you are infected with a pathogen such as the influenza virus (the flu) or streptococcus bacteria (strep throat), inform your clients and either postpone their appointments for a week or refer them to someone else. Avoid offering clients food or drinks that are not individually wrapped and sealed or that are not dispensed from sterile containers. For instance, homemade baked goods or a cup of hot tea may seem like a nice treat to offer clients, but you cannot be sure that they do not contain harmful pathogens that could cause illness. It is acceptable to offer individually wrapped mints, sports snacks, or granola bars. You can safely offer clean, disposable cups and water from a cooler that holds 5-gallon bottles that are sealed when you purchase them. Knowing the mechanisms for pathogen transmission can help you minimize the pathogenic risks to your clients.

Hand Hygiene

The CDC has shown that when hand hygiene procedures are followed, the spread of pathogens is reduced. Keep your fingernails short, as discussed above in this chapter, and avoid wearing artificial fingernails. The CDC makes no specific recommendations regarding jewelry, but because it can scratch or be uncomfortable to clients during a massage stroke and lubricant can accumulate in the jewelry and harbor pathogens, you should consider removing jewelry from your hands during massage. Make sure your hands are kept moisturized with lotions or creams to prevent them from cracking and increasing the risk of pathogen transmission. Above all, wash your hands properly.

The CDC has determined that handwashing is the single most important procedure for the prevention of infection. Thoroughly wash your hands immediately before and immediately after massaging your clients, immediately after contacting any bodily fluids, and immediately after taking off protective gloves. You can use traditional soap and water, antimicrobial soap and water, or alcohol-based hand rubs. It is safer to use pump dispensers for soap because, surprisingly, soap can harbor some pathogens. The following are the steps to proper handwashing, according to the CDC:

1. Wet your hands and apply liquid soap or clean bar soap. If you use bar soap, replace it on a rack that allows it to drain and dry.
2. Rub your hands vigorously together, scrubbing all surfaces, for about 15 seconds.
3. Rinse well with water and dry your hands thoroughly with a disposable towel.
4. Use the towel to turn off the faucet.
5. Dispose of the used towel in a trash receptacle.

In addition to washing with soap and water, the CDC has determined that healthcare workers can also use alcohol-based hand rubs as a suitable alternative. They significantly reduce the pathogens on your skin very quickly, and they are not as likely to cause skin irritation with repeated use. Before and after massaging each client, you can apply the alcohol-based hand rub (as directed on the product) to the palm of your hand, rub your hands together to cover all of your hands and fingers, and continue rubbing until your hands are dry. Antimicrobial disposable wipes are not as effective as handwashing or alcohol-based rubs and should not be used in their place.

Barrier Techniques

On the rare occasions when clients leave bodily fluids on your massage table or anywhere else in your practice, you need to know how to safely use barrier techniques. There are a number of protective physical barriers such as latex gloves, gowns, aprons, masks, or protective eyewear that can reduce the risk of acquiring pathogens on your skin or mucous membranes any time you contact blood or bodily fluids.

Wear latex gloves if you have to touch any bodily fluids except sweat, any surfaces that have bodily fluids on them, your clients' mucous membranes, and clients' skin that is not intact (has a cut or open wound). Remove gloves and properly disposed of them after contact with each patient or contaminated surface. You could accidentally be contaminated by small defects in the gloves or while you are removing the gloves, so you *must* wash your hands and other exposed skin surfaces immediately after removing the gloves. The use of gloves does not eliminate the need for hand hygiene, and the use of hand hygiene does not eliminate the need for gloves.

It is difficult to work with gloves on. They reduce the sensitivity of your hands, and many persons are allergic to latex. If you or your clients have latex sensitivities or latex allergies, there are substitutes you can use. Vinyl gloves are similar in cost to latex, but because they are not as durable, avoid wearing them for longer than 30 minutes. Gloves made of nitrile, neoprene, and thermoplastic elastomers are suitable alternatives whose durability and strength equal or exceed those of latex, but they are more expensive.

Cleaning and Sanitizing Procedures

Keep your massage room and office or home space clean, clear of debris, pests, trash, spills, or any other potential hazards. Decorative fountains are relaxing, popular accents to many massage practices, but they are potential reservoirs for microorganisms. If you use one, keep it out of the treatment room and disinfect it on a regular basis. Fish tanks are also good for creating a calming atmosphere, but they need regular maintenance, and keep them out of the treatment room. Clean and disinfect toilets, sinks, and other surfaces that are touched frequently: doorknobs, light switches, faucet handles, water dispenser handles, chairs, and desktops. The surfaces that need to be cleaned when they appear dusty or dirty include the walls, blinds, and window treatments.

Cleaning your equipment is critical.

> ⚠ *The massage table, face cradle, vinyl-covered bolsters, table extensions, and linens must be properly disinfected after every client.*

Even if you use disposable linens and face cradle covers, your equipment needs to be disinfected after every use. Antimicrobial and antibacterial products are not strong enough to eliminate most pathogens, so make sure the solution you purchase is labeled a disinfectant. Sodium hypochlorite is an EPA-approved disinfectant and is commonly available as household bleach (which is usually 5.25% sodium hypochlorite). You can mix household bleach and water in different concentrations, depending on the strength disinfectant you need. Household bleach is the least expensive, most readily available solution with which to make an appropriate disinfectant. The disadvantages to using bleach are that it degrades quickly, and it is a harsh, caustic, corrosive chemical. Bleach solutions must be mixed daily to guarantee their ability to disinfect, and the solutions must be mixed carefully in a ventilated room. Lysol spray is a phenolic disinfectant that is readily available, easy to use, and EPA-approved, but aerosol products are discouraged by the CDC.

The surfaces that need disinfection and the pathogens that need to be eliminated determine the steps required to prevent pathogen transmission. There are three generally recognized levels of infection control: high-level, intermediate-level, and low-level. Below is a list of the infection control levels and appropriate disinfection procedures you can use:

- **High-level** exposures include spills of bodily fluids.
    1. Put on latex gloves.
    2. Absorb the spill with disposable towels.
    3. Apply disinfectant to the area and let it sit for 20 minutes—sodium hypochlorite (household bleach) diluted 1:50, or about 2 tablespoons per quart of water (this is a strong and corrosive mixture, so be careful with it).
    4. Absorb the disinfectant solution with disposable towels.
    5. Dispose of all articles with bodily fluids and used disinfectant, including gloves, in plastic bags, and seal the bags.
    6. Wash hands.
    7. Allow the area to dry completely.
- **Intermediate-level** exposures include smooth, hard surfaces that come in contact with mucous membranes or broken skin.
    1. Apply enough disinfectant (identified as EPA-approved tuberculocides) to wet the entire surface and let it sit on the surface for about 10 minutes:
        a. 70–90% ethyl alcohol or isopropyl alcohol
        b. phenolic disinfectant (Lysol), per label instructions
        c. sodium hypochlorite (household bleach) diluted 1:50, or about 2 tablespoons per quart of water (this is a strong and corrosive mixture, so be careful with it).
    2. Absorb the disinfectant solution with disposable towels.
    3. Dispose of towels in trash receptacle.
    4. Wash hands.
- **Low-level** exposures include smooth, hard surfaces touched by intact skin.
    1. Apply enough disinfectant (labeled as EPA-approved hospital disinfectants) to wet the entire surface and let it sit on the surface for about 10 minutes:
        a. 70–90% ethyl alcohol or isopropyl alcohol
        b. phenolic disinfectant (Lysol), per label instructions

    c. sodium hypochlorite (household bleach) diluted 1:500, or about 2 teaspoons per gallon of water
    2. Absorb the disinfectant solution with disposable towels.
    3. Dispose of used towels in trash receptacle.

Laundry

The CDC has found that although soiled linens are a source of pathogens, there is negligible risk of transmission. It recommends hygienic and common sense processing and storage of linens. All of your linens, including your sheets, towels, pillowcases, and blankets require infection control and need to be laundered after every use. Soiled sheets should be handled as little as possible and stored in a closed receptacle such as a hamper. Unless there are bodily fluids on the linens, they can be laundered in hot water at 160°F for 25 minutes with regular detergent or at a lower temperature with a disinfectant such as bleach. Dry your linens completely in a dryer instead of outside in fresh air.

If your linens are contaminated with bodily fluids, you need to handle them carefully. Wear gloves, carefully place contaminated linens in plastic bags, seal the bags, and label the bags as contaminated laundry. Use ¾ cup of household bleach per wash load of contaminated laundry, and dry your linens completely in a dryer.

Clean sheets should be stored in a way that ensures and maintains their cleanliness. Keep them off the floor, away from food or drinks, and apart from used linens. For more detailed procedures and updates on sanitation and standard precautions, you can refer to the CDC at www.cdc.org or the American Red Cross at www.redcross.org.

SAFETY

The safety of your practice depends on sanitation as well as regular maintenance of all aspects of the business—parking lot, walkways, stairways, doors, windows, floors, furniture, electricity, and fire safety. In addition to current certification in First Aid and CPR, you need a first aid kit on the premises. Insurance coverage (discussed in the chapter on massage therapy business concepts) protects you against the legal and financial ramifications for any injuries clients sustain on your premises.

Fire safety is an important aspect of your practice. Check with your local fire department for specifics that detail the use of

- Candles
- Smoke detectors—placement and regular testing

- Evacuation plans
- Fire drills
- Fire extinguishers—instructions, approved types, inspections
- Electricity—fixtures, outlets
- Stairways, walkways, doors, locks
- Fire hazards

Chapter Summary

The equipment and environment of your massage practice are important considerations before you treat your first client. Spend some time looking over the endless equipment options to make sure you are comfortable adjusting and transporting equipment before you purchase it. Your school may recommend a specific type of lubricant or draping fabric, but you can still sample different lubricants and try different draping methods outside the school. The massage environment you create is more than just your personal approach to massage and the decorations in your treatment room. The location, privacy, sights, smells, and sounds of your treatment room, as well as the safety of the premises are all factors of the massage environment. To maintain a client-centered focus, you must pay attention to preparedness, sanitation, and safety.

 CHAPTER EXERCISES

1. Write a description of the locations of at least five different massage practices you have seen or visited. Compare and contrast the locations and your perception of the massage environment.

2. Write a description of your ideal massage treatment room, including the location, all of the equipment, and environment factors.

3. Massage equipment manufacturers typically offer equipment packages that include an adjustable massage table and some accessories such as a bolster and/or carrying case. Research the massage equipment packages offered by at least four different companies and write down the similarities and differences between them.

4. List at least five different aspects of fire safety.

5. List at least five different categories of noninfectious disease.

6. Describe each of the three different levels of infection control.

7. What temperature and wash cycle length are required for proper disinfection of your linens after every massage?

8. How much household bleach should you add to a wash cycle of laundry that has been contaminated with bodily fluids?

9. Describe the five steps of proper handwashing as outlined by the CDC.

10. Identify the four concepts of standard precautions you need to follow.

REFERENCES

1. http://www.osha-slc.gov/SLTC/healthguidelines/oilmist/recognition.html, U.S. Department of Labor web site, Occupational Safety and Health Guideline for Oil Mist/Mineral Oil, accessed 3/11/03.
2. http://www.preventcancer.com/articles/right.htm, accessed 8.24.03.
3. http://www.nlm.nih.gov/medlineplus/ency/article/002771.htm, Medline Plus Health Information web site, "Chalk," accessed 3/11/03.
4. http://www.nlm.nih.gov/medlineplus/ency/article/002719.htm, Medline Plus Health Information web site, "Talcum Powder," accessed 3/11/03.
5. Campbell D. The Mozart Effect. New York: Avon Books, 1997.

SUGGESTED READINGS

Boyce-Tillman J. Constructing Musical Healing. Philadelphia: Jessica Kingsley, 2000.
Brown J. Don't Touch That Doorknob!: How Germs Can Zap You and How You Can Zap Back. New York: Warner Books, 2001.
Campbell D. The Mozart Effect. New York: Avon Books, 1997.
Jackson R. Holistic Massage, The Holistic Way to Physical and Mental Health. New York: Sterling Publishing, 1987.
Pagliarulo, Michael A, PT. Introduction to Physical Therapy. 2nd ed. St. Louis: Mosby, 2001.
Ruud E. Music Therapy: Improvisation, Communication and Culture. Gilsum, NH: Barcelona Publishers, 1998.
Werner R. A Massage Therapist's Guide to Pathology. Baltimore: Lippincott Williams & Wilkins, 1998.
http://encarta.msn.com 1997–2003 Microsoft Corporation, "Human Disease," Microsoft Encarta Online Encyclopedia, 2003, accessed 8.20.03.
http://seattlepi.nwsource.com/national/cra30.shtml, accessed 3.11.03.
http://web-ukonline.co.uk/webwise/spinneret/edexcel/spcodi.htm, accessed 8.20.03.
http://www.apic.org/pdf/brdisin.pdf, accessed 8.30.03.
http://www.biotone.com, accessed 8.30.03.
http://www.britannica.com/eb/article?eu=119800, accessed 3.12.03.
http://www.cdc.gov/mmwr/preview/mmwrhtml/rr5116a1.htm, accessed 8.23.03.
http://www.cdc.gov/ncidod/hip/Blood/UNIVERSA.HTM, accessed 8.23.03.
http://www.cdc.gov/ncidod/hip/sterile/laundry.htm, accessed 8.29.03.
http://www.cdc.gov/ncidod/hip/sterile/sterilgp.htm, accessed 8.29.03.
http://www.cdc.gov/ncidod/op/handwashing.htm, accessed 8.29.03.
http://www.cdc.gov/niosh/hcwold5.html, accessed 8.29.03.
http://www.cdc.gov/od/oc/media/pressrel/fs021025.htm, accessed 8.29.03.

http://www.cinetwork.com/otero/cdc.html, accessed 8.29.03.

http://www.clorox/laundry.com/laund_qa_laundry.shtml#amount, accessed 8.30.03.

http://www.customcraftworks.com, accessed 8.30.03.

http://www.epa.gov/oppad001/list_b_tuberculocide.pdf, accessed 8.30.03.

http://www.earthlite.com, accessed 8.30.03.

http://www.factmonster.com, accessed 8.23.03.

http://www.geologyshop.co.uk/chalk.htm, accessed 3/11/03.

http://www.mansfield.ohio-state.edu/~sabedon/biol2050.htm, accessed 8.23.03.

http://www.nlm.nih.gov/medlineplus/ency/article/002719.htm, accessed 3/11/03.

http://www.nlm.nih.gov/medlineplus/ency/article/002771.htm, accessed 3/11/03.

http://www.nohsc.gov.au/OHSInformation/Databases/Exposure-Standards/az/Oil_mist_refined_mineral.htm, accessed 3/11/03.

http://www.nursingworld.org/AJN/2000/aug/Health.htm, accessed 8.30.03.

http://www.osha-slc.gov/SLTC/healthguidelines/oilmist/recognition.html, accessed 3.11.03.

http://www.preventcancer.com/alerts/talc.htm, accessed 3/11/03.

http://www.redcross.org/services/hss/tips/universal.html, accessed 8.29.03.

http://www.wdghu.org/topics/cd/cd_precautions.htm, accessed 8.30.03.

9

Client Positioning and Body Mechanics

UPON COMPLETION OF THIS CHAPTER, THE STUDENT WILL BE ABLE TO:

- Name the three client positions on the massage table
- Identify at least two places to bolster clients in each of the client positions
- Name the two primary reasons for draping clients during a massage
- Demonstrate draping techniques to expose at least three different areas of a partner's body on the massage table
- Name the two primary components of good body mechanics
- List at least three reasons to lean instead of push into clients
- Demonstrate the asymmetric stance while leaning into a partner on the massage table
- List at least five ways to minimize your risk for injury

KEY TERMS

Asymmetric stance (also called archer, bow, and lunge stance): standing position in which both feet are on the ground, shoulder-width apart, one foot is in front of the other, and the back foot is laterally rotated

Body mechanics: the careful, efficient use of your body by incorporating the principles of leverage and structural alignment to prevent injury and reduce fatigue

Laterally recumbent (also called side-lying): lying on one's side

Leverage: the mechanical use of your body as a rigid structure that can apply a lot of pressure without doing a lot of muscular work

Repetitive stress injury (RSI): an injury that occurs when a particular body movement is repeated often enough to damage the structures involved in the movement

Symmetric stance (also called the horse stance and warrior stance): standing position in which both feet are placed as if the toes are on a line, pointing forward, shoulder-width apart

The main considerations when performing massage are comfort and safety for both you and your clients. To relax, clients must feel safe, secure, and comfortable. Before clients get on your massage table, you must be familiar with the different body positions clients can use, different ways to drape their bodies to keep them warm and modestly covered, and the different ways to position and support them throughout the massage, using various bolsters. Appropriate client positioning, proper bolstering, and secure draping, which must all be considered before and during the session, are the topics discussed in this chapter.

Additionally, your own body should remain relaxed and comfortable to deliver massage techniques efficiently and effectively without injuring yourself. You can achieve this by learning the basic concepts of body mechanics and applying them as you learn how to practice massage. As you learn and practice your strokes and techniques, monitor your body to make sure that you establish nerve tracks that include good body movement habits. If you learn how to perform strokes carefully and efficiently in the first place, good body mechanics will become second nature, minimizing your fatigue and preventing work-related pain and injuries.

Client Positioning

Clients can lie on the massage table in three different positions to receive massage: prone (face down), supine (face up), or laterally recumbent (side-lying). Seated massage, an alternative to table massage, is covered below in Chapter 13, Special Techniques. Most therapists get in the habit of starting clients in the prone or supine position, but you must maintain a client-centered focus and modify your preferences and tendencies to fit your clients' needs and wants. Some clients determine their own positioning for the massage, asking to turn supine before you are ready for them to turn over or asking to remain in a side-lying (laterally recumbent) position for the duration of the session. Unless there are contraindications associated with the client's requests, it is appropriate to follow the client's lead.

You can make clients more comfortable during the massage by using bolsters and table extensions. These cushions, pillows, and platforms fit under and around clients' bodies for extra support and padding. Bolstering is intended to help clients' bodies relax with the natural curves of their bodies supported, but not all clients like to be bolstered. Position a bolster for support and ask if the client is more comfortable with the bolster in place. If not, remove the bolster. You can use pillows and vinyl-covered retail bolsters as shown in Chapter 8, Equipment and Environment, or you can fashion your own bolsters out of rolled or folded towels and blankets. Remember to properly disinfect bolsters after every use or place them inside a covering that can be removed and properly disinfected after every use. As an added layer of protection, you can slide bolsters underneath the sheet that covers the table. Proper sanitation and hygiene are as important to your practice as your massage.

Several factors govern how you position clients on the massage table, including their preferences, physical condition, and treatment goals and your preferred strokes, techniques, and flow. Flow, covered in more detail below in Chapter 10, is a routine-like sequence of steps that leads the massage from one body part to the next in a systematic, fluid pattern. A flow often includes directions for specific stroke sequences and techniques to use.

SUPINE POSITION

Supine is the term that describes someone lying on the back, or spine, face up. When clients are in the supine position, you have direct access to the anterior surface of their body, and you can incorporate a number of joint movements into the massage. A small bolster under the curve of the neck and a larger bolster under the client's knees support the spine in a more natural position (Fig. 9-1). There is a bolster that is specially shaped to elevate the lower legs, ankles, and feet that you can offer as an alternative. This position is preferred by clients who like to talk, who do not like confined spaces, whose heads are congested, or who are uneasy and nervous about being on the table.

For example, clients who come to the session with a lot of stress may be particularly interested in talking about the stress in their lives. Starting the massage in the supine position allows them to talk freely and use eye contact while speaking. It is easy to get swept into conversation when clients share their experiences and emotions, but your job is to treat the soft tissues, not the emotions. Listen to clients more than you talk, and stay focused on the soft tissues.

Clients with allergy and cold-related upper respiratory congestion may prefer being supine for the duration of the massage because lying in the prone position can aggravate congestion. Massage promotes the release of histamines, which are fluids the body secretes to flush out allergens and foreign particles. Making matters worse, gravity encourages extra fluids to drain into the sinuses, and pressure on the face from the face cradle restricts circulation altogether. In the supine position, gravity enhances the flow of deoxygenated blood and lymph out of the sinuses to reduce sinus congestion.

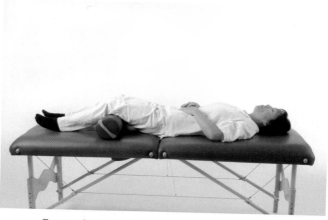

FIGURE 9-1   Supine with neck and knee bolsters.

Along with the advantages of the supine position, there are some considerations keep in mind. Ceiling light fixtures, directly over the massage table, can be bothersome to clients who are supine. Turn them off and use floor and table lamps, or dim the overhead lights, if possible. Aside from the massage environment's impact on clients who are supine, some physiological conditions influence client positioning. Just as the prone position aggravates a congested head, the supine position aggravates a congested chest. You can adapt the supine position to clients with chest congestion by using bolsters to elevate their head and shoulders. The supine position is contraindicated for women who are in their last few months of pregnancy, because the weight of the fetus can compress the aorta and cut off the mother's circulation. The side-lying position is the least dangerous to the mother and fetus, but some women find it uncomfortable. You can bolster these women in a semireclining position to let them relax comfortably and enjoy massage.

PRONE POSITION

Prone is the term that describes clients who are lying face down on the massage table. You have unrestricted access to clients' backs and gluteal areas when they are in the prone position, and you can incorporate many joint movements into the massage. Additional comfort is provided by a face cradle and bolsters. The face cradle allows the client's neck to remain neutral during the massage. Without the face cradle or a face hole in the table, clients can fold their arms on the table and rest the chin on the arms or they can turn the neck to the side. If clients choose to turn the head to the side, encourage them to turn the head to the other side once or twice during the prone

massage to avoid cramping. Sometimes they naturally turn the head when they get uncomfortable, but if you notice that about 10 minutes have passed without a head turn, you can suggest one. Most therapists offer clients a small bolster under the ankles (Fig. 9-2A), but clients with a large chest can be more comfortable with a soft bolster supporting the upper chest (Fig. 9-2B), and clients with low back pain may be more comfortable with a small bolster under the pelvis.

The prone position is preferred by clients who are shy, who are not interested in talking, or who are experiencing back pain. Back pain and tension are among the most common client complaints, making the prone position a good way to start the massage. By treating their back first and spending a lot of time working on it, you reassure clients that you heard them explain their condition. First-time clients may feel safer and more comfortable if the massage starts with the prone position because the genital areas are more protected.

There are some considerations involved in asking clients to lie prone. Anyone with head congestion should avoid this position, and one who is uncomfortable with confined spaces may not like using a face cradle. Clients who have large chests present a few challenges to using the prone position. First, their bodies are much higher off the table, making it necessary to lower your table for proper body mechanics. Second, you may need to bolster the upper chest to reduce the strain on the neck. And third, they may have to protract the neck an unreasonable amount to use a fixed face cradle. The tilting mechanism is not terribly helpful, either, because it only allows a client to rest the forehead on the face cradle. A face cradle with a telescoping mechanism that allows the whole face cradle to be raised is especially helpful for a client who has a large chest.

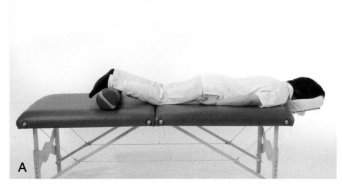
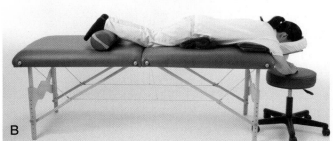

FIGURE 9-2 Prone position. **A.** Prone with ankle bolster. **B.** Prone with chest bolstering for a large chest and pelvic bolstering for low back pain.

SIDE-LYING (LATERALLY RECUMBENT) POSITION

The side-lying (laterally recumbent) position is lying on one's side. This position is not used as much as the prone and supine positions, but is sometimes the most effective position for treating some clients. It is excellent for working on neck and shoulder conditions because it presents all of the tissues and allows many different ranges of neck movement. To help clients be comfortable in the side-lying position, you need to have bolsters ready and you may need to give them specific directions such as

1. Straighten the bottom leg and keep it in line with the rest of the body
2. Flex the knee and hip of the top leg, bringing it forward in a bent position to rest on a large bolster
3. Flex the elbow and shoulder of the lower arm, and slide the hand under a pillow that supports the neck and head (Fig. 9-3)

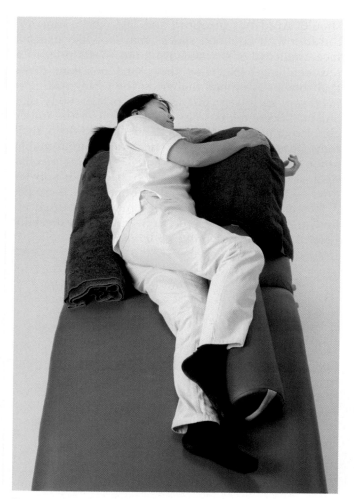

FIGURE 9-3 Side-lying position with bolsters for neck and head, top arm, and top leg and along back.

This position may be more comfortable for larger clients and for persons who do not like using a face cradle. It is also beneficial for working on women who are in the last few months of pregnancy. When a pregnant woman can no longer lie on her stomach, the side-lying position is appropriate for most, if not all, of the massage session. More-specific information on how to perform massage on pregnant clients is covered in Chapter 12, Special Populations.

Part of the reason the side-lying position is not as popular is because it is more awkward to drape and bolster clients properly and access different parts of the body. Since this position can be uncomfortable for clients without sufficient bolstering, you need to make sure that clients feel comfortable and secure when laterally recumbent. Try to keep your client's spine aligned along the midsagittal plane. The bolster under the neck and head should keep the client's head from laterally flexing in either direction. The bolster that supports the top leg should be large enough so that the top leg does not drop down significantly and strain the hip or back. Some clients cannot relax because they feel that they may roll off the table during the massage. You can roll up a towel or blanket and lay it at the base of the back to stabilize them and add a sense of security.

DETERMINING CLIENT POSITIONING AND BOLSTERING

Based upon the above information, ask yourself the following questions when determining how to position and bolster clients for their massage sessions:

- Does the client have a preferred position?
- What are the treatment goals for today's massage session?
- Does the client have any condition today that requires table adjustment?
- Does the client have any condition today that requires him or her to be in a different position from the one I usually use?
- Does the client have any condition today that requires additional bolstering or support?
- Where do I need bolsters or supports today?

Draping

Sheets and towels are draped over your massage table and your clients during the massage. This chapter focuses on draping, which is the process of using sheets and towels to keep clients covered to protect their modesty and keep them warm. Once clients are properly positioned and supported with bolsters, appropriate and modest draping helps them feel secure and comfortable throughout the massage. As the massage proceeds, you carefully expose only the specific part of a client's body receiving massage at that time. It may sound simple to keep clients completely covered during a massage, but it is more challenging than you think as you expose different body parts and ask clients to change positions. If you accidentally expose clients during a massage, which commonly happens during the learning process, cover them up, make a simple apology, and carry on. Draping helps you maintain ethical and professional boundaries during a massage session, and it helps clients feel safe and trusting enough to relax, even when they are undressed. Follow sanitation and hygiene standards by putting clean, disinfected linens on the table, and properly disinfect them after every use.

A particular amount of draping may be required by law in your locale or state, by the licensure or certification requirements, or as part of the professional standards of care governed by the professional organization with which you are affiliated. You are legally bound to adhere to the regulations, but they represent the minimum. If you feel that more draping is necessary or if your clients want more draping, you can ethically and professionally accommodate those situations. For example, you discover that under the law and professional standards of care, there are no requirements for draping whatsoever, and a male client wants only a small towel to cover his groin area. If you are not comfortable with that kind of exposure, how do you handle the situation? First, you can discuss your preference for more draping and educate your client about the drop in body temperature that results from massage. If the client wants to continue with treatment, he can agree to be covered with more draping. If he insists that he is perfectly comfortable with so much skin exposed and that you do not need to worry about his body temperature or modesty, you can refer him to another therapist for treatment.

Even though it is easiest to access all of the body parts of a client who is not covered with clothing, clients must not feel exposed or vulnerable. Reassure them that they should only take off the clothing they feel comfortable removing. As you step out of the room you can simply say, "I'll step out while you get undressed and get on the table, under the sheets. Please leave your underpants on as well as anything else you want to leave on. I'll knock on the door before I walk in to make sure you're under the sheets and ready." Clients may choose to wear shorts, swimsuit, or a sports bra during the massage, but you should still use draping. The most important goal of draping is to protect their modesty and comfort level, because clients who feel uncomfortable or compro-

mised in any way may be distracted, they may not be able to relax, and they may not get the best results from the massage session.

The core body temperature drops with the parasympathetic (relaxation) response to massage, making it a good idea to have extra blankets and towels on hand to cover clients who get cold. Being cold during a massage can cause muscles to remain tight, and it can distract clients from relaxing. On the other hand, clients may get hot during a massage session because of hormonal shifts that occur with pregnancy, menopause, and menstruation and after exercise. If so, you can uncover their feet, legs, and arms to dissipate heat and cool them off.

SHEET DRAPING

Sheets are larger than towels and, as long as they are opaque, they provide better and more secure coverage of the client's body than towels. This text focuses on the use of simple, two-sheet draping, but there are several different ways to drape with sheets. The examples here are only suggestions; your school or your instructor may have a preferred method of draping.

When clients step into your treatment room, the draping should be on the massage table, ready to be used. Sheet draping can be less intimidating than towel draping for clients because it is so similar to the way a bed is made. The familiar arrangement helps first-time clients feel comfortable about climbing onto the table and covering themselves with the top sheet, just as if they were getting into bed. Before you walk into the room, clients can cover themselves completely with the sheet, which gives them a sense of control and security.

A basic set of linens for two-sheet draping can include a fitted sheet to cover the table, a flat sheet to cover the client, and a pillowcase to cover the face cradle. A prepackaged set of twin sheets provides the basics for two-sheet draping, and it usually costs less. Purchase several sets, each of a different color or pattern, to have a variety of sheets on hand, and avoid light, see-through colors. It is easier to manipulate the top sheet for exposing and redraping when the flat and fitted sheets contrast. When you drape the table in preparation for a client, ensure that your flat and fitted sheets look different. Remember, avoid white or very light sheets, and purchase sheets with higher thread counts for better durability and comfort.

There is no single acceptable way to arrange your draping fabrics when you expose a body part to work on it, but your school or instructor may have recommendations or requirements. Basically, the goal is to uncover different areas of the body with-

PROCEDURE BOX 9-1
Draping Techniques for Uncovering Different Areas of the Body

A. Supine position, uncovering abdomen
   1. With the client supine, lay a pillowcase on top of the sheet, over the client's chest, with the client's hands on top of the pillowcase.

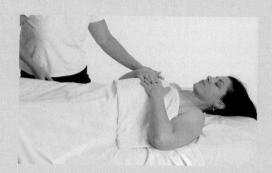

   2. Client holds the pillowcase while therapist pulls the sheet down to expose the abdomen.

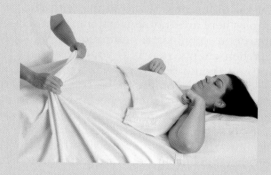

   3. Rest stroke on the client's abdomen.

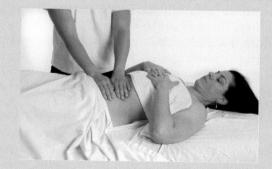

B. Prone position, uncovering leg
   1. With the client prone, push drape medial to the leg.

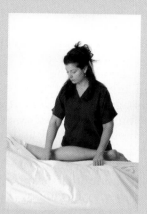

   2. Grasp the edge of the sheet and pull laterally with one hand while supporting and lifting the client's knee with the other, and tuck the sheet under the client's hip.

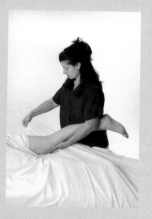

   3. Offer the client the edge of the sheet to hold for security, and rest your hands on the client's leg.

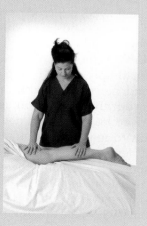

C. Side-lying position, uncovering back
   1. Standing at the client's back, make sure his or her top arm is on top of the sheet and tuck the drape into the armpit and under the chin to eliminate gaps in draping.

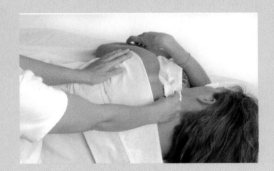

   2. Place your hand on the client's low back, around the waistband, while pulling the drape aside to expose the back.

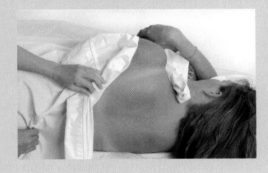

3. Rest your hands on the client's back.

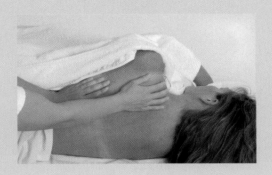

out exposing the genital area, the gluteal cleft, or women's breasts. In the process of uncovering parts of the body and redraping them, you can pick up the clients' arms and legs so the clients can stay relaxed, or you can ask clients to help you by lifting their own limbs. When you lift, make sure you use good body mechanics by using your legs to lift instead of your back and shoulders. Procedure Box 9-1 leads you through some steps to expose different areas of the body with two-sheet draping techniques. Several illustrations in Chapter 10, Massage Strokes and Flow, also show draping of different body parts during a massage.

There are some aspects of sheet draping to keep in mind. Flannel and jersey sheets tend to stick to each other, making it difficult to drape efficiently. If you insist on using them, use only one flannel or jersey sheet and one standard sheet. When the draping is pulled aside to expose an area of the body, make sure that the edge of the sheet is tucked firmly against the client's skin to give clients the feeling that they are securely covered. Clients with high levels of modesty can feel uncomfortable when they feel a breeze under the sheets if they suspect that you can see their body.

Sheet Draping for Position Change

Typically, clients change position at least once during the massage. They need your help to turn over safely without exposing the body. If clients are in the prone position and need to turn over into the supine position, you can follow the steps below (Fig. 9-4):

1. Remove bolsters.
2. If using a face cradle, ask clients to "scoot" toward their feet, out of the face cradle.
3. Reach across the table, gently scoop your fingers under the client's far shoulder, and lightly pull up on it, saying something like, "I'm going to hold the sheet up while you roll over this way, onto your back" (Fig. 9-4A).

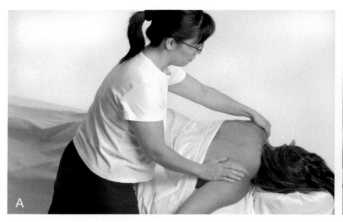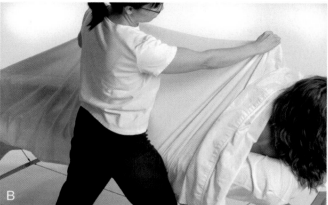

FIGURE 9-4   Sheet draping. **A.** Pull up on client's far shoulder to describe direction for turning over. **B.** Hold sheet up in a tent, pinning sheet to table.

4. Pick up the sheet with both hands into a tent, stand against the table to pin the sheet to the table, and ask the client to turn over (Fig. 9-4B).
5. Pull sheet down to expose the client's face.

The process of turning from the supine position into the prone position is similar; your position is not as critical during the turn. You can use the following sequence of steps:

1. Remove the bolsters.
2. Hold the sheet up like a tent, using both hands, and lean against the table to pin the sheet to the table.
3. Ask the client to turn over, onto the front.
4. If you use a face cradle, ask clients to scoot toward their heads and rest their faces on the face cradle.
5. Pull the sheet down to uncover the head.

TOWEL DRAPING

As in sheet draping, a fitted sheet covers the table, but clients are covered with one or more towels. There are various towel arrangements you can use to keep the genital area, gluteal cleft, and women's breasts covered to protect the ethical and professional boundaries of the session while working on different areas of the body. The simplest approach to towel draping is to use one large bath sheet with the same draping techniques you use for sheet draping (Fig. 9-5).

Towel Draping for Position Change

Turning clients over with towel draping is a little trickier because towels are smaller, and there is a greater chance of exposing your clients. When clients need to turn from prone to supine, you can follow the same steps that you used for sheet draping, but hold the towel tightly to avoid accidental exposure.

COMMUNICATION FOR CLIENT POSITIONING AND DRAPING

As part of promoting safety and comfort, you may want to explain the general positioning, bolstering, and draping of a massage session to clients who have never had a massage. A person who knows what to expect is better able to relax. Even for clients who have had massage before, but are new to you, it is good to clarify the positioning and draping techniques before or during the session. Box 9-1 presents one approach for explaining a massage session to new clients. This is only an example; with practice, you will develop your own way of familiarizing people with your massage.

On the other hand, the summary of an entire massage session can be too much for clients to comprehend all at once. You may find it more effective to explain your bolstering and draping techniques as you apply them during the massage. For example, as you start to uncover a client's back, you can say, "I am going to pull the sheet down to your waist so I can

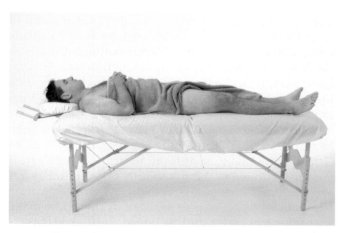

FIGURE 9-5   Towel draping showing exposed leg.

An Example of How to Describe a Massage Session to a New Client

"My goal is to have you comfortable and safe during your massage session. I will start the session with you lying face down on the table, underneath the top sheet, with your face in the face cradle. There is a hole in the face cradle so you can breathe comfortably. I will leave the room to wash my hands while you get undressed. You only need to take off the clothing you are comfortable removing, but know that your body will be covered by the top sheet throughout the massage, and only the body part I am working on will be exposed. I will knock on the door before I come in, just to make sure you are comfortably situated under the sheet. I will place a bolster under your ankles for comfort, and about halfway through the massage, I will ask you to turn over on your back. I will place bolsters under your knees and your neck for comfort, and I will massage your head and neck last. When I am finished, I will leave the room and give you time to get off the table and get dressed. There is a stool to use as you step down off the table, but if you need my assistance, let me know. Please tell me if you are uncomfortable at *any time* during the session, and I will make adjustments accordingly. For example, clients commonly feel a little cold during a massage, and I have extra blankets here if you need one. If you have any questions now or during the massage, please feel free to ask."

work on your back now." Or, as you finish working on the client in a supine position, you can say, "I'm going to hold the sheet up like a tent while you roll over onto your front and put your face in the face cradle. If you don't like the face cradle for any reason at any time, just let me know, and we'll continue without it."

When asking clients to change positions or actively participate in the massage, be aware that some directional terms are confusing for clients who are lying on the table. They may not be sure whether "up" means toward the ceiling or toward their head, or whether "down" means toward the floor or toward their feet. Instead of asking clients to move "up" on the table, ask them to move their whole body toward their head. Rather than ask clients to push "down," ask them to push toward the floor. When it is time for a client to switch from prone to supine, you can reach across the table to the client's far shoulder, scoop your fingers under it and gently pull up on it while you say, "Go ahead and roll over this way, onto your back." As clients roll over from prone to supine, it is safer if their back is toward you during the turn to prevent them from accidentally rolling off the table.

Assisting Clients On and Off the Table

Some clients may need assistance getting on and off the massage table if the table is too high or their physical condition makes it difficult or painful. You can have a footstool available for clients who have trouble with the height of the table, but sometimes that is not enough. Let your clients know that their safety is very important to you and that it is not a problem to help them get on and off the table. You can protect their modesty by showing them how to wrap the folded sheet around their body before you come into the room. If you want them in the prone position to start the massage, the free ends of the sheet should open to the front of their body, with the ends of the sheets overlapped in front. Conversely, if they are starting supine, the free edges of the sheet need to open to the back of their body, with the ends of the sheets overlapped behind them. After you have helped the client onto the table, and he or she is in the proper position, you can open the draping without exposing the client. (See Procedure Box 9-2 for an illustration of this process.)

Clients should be in the supine position for you to assist them off the table. If the massage ended in the prone position, ask clients to turn over to the supine position. Once in the supine position, you can use a "diaper drape" technique to help the client off the table while keeping the whole body completely covered. It is not terribly attractive, but it protects modesty. (See Procedure Box 9-3.) There is a simpler alternative to diaper draping, in which you tuck the sheet under the client's armpits, gather the sheet together at the back, and then help the client off the table. The problem with that technique is that the sheet is left to drag on the floor, which could easily trip someone who needs help getting off the table, such as the elderly, the injured, and those with balance problems.

Body Mechanics

Biomechanics is the study of how the movement of humans and living creatures is affected by both internal and external factors, including neurological input, muscle–tendon interactions, and physical strain on the body. The application of biomechanics to massage therapists is known as **body mechanics,** which is careful and efficient ways to move your body, incorporating the principles of leverage and efficient structural alignment of your body to minimize your fatigue and keep you from injuring yourself.

PROCEDURE BOX 9-2
Assisting a Draped Client into the Prone Position on the Table

1. Offer the sheet, folded in half, to your client, and demonstrate how you want him to wrap up in the sheet with the fold under his armpits and the free edges opening to the front. Leave the room and let the client undress and wrap himself in the sheet.

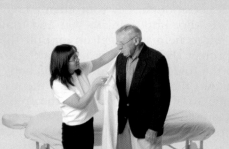

2. Offer the client your hand for support and stabilization while he uses a step stool to get on the table in a prone position.

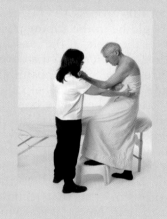

3. With the client prone and wrapped in the sheet, you pull the sheet out from under him.

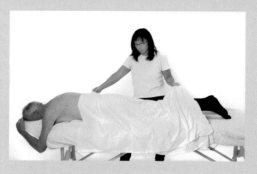

4. Unfold the sheets.

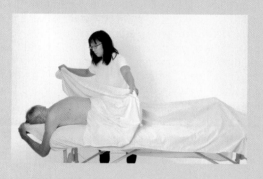

Holding and moving your body in less than efficient ways during a massage session can lead you to fatigue, increased discomfort, pain, and injury.

There are two primary components to good body mechanics, which includes the principle of leverage and efficient structural alignment. **Leverage** maximizes the amount of pressure you can apply with a minimum amount of muscular work by using your body as a rigid structure that leans into your clients with your body weight. In essence, leverage encourages you to keep your work close to your body to minimize the muscular work required to apply pressure or massage strokes. A quick demonstration of the principle of leverage in action is to hold up a book for several seconds with your arm outstretched, and then bring your arm close to your body and hold up the same book. It takes a lot more work to lift the book that is far away from your body than it does to lift that same weight when it is close to your body.

The concept of keeping your work close to your body to apply pressure is complicated by the muscles and joints of the human body. In addition to the use of leverage, you need to maintain efficient alignment of your skeletal structure to protect your muscles and joints from excessive stress and strain that can result in pain and injury.

1. Tuck the top edge of the sheet tightly under the client's armpits, and push the bottom corners of the sheet under the client's bent knees.

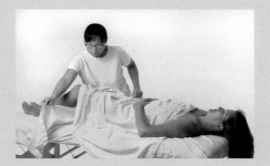

2. Ask your client to grab the bottom corners, lift the hips, and pull the sheet up to the waist.

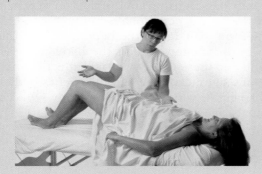

3. Take the corners of the sheet from your client and firmly tie them in front of the client's waist.

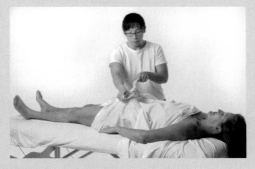

4. Lift the client's shoulder closest to you and tuck the sheet under it, pushing it toward the far shoulder.

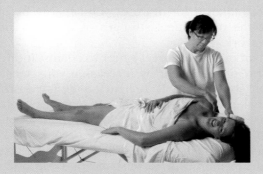

5. Walk to the other side of the table and gently lift up on the client's closest shoulder, ask your client to roll onto the side, and firmly tie the corners behind the client's back.

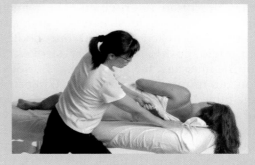

6. Walk to the other side of the table to face the client and
   a. slide one arm under the client's neck and your hand on the back.
   b. slide the other arm under the client's knees.

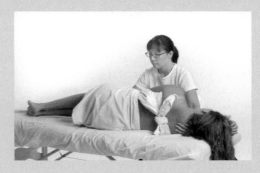

7. Lower your hips and pivot the client into a sitting position.

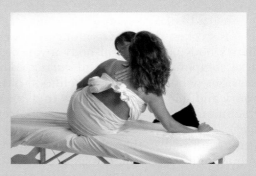

8. Offer your hand for support and stabilization as the client puts on socks and then steps off the table.

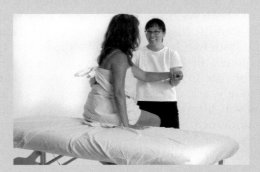

GOOD BODY MECHANICS

To minimize fatigue, we use leverage, and to prevent injury, we use good structural alignment. These concepts are not completely separate, and in fact, they are often intertwined. The principle of leverage applies to rigid structures, and although there are times when we hold our bodies in a straight, rigid position to deliver strokes, during most of the massage, we are moving. Besides leverage, you can minimize fatigue by making sure your massage table is set at the proper height, by leaning instead of pushing to apply pressure, and by using the strength and stability from your whole body, and you can apply the concepts of body awareness and proper breathing. It takes more work to stand than it does to sit, so take advantage of any opportunity you have to sit down while you give a massage, such as when you work on the face, the feet, or the hands.

As we use leverage and the other concepts for conserving energy, the alignment of our skeletal structures must not endanger any joint structures. For example, if you wanted to apply more pressure to a stroke, you could strictly follow the principle of leverage by moving your body directly over your hand. The problem with that approach is the resulting hyperextension of the wrist and compression on structures traveling through the carpal tunnel. There are general guidelines for minimizing injury and fatigue, and they pertain to your conservation of energy, proper alignment of your skeletal structure, use of the asymmetric (AY-sih-MET-rick) stance instead of a symmetric (sih-MET-rick) stance for strokes that travel along the length of the client's body, and general body awareness. Using these components before and during your massage sessions will decrease the likelihood of fatigue and injury and increase your ability to deliver massage techniques with more strength, power, and fluidity.

You may not realize that massage therapists do a fair amount of lifting during a massage. Draping, undraping, and joint movements generally require that you lift different parts of the body, and it is especially important to use good body mechanics for lifting. Keep the limb you are lifting close to your body, use your legs to lift instead of your back and shoulders, and use both hands to lift when you can. You can injure yourself lifting a limb, particularly if it is too heavy for you. In the interest of your own health, you can politely ask clients to help you lift by saying, "Could you lift your leg just a bit so I can slip this sheet underneath it?" Most clients are more than willing to help, and some even lift their limbs without a request, just to be helpful.

Proper Table Height

The position of your body in relation to the height of the table or, more importantly, to the height of the client's body on the table is a critical component of good body mechanics. The general rule, as discussed in Chapter 8, Equipment and Environment, is to set the height so that the top of the table is about at the middle of your index finger or the middle of your thigh, but again, that is only a starting place. If your table is too high or too low, you will have to adjust your posture to accommodate the height difference. A table that is too high can prompt you to elevate your shoulders, which can result in neck and shoulder tension, discomfort, and pain. Conversely, when a table is too low, you may find yourself bending at the waist to treat your client, which can result in low back tension, discomfort, and pain. Even if you are the only person using your table, you may need to adjust the height occasionally. As you stand next to a person on your table, the body of a very thin client can be a foot lower than the body of a very thick client, and these differences will affect your body mechanics significantly. When the client's body is at the right height, you can use your body with ease, and the massage can flow smoothly.

Leaning

The technique of leaning allows you to apply good pressure with the least stress on the body. If you have ever tried to push a heavy piece of furniture across the floor, your natural instincts probably led you to lean into the furniture with your arms straight, and your feet in a staggered position. You do not need to use those kinds of forces for massage, but the example shows how to maximize the work you do, with the least physical exertion. Leaning into the client's body with proper body mechanics creates a more fluid technique than pushing, it is less tiring, and feels better to the client. As you lean on your clients, gravity applies much of the pressure. Your body uses mostly the postural muscles to maintain the leaning position, requiring little additional effort or energy to provide pressure on the client. Pushing, on the other hand, takes a lot more of your energy because you use the mechanical strength of your muscles to do the work.

Not only does it feel better to clients, it offers them a sort of safety net by increasing your sensitivity to their soft tissues. If a client's body is resisting additional pressure, sometimes it twitches or jumps or tenses up nearby muscles. When you lean on clients, you are better able to feel the tissues resist. Therapists who push are less likely to feel the resistance and are more apt to push beyond the body's tolerance, possibly resulting in injury. The slow application of pressure that occurs with a lean allows the tissue to take more pressure without damage. For example, the femur, or thighbone, can withstand hundreds of pounds of pressure, if applied slowly and gradually. However, if a 20-pound weight falls on your femur, the bone will most likely break.

Symmetric Stance

The **symmetric stance,** also called the **horse stance** and **warrior stance,** has both feet placed as if the toes are on a line, pointing forward, a shoulder-width apart. Hips face forward, the knees are slightly bent, and your work is directly in front of you (Fig. 9-6). This stance is good for performing strokes in which your feet are fairly stationary, which happens when the stroke does not travel more than a few inches along the client's body and when the stroke travels directly across the client's body.

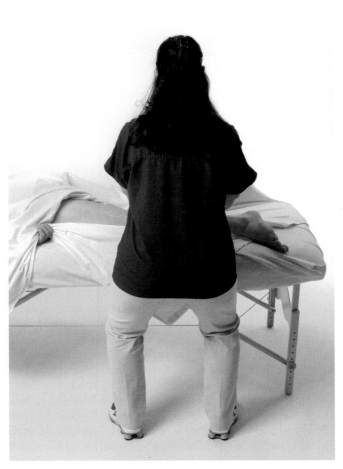

FIGURE **9-6** Symmetric stance.

Asymmetric Stance

The **asymmetric stance,** also called the **archer, bow,** or **lunge stance,** has both feet on the ground, a shoulder-width apart, one foot in front of the other, and the back foot laterally rotated. The front knee is flexed forward, and the back knee is just slightly flexed; the front foot is used more for balance than for support. Your weight is primarily supported by your back foot and the client's body at the contact point (Fig. 9-7A). This lunge position is most often used in massage therapy to provide the best leverage for strokes that require a lot of pressure or that travel along the length of a client's body. Again, leverage uses your body as a rigid structure to lean into your clients to apply pressure and does not use muscular work to push into clients' tissues. The same is true for pulling, when you can grasp your client's arm or hand, relax your elbows and shoulders, and lean backward rather than pull from your shoulders (Fig. 9-7B).

You can get more leverage from a longer lever, such as your straight body from head to back heel, than you can from a shorter lever, such as from the wrist to the shoulder. The asymmetric stance creates a longer lever than the symmetric stance. In terms of body mechanics, you can apply more pressure with the same amount of exertion if you lean from your back foot than if you lean from your waist. Given the principle of leverage, you can see how important it is to try to keep your ears, shoulders, hips, and back heel in a straight line. It minimizes unnecessary stress on your body and maximizes the pressure you can apply.

An open, asymmetric stance allows you to maintain the head-to-heel line as long as you are an appropriate distance away from the table. Typically, therapists keep their front foot less than 10 inches away from the table, but this is a general distance that is adjusted for different strokes and different applications. Standing too close to or too far from the table compromises the head-to-heel line. You can use the steps in Procedure Box 9-4 to take an asymmetric position next to a client on the massage table.

Using the Strength and Stability of your Whole Body

The body should move fluidly, using the movement and energy of the whole body instead of using the muscles of the upper body that move the shoulders, arms, hands, fingers, and thumbs. One of the keys to generating power and establishing stability behind your massage techniques is to direct the strength of your lower body and the energy of your entire body through your hands. Movement of the whole body improves the fluidity and rhythm of the massage. Especially when applying compression, you should use your whole body as leverage to deliver the pressure.

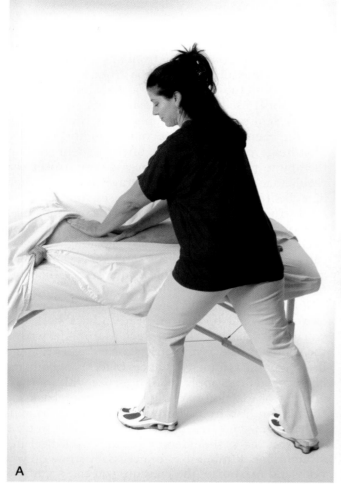
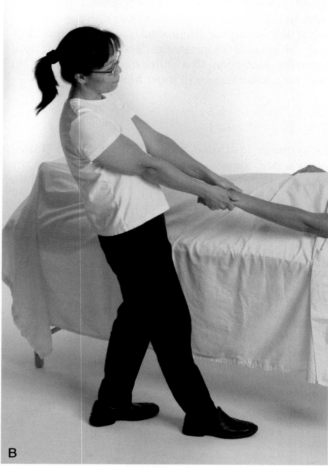

FIGURE 9-7   Asymmetric stance. **A.** Asymmetric lean. **B.** Asymmetric pull.

✓ PROCEDURE BOX 9-4
Taking an Asymmetric Stance Next to a Client on a Massage Table

1. Stand about 6 inches away from the middle of the massage table, with your head, hips, and toes all facing the center of the table.
2. Spread your feet shoulder-width apart.
3. Turn toward the client's head by pivoting on your toes. Your toes, hips, and face will all be facing your client's head, at an angle to the massage table, with one foot in front of the other.
4. Take a half step backward with your back foot to spread your feet apart. You may want to laterally rotate your back leg for stability.
5. Place the hand that is contralateral to (on the opposite side as) your back foot on the client's shoulder.
6. Lean on the client's shoulder and lift your weight off your front foot to rest your weight on the client's body and the floor under your back foot.
7. Place your other hand on the client for balance.

Stable, balanced structures are much more efficient than unstable, unbalanced structures. You can increase your stability by keeping your center of gravity low with bent knees. You can increase your balance with a shoulder-width stance. Slightly bent knees improve your balance as well, acting as shock absorbers.

Massage is a physically demanding career that requires strength and flexibility. If you do not keep your muscles healthy with sufficient exercise, water consumption, stretching, and massage, your body will be more susceptible to injury and fatigue. Strength will help you perform massage, and it comes in handy when clients need assistance getting on and off the table. Since massage involves a lot of muscular activity on your part, it is wise to stretch before and between massage sessions to keep your soft tissues flexible. Remember to breathe deeply, relax, stretch slowly to avoid the stretch reflex, and hold the stretch for at least 10 seconds to trigger the tendon reflex and comfortably enhance the stretch. If massage is going to be your career, you may want to consider strength training, yoga, tai chi, or stretching on a regular basis as part of your self-care regimen. Self-care for the massage therapist, including examples of stretches, is covered in more detail in Chapter 14.

Endurance is not necessary to perform one massage, but as you increase your practice to multiple massages each day and more than 10 a week, you will need endurance to sustain the practice. If your endurance is low, you may get tired easily, your body mechanics may suffer, and you may be more likely to suffer an injury. Along with developing strength and flexibility, it is also a good idea to develop your cardiovascular system to increase your endurance, which you can incorporate into your self-care regimen.

Efficient Structural Alignment

A critical component of good body mechanics is proper alignment of your body. When your joints are aligned efficiently, your physical work and the resulting stresses and strains are distributed evenly through-

out the body, allowing efficient motion and flow of energy. When the body is misaligned, which happens when you bend at the waist to apply a stroke or when you hyperextend your wrist to apply compression, the inefficient movement reduces the amount of energy you can deliver to the stroke. Strength, pressure, and control are compromised by poor alignment, and worse yet, your likelihood of injury increases.

The following guidelines can help you establish an efficient asymmetric alignment for applying most massage strokes (Fig. 9-8):

- Use an asymmetric stance, with staggered feet, when possible.
  Use the back foot to support your weight.
  Use the front foot for balance.
  Use the hand that is contralateral to the back foot to apply the stroke (use the right hand if the left foot is in back) to avoid twisting at the waist.

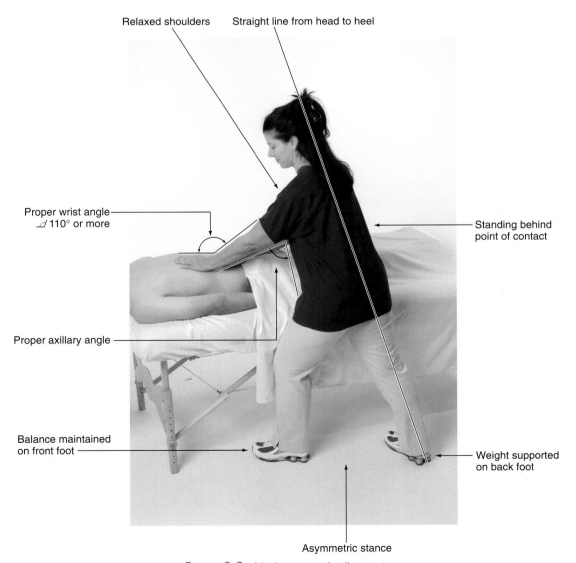

Relaxed shoulders   Straight line from head to heel

Proper wrist angle—
∠ 110° or more

Standing behind point of contact

Proper axillary angle

Balance maintained on front foot

Weight supported on back foot

Asymmetric stance

FIGURE 9-8   Ideal asymmetric alignment.

- Keep your ears, shoulders, hips, and the heel of your back foot in a line as much as possible, to provide the greatest amount of leverage by using the rigid structure of your body from head to toe as the lever.
- Point your feet and hips toward your work instead of twisting at the waist.
- The wrist angle, between the posterior surface of the hand and the forearm, should be no less than 110°
- The axillary angle, or the angle between your humerus and the side of your body, should not exceed 90°
- Position yourself behind your work instead of on top of it.

There should be enough floor space around your massage table so you can use an asymmetric stance and lean into your client without stepping on anything or running into a wall. If you do not have enough room around the table, your tendency will be to stand too close to your client's body and apply the pressure with muscular work or lose the proper alignment of your body and endanger your joints.

Maintaining the axillary angle of about 90°, or keeping your arm about perpendicular to your body, helps you maintain efficient alignment. When the angle is less than 90° or your arm is too close to your body, you may be applying pressure from above rather than from an angle, and your glenohumeral joint is susceptible to stress. When the angle exceeds 90° or your arm is too far away from your body, you have to use extra muscle strength to hold your body up, creating additional muscle strain and increasing the possibility of pain or injury. To maintain this angle while performing a long stroke that travels some distance along the client's body, you have to walk slowly and smoothly with the stroke (Fig. 9-9).

Your wrist should be kept relaxed, and the extension angle should not be less than about 110° (see Fig. 9-8). Actively extend your wrist and notice the limit of that range. That position is as far as you want to push your wrist when applying strokes. When the angle is less than that, the structures running through the carpal tunnel are compressed.

A general guideline is to have at least 3 feet of floor space around the edges of the table, if not more. With enough space to use a lunge position comfortably, you can position your body behind your work instead of positioning your body directly over your work. It is safer for clients if the pressure of your stroke is delivered at an oblique angle or from a somewhat sideways direction instead of vertically from above. When pressure comes from an angle, clients can roll away from pressure that is painful or uncomfortable, giving them a sense of control over the session. When the pressure comes from directly above the contact point, or the point where the massage stroke is applied to their skin, clients cannot roll away, and your structural alignment is inefficient.

Body Awareness

To use proper body mechanics, you must increase your body awareness, which is the ability to know where and how you are holding and moving your body. Body awareness helps you pay attention to your

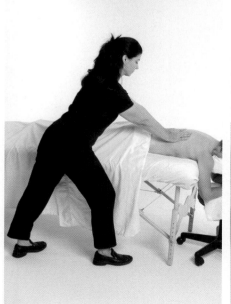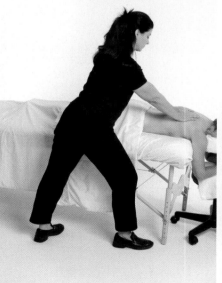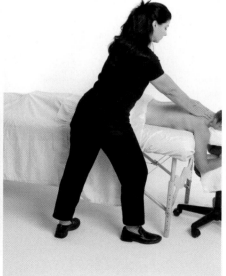

FIGURE 9-9   Walking with stroke.

body's signals and realize when your body mechanics are not as good as they could be. For example, it is common to shrug your shoulders as you give a massage, especially when you are learning and when you are tired. If you are aware of your body, you will feel the improper position of your shoulders and will have an opportunity to relax and drop your shoulders before pain and tension set in. With poor body awareness, you are apt to elevate your shoulders throughout the massage, and you could end up with very tight and sore shoulders by the end of the day.

Breathing is an important component of body awareness that is often ignored. Deep breathing increases circulation and decreases muscle tension. Using proper deep breathing techniques, you can draw in a maximum amount of air with the least amount of work. Minimizing your physical work and stress helps you conserve energy and helps you maintain a relaxed posture and good structural alignment while giving a massage. There is more information about breathing and an exercise for learning how to breathe from the diaphragm in Chapter 10, Massage Strokes and Flow.

You can train yourself to be more aware of your body by periodically asking yourself questions while you give a massage:

- Am I using my whole body?
- Does my body hurt anywhere as I apply this technique?
- Are my wrists, hands, and shoulders relaxed?
- Are any of my joints hyperextended?
- Am I breathing deeply?
- Are my hips between the line that goes through my head and heels?
- Are my hips and toes facing my work?

You may want to incorporate a body mechanics "check" into every massage when you hold the sheet and allow clients to turn over or when you redrape a particular area of the body. There is no doubt that at some point in your career you will experience some pain and discomfort, either in a massage session or as the result of performing several massages over time; increased body awareness will help you make the necessary adjustments to minimize your chance of injury.

IMPROPER BODY MECHANICS

Massage involves a lot of repetitive movements and static (stationary) compression, both of which are stressful on the joints. Using improper body mechanics can suddenly or gradually lead to fatigue and injury. A vicious circle of bad body mechanics begins as bad body mechanics lead to fatigue, fatigue often accentuates bad body mechanics, and so on.

The hands, fingers, thumbs, and wrists are used extensively in massage. Although the hands are the first things that come to mind when you think about giving a massage, the rest of your body supports your hands in the application of a stroke or technique. One massage performed with poor body mechanics may not cause much harm, but after several massages a day over months and years, bad body mechanics will undoubtedly cause trouble. You can develop chronic pain, injuries, and other uncomfortable symptoms in your hands, fingers, thumbs, wrists, shoulders, neck, back, and low back. In severe cases, these conditions can end your career.

Injury

Following the principles of leverage and proper alignment can keep injuries to a minimum, but massage puts undue stress on the muscles and joints even when you do use good body mechanics. Essentially, the body is not designed to constantly repeat motions for an extended period, which is what occurs in massage therapy. **Repetitive stress injuries** (RSIs) result when specific body movements are repeated enough to stress the structures involved in the movement to the point of damage, and massage therapists are prime targets for RSIs. There are a number of areas where massage therapists are prone to injury, and the following list identifies some of the possible causes:

- Neck and shoulders: hunched posture; table too high; shoulders shrugged; pressure being applied with pushing movements from the shoulder muscles instead of with the leverage of the whole body
- Wrist and hands: hyperextended wrists; standing directly over the work instead of behind the work; applying pressure with muscular gripping instead of with leverage of the whole body
- Fingers and thumbs: repetitive finger or thumb motions; using fingers or thumbs to press or squeeze instead of using leverage; insufficient support for fingers and thumbs when using them to apply strokes
- Back: bending and overreaching to perform techniques; lifting parts of the clients' bodies, without proper alignment
- Knees: hyperextending (locking) them while standing; twisting them by leaving toes pointed in one direction while the hips point in another direction
- Ankles and feet: standing for prolonged periods; working without supportive shoes

You can also hurt yourself by suddenly increasing your workload or decreasing the amount of rest you take between massage sessions. For example, your massage practice suddenly jumps from 3 to 5 clients a week, one or two massages per day, to 10 clients per week with 4 back-to-back massages in 1 day. This large clientele influx is financially appealing, but you will do yourself a long-term favor by pacing yourself and scheduling these clients over a 2-week period.

Muscles attach to bones via tendons. The musculotendinous unit can be injured when a muscle exerts excessive strain on its tendon, resulting in symptoms of inflammation, mild-to-severe discomfort or pain, decreased strength, and decreased range of motion. Examples of specific musculotendinous injuries include muscle strain, tendinitis, or tenosynovitis (tendon sheath inflammation) in the forearm, hands, fingers, thumbs, or rotator cuff (supraspinatus, infraspinatus, teres minor, and subscapularis muscles).

When nerves are compressed, they function abnormally, which results in symptoms such as burning, tingling, pins and needles (paresthesia), and radiating pain. Nerve compression injuries may include carpal tunnel syndrome and thoracic outlet syndrome. Briefly, the carpals of the wrist form a tunnel (the carpal tunnel) that serves as the passageway for nerves and tendons. Excessive pressure on the carpal tunnel can compress the median nerve, which serves the thumb and the first two fingers. Thoracic outlet syndrome is the result of restricted and tight soft tissues that compress the brachial plexus, which serves the shoulder, forearm, and hand.

Injury Prevention

To minimize your risk for injury, follow these guidelines:

- Use good body mechanics.
- Rest your body and your hands by scheduling clients far enough apart.
- Stretch before and after massage sessions.
- Use the appropriate table height.
- Make sure you have plenty of room to move around the table.
- Use a variety of techniques in your massage sessions.
- Be cautious with applications of sustained pressure.
- Increase your own physical fitness and endurance.
- Get enough sleep and rest.

Additionally, if you become aware of any soreness, aches, fatigue, pain, burning, numbness or numblike sensations, tingling, or signs of inflammation including redness, heat, swelling, or loss of function, you must change your technique, body position, or massage schedule. You could also visit the appropriate healthcare professional for evaluation and treatment for a specific condition. **Do not risk your career by living with pain and injury.**

There are some pieces of equipment that can reduce the physical stress of giving a massage, includ-

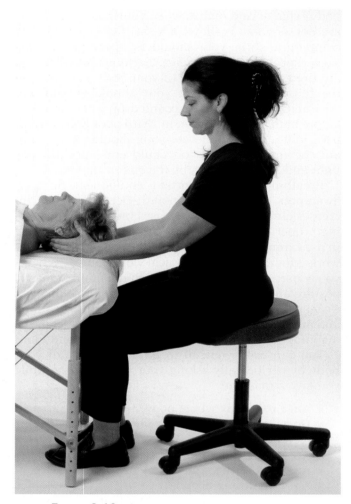

FIGURE 9-10 Sitting on a chair to conserve energy.

ing chairs, rolling stools, and massage gadgets discussed in Chapter 8, Equipment and Environment. Sitting uses less energy than standing, and there are times during the massage that you can sit in a chair and still maintain good body mechanics. Any time you work on a client's head, hands, or feet, it may be better to sit down (Fig. 9-10). Chairs and stools with wheels are especially easy to use, because you can easily move them around with your feet while your hands maintain contact with your client's body.

Body Mechanics for Additional Pressure

There are some effective and efficient ways to alter the pressure or depth of the stroke, making slight adjustments in the lean. In the asymmetric stance, your back foot supports your weight, your front foot is mostly for stabilization, and your hips are in line with your shoulders and back heel. In reality, as you apply massage strokes and move around the room, your front foot supports some of your weight during an asymmetric stance, and your hips are posterior to the head-to-heel line. To increase the pressure of a stroke, you can simply lift some or all of your weight off of your front foot or move your hips into the head-to-heel line. Additional pressure can be added by lifting the back heel to stand on your toes, essentially creating a longer lever. Leaning allows you to use the weight of your body instead of muscle strength to adjust the depth of pressure.

Chapter Summary

Client comfort and relaxation as well as the long-term success of your practice depend on your use of client positioning, draping, and body mechanics. Once you are adept at simple draping, you can explore adaptations and supplemental draping options with extra blankets, towels, or an additional sheet. It can be an awkward process at first, but with practice, you will develop your own draping techniques. The outcome will be good if the client's comfort level remains your primary intention.

Body mechanics are best learned in a classroom with an instructor to help you, but the concepts outlined in this chapter can serve as reminders outside the classroom.

There are various thoughts and opinions about which foot positions are best for minimizing stress on your body and maximizing your energy to practice massage. As you learn and practice the basic stances, your body awareness can guide you to postures and positions that are comfortable and do not create discomfort or pain in your body. A general rule for positioning your body is to find a position, relax your body, and begin to work. If you feel that you are developing muscle tension or you are fatigued at any point during a massage, change your position or change your technique. You *must* heighten your body awareness and develop good body mechanics as you learn the strokes and flow of massage so you can build a successful practice without damaging your body.

CHAPTER EXERCISES

1. Define the following terms:
   - Axillary angle
   - Body mechanics
   - Contralateral
   - Laterally recumbent
   - Leverage
   - Prone
   - Supine

2. Practice client positioning with a fully clothed partner on the massage table in the prone, supine, and side-lying positions, with and without a face cradle, and with and without the following bolsters:
   - Neck (prone, supine, and side-lying)
   - Chest (prone)
   - Pelvis (prone)
   - Ankles (prone)
   - Knees (supine)
   - Top leg (side-lying)
   - Along the length of the back (side-lying)

3. Practice draping with a partner on the massage table (the partner should be undressed and underneath the drape) to expose different areas of the body:
   - Prone position—back, leg, foot, arm
   - Supine position—arm, upper chest, abdomen, leg, foot
   - Side-lying position—back, top arm, top leg, bottom leg

4. Practice helping undressed clients on and off the massage table, maintaining modesty by keeping them covered with the drape.

5. Practice walking with your stroke. Ask a partner to lie prone on the massage table, and put your relaxed hand on his or her low back. Move the stroke toward the partner's head without changing the axillary angle by walking with the stroke.

6. Familiarize yourself with the safe wrist position. Perform active wrist extension, and notice the limit of the range of motion. Rest your hand on a desk top, table top, or massage table, and lean on that contact hand. Without moving your feet, slowly shift your weight so your shoulders move closer to the table top and are eventually positioned directly over your hand, and then shift in the opposite direction, away from the table top. Notice your wrist angle, axillary angle, and the stress on your shoulder joint as your body moves too close and too far away from your contact hand.

7. Describe at least five areas of a massage therapist's body that are prone to injury, and list at least one possible cause for each area listed.

8. Practice efficient alignment with a partner. Lean on a variety of objects of different heights, and try to maintain the head-to-heel line using the

asymmetric stance. You can try leaning on the seat of a chair, the top of a massage table, a doorknob, a windowsill, or a bookshelf.

9. There are client circumstances for which certain client positions are recommended. Describe at least two reasons why you would put a client in each of the three client positions.

10. Relaxed wrists and hands deliver a more comfortable stroke than tight, tense wrists and hands. Ask a partner to rest his or her arm on the desk top, table top, or massage table. Clench your hand into a tight fist and use the tightened forearm to lean on your partner's arm. Relax your arm, wrist, and hand and lean on your partner's arm. Ask your partner for feedback: how did the two pressures differ, which one was more comfortable, which one hurt.

SUGGESTED READINGS

Aslani M. Massage for Beginners. New York: Carroll & Brown, 1997.

Bruder L. Navigating the pathway to phenomenal touch: 10 steps to transform your massage. Massage Magazine 2002:March–April.

Frye B. Body Mechanics for Manual Therapists: A Functional Approach to Self-Care and Injury Prevention. Stanwood, WA: Freytag Publishing, 2000.

Greene L. Save Your Hands!: Injury Prevention for Massage Therapists. Seattle: Infinity Press, 1995.

Latchaw M, Egstrom G. Human Movement with Concepts Applied to Children's Movement Activities. Englewood Cliffs, NJ: Prentice-Hall, 1969.

Lidell L, Thomas S, Cooke CB, Porter A. The Book of Massage. New York: Simon & Schuster, 1984.

Lindsey R, Jones BJ, Whitley A. Body Mechanics, Posture, Figure and Fitness. 4th ed. Dubuque, IA: Wm. C. Brown, 1979.

Maxwell-Hudson C. Complete Massage. New York: Dorling Kindersley, 2001.

Nordin M, Frankel VH. Basic Biomechanics of the Musculoskeletal System. 3rd ed. Baltimore: Lippincott, Williams & Wilkins, 2001.

Rattray F, Ludwig L. Clinical Massage Therapy: Understanding, Assessing and Treating over 70 Conditions. Toronto: Talus Incorporated, 2000.

Seedor MM. Body Mechanics and Patient Positioning. New York: Teachers College Press, 1977.

Souriau P. The Aesthetics of Movement (Souriau M, transl and ed.) Amherst, MA: The University of Massachusetts Press, 1983.

Trager M, with Hamond C. Movement as a Way to Agelessness: A Guide to Trager Mentastics. Barrytown, NY: Station Hill Press, 1995.

10

Massage Strokes and Flow

- Explain the effects of massage on at least five organ systems of the body
- Name the three stationary massage "strokes"
- Identify the six basic massage strokes
- Explain at least two effects of each basic massage stroke
- Demonstrate each stroke presented in this chapter
- Explain the effects of joint movement
- Follow a basic relaxation massage flow
- Describe how to follow a flow during a therapeutic massage

KEY TERMS

Centering: a technique that helps you focus your attention on your clients

Compression: a stroke that applies pressure to soft tissues to squeeze them together without any slip

Deep fiber friction: a stroke that is applied with deep, localized pressure without any slip on the skin to break up fascial adhesions and separate the muscle fibers

Effleurage (EF-lur-ahzh): a slow, gliding stroke along the client's skin

Excursion: the physical length of one stroke along the client's skin

Flow: a routinelike sequence of steps that leads the massage from one body part to the next in a systematic, fluid pattern that often specifies stroke sequences

Friction: the physical resistance between two surfaces as they rub against each other and create heat

Grounding: a technique you can use to establish an emotional and energetic boundary between you and your clients

Passive contraction: a stationary muscle position created when you move the origin and insertion of a client's muscle closer together while the client relaxes

Petrissage (PET-rih-sahzh): a stroke that kneads soft tissues with a grasping and lifting action

Resting stroke: a stroke that requires you to stop moving and lightly rest your relaxed hands, fingers, or arms on your client for several seconds

Slip: the sliding of your skin over the surface of the client's skin

Superficial friction: a brisk variation of light effleurage that increases circulation in the superficial tissues and dissipates body heat

Tapotement (tuh-POHT-ment): a fast rhythmic stroke that uses both hands, like rapid drumming

Vibration: a stroke that involves high-frequency shaky hand movements and is capable of deep effects

Massage is both art and science. There are individual nuances to every massage that make it impossible to perform the exact same massage twice. This artistic aspect of massage encompasses the personal and unique characteristics of touch:

- The intent of the touch
- The delivery of the touch
- The attitude of the person delivering the touch
- The focus of the person delivering the touch
- The mental condition of the person receiving the touch
- The physical condition of the person receiving the touch
- All of the factors of the massage environment

Touch can be obvious or subtle, significant or meaningless. For example, a very light caring touch is vastly different from an accidental brush against a stranger in a crowded store. As a massage therapist, you have the ability to use the power of touch to affect another human being. The trick, therefore, is to know how to tailor the massage session to the needs and wants of your clients. You must know how to perform the basic massage strokes, but it is equally, if not more important to know where and when to use them. The scientific aspect of massage includes all of the anatomy and physiology involved in massage, as well as the organized approach to assessments and treatment plan. Along with effective communication skills and your academic knowledge of anatomy and physiology, the physiological effects of massage presented in this chapter will help you determine which strokes are appropriate. Combining your scientific knowledge with an artistic and individualized approach to touch creates a unique massage every time.

Despite the fact that each massage is different, there are some aspects to many massages that are similar. The massage **flow** is a routine-like sequence of steps that leads the massage from one body part to the next in a systematic, fluid pattern. Similar to a recipe, a flow can specify the parts of the body you treat, the order in which you treat them, and the strokes you apply. Some flows start with clients in the prone position (face down), while others begin with clients in the supine position. Some flows are designed for clients who remain in a laterally recumbent (side-lying) position throughout the entire massage, and others are designed for clients in a seated position. With practice, your flow becomes second nature and lets you think about which strokes and techniques you apply instead of which body part to work on next.

Effects of Massage

Without question massage affects the physiology of the human body. You may recall Dr. John Kellogg's determination of the mechanical, reflexive, and metabolic effects of massage. A more practical way to learn how massage affects the body is to understand how massage affects the physiological functions of different organ systems:

- Integument
- Skeletal system
- Muscles
- Nervous system
- Circulatory system
- Respiration
- Digestion
- Thermoregulation

INTEGUMENT

The skin is loaded with sensory receptors and is the point of contact between you and your clients. Mechanically, massage warms the skin with friction and increases circulation of blood and lymph in the skin. The enhanced heat and circulation stimulate the sebaceous glands to produce more secretions that make the skin more supple and pliable, and increase sweat production, which has a cooling effect on the body when it evaporates. Adhesions in the subcutaneous layer, or superficial fascia, can constrict the circulatory vessels, reducing the local flow of blood and lymph and restricting movement of muscles and nearby tissues. Massage is one of the most effective treatments to break down fascial adhesions to restore circulation and movement.

SKELETAL SYSTEM

Even though massage is not intentionally used as treatment for the bones and joint structures, they do benefit. Massage therapists may incorporate joint movement into their treatment when evaluating ranges of motion. In response to joint movement, the body produces synovial fluid, which cushions and lubricates the synovial joints to help keep them healthy. Massage increases the number of red and white blood cells in the blood, which increases the body's ability to deliver oxygen to cells and fight germs. The bones house the red marrow, which is the site for red blood cell production, and higher numbers of blood cells benefit all of the tissues and organs of the body.

MUSCLES

The skeletal muscles, which make up about half of our body weight, are the primary focus of massage therapy. In fact, sometimes massage is the best treatment for muscles, tendons, and fascia, capable of benefiting muscle tissue in many ways.

First, massage increases the nutrition and development of muscles by enhancing the delivery of oxygenated blood and removal of cellular waste. Exercise, which can also increase circulation within muscle tissue, results in higher blood pressures and faster pulse rates. Since these stressful physiological conditions do not accompany relaxation massage, the effects of massage are especially beneficial. Inactive and paralyzed muscles benefit greatly from massage because it delivers oxygen and nutrients to muscle cells to keep them healthy.

Massage increases the excitability of muscles, making them more sensitive to nerve impulses. Faster reaction times, more effective movements, and better coordination can all result from massage. Physical exertion is often followed by muscular fatigue, and massage is one of the most practical and beneficial treatments for muscular fatigue. Massage helps to speed up the recovery of fatigued muscles by encouraging lactic acid, the chemical responsible for the symptoms of muscular fatigue, out of the muscles and into the bloodstream.

 It is possible to create fatigue-like symptoms with massage techniques that are too aggressive.

Manipulation of the muscles also produces heat, partly as a result of the increased circulation, partly because of increased chemical activity in muscle cells, and partly because of the heat generated when fascia is subjected to pressure. Muscle contractions produce heat as a byproduct of chemical reactions, and manipulation of the muscles increases these chemical reactions. In the anatomy and physiology chapter, we discussed the thixotropic property of deep fascia. Without movement, fascia can thicken, contract, and become less pliable, restricting muscle movement and circulation within the muscles. Manipulation of the muscles deforms the fascia, which creates heat, similar to how bending a paperclip back and forth heats up the area being deformed.

NERVOUS SYSTEM

All of the sensory input of your massage environment can affect the nervous system as well as the mental condition of the client, so be aware of your surroundings and be sensitive to client responses. Initial contact with the skin reflexively stimulates a sympathetic nervous response to prepare us for flight or fight in case the contact turns out to be a real or perceived threat. When the body has determined that the sustained touch does not pose any danger, it stops the sympathetic nervous response. In about 10–15 minutes, sustained touch and massage actually activate the parasympathetic nervous response of relaxation. Massage can soothe the nervous system, changing the blood levels of several neurochemicals and hormones associated with pain:

- Increases dopamine (DOH-pah-meen)—a pain-relieving chemical involved in voluntary movement and clear thinking
- Increases endorphins (ehn-DOR-finz)—very strong pain-relieving chemicals that suppress all nerve functions to some degree
- Increases enkephalins (ehn-KEHF-uh-lihnz)—strong pain relievers involved in sensory integration
- Increases oxytocin (AHK-sih-TOH-sihn)—a chemical that increases the pain threshold, stimulates smooth muscle contractions, decreases sympathetic nervous response, and has sedative effects
- Increases serotonin (SAIR-uh-TOH-nihn)—a chemical that generally diminishes pain and appetite, regulates moods and sleep patterns, and stimulates smooth muscle contraction
- Decreases cortisol (KOR-tih-sohl)—a natural antiinflammatory produced in response to stress that can accelerate the breakdown of tissues and prevent tissue repair, both of which can cause pain
- Decreases substance P—a neurotransmitter that triggers the pain response

CIRCULATORY SYSTEM

The effects of massage on circulation are determined by where and how strokes are applied. The sympathetic nervous system can accomplish the task, but at the expense of increased blood pressure and heart rate. Initially, the reflexive effects of percussive massage strokes cause local vasoconstriction (blood vessel constriction). Sustained percussion, however, can result in vasodilation (blood vessel dilation) in surrounding areas.

Mechanically, pressure on the blood and lymph vessels increases circulation. The inactive or dormant capillaries and the capillaries with poor blood flow respond to this kind of mechanical pressure remarkably well and can then supply oxygenated blood to local tissues that were previously suffering from ischemia. Massage increases the permeability of the capillary walls, enhancing the delivery of oxygen and nutrients.

Massage is especially beneficial to the lymphatic system. Without a pump behind it, the lymphatic system of vessels and valves is aided by rhythmic contraction of the skeletal muscles and gravity. The diaphragm muscle is particularly helpful to the lymph system. There are a lot of lymph vessels in the central tendon of the diaphragm, so when it contracts, lymph is pushed through the one-way valves. Also, contraction of the diaphragm creates a vacuum in the thoracic cavity that pulls both lymph and venous blood through their respective vessels and one-way valves.

Numerous lymph vessels travel through the superficial and deep fascia, and the mechanical pressure of massage strokes on these vessels increases the flow of lymph through them. Similarly, skeletal muscle contractions put pressure on the lymph vessels and pump lymph through the one-way valves. Joint movement and passive contractions applied during a massage activate this skeletal muscle pump, though not as effectively as active contractions.

RESPIRATION

The process of cellular respiration is enhanced by massage and manipulation of the tissues, partly as a result of the increased circulation. As muscles are massaged, the heat and oxidation of glycogen creates additional amounts of carbon dioxide that the body has to expel to maintain homeostasis. We eliminate carbon dioxide by exhaling it through the lungs and can eliminate unusually high amounts by breathing deeply and more effectively. Furthermore, massage that lasts longer than 10–15 minutes activates the parasympathetic nervous response, which encourages slow, deep contractions of the diaphragm.

DIGESTION

Massage generally stimulates cellular metabolism and increases the delivery of nutrients to cells and tissues. As the nutrients are used up, the body recognizes the need for more nutrients by triggering the appetite. In other words, we feel hungry as a reflexive effect of massage. Likewise, the production and activity of digestive enzymes increases as circulation and metabolism increases, hastening the process of digestion. Massage can mechanically push the indigestible waste through the intestines, but massage also evokes the parasympathetic nervous response that encourages digestive activity.

THERMOREGULATION

Muscle contractions create heat. Even when muscles are "at rest," some of the muscle cells in a muscle are contracting to maintain muscle tone. The primary mechanism for producing body heat is muscle contraction. Heat is similarly produced when muscles are kneaded, but the increased temperature of the muscles does not raise the body temperature significantly. Brisk, superficial massage on the skin, sometimes called superficial friction, creates vasodilation in the skin. As a result, body heat is dissipated, and the core temperature can drop. Basically, kneading strokes can increase heat production, and superficial friction strokes can increase heat reduction.

Stationary Massage "Strokes"

There are several techniques and strokes that you incorporate into the basic massage. Some do not require any pressure or manipulation of soft tissues, and others do. Grounding, centering, and resting strokes require no lubricant because there is no **slip,** which is the sliding movement of your skin across the surface of the client's skin.

GROUNDING

Grounding is a process that is typically used before the massage to create a kind of boundary between yourself and your clients. Massage therapists who regularly give several massages a day sometimes feel drained or exhausted after a particular client, suggesting that some people "take" more of our core energy than others. Instead of thinking that you are "giving" clients your energy, slightly change your frame of mind and think of yourself as a conduit for energy, a mechanism that redirects and refocuses the client's energy. You are more effective as a conductor of energy than as a source of energy. By changing the perception of your work, you may not feel the exhaustion that results from conceptually giving away your own energy. Grounding is an intangible screen of protection that helps you keep your energy separate from your client's energy.

Spending time with people who are laughing and happy can raise our spirits, just as people who are sad and depressed can make us feel gloomy. Basically, we are susceptible to other people's emotions. A similar phenomenon sometimes occurs with a client's symptoms. There are occasions when, following a massage, your client's original complaints seemingly manifest themselves in your own body. Although it may sound incredible, it does happen, and the experience can be unsettling and unpleasant. Grounding techniques used before and during a massage can prevent such situations.

Generally, you ground yourself as you establish initial contact with a client at the beginning of the massage. The following visualization technique is an easy way to ground yourself while establishing contact with a fully draped client on the massage table:

1. Stand next to the massage table and direct your thoughts to your feet and their contact with the floor.
2. Imagine your feet as the roots of a tree, giving you stability and acting as a sort of drain for any unwanted tensions or stressful energy.
3. Establish contact by gently resting your hands on top of the sheets, on your client:
   a. If the client is supine, rest your hands on the shoulders or feet.
   b. If the client is prone, rest your hands on the back, shoulders, or feet. (See Fig. 10-1 for different hand positions for resting strokes.)
4. Close your eyes and take a few deep breaths as you clear your mind and focus on your client.

Grounding techniques can be used before the massage, either outside or inside the treatment room, and they can be used during a massage if you feel distracted or as if you are running out of energy. You can ground yourself anytime, any day, in your personal life as well as your professional life.

CENTERING

Centering is the process of focusing your attention on the massage session and being present in the moment. It should be done before every massage session and can be combined with your grounding technique. You may get frustrated with the process of clearing your mind, particularly if you tend to have a lot of things on your mind. Instead of paying attention to the distractive thoughts you want to forget, such as schedules, grocery lists, errands, finances, or social commitments, you can start centering yourself by focusing on your breath.

Close your eyes and focus on deep breathing in an attempt to quiet your mind and eliminate any stray thoughts or concerns. Listen to the air as it moves through your airway. Feel the expansion of your ribcage while you relax the muscles in your shoulders and your pelvic floor. Focus on a few deep breaths to clear your mind, and as you feel yourself calm down, start turning your attention to your client. Think about the client's concerns and consider how his or her life is being affected. By giving clients your full attention, you can better respond to, and be guided by, their needs and your intuition. The purpose of centering is to put your own concerns aside and focus on the client's needs and wants.

Diaphragm Breathing

The process of breathing involves the antagonistic actions of inhalation and exhalation. Inhalation occurs in two phases. In the first phase of proper, natural breathing, the diaphragm contracts and pulls downward until it rests on the abdominal organs. The abdomen expands as the diaphragm pulls air down into the lungs. Once the organs stop the diaphragm, the second phase of inhalation begins. The diaphragm continues to contract and pull air into the lungs, resulting in an upward expansion of the rib cage. With palpation, you can feel your belly expand during the first phase of inhalation and your sternum rise up in the second phase. Normal, natural exhalation occurs in the opposite sequence, with the chest deflating first, and the abdomen contracting second.

To take a full, deep breath, you need to use your diaphragm muscle instead of the scalenes and other accessory muscles. First, make sure your waistband or belt is loose to give your abdomen room to expand. Place one hand on your abdomen, and the other hand on your sternum. Sit or stand up straight, drop your shoulders, and slowly inhale through your nose and feel the expansion of your belly followed by the rise in your ribcage. You can look in the mirror or use a partner to monitor your shoulders while you take a deep breath. Watch to make sure that the shoulders do not elevate significantly and that the scalene muscles do not tense up. Slowly exhale through your mouth, feeling the deflation of your ribcage followed by the contraction of your abdomen. Full, deep diaphragm breathing is more efficient than quick, shallow breathing because it provides more oxygen with less energy expenditure. Now try to make yourself yawn while you keep your hands in position to monitor the expansion and contraction that occurs. Notice how your body naturally breathes properly during a yawn, straightening the back, lifting the head on top of the spine, and using the diaphragm to breathe in and out.

RESTING STROKE

The **resting stroke** involves no movement, no slip, and no application of pressure, but it requires that you touch your client with a therapeutic intent. When you stop moving and lightly rest your relaxed hands, fingers, or arms on clients for several seconds, it is considered a resting stroke. It is a good stroke to use at the beginning of the massage, as a sort of greeting to the client's body, but it can be used just as effectively anytime during the massage.

When applied at the beginning of the massage, a resting stroke establishes your initial contact with the client and lets their nervous system recognize your touch as safe and nonthreatening. Figure 10-1 illustrates some different hand positions for resting strokes. Besides using the resting stroke to signal the nervous system that you present no danger, you can use the resting stroke as an initial palpation assessment tool to evaluate body rhythms and temperature, texture, and fullness of the tissues under your relaxed hands.

In addition to using it at the beginning of your massage, you can use the resting stroke periodically throughout the massage. You can use it to ground or center yourself or to reevaluate the client's tissues to help you choose the appropriate technique at any given moment. After you work on a specific area for a long time or use a lot of therapeutic techniques on one area, your touch can be perceived as a source of aggravation that stimulates the sympathetic nervous response. Avoid that situation by using a resting stroke to settle the nervous system and allow relaxation to continue.

Another way to use a resting stroke during the massage is to use it as a connecting stroke. You want to minimize the number of times you break contact with the body because every time you break contact, you have to reinitiate contact, and initial contact can be stimulating. To move from one area of the body to another without breaking contact, you can leave one hand on the area that you have just finished massaging, and place the other hand on the area that you will start working on. Essentially, your resting stroke connects the area that has been massaged with the area that will be massaged.

Basic Massage Strokes

The six basic massage strokes involve the application of pressure in some form, and they all have mechanical and reflexive effects. Some strokes incorporate slip on the client's skin, and others do not. Compression is a variation of a resting stroke, but because pressure is applied, it is considered a basic massage stroke. The fundamental massage techniques that arise from Per Henrik Ling's Swedish Movements include effleurage (EF-lur-ahzh), petrissage (PET-rih-sahzh), tapotement (tuh-POHT-ment), friction, and vibration. A Swedish massage, also called a relaxation or wellness massage, is one that generally includes these basic strokes and no specific therapeutic techniques.

COMPRESSION

The **compression** stroke applies pressure to soft tissues to squeeze them together without any slip. The tissues can either be pressed against the underlying bone, or they can be manually squeezed together with your own hands or fingers. Compression can be used to increase circulation, warm the tissues, de-

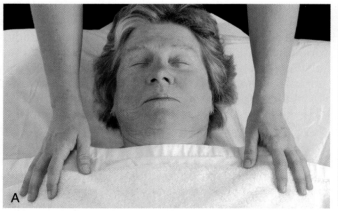
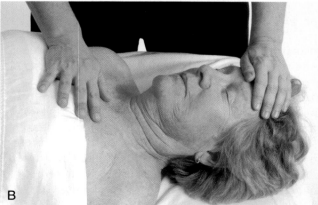

FIGURE 10-1 Resting strokes. **A.** Shoulders of supine client. **B.** Forehead and heart.

crease muscular tension, and reduce pain. You can apply compression with your thumbs, finger pads, the palm or heel of your hand, the knuckle portion of a fist, or your forearm. In a special form of bodywork called shiatsu, therapists also use their feet and knees to apply compression. (Fig. 10-2 shows some examples of compression.)

Effects of Compression

With your knowledge of anatomy and physiology of circulatory vessels, you can understand how compression is useful for increasing circulation and warming tissues. Blood is pushed through the arteries with the forceful contractions of the heart. By compressing the arteries and arterioles and stopping the flow of oxygenated blood, pressure builds behind the blockage as the heart continues to pump blood. When the compressed artery is released, a larger amount of blood rushes forth with a higher force than usual, warming the tissues supplied by that artery.

The veins and lymph vessels are equipped with valves that force their contents to flow in only one di-

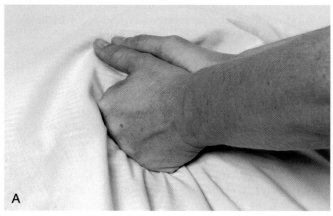

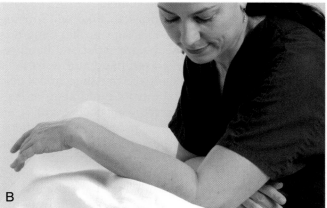

FIGURE 10-2 Compression strokes. **A.** Back of knuckles (fist). **B.** Forearm to gluteals.

rection. Compression strokes force blood out of the veins and through the one-way valves toward the heart. Likewise, compression on the lymph vessels forces lymph toward the lymph ducts that drain into the heart. There are better strokes for enhancing venous and lymph flow, but manual compression works as effectively as the active muscle contractions of the skeletal muscle pump.

Because of the thixotropic property of fascia, compression strokes can soften the fascia to restore movement and circulation to the muscles. Thus, compression can reduce muscular tension.

Muscles are composed of organized groups of muscles cells bundled together with fascia. Nerves and nerve cells travel through that fascia, carrying nerve impulses to and from the skeletal muscles. Compression on the soft tissues puts pressure on the nerves as well as the blood vessels and can reduce the nerve impulses transmitted by pain receptors. Consider the many ways people instinctively use pressure for pain relief:

- People put pressure on the cheek when they have a toothache.
- People press on their temples when they have a headache.
- People press on muscles that are sore.
- People press on their "shin" when they bump it.
- People squeeze the abdomen when they have abdominal pain.

Application of Compression

Thumbs, finger pads, palms or heels of the hand, fists, and forearms can be used to deliver compression. The stroke requires no slip on the skin, making it easier to apply compression without lubricant. You can squeeze tissues together to compress them, but that form of compression requires muscular work from your hands, which should be avoided when possible. To apply compression with less work, simply touch the client and gradually apply pressure using proper body mechanics such that your compression slowly sinks into the client's tissues. You can use your fingers to press on the tissues of the face or phalanges, but for the larger leg or gluteal muscles, you need to use good body mechanics with a proper lean to compress the tissues against underlying bones. If you are leaning instead of pushing into the large muscles, you will sink farther into the tissues as they soften up, without any extra effort. You can support your hand, finger pad, or thumb with the other hand when you need to maintain the compression for extended periods.

There is a variation of compression called rolling. Like the method you use to roll a pencil back and forth on a table, you can use rolling on the arms, legs, fingers, and toes by applying compression and rolling the structure back and forth under the pressure. There is no slip on the skin, so it does not matter whether there is lubricant on or not. The amount you can roll a body part varies with the size of the body part, the joint structure, and the soft tissue restrictions. Move slowly enough to sense a joint's end feel and stop the movement.

EFFLEURAGE

Effleurage is an elongated, slow stroke that slides across the surface of the client's skin with minimal drag. It benefits the skin by warming it with friction and increasing its circulation of blood and lymph, stimulating the sebaceous glands that make the skin soft and pliable. It is used to apply and spread lubricant, assess the client's soft tissues, create heat, increase circulation of blood and lymph, decrease muscle tension, relieve pain, and encourage relaxation and for connecting strokes. Your forearm, the palm or heel of your hand, your knuckles, thumbs, or finger pads can deliver effleurage strokes, but you need to use common sense. It is obviously inappropriate to use a forearm to apply effleurage to someone's face. The pressure varies from superficial to deep, and you need to keep your hands and wrists relaxed so they can gently encompass or mold to the client's body throughout the stroke. During the stroke, make palpation assessments regarding the quality of the client's tissues.

Effects of Effleurage

Most often, effleurage is used to apply and spread lubricant, and it is one of the best strokes for assessing the quality of superficial and deeper layers of tissue. You can feel the movement, fullness, texture, temperature, and body rhythms as your stroke travels across the tissues. When the effleurage stroke is directed toward the heart, it assists the return of blood and lymph through the valve system in the veins and lymph vessels, making it the best stroke for circulatory enhancement. As the effleurage stroke compresses tissues, it increases arterial circulation and cellular metabolism, including glycolysis, the heat-producing chemical reaction that occurs in muscle cells. Additional heat is created with the deformation and softening of the thixotropic fascia, which decreases muscular tension.

Ischemic tissues, or tissues that have a poor blood supply, are often painful as they suffer the effects of insufficient oxygen. Effleurage can restore circulation to ischemic tissues to improve the health of those tissues and reduce pain. With less pain, people are better able to relax.

Application of Effleurage

You must use lubricant for effleurage because the stroke travels across the surface of the client's skin. The lubricant reduces drag and increases slip to make the stroke more comfortable for clients. Be that as it may, too much slip is disadvantageous. It reduces your ability to assess the movement and texture of tissues, and you may need to compromise your body mechanics to resist the slip. Clients who have a lot of body hair present a special challenge. You can use more lubricant or use lubricants with a lot of slip, such as oil or gel, to keep from pulling their body hair. Some people find it uncomfortable to be rubbed "against the grain" of their body hair, so you may want to move in the same direction the hair lays, but some clients are not bothered if you use enough lubricant. Generally, effleurage strokes are performed at a rate of about 1–2 inches per second, and the **excursion,** or length of the stroke along the client's skin, is about 10–15 inches.

The amount of pressure that accompanies the effleurage stroke depends on where and why you apply it. Effleurage on the face typically uses very little pressure; effleurage on the back and shoulders usually requires more pressure. With that in mind, massage is a client-centered art that requires you to be aware of the needs of each client and treat accordingly.

Body mechanics must be incorporated with every stroke, but because effleurage is used so much, it is especially important to learn to use proper body mechanics with effleurage strokes. Keep your wrist and hand as relaxed as possible to minimize your own muscular tension and maximize your palpation sensitivity. Keep your joints stacked as much as possible and use a proper lean. Avoid twisting and bending, and maintain an asymmetric stance.

There are a few precautions to take when using your forearm to apply any massage stroke. First, it is especially important to keep your wrist and hand relaxed. A forearm with a relaxed hand and wrist feels better to the person receiving the massage, and it also benefits you. It prevents you from building up excess tension, it helps you conserve your energy, and it increases your sensitivity for palpation assessment. Second, although some persons recommend using your "elbow" to deliver pressure, you must use the proximal part of your forearm and not the point of the olecranon process. The ulnar nerve, which is often referred to as the "funny bone," is relatively unprotected as it runs through the cubital tunnel of the elbow, making it susceptible to damage if you use your olecranon process to apply pressure.

 To protect the ulnar nerve from damage, use the proximal part of your ulna to deliver pressure instead of the olecranon process.

(Fig. 10-3 shows various applications of effleurage, including proper use of the forearm.)

Superficial Effleurage

Superficial effleurage strokes can be performed with short, long, or circular motions with the thumbs, fingertips, or palms of the hands. Short and circular superficial effleurage can be applied to the face and other small areas of the body.

Nerve strokes are very light, feathery effleurage strokes applied in long, sweeping motions that are slow or fast (Fig. 10-4A). You can use them to "brush down" an area of the body after massaging it, giving the client's nervous system an opportunity to recognize that the invasive work is finished and that there is no need to stimulate sympathetic nervous activity.

Massage can cause a client to feel "disconnected" toward the end of the massage because each part of the body receives what can seem like a separate massage. For example, you spend some time massaging the client's back, spend a few minutes on the right arm, spend a few more minutes on the left arm, move to the left leg and devote several minutes to it, and then spend several minutes on the right leg, and so on. Nerve strokes can be used as connecting strokes during the massage, sweeping from the area that you just finished to the area you plan on massaging next. They signal a transition from one area to the next to help the client know what to expect. Remember, more relaxation is possible when the sympathetic nervous response is not stimulated. Clients who are comfortable and who know what to expect are more likely to relax throughout the massage, and nerve strokes are a nonverbal way to let clients know what you are doing.

Slow nerve strokes that run from head to toe can also be used at the end of the massage to conceptually and proprioceptively reconnect all of the separate body parts. The proprioceptors are the sensory receptors responsible for the position and tension of the muscles and joints to tell us where we are in physical space and to help us coordinate our movements. Nerve strokes that run the length of the body serve as gentle proprioceptive reminders of the position of all the body parts in space. The head-to-toe nerve stroke should last between 5 and 10 seconds, and as you move toward the client's feet, you take steps as necessary to maintain proper body mechanics:

1. Stand next to the massage table, at the client's shoulder, facing the client's head.
2. Gently rest the fingertips of both hands on the top of the client's head.
3. Apply a nerve stroke with your fingers from head to toe via:
   a. Top of the head
   b. Shoulders
   c. Elbows
   d. Hands
   e. From the hands onto the client's legs
   f. Knees
   g. Feet

If you always end massages with this full-body nerve stroke, your returning clients will learn that this stroke signals the completion of the massage.

Deep Effleurage

The deeper strokes are often applied with your thumb, your knuckles, the heel of your hand, interlaced fingers, or forearm. (Fig. 10-4B shows deep effleurage strokes applied with the thumbs.) You want the client's body to relax during deep effleurage so you can assess and treat the deeper tissues, thus you *must* apply the stroke slowly to avoid triggering protective muscular tension.

Again, you need to maintain proper body mechanics during effleurage. The asymmetric stance is usually better, since the stroke tends to travel along the client's skin. Apply deep effleurage strokes by leaning into tissues so that your stroke runs uphill rather than downhill. The compression is more effective when you lean into uphill tissues, and you tend to move more slowly and carefully. Gravity can accelerate a downhill stroke, and you may have to hold your body back to avoid sliding too fast. Resisting gravity requires unnecessary work and can create excess stress, so direct your deep effleurage strokes uphill.

PETRISSAGE

Petrissage is directly translated from French as "the act of kneading." It is delivered as a rhythmic series of intermittent compressions combined with a grasping and lifting action that pulls the tissues away from the bones. The tissues can either be compressed against the underlying bones or manually squeezed with your hands, but you must use proper body mechanics in either application. The benefits of effleurage also pertain to petrissage, but petrissage is

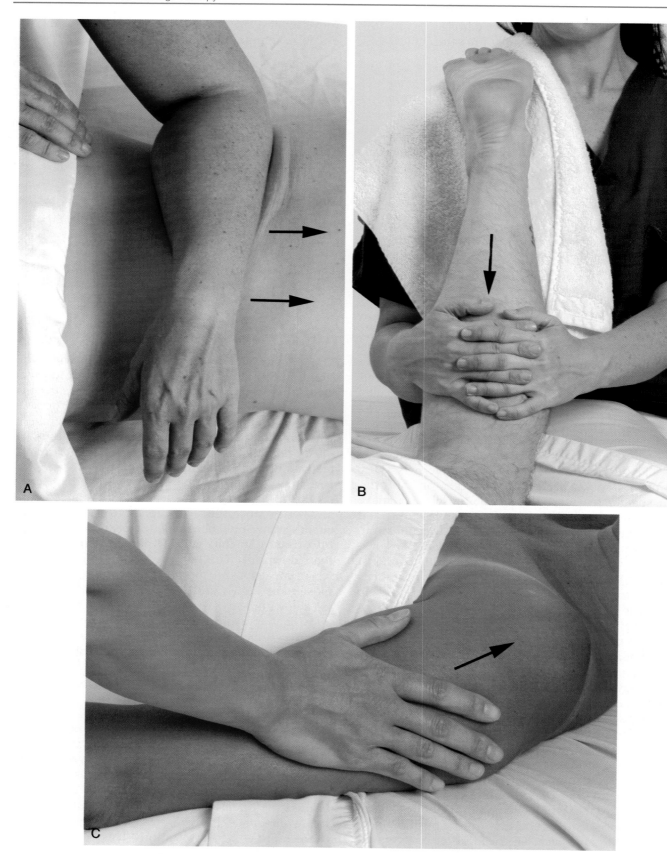

FIGURE 10-3 Effleurage strokes. **A.** Forearm. **B.** Interlaced fingers. **C.** Palm.

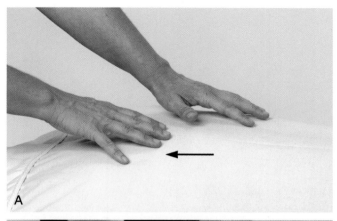

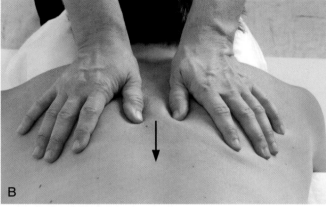

FIGURE 10-4 Types of effleurage. **A.** Superficial effleurage, also called nerve strokes. **B.** Deep effleurage.

more effective at improving muscle tone, increasing the elasticity of muscle tissue, and increasing muscle contractility.

Effects of Petrissage

The pressure of petrissage strokes increases the circulation of blood and lymph, stimulates sebaceous gland activity to soften the skin and keep it supple, warms the soft tissues, makes the muscles and fascia more pliable, decreases muscular tension, relieves pain, and encourages relaxation in the same way effleurage does. Petrissage is very effective at improving the health of muscle tissue. The deep kneading increases circulation and metabolism of all of the cells and tissues within a muscle, including the blood vessels, lymph vessels, nerve cells, and muscle cells. Studies have shown that muscles respond to massage with better muscle tone, more elasticity and pliability, and greater sensitivity to nerve impulses for contraction, or contractility. Muscles also demonstrate faster reaction times and more coordinated movements.

The focus of superficial petrissage is to soften the thixotropic fascia and increase circulation to the superficial fascia. Deep petrissage focuses on the muscle tissues and deep fascia. It deforms the deep fascia and improves the circulation of blood and lymph to the deepest layers of muscles, which increases the elasticity and health of the muscle tissue.

Application of Petrissage

The amount of force you put into your petrissage varies, but generally, thicker tissues take more pressure. Superficial applications of petrissage are very much like skin pinches and require little or no lubricant because the strokes only treat the superficial fascia and subcutaneous fat. The strokes can be effective when applied to general areas of the body, both localized and broad, because the focus is on the continuous sheet of superficial fascia.

Because of the effects of deep petrissage on the muscle tissues, these strokes are often applied to an individual muscle or a group of synergistic muscles rather than a general area of the body. For deeper applications of petrissage, you may need a small amount of lubricant to prevent the stroke from pinching, to ensure that the strokes are comfortable, and to help put the muscle or group of muscles into passive contraction. When muscles are stretched out, the aligned muscle fibers get closer together and become taut, like the way a rubber band acts when it is pulled tight. In a **passive contraction,** you bring the origin and insertion of a client's muscle closer together while the client relaxes. Again, like a rubber band, the muscle fibers are more flexible and pliable in this position, allowing you to work deeper with less effort. If you attempt to resolve deep muscle tension in muscles that are stretched tight, you waste energy and can hurt the client. The stroke has no true excursion; you apply a series of individual strokes all over the area you are treating. Each stroke should move to a slightly different spot so that you do not grasp the same exact tissues twice in succession. As you apply petrissage in an attempt to reach the deeper tissues, slowly increase your pressure to allow the tissues time to adjust and soften enough to let you in. Petrissage is generally applied with soft hands that squeeze, lift, and release the client's tissues in an alternating rhythm of left and right hands. A typical rhythm for petrissage is about one stroke per second, but the rhythm is faster for smaller or thinner tissues such as the face and hand, and slower for the thicker or larger tissues like the thigh and scapular area.

Try to keep your fingers together and use them as one large surface to scoop the tissues into the fleshy part at the base of the thumb called the thenar eminence (THEH-nahr EHM-ih-nents), grasp and squeeze those tissues gradually, and then release them. By pulling the tissues up and away from the bone, you mechanically deform and separate the layers of superficial and deep fascia more than you can with rhythmic compression or effleurage strokes. Some variations of petrissage use your thumb and finger pads, and others use a soft fist to push the tissues into the relaxed, cupped palm of the other hand. (Fig. 10-5 illustrates different forms of petrissage.)

Petrissage is one of the more challenging strokes when it comes to maintaining good body mechanics. The hand muscles are required to work harder than normal to squeeze and lift tissues. Also, excessive strain occurs in the muscles that move the forearm and wrist because you use so much active supination, pronation, and wrist extension. As you repeatedly compress and lift the tissues, it is easy to forget about leaning properly. Make sure you maintain the straight line between your head and back toe when you lean and lift to avoid stress on your low back. Try to minimize the amount of petrissage you use because it requires so much muscular work, and when you do use it, watch your body mechanics.

Variations of Petrissage

Deep petrissage is occasionally applied without the grasping and lifting component, which makes it resemble circular deep effleurage. Because the focus is still on intermittent and rhythmic compression of the tissues, the stroke is still considered petrissage. There is minimal slip on the skin, just as with standard petrissage, but instead of grasping the tissues, you push them aside and out of the way, which causes them to lift up to some extent.

During a massage, you may cross an area of restricted superficial fascia, which can feel as if your massage stroke is skidding along the client's skin or has come to a stop. In other words, the slip turns into drag. There are several forms of petrissage that you can use to loosen these restrictions. Wringing is a slow application of petrissage that does not include the lifting component. The hand movement of this stroke mimics the act of wringing out a wet towel and is very similar to an "Indian burn" that children give each other, except there is no friction or slip on the client's skin. You grasp a limb with both hands and simultaneously rotate your hands in opposite directions without any slip on the skin. One stroke lasts 2 seconds, making it more like a very slow moving compression stroke that primarily deforms the superficial fascia.

Skin rolling is a variation of petrissage that primarily lifts the superficial fascia to deform and loosen it.

 Skin rolling can be fairly uncomfortable to clients, so move slowly and pay attention to their response.

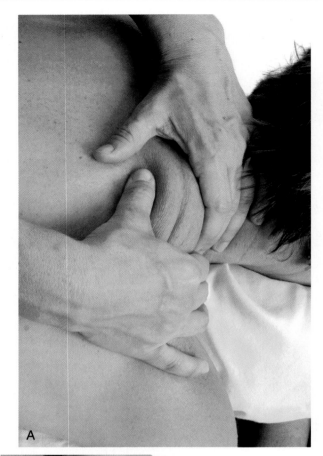

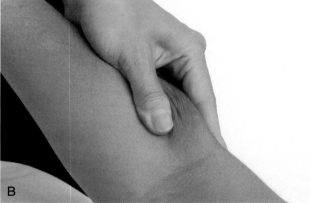

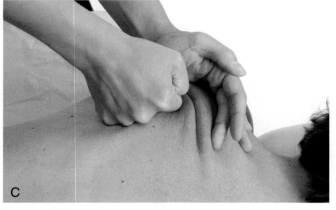

FIGURE 10-5 Different kinds of petrissage. **A.** Whole hand. **B.** Thumb and fingers. **C.** Into cupped hand.

Grasp a large section of skin and superficial fascia with your thumbs and finger pads. Pinch it together and lift it up, away from the body. With the roll of tissue in your grasp, you *very slowly* walk your fingertips and thumbs away from you while keeping the roll of tissue elevated (Fig. 10-6). The rate of movement tends to be about 1 centimeter per second, but looser fascia can be rolled faster, and more restricted fascia must be rolled more slowly. The excursion of the skin roll should travel across the area of the restriction, which can be anywhere between 3 and 12 inches or longer. Make sure that there is no lubricant on the skin because you need to have a firm hold on the tissues, which is impossible with lubricant. If you find an area of restricted superficial fascia in the middle of a massage and have already applied lubricant, you can use a towel to wipe off the excess. This technique can be applied therapeutically if you perform specific assessments prior to using a skin roll. (See the chapter on therapeutic techniques for more detail.)

TAPOTEMENT

Tapotement is a fast rhythmic stroke that uses both hands, like rapid drumming. In fact, sometimes tapotement is referred to as percussion, and it can be applied with cupped hands, flat hands, the medial side of open hands, the medial side of the relaxed fists, or the fingertips. See Figure 10-7 for different examples of tapotement. Initial and very light tapotement strokes stimulate the sympathetic nervous system and cause superficial vasoconstriction. Conversely, sustained and heavy tapotement results in superficial vasodilation, pain relief, and relaxation.

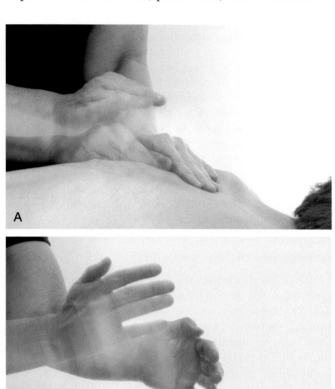

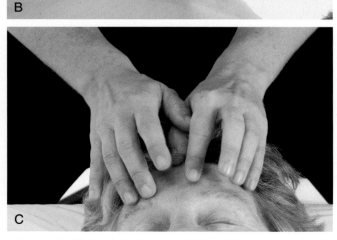

FIGURE 10-6 Skin rolling.

FIGURE 10-7 Tapotement. **A.** Cupping. **B.** Hacking. **C.** Tapping.

Effects of Tapotement

The different effects of tapotement are determined by its application. Consistent with the general physiological effects of touch, initially tapotement is more stimulating than relaxing, whereas prolonged applications encourage relaxation. In addition to stimulating the parasympathetic nervous response, research shows that several minutes of tapotement has an anesthetic effect on hypersensitive nerve endings.[1] When applied with more force, the effects of tapotement are similar to those of compression, including vasodilation, increased circulation, and increased tissue temperature. Firm, abrupt applications of tapotement, especially when applied near the musculotendinous junction, stimulate muscle contractions with the tendon reflex. The response to very light fingertip tapotement is quite different, however, as the body reacts with a more protective mechanism. Vasoconstriction of the superficial blood vessels pulls them away from the surface of the skin to keep them from being damaged. Therapeutically, tapotement with cupped hands can be used to break up congestion in the lungs of people with cystic fibrosis. This stroke can be very effective, but you need a thorough understanding of the pathological condition, you need to know the specific technique, and the client will benefit more if you can work with the client's physician.

Application of Tapotement

There is no slip with any form of tapotement, so the stroke can be performed with or without lubricant. The rhythmic percussive strokes are delivered very quickly, somewhere around five beats per second, but they can be applied faster with the fingertips and more slowly with the fists. There is a critical elastic component of tapotement that allows the stroke to affect the deeper layers of tissue without damaging the more superficial layers, and it can only be accomplished by keeping your wrists and hands relaxed. In addition to being safer for the client's tissues and being less stressful for your body, tapotement delivered with a relaxed, springy rebound feels better. As in petrissage, there is no excursion with the stroke. You apply a series of individual strokes over the area you are treating.

The different variations of tapotement can be applied as follows (Fig. 10-7 illustrates some of these):

- To use cupped hands (cupping), your wrists must stay relaxed, but you need to hold your fingers loosely in the cupped position. When you strike the client's skin, the cupped hand should make a resounding kind of hollow noise.
- To use the flat surface of your finger pads (slapping), keep your fingers together but keep your wrists and fingers relaxed and loose. When your hand strikes the client's skin, it should sound and feel like a light smack.
- If you use the medial edge of your open hands for tapotement (hacking), keep your hands relaxed so that your fingers are comfortably spread apart. Upon striking the client's skin, your relaxed fingers "squish" together to absorb some of the shock.
- To use your fists for tapotement (pummeling or beating), keep your fists and wrists loose, and only use this stroke on the fleshy areas of the body such as the hips, thighs, and gluteal areas. There is almost no sound when your fist strikes the client's skin.
- If you use your fingertips for tapotement (tapping), the superficial fascia should be thin to create the appropriate effect. No sound occurs with fingertip tapotement because you use hardly any pressure, and you keep your fingers relaxed to absorb what little rebound there is.

As you apply tapotement, constantly move around to avoid striking the same spot repeatedly and be careful of areas where nerves and organs are relatively unprotected.

> ⚠ *Do not use tapotement directly over the spine, bruises, or varicose veins and be very careful when applying it to the back over the kidneys.*

The kidneys are relatively unprotected and are suspended in a fatty mass called the adipose capsule, and although it is not likely that you will shake them loose with tapotement, you need to ensure that you do not traumatize or injure them. The kidneys are located on either side of the spine, at the level of the superior lumbar vertebrae, just beneath the ribcage.

Watch your body mechanics when you use tapotement. Besides keeping your wrists and hands relaxed, use your legs with your knees slightly bent as you move around to apply tapotement instead of bending and twisting at the waist.

FRICTION

Friction is a stroke that can be applied superficially or deep with completely different methods and effects. **Superficial friction** is a brisk variation of light effleurage intended to increase circulation in the superficial tissues and dissipate body heat. The application of **deep fiber friction** (also called **cross fiber friction** and **transverse friction**) resembles the variation of compression called rolling. It is a deep, localized application of pressure, without any slip on the skin, primarily used to break up fascial adhesions and separate the muscle fibers.

Effects of Friction

Heat is created by friction, which is the physical resistance between two surfaces as they rub against each other. The massage stroke called superficial friction is applied by briskly rubbing the client's skin to create heat. It mechanically enhances the flow of blood and lymph and reflexively causes vasodilation in the skin, which increases circulation in the skin, increases the temperature of the skin and superficial fascia, and dissipates body heat from the skin. The general purpose of superficial friction is to create heat and increase the blood flow to the treated area, or local hyperemia (HAHY-per-EE-mee-ah).

Deep fiber friction is quite different from superficial friction. The pressure of the stroke increases circulation in the deep fascia and muscle tissues, breaks up fascial adhesions and scar tissue, and separates the different components within a muscle. Chronically hypertonic muscle tissue is often accompanied by restrictions in the deep fascia. When people "stretch" their connective tissues, the elongation of the tissues also causes the muscle fibers and surrounding fascia to get closer together. Deep fiber friction, especially when applied perpendicular to the relaxed muscle fibers of a passive contraction, is uniquely able to separate those fibers, increase local circulation, and restore movement.

Application of Friction

More heat is created when there is more resistance between your and the client's skin, so if you are applying superficial friction to warm the tissues, less lubricant is better. The rate of the strokes is moderately fast, somewhere around 1–3 strokes per second, and the length of the stroke along the skin, or excursion, is a few inches. You can use your thumbs, finger pads, or palms to apply superficial friction with just enough pressure to feel the surface resistance as you briskly rub the client's skin. When you vigorously rub your palms together to warm them up, you are using superficial friction. To maintain proper body mechanics for superficial friction, keep your arms, wrists, and hands as relaxed as possible and minimize the use of superficial friction because it requires vigorous activity on your part.

Deep fiber friction is applied without any slip on the skin, so again, little or no lubricant is better. It can be applied perpendicular to the length of the muscle fibers with a strumming action, or it can be applied in a circular motion over the muscle fibers. Typically, deep fiber friction strokes take about 3 sec-

onds to travel across 1 inch of muscle tissue, without any slip on the skin. You can use your thumbs, finger pads, the knuckle portion of a fist, or your forearm, but it is wise to always remember the body mechanics rules of keeping your joints stacked, keeping your shoulders down, and maintaining a proper lean. See Figure 10-8 for deep fiber friction over the erector spinae muscles. Because deep fiber friction can be perceived as an invasive technique, you must prevent the guarding response by warming up the tissue with other techniques prior to applying it.

VIBRATION

Vibration is a stroke that involves high-frequency shaky hand movements. Vibrations can travel through our bodies, affecting everything from the surface of the skin to the deepest organs. A common misconception in massage is that deep tissue work requires a lot of pressure or manipulation, but vibration demonstrates just how incorrect that is. Consider how the ground shakes when a large trailer truck rumbles by or how you *feel* the booming bass of a nearby car stereo sometimes more than you hear it. Vibration can be used to stimulate the nerves, muscles, and organs, to increase circulation and temperature of local tissues, and as a form of anesthesia. Some variations of vibration, including rocking, shaking, and jostling, are generally used for relaxation.

Effects of Vibration

Muscle contractions can be sustained when the muscle receives 10–20 nerve impulses per second. Vibration can stimulate muscle contractions when the frequency of the vibratory movements matches or exceeds the frequency of the nerve impulses for muscle contraction. Unfortunately, our hands can move

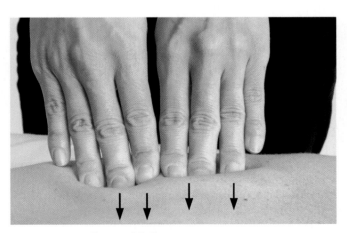

FIGURE **10-8** Deep fiber friction.

at a rate of about 10–12 movements per second, which is not usually fast enough to stimulate muscle contraction. If you or your clients want the stimulating effects of vibration, you can consider using a machine that is more effective at delivering the necessary high frequencies. Like the other initial reflexive effects of touch, vibration initially stimulates the nervous system and organ activity. The effect is very similar to being shaken awake or shaken to pay attention. After several minutes of vibration, the reflexive effects of relaxation begin: pain sensitivity is decreased, circulation increases, the temperature of the tissues increases, and muscle tension decreases.

Application of Vibration

Some people find it difficult to learn how to apply vibration because you have to keep your shoulder, arm, wrist, and hand very relaxed while moving them very fast. Without loose joints and muscles, you will create excessive strain on your muscles and you lose the effectiveness of the stroke. Rest your relaxed fingertips or finger pads on the client's skin and start moving your wrist and hand with a gentle, nervous trembling motion. Again, maintain proper body mechanics by staying as relaxed as possible, from your shoulders through your fingertips. Your fingers can remain stationary on the client's skin or you can lightly slide your fingertips along the surface of the client's skin while applying vibration.

Variations of Vibration

Rocking is a technique for which you use smooth, rhythmic, intermittent pushes to slowly rock a client's limb or entire body. Slow and gentle rocking movement is a well-known way to soothe and relax babies and adults, alike. Rocking is accomplished by maintaining the back-and-forth rhythm of the client's body with well-timed series of pushes and releases. You can put pressure on the client's arm, leg, or pelvis to create the rocking motion. You must tune into the client's natural rhythm when rocking to allow the body to relax. Once you start rocking the client, make sure that you push at exactly the same time the client's body is starting to roll away from you. If you push while the body is still rolling toward you, there will be an irregularity and awkwardness to the rocking that is more bothersome than relaxing. The main purpose of rocking is to encourage relaxation.

Jostling moves the client's limbs back and forth in a wavelike snaking motion. As with shaking, the purpose of jostling is to confuse the nervous system and induce relaxation. It is applied by grasping an arm or leg, providing a small amount of traction, and then moving the extremity by wiggling it side to side (Fig. 10-9).

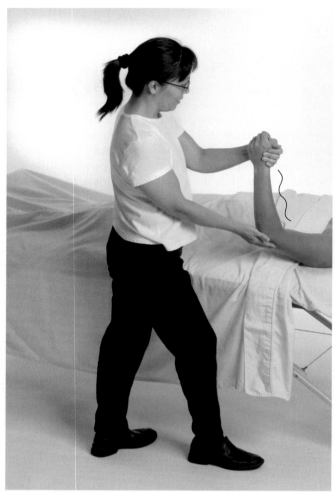

FIGURE 10-9 Jostling.

Joint Movement

All of the movements of the synovial joints are listed in the special muscle section at the end of the anatomy and physiology chapter. Movement of the synovial joints, whether active or passive, encourages the production of synovial fluid, which nourishes and protects the joint structures. Joint movement also encourages the circulation of lymph by activating the skeletal muscle pump mechanism. Joint movements are easily incorporated into a massage and are very beneficial for the client. Passive movements require that you hold and move your clients gently and securely. Figure 10-10 illustrates passive lateral flexion of the neck. It takes more work on your part but allows clients to relax while you evaluate the quality and quantity of the movement. Active movements allow you to save your own energy because the client does the work while you visually evaluate the quality and quantity of the movement. Some clients do not

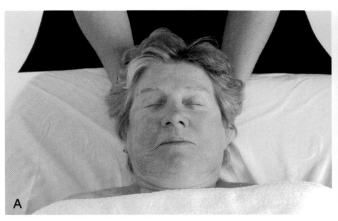 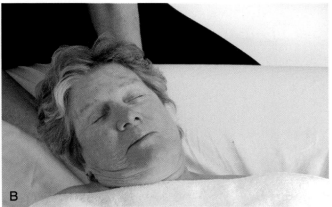

FIGURE 10-10   Passive lateral flexion of the neck. **A.** Starting position. **B.** Final position: at limit.

like to participate during the massage session, but you can still incorporate active joint movements during the pretreatment and posttreatment assessments.

Flow

You are now faced with the challenge of putting all of your academic knowledge and artistic skill into a massage. The first time you stand beside a client who is lying on a massage table, waiting for a massage, you may wonder whether it is possible to spend an hour massaging one body. Where do you start? What strokes do you use? Should the client start supine or prone? What position should the client be in? You will find the answers to these questions by learning and understanding massage flow, which is a routine-like sequence of steps that leads the massage from one body part to the next in a systematic, fluid pattern.

Similar to a cooking recipe, a flow is a set of step-by-step directions for your massage. It usually specifies the client's position on the table and tells you which body parts to work on and in what order. A flow can also suggest massage strokes to use on the different areas of the body. With practice, a flow becomes second nature and lets you evaluate the tissues throughout the massage instead of focusing on which body part to work on and what strokes to use. Good cooking recipes present their directions in a logical order that can be followed easily and efficiently. In the same way, a good massage flow guides therapists through a fluid, logical order from body part to body part without a lot of wasted time or energy. For instance, a good flow might direct you to massage the client's right hand, work up the right arm to the right shoulder, connect the right and left shoulder with a resting stroke in which one hand is on each shoulder,

and with a nerve stroke, move down to the client's left hand to begin work there. A bad flow might instruct you to massage the client's right hand, then move to the left hand, then the right shoulder, and then to the client's left shoulder. As a recipe is written to help us prepare edible and presentable food that people enjoy and does not make people sick, the massage flow is designed to accomplish the long-term treatment goal without endangering the client's health.

FLOW SEQUENCES FOR DIFFERENT CLIENT POSITIONS

There are general flows for clients in the supine position, prone position, laterally recumbent (side-lying) position, and seated position. Each position limits your access to some part of the client's body, which is why most therapists prefer asking a client to assume two or three different body positions during the massage. The flow sequences for these different positions outlined below are very general directions that guide your movement around the client's body to access all the different body parts smoothly and efficiently. The accompanying illustrations provide suggestions for exposing the body parts with your draping techniques. As you gain experience, you will develop your own combination of strokes and techniques, but as a place to begin, the following section includes suggestions for sample flows for specific body parts.

Supine Position

The supine position is a good position to access the anterior side of the body—the face, the chest, the abdomen, and the anterior aspect of the legs. Unfortunately, it is difficult to reach the posterior portions of the body. Persons with sinus congestion, those who do not like confined spaces, and those who are very talkative during a massage may prefer the supine

PROCEDURE BOX 10-1
Supine Massage Flow

1. Stand or sit at the head of the massage table, facing the client to massage the
   - Face
   - Ears
   - Scalp
   - Neck
   - Upper chest
   - Shoulders

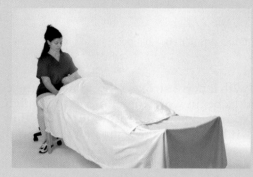

2. Walk to the client's left side, undrape the left arm and massage the client's left hand, forearm, upper arm, and shoulder, and redrape the arm.

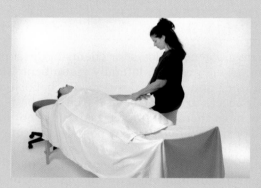

3. Use connecting strokes to walk toward the client's left foot.

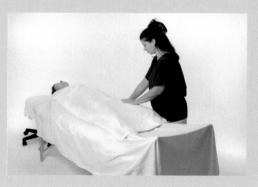

4. Sit or stand at the client's feet, undrape the left foot and massage the

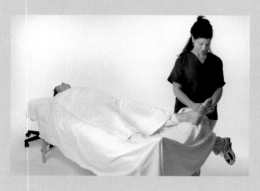

   - Sole
   - Ball of the foot
   - Toes
   - Top of the metatarsals
   - All around the ankle and heel

5. Stand at the client's left side, expose the left leg, and massage the

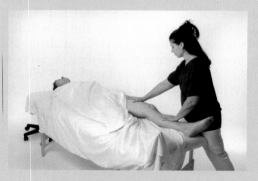

   - Lower leg
   - Upper leg

6. Redrape the left leg and move to the client's feet.

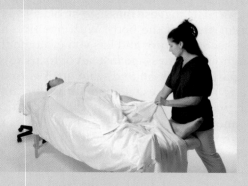

7. Undrape the client's right foot and massage the sole of the foot, ball of the foot, toes, and all around the ankle and heel.

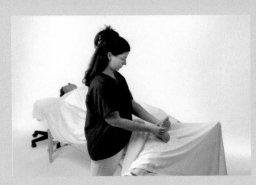

8. Stand at the client's right side. Expose the right leg and massage the lower leg and upper leg.

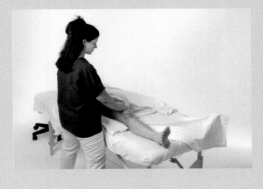

9. Redrape the right leg, undrape the right arm, and massage the
   - Hand
   - Forearm
   - Upper arm
   - Shoulder

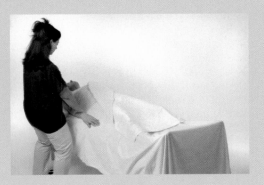

10. Redrape the arm and apply head-to-toe nerve strokes to reconnect the entire body.

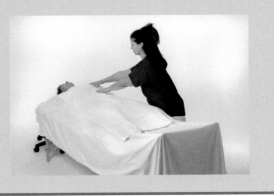

position. Procedure Box 10-1 includes an illustrated series of steps for a general supine massage flow.

Prone Position

Clients who are not interested in having a conversation or who are suffering back pain may prefer the prone, or face-down, position. In this position, you have particularly good access to a client's back, gluteal muscles, and the posterior aspects of the legs, but your access to the anterior aspect of the body is limited. If a client uses the face cradle to maintain a neutral neck position while lying in the prone position, the entire neck and shoulder region is easily accessible to you. Procedure Box 10-2 includes a sample flow for massaging clients in the prone position.

Side-lying Position

The side-lying position is not as popular as the others because it requires additional bolstering and because the draping can be challenging and awkward.

Many therapists do not incorporate this position into their massages, but there are times when a client is better served in the side-lying position. For example, it is dangerous to keep a pregnant woman supine during her last few months of pregnancy because the fetus can put excessive pressure on her descending aorta. Since massage is very beneficial during pregnancy, these clients can safely receive massage in the side-lying position as long as there are no systemic contraindications. Prenatal or pregnancy massage is covered in more detail in Chapter 12, Special Populations. Additionally, when a client has a lot of neck and shoulder restrictions, you have excellent access to the entire region when the client is in the side-lying position. It also gives you a unique ability to maneuver the client's neck and shoulders through all of the possible joint movements, so if you find that many of your clients are complaining of neck and shoulder problems, you should incorporate the side-lying position. Procedure Box 10-3 includes an example of a massage flow

PROCEDURE BOX 10-2
Prone Massage Flow

1. Standing at the client's left side in an asymmetric stance, place your hands on top of the drape and apply a resting stroke to the client's low back.
2. Expose the client's back and, working only on the client's left side, massage the
   - Back
   - Scapular area
   - Shoulder area
   - Neck area
3. Use connecting strokes to walk around the client's head to the client's right side and massage the right side of the client's back, scapular area, shoulder area, and neck area.
4. Redrape the back and use connecting strokes to move to the client's right gluteal area.
5. Massage the right gluteal muscles on top of the sheet, with compression and possibly some petrissage.
6. Expose the client's right leg and massage the
   - Upper leg
   - Lower leg
7. Redrape the right leg, leaving the right foot exposed, and sit or stand at the end of the table to massage the client's right foot.
8. Redrape the right foot and use connecting strokes to walk around the table to the client's left gluteal area.
9. Massage the left gluteal muscles on top of the sheet with compression and possibly some petrissage.
10. Expose the client's left leg and massage the upper leg and lower leg.
11. Redrape the left leg, leaving the left foot exposed, and sit or stand at the end of the table to massage the client's left foot.
12. Redrape the left foot, and place one hand on each of the client's feet as a resting stroke.

PROCEDURE BOX 10-3
Side-lying Massage Flow (client positioned as in Fig. 9-3)

1. Stand at the side of the table, facing the client's back, and rest your hands on the client's left shoulder and hip.
2. Expose the client's back and massage the left side of the
   - Back
   - Scapular area
   - Shoulder
   - Neck
3. Redrape the back and maintain contact with your client as you walk around his or her head to the other side of the table.
4. Facing your client, expose the left arm and massage the
   - Hand
   - Forearm
   - Upper arm
   - Shoulder
   - Neck
5. Redrape the left arm, and use connecting strokes to move to the legs.
6. Expose the left leg (top leg) and massage the
   - Upper leg
   - Lower leg
   - Foot
7. Redrape the left leg and use connecting strokes as you move around the client's feet to the other side of the table and stand beside the right leg.
8. Expose the right leg and massage the
   - Upper leg
   - Lower leg
   - Foot
9. Redrape the right leg and use a head-to-toe nerve stroke to reconnect the body.

for a client who is lying *on* her right side, properly positioned and bolstered.

Seated Position

Although it does not happen often, you may need to give a complete relaxation massage to a client who is seated. If someone is unable to climb onto your table, is not comfortable lying down, or is bound to a wheelchair, a seated massage may be appropriate. This seated flow is designed for relaxation, making it different from the stimulating focus of chair and corporate massages with a short duration. Since clients remain clothed for the massage, there are no draping considerations, but if they wear shorts and tank tops or short sleeves, you have better access to their tissues and can apply more strokes that offer clients more benefits. You can easily apply compression, tapotement, and vibration through clothing, and pos-

sibly some petrissage or deep fiber friction. Effleurage, which is such a good stroke for assessing the condition of the client's tissues, is not appropriate for clients who are clothed. You can deliver a seated massage to a client in a chair by following the steps in Procedure Box 10-4.

Full-Body Massage Flows

The sample flows do not provide directions for a full body massage because of the individualized aspect of each massage. Your artistic combination of strokes and techniques, the speed at which you apply them, and the length of time you keep the client in any one position creates a unique massage every time. Using the sample flows, you can combine them in any order to accomplish a full body or partial body massage. Most massage therapists use the prone and supine positions, in either order, but you should try several

PROCEDURE BOX 10-4
Seated Relaxation Massage Flow (client fully clothed)

1. Stand behind the client's chair, and gently rest your hands on the client's shoulders.
2. Slowly move your hands to the top of the client's head and massage the
   - Scalp
   - Neck
   - Shoulders
   - Scapular areas
   - Any areas of the back you can access easily, which depends on the chair
3. Maintain contact with the client as you move to the client's left side.
4. Sit or kneel next to the client to massage the left hand.
5. Stand up to massage the
   - Forearm
   - Upper arm
   - Shoulder
6. Use connecting strokes as you move around to the client's right side and sit or kneel next to the client to massage the right hand.
7. Stand up to massage the forearm, upper arm, and shoulder.
8. Sit or kneel next to the client's right foot and massage the
   - Right foot
   - Right lower leg
   - Right thigh
9. Move to the client's left foot and massage the left foot, left lower leg, and left thigh.
10. Stand up, facing the client, and use a head-to-toe nerve stroke to reconnect the body.

different combinations to get comfortable with the change of positions and the draping considerations:

- Clients start supine, then turn over, finishing in the prone position
- Clients start prone, then turn over to finish in the supine position
- Clients start prone, assume a side-lying position on their right side, turn to lie on their left side, then turn onto their back, finishing in the supine position
- Clients start supine, lie on their left side, turn over to their right side, then flip once more to finish in the prone position
- Clients start in the side-lying position on one side, then flip over to finish in the side-lying position on the other side

It takes time for clients to change positions during a massage, so you may want to keep the number of positions to a minimum. Also, some clients do not like to have to move during the massage and do not

appreciate having to flip over more than once during the massage. On the other hand, therapeutic massage is intended to treat soft tissue conditions that you discover before and during treatment, and it may serve the client best to use more than two positions during a massage. If you discover that the client will benefit from multiple positions, educate them on your plan and why you will be moving them around during the session.

SAMPLE FLOW SEQUENCES FOR SPECIFIC AREAS

Below are some suggested flows to familiarize you with the process of combining basic massage strokes with resting strokes and connecting strokes. These flows are only a guide to get you started. Once you are comfortable holding and touching clients and you can use different massage strokes effectively, use the strokes you think are most appropriate, and treat the client's body parts in the order that makes sense to you. In all of the following flows, clients start fully draped in the position indicated, and you have performed your grounding and centering techniques. There are no specific directions for lubricant application because it is up to you to determine how much is necessary to make your strokes comfortable with the right amount of slip.

Supine: Chest, Neck, and Head

A supine client's chest, neck, and head can all be accessed from one position, as you stand at the head of the massage table.

> ⚠️ When massaging the chest and neck area, do not put pressure over the endangerment sites of the anterior triangle of the neck, the jugular vein, and the brachial plexus.

Procedure Box 10-5 illustrates a massage sequence for a supine client's chest, neck, and head.

Supine: Arm

It is possible to massage the client's arm in both the prone and supine positions. The shoulder, however, is capable of more joint movements when clients are supine. The massage sequence in Procedure Box 10-6 describes how you can massage the arm of a client who is in the supine position.

Supine: Abdomen

The abdomen can only be accessed in the supine position. The client's knees must be bent to keep the abdominal area soft enough to let you apply pressure,

PROCEDURE BOX 10-5
Massage Flow for a Supine Client's Chest, Neck, and Head

1. Standing at the client's head, uncover the client's upper chest, tuck the drape underneath the client's armpits, and perform a resting stroke with one hand on each shoulder.

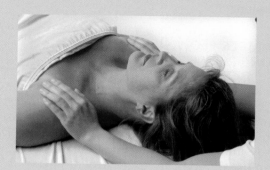

2. Effleurage the client's chest, from the sternum to the shoulders, with both palms simultaneously, 2–3 times.

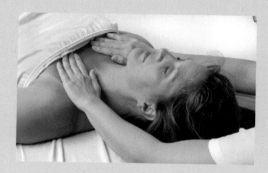

3. Effleurage the back of the client's shoulders, from the deltoids to the neck, using both palms simultaneously, 2–3 times.

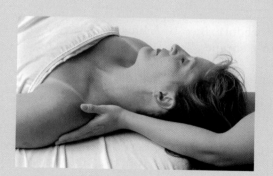

4. Redrape the upper chest and slide both hands under the shoulders to cradle the client's upper thoracic spine with both hands. Using your finger pads, effleurage and petrissage the muscles just lateral to the spine, all the way up to the occipital ridge, about 20 seconds.

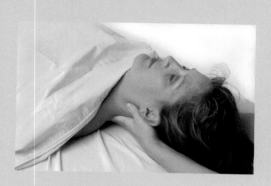

5. Cradle the client's head and perform passive joint movements:
   - Neck flexion
   - Neck rotation to the left and to the right
   - Lateral neck flexion to the left and to the right

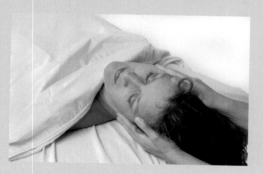

6. Petrissage the entire scalp and external parts of the ear with your fingertips and thumbs, 20 seconds.

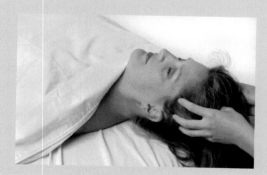

7. Starting medial and moving laterally, use your thumbs and fingertips to effleurage once or twice each:
   - Along mandible
   - Along maxilla
   - Along inferior surface of zygomatic process to temples
   - Along eyebrow ridge
   - Along the top of the forehead

9. Apply nerve strokes from the chin to the temples, twice.

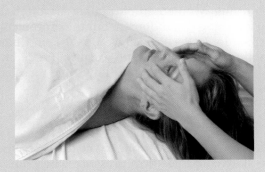

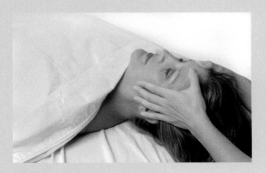

10. Loosely cradle the client's head.

8. Use your fingertips to apply tapotement lightly to the face, 10 seconds.

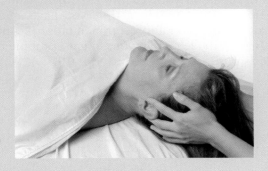

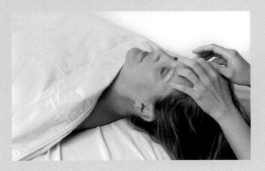

 Procedure Box 10-6
Massage Flow for a Supine Client's Arm

1. Stand at your client's right side, facing your client.
2. Push the drape aside to take hold of the client's right hand and expose the arm, tucking the edge of the sheet under the client's arm and under the armpit, and place the arm on top of the sheet.
3. Effleurage and petrissage the palm and the back of the client's hand and each finger individually, using your thumbs and finger pads, about 20 seconds.
4. Perform joint movement by passively extending client's wrist and fingers in pairs:
   - Pinky and thumb
   - Ring finger and index finger
   - Middle finger and wrist
5. Jostle the client's arm while grasping the client's hand and supporting the elbow.

6. Effleurage and petrissage the forearm, maintaining your grasp of the client's wrist with one hand for stability while you apply a stroke with your other hand, and then alternate hands to apply strokes, proximally from wrist to elbow, about 20 seconds.
7. Rest your client's arm on the table for support while you apply effleurage and petrissage with alternating hands, proximally from elbow to shoulder and over the deltoids, about 20 seconds. You can abduct your client's arm to put the deltoids into passive contraction, which allows you to get deeper into the tissues with less work.
8. Apply nerve strokes from shoulder to wrist.
9. Redrape the arm and apply nerve strokes from shoulder to hand.
10. Connect the client's wrist and shoulder with a resting stroke.

so you can use a bolster to hold the knees up. Many people are uncomfortable with abdominal massage, but it is beneficial for the digestive system and is worth trying. Women, in particular, are often uneasy about exposing the abdomen, but the draping process described in earlier Procedure Box 9-1, in Chapter 9, maintains their modesty and warmth. Procedure Box 10-7 includes a suggested flow for massaging a client's abdomen.

Supine: Leg and Foot

The feet are especially prone to the ticklish sensation. Move slowly and use firm pressure when massaging feet to avoid that response. The legs and feet can be treated in both the supine and prone positions, and whether you use one or both positions in your massage depends on your client's treatment goals, your preference, the amount of time you have, and your instructor or school's recommendations. Applying massage to the leg when your client is supine can be done as outlined in Procedure Box 10-8.

Prone: Back

The prone position allows you access to the entire back, and also gives you a good opportunity to make visual assessments. As you apply massage to the back, remember that the kidneys are relatively unprotected.

 Use light applications of tapotement over the kidneys so you do not traumatize or injure them.

PROCEDURE BOX 10-7
Massage Flow for a Supine Client's Abdomen

1. Make sure client's knees are bent, and expose the abdomen (for a female client, follow the instructions in Procedure Box 9-1).
2. Use a symmetric stance to face directly across the table at the client's side and effleurage with both hands crossing the abdomen in an alternating pattern, 8 strokes.
3. Change to an asymmetric stance beside the client's femur, angled toward the client's head, and effleurage the abdomen with the flats of your alternating hands, in a clockwise pattern, 8 strokes.
4. Apply a resting stroke with both palms on the client's abdomen.
5. Redrape the abdomen, and apply a resting stroke on top of the drape, connecting the abdomen to the upper part of the client's sternum.

PROCEDURE BOX 10-8
Massage Flow for a Supine Client's Leg and Foot

1. Stand, kneel, or sit at the foot of the table, or sit on the end of the table, expose the client's foot, and apply compression by squeezing both sides of the client's foot, about 5 times.
2. Deep effleurage the sole of the foot, distally with your thumbs, 3 times.
3. Apply circular friction to the ball of the foot with your thumbs, about 20 seconds.
4. Apply deep effleurage with your thumbs or finger pads around the ankles, and along the tops of the metatarsals and each toe, moving distally, 2–3 times.
5. Perform joint movements by passively
   ■ Extending each toe
   ■ Moving the ankle through a circular motion from dorsiflexion, to eversion, to plantarflexion, to inversion
6. Hold the client's foot for a resting stroke.
7. Expose the leg and stand near the client's foot in an asymmetric stance, facing the client's head.
8. Effleurage and petrissage the anterior and lateral aspects of the lower leg, in a proximal direction, using your thumbs and the heels of your hands, about 30 seconds.
9. Effleurage and petrissage the anterior, medial, and lateral aspects of the client's thigh, using your palms, the heels of your hands, or your fists, about 30 seconds.
10. Redrape the leg and apply nerve strokes from the client's hip to toes, 2 times.

Prone clients are easily startled when you establish initial contact. To minimize the stimulation, you can tighten the draping near the area where you will contact the body, and use that sensory input to ease clients into your touch. You can apply massage to the back as described in Procedure Box 10-9.

Prone: Leg and Foot

By using both prone positions to massage a client's legs and feet in addition to the supine position, you can easily access all the soft tissues of the legs.

 Do not apply direct pressure over the endangerment site at the popliteal fossa behind the knee.

The steps in Procedure Box 10-10 can be used to apply massage to the client's legs and feet in the prone position.

PROCEDURE BOX 10-9
Massage Flow for a Prone Client's Back

1. Stand with an asymmetric foot position at the client's left side, facing the client's head, and expose the client's back.
2. As you tuck the sheet near the hips, leave your hand on the sheet and transition onto the client's skin to minimize the stimulation of initial contact. Apply effleurage to the left side of the client's back, using flat hands or the heels of your hands, first to spread lubricant and then progressively deeper, about 6 times.
3. Apply effleurage and petrissage, using the heel of your hand or your thumbs all over the left side of the client's back, from the iliac crest to the occipital ridge and from the spine all the way out to the muscular attachments at the proximal humerus.
4. Use the hacking form of tapotement over the left rhomboids, 10 seconds.
5. Apply gentle effleurage over the left side of the client's back, using flat hands in a superior direction, about 4 times.
6. Maintain contact with client's left shoulder as you walk around the client's head to the client's right side, and repeat steps 2–5 on the right side of the client's back.
7. Redrape the back and apply a resting stroke on top of the sheet with one hand on the middle of the client's back, and the other hand over the sacrum.

PROCEDURE BOX 10-10
Massage Flow for a Prone Client's Leg and Foot

1. Stand beside the client's leg, undrape the leg, and give a little tug on the sheet at the client's hip as sensory input to minimize the stimulation of your initial contact as you apply a resting stroke to the client's thigh.
2. Apply effleurage strokes in a proximal direction, first to spread lubricant on the client's thigh, and progressively deeper, about 20 seconds.
3. Effleurage and petrissage the upper leg, using your fists and the heels and palms of your hands, from the knee to the ischial tuberosity, making sure to address the lateral and medial aspects of the thigh, about 30 seconds.
4. Support the client's ankle on a bolster and apply effleurage and petrissage to the lower leg in a proximal direction, using your palms and thumbs, making sure to address the lateral aspects of the lower leg and the entire gastrocnemius muscle, which goes past the knee joint, 20 seconds.
5. Redrape the leg and apply nerve strokes, hip to heel, 2 times.
6. With the bolster still supporting the client's foot, expose the foot and apply compression to the sole of the foot.
7. Apply deep effleurage to the sole of the foot in a distal direction, using your thumbs or the heel of your hand, 3 times.
8. Redrape the foot and apply a resting stroke to the sole of the client's foot.

Closing Sequence

One way to finish a massage is to reconnect all the parts of the body and apply a last resting stroke to signal the end of the physical contact. Whether a client is supine, prone, or side-lying, the following steps can be used as a closing sequence:

1. Apply one or two slow nerve strokes from head to toe.
2. Apply a series of resting strokes:
   a. Both feet
   b. Both knees
   c. Both hips (ASIS if supine, PSIS if prone, or the protruding greater trochanter if side-lying)
   d. Head

CONSIDERATIONS FOR THERAPEUTIC MASSAGE

A routine massage that strictly follows a given flow applies the same number of strokes in the same order and treats the body parts in the same order for every client. The benefit to using a routine is that you do not need to think about what to incorporate into the session. Unfortunately, it also seriously limits your capability to provide a client-centered massage.

Going back to the recipe analogy, people commonly substitute ingredients or alter the directions of a recipe with excellent results. Consider a good cook who can make delicious food without a recipe, using everyday cooking tools and whatever ingredients are in the house. Often, those creations are better than a cookbook recipe because the cook can add special ingredients or combine the ingredients in interesting ways to make the dish a success. In the same manner, you can make adjustments to a massage flow by tailoring the session to each client with different strokes or techniques. Flow can be varied to accommodate your equipment, the client's body position, or the condition of the client's soft tissues. For example, a client who complains of excessive shoulder pain may want you to spend extra time working on the shoulder area with therapeutic techniques. Follow a flow loosely to allow the massage to fit the needs of the client.

Throughout the flow of the massage session, you should "listen" and respond to the client's tissues, traveling only as fast as the tissues allow. In general, the more tense the muscle, the more slowly you should move. If you move too quickly or with too much pressure, the client might hold his or her breath, the client's body might resist the work, or it might tense up and effectively push you out. When there are any indications that the body is tensing up, you need to adjust your stroke, the pace, or the intention of the massage. You must remain psychologically flexible about the flow instead of approaching your massage with a determined and uncompromising attitude.

By combining techniques and strokes and applying them to different body parts in different orders, you can create thousands of different flows. As a result, therapists often develop their own unique general flow for a massage session. The key to a good massage lies in blending rhythm and pressure with continuity and focused contact. Once you have learned the basic massage strokes and are comfortable applying them, your flow will become natural and effortless.

Chapter Summary

Massage has many physiological benefits, but you must assess your clients before and during treatment to make sure there are no contraindications. You can educate clients about their conditions and how massage might benefit them. Massage that lasts for 10 minutes or longer can improve circulation of blood and lymph, increase the warmth of the tissues, decrease pain, induce the relaxation response, decrease muscular tension, and normalize the activity of the nervous system. Throughout the massage, you must maintain good body mechanics, and you must stay grounded and centered.

To be successful you must practice massage strokes and flows and get constructive feedback. You must also receive massage from others to better understand how touch differs from person to person and to experience different flows to understand how they can influence a client's response to your work. The basic techniques mean nothing without knowing how to apply them effectively and comfortably. With a lot of experience, the distinct differences between the individual strokes become less defined. For instance, you could be applying an effleurage stroke when you come across a fascial restriction, and instantly turn the effleurage stroke into a compression stroke. The compression may lead you into an application of vibration or any one of the therapeutic techniques. As you get more comfortable with applying the different strokes and knowing when to use them, they will run together, and your massage will become more fluid and efficient.

 CHAPTER EXERCISES

1. Explain at least one effect that massage has on each of the following body systems:
   a. Integument
   b. Skeletal
   c. Muscular
   d. Nervous
   e. Circulatory
   f. Respiratory
   g. Digestive
   h. Thermoregulatory

2. Explain the importance of grounding and centering before a massage session.

3. Describe the process of diaphragmatic breathing.

4. Explain the purpose of using a resting stroke.

5. List and describe the six basic massage strokes.

6. Practice each of the six strokes on a partner. Ask your partner to watch your shoulder, elbow, wrist, and hand as well as your head-to-heel line while you apply the strokes. Ask your partner to let you know if any part of your arm looks tight and tense or if you have abandoned the head-to-heel line.

7. Describe the difference between superficial and deep effleurage.

8. Describe at least one effect of each basic massage stroke:
   a. Compression
   b. Effleurage
   c. Petrissage
   d. Tapotement
   e. Friction
   f. Vibration

9. Describe the benefits of using joint movement during a massage session.

10. Write a flow for a relaxation massage, including step-by-step instructions for client positioning, bolstering, draping and redraping of specific areas of the body, and specific strokes and techniques.

REFERENCE

1. Russell WR. Percussion and vibration. In: Licht S, ed. Massage, Manipulation and Traction. Huntington, NY: Robert E. Krieger Publishing, 1976.

SUGGESTED READINGS

Aslani M. Massage for Beginners. New York: Carroll & Brown, 1997.

Bruder L. Navigating the pathway to phenomenal touch: 10 steps to transform your massage. Massage Magazine 2002: March–April.

Claire T. Bodywork: What Type of Massage to Get—and How to Make the Most of It. New York: William Morrow, 1995.

Cyriax JH. Clinical applications of massage. In: Licht S, ed. Massage, Manipulation and Traction. Huntington, NY: Robert E. Krieger Publishing, 1976.

DeVane CL. Substance P: A New Era, A New Role. http://fmscommunity.org/subp.htm, accessed 9.2.03.

Dickson FD. Posture: Its Relation to Health, Philadelphia: JB Lippincott, 1930.

Françon F. Classical massage technique. In: Licht S, ed. Massage, Manipulation and Traction. Huntington, NY: Robert E. Krieger Publishing, 1976.

Frye B. Body Mechanics for Manual Therapist: A Functional Approach to Self-Care and Injury Prevention. Seattle, WA: Consolidated Press, 2000.

Kellogg JH. The Art of Massage. Reprinted. Mokelumne Hill, CA: Health Research, 1975.

Latchaw M, Egstrom G. Human Movement with Concepts Applied to Children's Movement Activities. Englewood Cliffs, NJ: Prentice-Hall, 1969.

Licht S. Mechanical methods of massage. In: Licht S, ed. Massage, Manipulation and Traction. Huntington, NY: Robert E. Krieger Publishing, 1976.

Lidell L, Thomas S, Cooke CB, Porter A. The Book of Massage. New York: Simon & Schuster, 1984.

Lindsey R, Jones BJ, Whitley A. Body Mechanics, Posture, Figure and Fitness. 4th ed. Dubuque, IA: Wm. C. Brown, 1979.

Maxwell-Hudson C. Complete Massage. New York: Dorling Kindersley, 2001.

Russell WR. Percussion and vibration. In: Licht S, ed. Massage, Manipulation and Traction. Huntington, NY: Robert E. Krieger Publishing, 1976.

Seedor MM. Body Mechanics and Patient Positioning. New York: Teachers College Press, 1977.

Souriau P. The Aesthetics of Movement (Souriau M, transl and ed.) Amherst, MA: The University of Massachusetts Press, 1983.

Stryer L. Biochemistry. 2nd ed. New York: WH Freeman, 1981.

Trager M, with Hamond C. Movement as a Way to Agelessness: A Guide to Trager Mentastics. Barrytown, NY: Station Hill Press, 1995.

Wakim KG. Physiologic effects of massage. In: Licht S, ed. Massage, Manipulation and Traction. Huntington, NY: Robert E. Krieger Publishing, 1976.

http://www.miami.edu/touch-research/references.html, accessed 9.2.03.

11

Therapeutic Applications

UPON COMPLETION OF THIS CHAPTER, THE STUDENT WILL BE ABLE TO:

- Describe what happens in each of the three phases of healing
- Explain the three stages of the pain cycle
- Identify the four signs of inflammation
- Explain the difference between lengthening and stretching
- Correctly perform at least three proprioceptive neuromuscular facilitation techniques on a partner
- Correctly perform at least one connective tissue technique
- Correctly perform at least one trigger point release technique
- Write an effective therapeutic massage treatment plan

KEY TERMS

Direct manipulation (DM): a proprioceptive neuromuscular facilitation (PNF) technique in which you use the muscle spindles and Golgi tendon organs to relax a hypertonic muscle

Direction of restriction: the direction in which tissues resist movement the most

Hypertonic (HAHY-per-TAHN-ik)**:** excessively tense or tight

Lengthening: the neurological process that lengthens myofibrils and results in a longer muscle

Muscle energy techniques (MET): massage applications that use the nervous system to change a muscle's resting length, also called proprioceptive neuromuscular facilitation

Muscle guarding: hypertonic muscles stabilizing or splinting an injured area

Positional release (PR): a PNF technique that relieves hypertonicity by holding the body in a painless position and waiting for the nervous system to trigger relaxation, also called strain/counterstrain

Post-isometric relaxation (PIR): a PNF technique that uses active contraction and relaxation of the target muscle to lengthen the muscle

Proprioceptive neuromuscular facilitation (PROH-pree-oh-SEP-tive NOO-roh-MUSS-kyoo-lar fah-SIHL-ih-TAY-shun) **(PNF):** bodywork applications that use the nervous system to change a muscle's resting length, also called muscle energy techniques

Reciprocal inhibition (RI): a PNF technique in which the client contracts a target muscle's antagonists to reflexively relax the target muscle

Resting length: the length to which a relaxed, inactive muscle can be safely extended

Strain/counterstrain (SCS): a PNF technique that relieves hypertonicity by holding the body in a painless position and waiting for the nervous system to trigger relaxation, also called positional release

Stretching: an elastic deformation of the fascia that extends its length

Target muscle: the muscle being treated in a therapeutic technique

Tender point: a small, painful area of hypertonicity, also called a tender spot

Trigger point: a localized area of hypertonicity at the motor end unit, or neuromuscular junction, that refers symptoms to other areas of the body

Unwinding: the process in which soft tissues move in different directions, circles, or wavy lines as the collagen fibers change shape and the fascia softens

This chapter focuses on massage applications with therapeutic and rehabilitative techniques. In addition to providing the general benefits of the basic massage strokes, including relaxation, pain relief, enhanced circulation, and decreased muscular tension, you can use therapeutic applications to treat specific soft tissue conditions with less time and energy. Clients often complain of tightness in a particular muscle, a "knot" or localized area of tight muscle tissue, pain or discomfort in a specific muscle, restricted movement, and specific soft tissue injuries. You must understand the body's tissue repair mechanism so you can appreciate how massage affects the healing process to prevent further injury and promote healing.

There are principles for applying therapeutic techniques that can maximize the efficiency of your work. It makes sense to want to work with the body rather than against it, but sometimes that means you accentuate the client's problem before you resolve it. Second, you must incorporate both lengthening and stretching of soft tissues into therapeutic massage because without both, the results of the massage could be short-lived. If your treatment does not change their condition, clients can lose interest or question your skills.

Three main categories of therapeutic applications are introduced in this text: proprioceptive neuromuscular facilitation (PNF), myofascial techniques, and trigger point techniques. PNF works through the nervous system to create reflexive changes in the length of muscles. Myofascial techniques concentrate on the fascia in and around the muscles mechanically changing the shape or structure of soft tissues. There are mechanical and reflexive techniques for relieving trigger points. Sometimes a combination of therapeutic techniques is more effective than a single approach. Practice all of the advanced techniques and use them carefully in a massage session.

Another difference between wellness massage and therapeutic massage is the depth of the treatment plan. Sometimes therapeutic massage is referred to as treatment-oriented massage. For professional consistency, include a treatment plan for all of your clients, but when clients are looking for specific results for a particular condition, incorporate more details in your plan for future treatment. Specify the duration and frequency of future sessions, suggested techniques, client likes and dislikes, self-help suggestions, and, when appropriate, professional healthcare referrals. With all of the specific information in a therapeutic treatment plan, a standard SOAP note or other medical charting method is more appropriate than a shortened health form or history form.

Therapeutic techniques are nothing more than the basic massage strokes. Compression, effleurage, petrissage, tapotement, friction, joint movements, palpation skills, and the principles of proper body mechanics are your foundations for therapeutic applications.

Mechanisms of Injury and Tissue Repair

When tissues are injured, the body automatically repairs the damage with regeneration, or replacement of destroyed cells, and with fibrosis, the production of fibrous connective tissue. Bones, epidermis, and mucous membranes can successfully regenerate and be repaired with connective tissue. Muscle cells and nerve cells, however, cannot be replaced. Injured muscle tissues and nervous tissues can only be repaired with connective tissue. The extent to which any given tissue undergoes regeneration or fibrosis depends on the types of cells, the severity of the injury, and the local supply of blood via the circulatory vessels. The healing process occurs in three physiological phases, as described below for a typical skin wound. In phase I, the bleeding stops and inflammation occurs. During phase II, tissue regeneration occurs, if possible, and in phase III, the remodeling of tissues is completed.

HEALING: PHASE I

When tissues are torn, the first phase of injury repair begins immediately and usually lasts a few days. Phase I is also known as the inflammatory phase, as it involves inflammation. The process starts with hemostasis (HEE-moh-STAY-sis), which forms a blood clot and stops the bleeding. Inflammation occurs next, flooding the area with oxygen-rich blood and neutrophils and constructing a framework for tissue repair. Finally, macrophages, attracted by the neutrophils, help digest and eliminate debris and then attract fibroblasts to synthesize collagen fibers.

Hemostasis

The body's automatic response to stop blood loss is a process called hemostasis, which is discussed in the circulatory system section in Chapter 4. It starts as a result of chemicals that are released when the surface of the tissues is disrupted. The chemicals cause the blood vessels to narrow, called vasoconstriction (VAY-zoh-kuhn-STRIHK-shun), which restricts blood flow to the area.

Inflammation

After blood loss has been stopped, inflammation occurs, increasing circulation to the injured area, preventing further damage to the injured area and the immediate surroundings, and setting the stage for repair processes. **Without inflammation, healing will not occur.** Inflammation is the body's second line of defense and can be identified by the following characteristics:

- Redness
- Swelling
- Heat
- Pain

Chemicals in the blood cause vasodilation (VAY-zoh-dahy-LAY-shun); the blood vessels widen and flood the area with red blood cells that carry oxygen and white blood cells that fight infection. The increased amount of blood circulating through the area increases the temperature of the skin and creates redness in the area that is healing. Increased circulation transports platelets, red and white blood cells, macrophages, and proteins to the area.

The capillaries become thinner and leaky, allowing extra interstitial fluid to seep into the surrounding tissues as lymph. The resultant edema (eh-DEE-muh), or swelling, puts extra pressure on the nerves, causing pain. When persons experience swelling and pain, the natural response is to minimize movement of that area or minimize any movements that increase the pain. Not only does reduced movement prevent further damage to the original injury, it also keeps the surrounding areas from being flooded with the chemicals that induce vasodilation and leaky capillaries.

Phagocytosis

Swelling restricts circulation, and the body's third line of defense, the immune response, is activated. The increased temperature of the area amplifies chemical reactions for increased immune activity that destroys pathogens and that breaks down cellular debris. Neutrophils, which are special white blood cells, pass through the capillaries more easily to destroy any pathogens that might have entered the wound. Neutrophils attract even more leukocytes to the area. Macrophages gravitate toward the neutrophils to destroy and digest cellular debris and pathogens.

Finally, fibrin protein strands tangle together at the injury site and trap other blood cells with a platelet plug, further decreasing blood flow and blood loss. The platelet plug, or scab, shrinks and pulls the edges of the wound together, creating a framework for tissue repair. Inflammation subsides, leading to the next phase of the healing mechanism. Since the many factors of a person's healing environment influence the speed at which the body accomplishes each phase of healing, phase I can last anywhere from 2–3 days to 2–3 weeks.

HEALING: PHASE II

The second phase of healing, also called the proliferation phase, typically begins 2–3 days after the injury and lasts about 6 weeks. During this process many new blood vessels and capillaries develop, bringing nutritious, oxygenated blood to the area. The macrophages continue to remove damaged tissue, pathogens, and other cellular debris, and they attract fibroblasts, which serve as precursors for collagen fibers. The first strands of collagen are laid down randomly, forming a tangled web of fibers that serves as the foundation for replacement tissues.

Fibroblasts continue to migrate across the injury to provide the collagen framework for replacement tissue. Once the fibroblasts have covered the entire wound and epithelial cells have grown into the framework to create a layer of epithelial tissue, tension gradually pulls the edges of the wound together.

When the cells cannot be regenerated, as occurs with nervous and muscle tissue, only connective tissue is produced. When a lot of fibrous connective tissue is deposited without the appropriate replacement cells, the result is scar tissue. The problem with scar tissue is that as it is laid down, it can attach to overlaying tissues. These connective tissue adhesions, or fascial restrictions, can interfere with normal function of the tissue. **A fascial restriction in one area of the body can restrict movement in other parts of the body, depending upon how long the restriction has existed.** Massage therapists *must* understand the development of scar tissue because of its impact on muscle tissues and skeletal movement.

HEALING: PHASE III

The third phase of healing, also called the remodeling phase, starts about 6 weeks after the original injury, and it can last a year or longer. The collagen fibers that were laid down in the previous stages of healing are steadily replaced with another, more organized form of collagen. The blood vessels that developed during phase II are no longer necessary, and little by little, they break down. As they recede, the scar loses some of its redness.

Remodeling is a dynamic process in which the replacement tissue gradually gains tensile strength and the collagen fibers can be rearranged until they are aligned like the fibers of the surrounding tissue. You must understand this process because muscle tissue is repaired primarily with collagen and connective tissue. During this phase, you must use either active and passive ranges of motion without weights or electrical stimulation to keep the collagen fibers from adhering to surrounding tissues.

> **!** *Using weights or electric stimulation is generally not in the scope of practice for a massage therapist; however, the client may be under concurrent treatment with another healthcare professional. You must know what kind of treatment is being administered, so you do not overtreat the client.*

As long as the scar remains mobile, the fibers can still be realigned. Gentle movement of the healing muscle tissues also encourages the collagen fibers into the same alignment as the original muscle fibers. This functional linear alignment provides greater strength and flexibility to the healing tissue. Without mobility, the repair process can result in tough, nonelastic scar tissue that is more easily reinjured.

The permanence of scars depends on the individual's healing capacity as well as the kind of movement the scar is subjected to. Several factors can increase or decrease the effectiveness of the body's natural healing mechanism:

- Injury—the extent and location of tissue damage
- Client—time lapse before treatment, general health, smoking habit, age, prior injuries, cooperation with self-help suggestions, nutrition, amount of rest/sleep, stress levels
- Treatment—improper self-care, inactivity, excessive activity, medicine, therapeutic interactions

Because the tissue repair process requires additional resources from the body, adequate amounts of rest, hydration, nutritional protein, and vitamins are necessary to facilitate healing. For example, vitamin C is needed for fibroblasts to be converted into collagen fibers, which is why vitamin C is so critical to health and healing. The speed of healing varies with the individual's age, health, nutrition, emotional and environmental stressors, and self-care. Massage can facilitate the healing process by restoring movement,

creating functional scar tissue, and increasing the circulation of blood and lymph, which delivers nutrients and removes waste from the cells and tissues.

Pain/Spasm/Ischemia Cycle

Pain can occur in a vicious circle that involves the muscles and circulation. A **hypertonic** (HAHY-per-TAHN-ik) muscle is an excessively tight muscle. Hypertonicity results when many of the muscle's individual muscle cells remain in a contracted, shortened state and do not relax, even when the muscle is inactive. Even when a hypertonic muscle is relaxed, it has a shorter **resting length,** or the length to which a relaxed, inactive muscle can be extended, because so many of its muscle cells are shortened. Like a spring that has been wound tighter and gets shorter, a muscle that becomes hypertonic develops a shorter resting length. The myofibrils within a muscle cell are tightly packed together, reducing circulation within a hypertonic muscle. **Insufficient oxygen supply can result in pain, discomfort, compensation patterns, and restricted functional movement.** Restricted movement then leads to reduced circulation, reducing the amount of oxygen available to cells, and so on. This is an interconnected pattern called the pain-spasm-ischemia cycle, also known as the pain cycle (see Fig. 4-76):

1. Pain causes a person to tense up, resulting in hypertonicity.
2. Hypertonicity causes decreased movement and also reduces local circulation of oxygen and other nutrients.
3. Reduced amounts of oxygen, or ischemia, can cause tissue degeneration and pain, returning the person to step 1.

A variation of this cycle begins with an injury. The body responds to an injury by minimizing movement of the injured area in an effort to minimize pain. The decreased activity requires less oxygen and nutrition, so local circulation is reduced. Nerve impingement may occur as well. When the blood supply to a localized area is insufficient, the supply of oxygen is decreased. The condition, called ischemia (iss-KEE-mee-uh), prevents efficient healing of an injury and causes more pain. **Without oxygen, cells suffer and eventually die.** The resulting pain often causes a person to tense up or reduce movement of the injury, and the cycle keeps repeating.

Being caught in the pain cycle can have significant effects, such as muscle imbalance, joint stress, muscular and skeletal compensation patterns, chronic ischemia, and tissue degeneration. Fortunately, the cycle can be broken anywhere along the way, using several different methods of intervention. The first step is to recognize this pattern and intervene to break it. Then, methods involving pain reduction, increased circulation, and increased exercise and stretching can all help break the cycle. Massage can relieve pain, reduce hypertonicity, and increase circulation. Better yet, specific therapeutic massage techniques can reflexively trigger the shortened muscles to lengthen.

Principles of Therapeutic Techniques

Sometimes called rehabilitative or treatment-oriented massage, therapeutic massage is based on the assessment, palpation, and treatment of specific injuries or compensation patterns in soft tissue structures of the body with therapeutic techniques. When using a therapeutic technique, the muscle you are addressing is called the **target muscle.** In other words, if a client complains of pain and tension in the calf, one of your target muscles is the gastrocnemius, and you could apply one or more therapeutic techniques to relax and lengthen it. Applications of therapeutic techniques are based on the core principles listed in Box 11-1. The pain and swelling that occur in the process of injury repair can develop into a compensation pattern. To avoid pain and discomfort, movement of the injured area is minimized. To reduce movement even further, the body can develop hypertonic muscles to stabilize or splint the injured area. Also called **muscle guarding,** the splinting is exaggerated further when clients hold the body in positions that ease the pain. The compensation pattern is the limited movement or an unnatural body position that attempts to correct an imbalance or protect a primary dysfunction or injury. In the third phase of injury repair, the client's compensation patterns or movements can establish nerve tracks that cause those unnatural positions to become habit.

When a client has developed compensation patterns because of an injury, always be aware of tissue resistance and acceptance. The longer a person has held the pattern, the more it will resist change. If your technique exceeds the tissue's tolerance, the client's body may react adversely by increasing the muscle guarding, which reinforces the compensation patterns and can cause further injury. Use good body mechanics, including the proper leaning technique, to avoid pushing into tissues that are resistant, so you can better follow the tissue's lead. With practice, you will be able to feel the difference between when tissues are resistant and when the client's tissues soften up to allow deeper or more invasive work.

Treating soft tissue injuries and compensation patterns is like peeling the layers of an onion. You begin treatment with the outside layer, making necessary changes and adjustments according to the client's condition. Then move, layer by layer, to the core, treating tissue layers appropriately along the way and encouraging the body to restore itself to its most functional state. Go slowly, pay attention to the tissue's resistance, and wait for tissues to accept your work. This allows the client's tissues to lead the treatment.

Following the tissues' lead is not the only way to use massage therapy, but it will help you work with the body instead of against it, using an approach that is gentle instead of forced. The technique that uses the least energy from both client and therapist is more effective than one that uses more energy and creates more pain.

Several other principles are important, and at first, some may seem illogical. **Too often, when it comes to massage treatment, people think that more is better. In reality, more is usually not better; more treatment can create more inflammation, more injury, or more compensation. Follow the principle that less is more.** Slowly and carefully palpate tissues to make your way through "the layers of the onion" with the appropriate amount of treatment to facilitate healing and restore normal structure and function. Overtreatment is not optimal, and the same is true for undertreatment. Always remember that each client is unique and that a technique that was effective for one client with a particular condition may not work on another with the same condition.

Another concept to keep in mind is the antagonistic activity of muscles and muscle groups. To create movement, one group of muscles contracts and gets shorter while the antagonistic muscles relax and get longer. If there is a restriction in either muscle or muscle group that prevents a length change, movement will be limited in varying degrees. Both lengthening and stretch-

---

Box 11-1

Principles of Therapeutic Massage

- Respect the client and his body
- Work within the client's tolerance
- Follow the tissue's lead
- SLOW DOWN . . . and wait for the tissues to respond
- Less is more
- Overtreating can be worse than not treating at all
- Sometimes the lightest work can create the deepest effect
- Massage is essentially the application of pressure moving across the skin

ing are critical to therapeutic massage, and although the terms are mistakenly interchanged, they are very different techniques with very different results. This is explained in detail later in this section.

DIRECTION OF EASE

The direction of ease concept can be applied to massage by working with the body instead of against it. If you accentuate a compensation pattern and then slowly lead the client's body out of the compromised position, you are working in the direction of ease. For example, a client's right sternocleidomastoid muscle could be hypertonic, giving the client a stiff neck that is slightly flexed and slightly rotated to the right. To relax and lengthen the sternocleidomastoid muscle, you can move in the direction of ease by first shortening the muscle even further with a passive contraction that increases the client's neck flexion and rotation to the right. Accentuation of the body's compensation pattern usually reduces the pain. By assuming the position slowly and safely without endangering the tissues, the nervous system perceives no threat or danger and can neurologically allow the sternocleidomastoid muscle to relax.

A different example of using the direction of ease in therapeutic massage illustrates how to work with the body rather than against it. A client who has right shoulder pain may find it uncomfortable to flex the right shoulder. Your assessment determines that the coracobrachialis muscle, which is partially responsible for flexing the shoulder, is hypertonic. To treat it, you want to put the coracobrachialis into passive contraction, but flexion is painful for the client. Rather than making the client uncomfortable by moving the shoulder directly into flexion, you can work in the direction of ease and position the coracobrachialis in a passive contraction from a different, less painful direction. You could try abducting the shoulder to bring the client's arm overhead, and then lower the client's arm to the position of passive contraction of the coracobrachialis.

LENGTHENING AND STRETCHING

You must understand the difference between lengthening and stretching in treatment-oriented massage. These are two very distinct and different mechanisms and involve different structures. **Lengthening,** the technical term for muscle relaxation, is a neurological process that elongates myofibrils and results in a longer muscle. **Stretching** is an elastic deformation of the fascia that extends its length. When muscles are stretched, the elastic connective tissues in and around the muscle cells are pulled into a longer form. As with a rubber band, though, the stretch is tempo-

rary, and the resting length of those muscles is basically unchanged. Both lengthening of the muscle and stretching of the fascia must be accomplished to create an effective and lasting change in muscle length.

Lengthening

Each muscle has a normal resting length. When it is too short or too long, there is an imbalance that leads to dysfunction. The resting length can be shortened actively by excessive, repetitive, or atypical kinds of muscular activity. The resting length can also be shortened passively if the muscle is held in a contracted state for an extended time. For example, a person who sits for long periods is putting the psoas major in passive contraction. Eventually, the psoas major will have a shorter resting length, which may cause low back pain and other symptoms.

With the appropriate techniques, the muscle's resting length can be reset through the body's neurological system. Lengthening restores a normal resting length to a muscle or the most functional resting length for the individual client. Simply, lengthening is a true, neurological relaxation of the muscle.

Stretching

The elastin proteins in soft tissues allow soft tissues to be stretched without being torn, but the elasticity also returns those tissues to their original length. A stretch pulls the fascia, the muscles, and their tendinous attachments. A stretch does not change the resting length of a muscle, but once a muscle has been neurologically lengthened, a stretch can help maintain the new length, increase flexibility, and enhance the fluidity of movement. The proprioceptors that sense tension in the muscle or tendons can trigger the stretch reflex, which is a protective muscle contraction that occurs when the tissues are stretched too far and/or too fast. The stretch reflex defeats the purpose of a stretch and can even put the muscle farther into spasm. The tendon reflex, on the other hand, is triggered when the proprioceptors sense a slow, gradual, sustained stretch at the musculotendinous junction. When a stretch does not threaten the muscle's integrity, the nervous system responds by allowing the muscle to relax and lengthen. Therefore, it is recommended that stretches be performed slowly and gradually rather than quickly or with a bouncing action, and they should be held for at least 5–10 seconds to achieve the tendon reflex.

The concept of lengthening and stretching can be likened to a loaf of bread (the muscle) in a plastic bag (the fascia). The individual pieces of the loaf of bread are like the myofibrils of the entire muscle. When myofibrils are lengthened, the entire muscle becomes longer than it used to be, just as thicker pieces of bread make a longer loaf. Fitting the longer loaf into its old, short bag would require "squishing" the bread into a shorter loaf. But if the longer loaf is put into a bag that has been stretched, it could retain its new length. The same is true of muscles. If the muscle is lengthened but the fascia is not stretched, the muscle will cramp back down to fit within the contracted fascia. First, the muscle must be lengthened, and then the fascia must be stretched. This lengthening can be accomplished effectively by many of the therapeutic techniques in this chapter.

Proprioceptive Neuromuscular Facilitation Techniques

Proprioceptive neuromuscular facilitation (PROH-pree-oh-SEP-tive NOO-roh-MUSS-kyoo-lar fah-SIHL-ih-TAY-shun), commonly called PNF, uses the nervous system to reset a muscle's resting length. PNF is a general term for a set of techniques. Remember, the muscle spindles and Golgi tendon organs are proprioceptors of the nervous system that recognize stretch and tension in the muscles and tendons. These massage techniques manipulate the *proprioceptors* of the *nervous* and the *muscular* systems to *facilitate* a reflexive change in the resting length of a muscle. These techniques are also called **muscle energy techniques,** or METs. The terms PNF and MET are often interchanged. PNF techniques can reduce pain, relax a hypertonic muscle, realign postural deviations, and restore range of motion. Some of the more common PNF techniques are direct manipulation, positional release (PR), post-isometric relaxation, and reciprocal inhibition.

Some persons respond well to PNF, and others do not. Some respond better to one particular PNF technique than to another. The results depend on the length of time the target muscle has been affected, the synergists that are involved, any compensation patterns that are present, and the factors that influence the client's health and healing. Sometimes the results can be immediate and permanent, and other times, PNF can be unsuccessful. Most of the time, PNF is an effective and efficient approach to specific areas of hypertonicity that plainly demonstrates some of the benefits of massage.

MUSCLE MOVEMENT AND STABILITY

Performing PNF requires a basic understanding of muscle movement and stability. In addition to creating movement, muscles also function to stop movement and to stabilize joints. The muscle or group of muscles that creates a certain movement is called the agonist (prime mover). The muscle or group of mus-

cles that performs the opposite work is called the antagonist. **In normal, concentric movements, the antagonist must relax for the agonist to contract.** For example, when the biceps brachii muscle contracts and shortens to create flexion, the triceps brachii muscle must neurologically relax and lengthen. PNF techniques often use the antagonistic mechanism of muscle contraction to create reflexive changes in muscle length. Muscles called synergists assist the agonist to create the desired motion. The synergists help by contracting in the same direction as the agonist or by stabilizing the joint to prevent another motion from occurring during movement.

If you are trying to relax and lengthen the biceps brachii muscle, the biceps brachii is your target (agonist) muscle. You can use a contraction of its antagonist, the triceps brachii muscle, to neurologically relax the biceps brachii. Knowing the major skeletal muscles of the body and their actions, antagonists, and synergists is important for using therapeutic techniques. For that reason, massage students must learn antagonistic muscle movements and the muscles responsible for those movements (Table 11-1).

DIRECT MANIPULATION

Direct manipulation (DM) is a PNF technique in which your fingers *directly manipulate* the muscle spindles and Golgi tendon organs of a hypertonic muscle to trigger relaxation. The muscle spindles are found between the muscle fibers and respond to tension in the muscles. The Golgi tendon organs are located between collagen fibers in the tendons and also respond to tension. These proprioceptors are components of such reflex arcs as the stretch reflex and the tendon reflex, which are protective mechanisms that help us to avoid injury. You can use these proprioceptors to fool the body into thinking that a muscle is too short or too long. If the proprioceptors sense that a muscle is too short, the nervous system can stimulate muscle lengthening, or relaxation. You can accomplish this with the following steps:

1. Determine the target muscle. Position the target muscle in a partial passive contraction.
2. Use your thumb and fingers to effleurage the target muscle with a pinching or gathering action, which addresses the muscle spindles.
3. Effleurage the tendons toward their bony attachments, which addresses the Golgi tendon organs.
4. Slowly extend the target muscle to its new length, stopping at the end feel. Hold the new length for at least 5–10 seconds. During this period, be prepared for a possible tendon reflex that allows the muscle to lengthen a bit further. If so, hold it at its new length.

TABLE 11-1

Antagonistic Actions

MUSCLES	ANTAGONISTIC ACTIONS		MUSCLES
Levator scapula, rhomboid major, upper trapezius, middle trapezius	Elevation	Depression	Serratus anterior, subclavius, lower trapezius, pectoralis minor

Scapula

MUSCLES	ANTAGONISTIC ACTIONS		MUSCLES
Serratus anterior, pectoralis minor	Protraction	Retraction	Rhomboid major, middle trapezius, lower trapezius
Serratus anterior, upper trapezius, lower trapezius	Upward rotation	Downward rotation	Levator scapula, pectoralis minor, rhomboid major

Shoulder

MUSCLES	ANTAGONISTIC ACTIONS		MUSCLES
Coracobrachialis, anterior deltoid, pectoralis major, biceps brachii	Flexion	Extension	Posterior deltoid, latissimus dorsi, teres major, triceps brachii
Deltoid, supraspinatus, biceps brachii	Abduction	Adduction	Latissimus dorsi, pectoralis major, teres major, triceps brachii, coracobrachialis, pectoralis minor
Posterior deltoid, infraspinatus, teres minor	Lateral rotation	Medial rotation	Anterior deltoid, latissimus dorsi, pectoralis major, subscapularis, teres major
Medial deltoid, posterior deltoid, teres minor, infraspinatus	Transverse abduction (laterally rotated humerus moves horizontally out to sides)	Transverse adduction (laterally rotated humerus moves across chest)	Pectoralis major, coracobrachialis
Pectoralis major, deltoids, coracobrachialis, biceps brachii	Transverse flexion (medially rotated humerus moves across chest)	Transverse extension (medially rotated humerus moves horizontally out to sides)	Posterior deltoid, infraspinatus, latissimus dorsi, teres minor

Elbow

MUSCLES	ANTAGONISTIC ACTIONS		MUSCLES
Biceps brachii, brachialis, brachioradialis	Flexion	Extension	Triceps brachii, anconeus
Pronator teres, pronator quadratus, anconeus, brachioradialis	Pronation	Supination	Biceps brachii, supinator

Wrist

MUSCLES	ANTAGONISTIC ACTIONS		MUSCLES
Flexor carpi radialis, flexor carpi ulnaris, palmaris longus, flexor digitorum superficialis, flexor digitorum profundus	Flexion	Extension	Extensor carpi radialis brevis, extensor carpi radialis longus, extensor carpi ulnaris, extensor digitorum, extensor pollicis longus, extensor indicis
Extensor carpi radialis brevis, extensor carpi radialis longus, flexor carpi radialis, extensor pollicis brevis	Abduction (radial deviation)	Adduction (ulnar deviation)	Extensor carpi ulnaris, flexor carpi ulnaris

Fingers

MUSCLES	ANTAGONISTIC ACTIONS		MUSCLES
Flexor digitorum profundus, flexor digitorum superficialis, flexor digiti minimi	Flexion	Extension	Extensor digiti minimi, extensor digitorum, extensor indicis
Dorsal interossei, abductor digiti minimi, extensor digitorum, extensor digiti minimi, extensor indicis	Abduction	Adduction	Palmar interossei, flexor digitorum superficialis, flexor digitorum profundus

Thumb

MUSCLES	ANTAGONISTIC ACTIONS		MUSCLES
Abductor pollicis brevis	Abduction	Adduction	Adductor pollicis
Flexor pollicis brevis, flexor pollicis longus	Flexion	Extension	Extensor pollicis brevis, extensor pollicis longus

Hip

MUSCLES	ANTAGONISTIC ACTIONS		MUSCLES
Adductor brevis, adductor longus, iliacus, pectineus, psoas major, rectus femoris, sartorius, tensor fascia latae	Flexion	Extension	Adductor magnus, biceps femoris, gluteus maximus, semimembranosus, semitendinosus

TABLE 11-1

Antagonistic Actions (continued)

MUSCLES	ANTAGONISTIC ACTIONS		MUSCLES
Hip (continued)			
Gemellus inferior, gemellus superior, gluteus maximus, gluteus medius, gluteus minimus, piriformis, tensor fascia latae	Abduction	Adduction	Adductor brevis, adductor longus, adductor magnus, biceps femoris, gluteus maximus, gracilis, pectineus, psoas major
Gluteus medius, gluteus minimus, tensor fascia latae	Medial rotation	Lateral rotation	Adductor brevis, adductor longus, adductor magnus, biceps femoris, gemellus inferior, gemellus superior, gluteus maximus, gluteus medius, obturator externus, obturator internus, piriformis, quadratus femoris, sartorius
	Knee		
Biceps femoris, gastrocnemius, gracilis, popliteus, sartorius, semimembranosus, semitendinosus	Flexion	Extension	Rectus femoris, tensor fascia latae, vastus intermedius, vastus lateralis, vastus medialis
Gracilis, popliteus, sartorius, semimembranosus, semitendinosus	Medial rotation	Lateral rotation	Biceps femoris
	Ankle		
Extensor digitorum longus, extensor hallucis longus, peroneus tertius, tibialis anterior	Dorsiflexion	Plantarflexion	Flexor digitorum longus, flexor hallucis longus, gastrocnemius, peroneus brevis, peroneus longus, plantaris, soleus, tibialis posterior
Extensor digitorum longus, peroneus brevis, peroneus longus, peroneus tertius	Eversion	Inversion	Flexor digitorum longus, tibialis anterior, tibialis posterior
	Spine		
External obliques, internal obliques, rectus abdominis	Flexion	Extension	Iliocostalis, longissimus, multifidi, rotatores, spinalis
Multifidi, quadratus lumborum, rotatores	Lateral flexion		
External obliques, iliocostalis, internal obliques, multifidi, quadratus lumborum, rotatores	Rotation		
	Diaphragm		
External obliques, internal intercostals, internal obliques, rectus abdominis, transversus abdominis	Exhalation	Inhalation	Diaphragm, external intercostals, internal intercostals, scalenus anterior, scalenus medius, scalenus posterior
	Neck		
Scalenus anterior, scalenus medius, scalenus posterior, sternocleidomastoid	Flexion	Extension	Iliocostalis, levator scapulae, longissimus, multifidi, rotatores, semispinalis, spinalis, splenius capitis, splenius cervicis, upper trapezius
Levator scapulae, longissimus, semispinalis, splenius capitis, sternocleidomastoid, middle trapezius	Lateral flexion		
Multifidi, rotatores, splenius capitis, splenius cervicis, sternocleidomastoid	Rotation		
	Temporomandibular joint (or jaw)		
Masseter, medial pterygoid, temporalis	Elevation	Depression	Lateral pterygoid, platysma, suprahyoids
Lateral pterygoid, masseter, medial pterygoid	Protraction	Retraction	Temporalis

Procedure Box 11-1 illustrates these steps with the biceps brachii as the target muscle.

This technique leads the nervous system's proprioceptors into perceiving that the muscle is dangerously hypertonic. When a muscle is strongly contracted and too short, it is in danger of being torn. Pushing the muscle spindles together sends a message that the muscle fibers are too close, or that the muscle is contracted too much. Pushing the Golgi tendon organs away from the muscle conveys a message that the musculotendinous junctions are being stressed, or that the muscle is contracted too much. The nervous system will respond by protectively relaxing and lengthening that muscle.

These are reflexive responses in which the massage application causes the nervous system to create a physical change. Once the muscle has been lengthened by the nervous system, the surrounding fascia must be stretched for the treatment to retain its effect. The extended hold at the end of the DM procedure provides the stretch for the fascia at the same time it allows the proprioceptors to recognize the new length that should be maintained. All stretching must be done carefully to avoid a protective spasm.

DM is a good technique to use on painful muscles and muscles that are not attached to the limbs, such as the trapezius or rhomboids. Clients who hurt with any kind of movement and clients who are not interested in actively moving or participating in the massage may prefer DM to some of the other PNF techniques.

POSITIONAL RELEASE

To perform PR, also called position release and **strain/counterstrain** (SCS), you hold the client's body in a position that reduces the hypertonic muscle pain and wait for the nervous system to trigger relaxation. This technique takes advantage of the body's inherent ability to reduce pain and release hypertonic muscles. When a muscle develops a shortened resting length, the body finds a position that relieves the associated discomfort. Unfortunately, the hypertonicity that reduces the movement and use of a muscle can start the pain cycle. Using the direction of ease concept, you can follow the body's lead rather than work against it. To perform PR, you apply pressure to a localized hypertonic or painful spot and move the client's body into a position that reduces or eliminates that pain. Basically, PR puts the client's body into a position that it may have been in before a protective spasm resulted from stress or strain. When the body senses that the position is nonthreatening, the nervous system may respond by relaxing the protective spasm. Physical therapists, osteopaths, and chiropractors frequently use this technique.

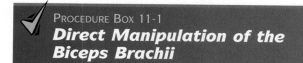

PROCEDURE BOX 11-1
Direct Manipulation of the Biceps Brachii

1. Determine the target muscle: biceps brachii.
2. Put the biceps brachii into a partial passive contraction.

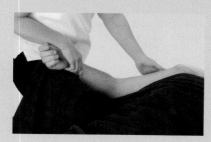

3. Use your thumb and fingers to effleurage the biceps brachii with a pinching or gathering action.

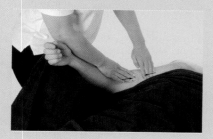

4. Effleurage the tendons toward their bony attachments at the radial tuberosity and the glenohumeral joint.

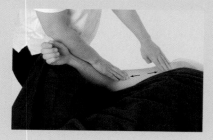

5. Slowly extend the biceps brachii to its new length by extending the elbow and the shoulder, stopping at the end feel. Hold the new length for at least 5–10 seconds. During this period, be prepared for a possible tendon reflex that allows the muscle to lengthen a bit further. If so, hold it at its new length.

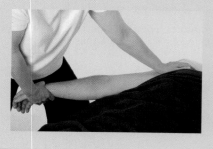

The very small area of pain or hypertonicity is referred to as a **tender point,** tender spot, or knot. It is often found during the massage in the midst of an effleurage stroke. Sometimes the client will express discomfort as you pass over it; other times you may feel a difference in the tissue quality and should ask the client if there is any associated discomfort. With enough experience, you will be able to find tender points without any input from the client, but until then, verbally communicate with the client.

Monitoring the Tender Point

The tender point is monitored with your finger, forearm, or thumb throughout the process, so you need to use good body mechanics while you maintain pressure on it. You should put enough pressure on the tender spot that clients notice the discomfort, but not so much that they are distracted by it. You can ask clients to rate the pain or discomfort on a scale of 0 to 3, where 0 indicates no pain and 3 indicates severe pain, or a scale of 0 to 10, where 0 indicates no pain and 10 indicates severe pain. For clients who do not like to use a rating scale, you can ask them to indicate whether the discomfort is absent, mild, moderate, or severe. With experience, you will be able to feel resistant tissues soften up when you apply the appropriate amount of pressure with proper body mechanics and palpation skills.

Positioning the Body

Once the correct pressure and body mechanics have been found, start moving the client's body to minimize the discomfort. Based on your knowledge of the major skeletal muscles and their attachments and actions, you can begin positioning the client by putting the target muscle into a passive contraction. Occasionally this passive contraction of the target muscle eliminates the pain, but most of the time, you have to fine-tune the position by moving other body parts or changing the position slightly. Since the three-dimensional fascial pulling can be a component of the client's discomfort, the process of positioning can sometimes require you to move a part of the client's body that is seemingly unrelated to the target muscle. For example, you may flex the client's other elbow, laterally rotate a leg, or rotate the neck to reduce the pain further.

When moving in the primary direction of ease does not decrease the discomfort, continue to adjust the position until the pain diminishes. Since the body has an inherent tendency to find the most comfortable position in any given situation, you can also ask the client to try to find the right position. At times, however, the pain does not seem to diminish in any position. In these cases, another PNF technique may be the better option.

Once you find a position that significantly diminishes or eliminates the pain, hold the client's body in that position for at least 90 seconds. It is not critical to maintain the same amount of pressure with your monitoring finger, but this is a good practice. If you vary the pressure, the client may suspect the pain is gone because you are not pressing as hard. Because you must hold the client's body in position, you *must* maintain good body mechanics.

Releasing the Tender Point

During the hold, your monitoring finger may feel a difference in the tissues as the tender point is released. It can feel like the tissues are melting or softening under your pressure. Sometimes the release is accompanied by a change in the client's breathing pattern or a sigh. Whether or not you notice the release, you need to hold the position for 90 seconds.

After the 90-second hold, slowly and gently return the client's body to the anatomical position. With your monitoring finger on the tender point, ask the client to rate the discomfort level following PR. If the tender spot has been released, there will be no discomfort. If pain is still present but is reduced, you may want to repeat the process. If there is no change, you can try PR with a different position or you can try another technique.

Once the target has been satisfactorily relaxed, the fascia in and around the target muscle needs to be stretched. Slowly extend the target muscle until you reach the end feel. You will sense the end feel better with good body mechanics and proper lean technique. Were you to push the client's body with your own strength, you would be more likely to pass through the client's comfort barrier and the end feel, possibly causing injury. Once you reach the barrier, hold the extension for at least 5 seconds, waiting for a possible tendon reflex to relax the target even farther.

PR is a good technique to use with clients who are not interested in actively moving or participating during the massage. As always, use good body mechanics with PR, especially if your clients are large or heavy because of the physical work required to lift and hold their limbs or body parts. The process is described in Procedure Box 11-2.

POST-ISOMETRIC RELAXATION

Post-isometric relaxation (PIR) is a PNF technique that can reduce hypertonicity in a muscle by actively contracting and relaxing the target muscle. Also

PROCEDURE BOX 11-2
Positional Release of the Lower Trapezius

1. Apply a small amount of pressure to a tender point or small knot in the trapezius muscle. Ask the client to rate the discomfort on a scale of 0 to 3 (where 0 is pain free and 3 is very painful). Adjust the pressure of your monitoring finger using good body mechanics until the pressure elicits a pain rating of 1 or 2.

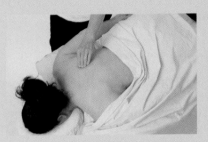

2. Maintain the contact and pressure on the tender point and move the client's body into a position that eliminates or significantly reduces the discomfort.
3. Hold the client's body in this position for at least 90 seconds with your monitoring finger still in place. Ask the client to take a few deep breaths.

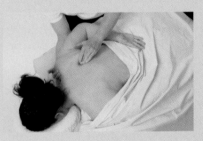

4. Slowly return the client's body to the original position, maintaining contact with your monitoring finger. Ask the client to rate the discomfort again, using the same scale.

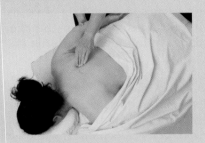

5. After the tender point has been relieved, extend the target muscle to its new length. Hold the new length for at least 5–10 seconds to see if the tendon reflex will allow the muscle to lengthen a bit farther. If so, hold it at its new length.

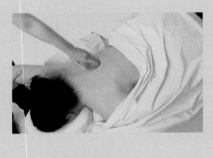

---

known as tense and relax (T&R), it requires work from the client and is often more effective and longer lasting than DM or PR. PIR uses an *isometric* contraction of the target muscle *followed by* slow *relaxation* and elongation. Isometric contractions use active muscle contraction without producing any movement. For example, if you squeeze your knees together, the adductor muscles are all actively contracting, but no movement occurs because the opposite knee acts as a physical barrier. The PIR technique involves the following steps:

1. Determine the target muscle and its action.
2. Extend the muscle to its end feel.
3. Pull back from the barrier by a few degrees, or a small amount.
   a. Stabilize the client's body in that position to provide a physical, immovable barrier to the target muscle's contraction.
   b. Ask the client to gently push against the barrier, using only about 10% of his or her strength, and hold the push.
4. After 5 seconds, clearly explain that you want the client to *slowly* relax and let go of the push.
   a. Gently extend the target muscle to the muscle's new length.
   b. Hold the position for at least 5–10 seconds, waiting for a tendon reflex to lengthen the muscle further. If it does, hold it at its new length.

Procedure Box 11-3 demonstrates PIR applied to the gastrocnemius.

Positioning the Body

Because a fully extended muscle has very little leverage and cannot contract efficiently, synergists are often recruited to perform the desired movement. In an effort to isolate the muscular contraction for PIR, the target muscle is positioned with a slight contraction. To position the target muscle for PIR, you passively extend it, stretching the muscle to its end feel, and then relieve some of your pressure and back away from the end feel, allowing the muscle to rest just short of full extension.

Stabilizing the client's body requires some practice to incorporate good body mechanics. Use a solid lean, either into or away from the client's body, with as little arm or back strength as possible. You may need to remind clients that this technique is not a strength contest, and tell them simply to "hold against my pressure" or to use only 10% of their strength during the contraction—just enough to signal some of the muscle fibers to contract. If you do not, you may get pushed or pulled off balance. Then ask the client to push or pull against the physical barrier and hold the isometric contraction.

Relaxing the Target Muscle

After about 5 seconds, ask the client to slowly relax the muscle. This works best if you slowly relieve the counterpressure. As the client relaxes the target muscle, the nervous system relaxes and lengthens the muscle. Slowly take the target muscle into extension, using good body mechanics, and stop at the end feel. Hold the stretch for at least 5 seconds, allowing the proprioceptors to integrate the new muscle length while you wait for a possible tendon reflex. The tendon reflex will lengthen the muscle even more, and the increased extension provides the connective tissue stretch.

The client must relax the target muscle slowly to prevent a sudden, complete absence of muscular tension. Abrupt relaxation may cause your counterpressure to quickly push the muscle into a stretch, activating the stretch reflex and a protective spasm.

This technique requires the target muscle to contract. By using the neuromuscular communication path for contraction and relaxation of the target muscle, PIR can be very effective for muscles that have been hypertonic for more than 3 weeks. Contracting a muscle involved in a situation of protective muscle guarding or splinting may be painful or make the original condition worse.

> ⚠️ Any time there is muscle guarding, which often happens with conditions that have been present for less than 3 weeks, or any time there is pain upon contraction of the target muscle, you should avoid PIR.

PROCEDURE BOX 11-3
Post-isometric Relaxation Technique

1. Determine the target muscle and its action: the gastrocnemius is responsible for plantarflexion.

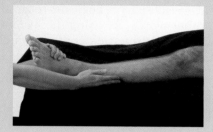

2. Extend the gastrocnemius to its end feel.

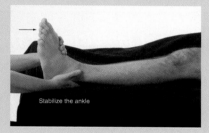

Stabilize the ankle

3. Pull back from the barrier by a few degrees, or a small amount.
   a. Stabilize the client's body in that position and provide a physical, immovable barrier to plantarflexion.

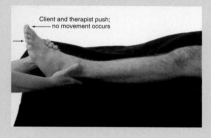

Client and therapist push; no movement occurs

   b. Ask the client to gently plantarflex against the barrier, using only about 10% of his or her strength, and hold the push.
4. After 5 seconds, clearly explain that you want the client to *slowly* relax and let go of the push. Gently extend the target muscle to the muscle's new length. Hold the position for at least 5-10 seconds, waiting for a tendon reflex to lengthen the muscle farther. If it does, hold it at its new length.

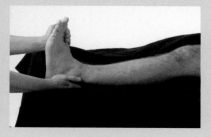

RECIPROCAL INHIBITION

The PNF technique called **reciprocal inhibition** (RI) is based on the agonist/antagonist principle. Movement can only be created by the agonist, or prime mover, if its antagonists relax to some degree. During the process of RI, the client contracts the opposing or antagonistic muscles to reflexively relax the target muscle. In other words, by using the *reciprocal* muscle action, the target muscle's contraction can be *inhibited*. RI is performed as follows:

1. Determine the target muscle, its action, and the antagonistic action.
2. Position the target muscle in a partial contraction.
3. Stabilize the client's body in that position.

   a. Provide a physical, immovable barrier to the antagonistic action.
   b. Ask the client to gently push against the barrier contracting the antagonist muscle, using only about 10% of his or her strength, and hold the push.

4. After 5 seconds, tell the client to slowly relax and let go of the push.
   a. Gently extend the target muscle to the end feel at its new length.
   b. Hold the stretch for 5–10 seconds, waiting for a possible tendon reflex that lengthens the muscle a bit farther. If so, hold it at its new length.

Procedure Box 11-4 illustrates how to apply reciprocal inhibition to the quadriceps femoris.

PROCEDURE BOX 11-4

Reciprocal Inhibition of the Quadriceps Femoris

1. Determine the target muscle, its action, and the antagonistic action: the quadriceps femoris is responsible for hip flexion and knee extension. Antagonistic actions are hip extension and knee flexion.

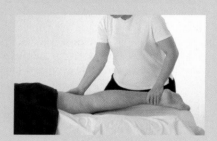

2. Position the quadriceps femoris in a partial contraction.

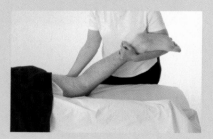

3. Stabilize the client's body in that position by placing a hand near the knee.
   a. Provide a physical, immovable barrier to the antagonistic action of knee flexion by leaning into the client's Achilles tendon.

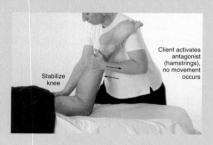

Stabilize knee

Client activates antagonist (hamstrings), no movement occurs

   b. Ask the client to gently flex the knee, pushing against the barrier, using only about 10% of his or her strength, and hold the push.

4. After 5 seconds, ask the client to slowly relax and let go of the push.
   a. Gently extend the quadriceps to the end feel at its new length by flexing the client's knee.

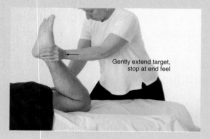

Gently extend target, stop at end feel

   b. Hold the stretch for 5–10 seconds, waiting for a possible tendon reflex that lengthens the quadriceps femoris a bit farther. If so, hold it at its new length.

Positioning the target muscle for RI is not a precise step. As long as the muscle is held toward the end of its range of motion, the position should be adequate for RI. Understanding the action of the target muscle and its antagonistic action is important. Often, if you can determine the target's action, the antagonistic action is second nature.

Stabilizing the client's body and providing a physical barrier to the antagonistic action requires good body mechanics. The barrier must not move when pushed by the client, because the muscle contraction must be isometric. With experience, you will develop techniques that work well. As with PIR, ask clients to push against the resistance using only about 10% percent of their strength and hold the isometric contraction. Ask clients to slowly relax the muscle after about 5 seconds. Once the neurological lengthening (relaxation) has occurred, the surrounding connective tissues must be stretched to maintain the change in length. Relieve the counterpressure slowly to facilitate smooth relaxation and avoid the protective spasm of a stretch reflex.

RI requires the client to actively participate in the massage but does not require the target muscle to do the work. In conditions that involve an extremely hypertonic or painful target muscle, RI is especially useful. As with all other PNF techniques, there is a wide variation in the amount of neurological relaxation that occurs as a result of RI. Chronically hypertonic muscles generally require more time and treatment to be restored to their normal resting length because of the fascial restrictions that develop, the compensation patterns that develop, and the nerve tracks that make the compensation patterns habitual. Stretching is important for reinforcing and maintaining RI work on chronically hypertonic muscles.

Myofascial Techniques

Myofascial techniques manipulate the fascia that runs throughout the musculature. Fascia is so pervasive that any restrictions, adhesions, or buildups of fascia can create problems for the musculature. Fascial restriction can often be felt during an effleurage stroke because it causes an irregularity in the speed or quality of the stroke. Sometimes the effleurage stroke will seem to skid across the tissue or get stuck and be difficult to move across the tissue.

Fascia is thixotropic (THIK-soh-TROH-pihk), which means that with deformation and mechanical manipulation, fascia becomes warmer and more liquid. This is primarily a result of the piezoelectric (pee-AY-zoh-ee-LEHK-trihk) quality of collagen. When collagen is mechanically compressed or squeezed, it develops an elec-

tric charge on its surface that liquefies the collagen to some degree, and the components of the tissue are rearranged. Recall that connective tissue is made of living cells suspended in a matrix of proteins that are secreted by those cells. The proteins, including collagen, elastin, and reticular fibers, provide strength, elasticity, and structural support. **Without sufficient movement, nutrition, and hydration, fascia stiffens and dries out.**

Myofascial techniques take advantage of the thixotropic nature of fascia to mechanically change the shape and position of restricted tissues. Due to the three-dimensional structure of fascia, the tissues might move in different directions, circles, or wavy lines as the collagen fibers change shape and get rearranged. This slow process is sometimes referred to as **unwinding** or **myofascial unwinding.** These techniques require that you maintain your original point of contact on the client's skin without slipping, so little or no lubrication is used. Because these techniques are sometimes uncomfortable, you should perform them slowly and with care. There are general connective tissue applications as well as specific techniques, including scar release, craniosacral therapy, and friction techniques.

CONNECTIVE TISSUE TECHNIQUES

Connective tissue techniques (CT) make the fascia more fluid, break up fascial adhesions, and can reduce scar tissue. **CT techniques specifically soften the fascia to create more space and allow more movement within the tissues.** You can feel the resistance of the tissues slowly melt away as the fascia softens. CT techniques include the 45° stroke, skin rolling, and variations of skin rolling.

45° Stroke

The most general connective tissue stroke is called the 45° stroke. The degree indicates the direction of pressure applied to the client's skin. The effleurage stroke, which moves along the surface of the client's skin, is considered to be applied at 0°. Compression, which pushes directly into the client's tissues, is considered a 90° stroke. The 45° stroke uses a pressure midway between that of effleurage and compression.

Once a restriction is found, you can alter your body position slightly to change the direction of your stroke to apply pressure at 45°. As you contact the client at this angle, the slip across the client's skin will almost disappear (Fig. 11-1). Maintain your contact point, continue the 45° pressure, and wait for the client's connective tissue to soften and unwind. In a variation of the stroke, you use one hand to stabilize tissue with compression while the other hand applies the 45° stroke.

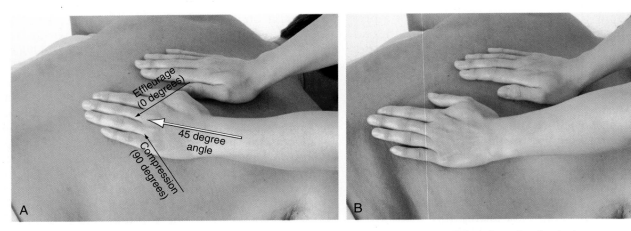

FIGURE 11-1 45° stroke **A.** Establish contact points and direct pressure at a 45° angle to the client's tissues without any slip on the skin. **B.** Maintain pressure as the connective tissue softens and spreads out.

This general 45° CT stroke can be applied with the fingers, thumbs, heel/s of the hand/s, whole hand, or even forearm. The restricted area on the client's body determines whether you use your fingers or forearms. For a large area, you may use your forearms, but to release a localized point, the fingers may work better.

Skin Rolling

Skin rolling is used mainly to break up adhesions in the superficial fascia. Restrictions in the fascia may be felt during an effleurage stroke as a skidding motion across the tissue or resistance to the stroke moving across the skin. When a large area of fascial restriction is found, skin rolling can be effective. Establish a contact point in the restricted area and palpate the tissues for restricted movement. Without any slip on the client's skin, push the tissues away from you, toward you, to your left, and to your right to determine the **direction of restriction,** which is the direction in which the tissues resist movement the most.

First, you work in the direction of ease, grasping and lifting the client's tissues into a roll, gently pulling it in the direction that it moves easily. Slowly, you change directions to pull the roll of tissues in the direction of restriction. Going along with the body's tendencies and then slowly moving in a therapeutic direction is usually more effective than immediately pushing the body in the direction of restriction. Tissues that are more restricted or dehydrated are more difficult to pick up, roll, and move. Skin rolling is especially uncomfortable when the client has considerable fascial restriction and therefore must be performed slowly and carefully, paying close attention to the client's body language. You may tell clients that if the work becomes too uncomfortable, you can slow down or back off a bit. Encourage clients to tell you

if the work is beyond their tolerance. People can manage pain better when they can breathe easily without bracing, recoiling, or wincing.

After the skin has been rolled for some distance, the tissues will feel less resistant. At that point, you can slowly release the roll. Use a resting stroke to allow the body a moment to relax and readjust to the reorganized tissues. Then return to the close vicinity of the original contact point and reevaluate the restriction by pushing the tissue in various directions to determine whether a change has occurred. Procedure Box 11-5 demonstrates the skin rolling technique.

C-Stroke, S-Stroke

You may find it difficult to lift the tissues enough to grasp them in a roll and even more difficult to keep the roll elevated while transporting it across the client's body. In these situations, you can try one of the variations of skin rolling, such as the C-stroke or the S-stroke.

The C-stroke is a variation of skin rolling in which you still lift a roll of tissue, but instead of transporting the elevated roll, you bend the rolled tissue into the shape of a C. The S-stroke is yet another variation in which you deform the roll of tissue into the shape of an S (Fig. 11-2).

SCAR RELEASE

When soft tissues are compromised or injured, the body automatically responds to repair the damage. In phase II of the healing mechanism, collagen fibers are produced to splint the area and prevent further damage. New collagen fibers are relatively easy to align with the fibers of the original tissue, given gentle movement throughout phase III. Collagen fibers continue to be produced during phase III, and with-

1. Establish the contact point and check the tissue for the direction of restriction while maintaining contact.

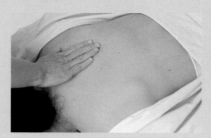

   a. Push the tissue away from you.

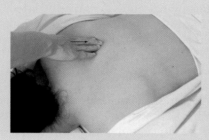

   b. Pull the tissue toward you.

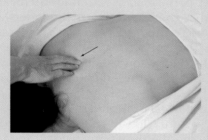

   c. Push the tissue to your left.

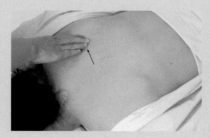

   d. Push the tissue to your right. Tissues do not move easily in this direction, making this the direction of restriction.

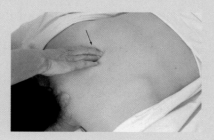

2. Grasp the tissue in a roll, pulling it slightly in the direction of ease, toward the client's spine.

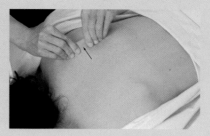

3. Gently change direction, pulling the rolled tissue into the direction of restriction.

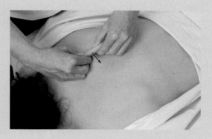

4. Slowly transport the rolled tissue in the direction of restriction by gathering the tissue with your fingers and feeding it into your thumbs, keeping the roll of tissue elevated. Continue the skin roll for several inches, or until the restriction diminishes.

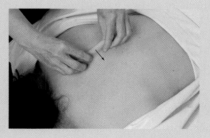

5. Release the roll of tissue carefully. Apply a resting stroke to allow tissues to reorganize. Return to the original contact area and reevaluate the tissue for restriction.

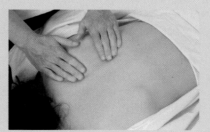

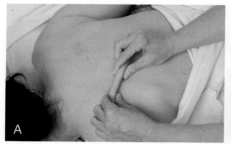
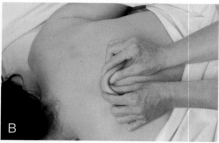
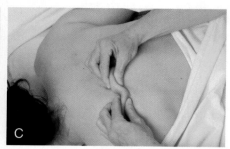

FIGURE 11-2   Variations of skin rolling: C-stroke and S-stroke. Lift tissue into a roll **(A)**. Then deform it into a C-stroke **(B)** or an S-stroke **(C)**.

out sufficient movement, they become sticky and hard. As a result, the collagen fibers are difficult to re-align and they easily develop into connective tissue adhesions, or scars, with far-reaching effects. The scars are visible when the integument is injured, but tissues beneath the surface of the skin can also develop scars. Invisible scars are equally capable of affecting structures in other areas of the body.

Once a scar or adhesion is created in one area, it begins to pull on the fascia throughout the body. The quicker the adhesion is treated, the less likely it is to affect the rest of the body. Because of its patchlike nature, there is a tendency for all other tissues to pull in the direction of the scar, which can lead to more compensation patterns and fascial restrictions.

The above connective tissue techniques are appropriate if the scar is not sensitive. If the client's scar tissue is sensitive, use a gentler technique that promotes the body's self-correcting mechanism and unraveling of the scar tissue. Although it is very similar to the other connective tissue strokes, the scar release technique uniquely combines palpation, connective tissue deformation, and direction of ease. You anchor one end of the scar with a finger, knuckle, or palm, hold another point on the scar, and apply a gentle 45° pressure in the direction of restriction. The scar, held in a passive stretch, may start to deform as the tissues are loosened and collagen rearranged.

Maintain your contact point and avoid slipping on the client's skin while you apply sustained 45° pressure. You may feel your finger start to move as the underlying tissues soften and spread out. Massage can help create more functional and mobile scar tissue, but the number of treatments depends upon how severe the scarring is and how long the client has had the scar. Procedure Box 11-6 illustrates the steps of scar release.

CRANIOSACRAL THERAPY

In the 1940s, William G. Sutherland, DO, developed a technique he called cranial osteopathy. It is based on his observations of cranial bones moving very slightly in a unique rhythm, distinct from the pulse or breath-

ing pattern. He suggested that restrictions of the cranial movement can negatively affect a person's health. Cranial osteopathy treats an imbalance or interrupted rhythm by manipulating the cranial bones.

John E. Upledger, DO, OMM, born in 1932, further advanced the practice and developed his own form of craniosacral (KRAY-nee-oh-SAY-kruhl) therapy (CST). Using the same basic theory and principles as cranial osteopathy, CST works more with the fascial component of the dura mater and dural tube that encase the brain and spinal cord. From 1975 to 1983, Dr. Upledger performed research at Michigan State University that confirmed the rhythmic movement of the cranial bones and clarified the craniosacral mechanism as the cause for the cerebrospinal fluid (CSF) pulse. His theory suggests that restrictions in the flow of the CSF affect the function of the central nervous system, including sensory and motor dysfunctions and neurological disabilities.

The rhythmic flow of CSF is conducted throughout the body via the three-dimensional fascia, making it possible to feel the movement almost anywhere on the body. Like the cardiac pulse, it is very subtle and difficult or nearly impossible to feel when you apply too much pressure. Although some persons learn to see this slow and very slight movement, most persons can learn to feel it using a very light touch, with no more force than the pressure applied by a nickel resting on your skin. The rate is much slower than the breathing rate, as it generally takes about 10 seconds to complete a cycle. It can be felt as a 4-second outward expansion of the body, followed by a 2-second pause, and then about a 4-second inward contraction or shrinking of the body.

CST practitioners first evaluate the craniosacral rhythm at different key points on the body for smoothness, amplitude, and bilateral evenness. Restricted movement can indicate an obstruction of the CSF flow. By applying very small amounts of pressure to the cranial bones or other areas on the body, you can manipulate the movement, which helps the body restore and regulate the flow of CSF. Theoretically, improving the flow of CSF can relieve a number of asso-

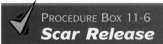

PROCEDURE BOX 11-6
Scar Release

1. Palpate the scar to determine the direction of restriction. Anchor one end of the scar with a finger or thumb.

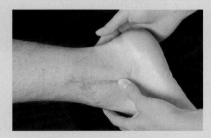

2. Using your other hand, apply 45° pressure with a finger or thumb in the direction of restriction while maintaining the pressure and your contact point. Follow the tissue as it softens and deforms.

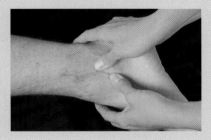

3. Continue to follow the tissue as the fascial adhesions release.

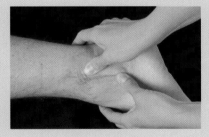

4. Slowly relieve your pressure when you feel the resistance fade away.

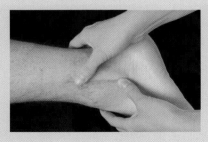

ciated health conditions such as headaches, autism, tinnitus, poor eye–hand coordination, and vertigo.

The techniques are taught at clinics and workshops worldwide. The Upledger Institute, located in Florida, is one of the foremost authorities on CST and offers courses and certification programs for massage therapists, osteopaths, chiropractors, physical therapists, and other healthcare professionals. See the Upledger Institute web site (www.upledger.com) for more information.

FRICTION TECHNIQUES

The fascial layer surrounding the muscles can become sticky or adhesive for several reasons, primarily insufficient hydration, poor nutrition, and inadequate activity. When an adhesion or scar tissue forms, collagen fibers are deposited in a random pattern with the fibers going in multiple directions. Friction is the main form of myofascial work specifically intended to disrupt and break down adhesions and scar tissue in soft tissue structures with linear fiber alignment such as muscles, tendons, and ligaments. The three basic types of friction are cross-fiber friction, circular friction, and longitudinal friction. The mechanism of friction actually reinjures the affected tissue to initiate phases II and III of the healing mechanism, which involve the production and proper alignment of collagen fibers. Understanding the process of collagen fiber alignment in phase III, you can help the original injury heal with a more mobile and functional scar.

The recovery period following a friction treatment is as important as the treatment itself. Make sure that the client uses the frictioned muscle regularly and without resistance or weight. The activity should be slow and careful, and it should move through the full range of motion to create a functional scar. Without this gentle activity, a connective tissue adhesion is likely to return.

James H. Cyriax, MD, MRCP, was an orthopedic doctor whose approach to musculoskeletal disorders included three principles:

1. Every pain has a source.
2. Treatment must reach the source.
3. Treatment must benefit the source to relieve the pain.

Starting at the location of a person's pain, he followed the myofascial lines of tension back to the site of the initial adhesion and was able to treat the pain by applying cross-fiber friction (XFF) to the adhesion. His work was so successful that Dr. Cyriax is credited with reintroducing manual therapy to the medical community. Because XFF can

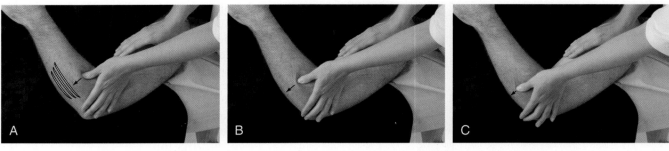

FIGURE 11-3   Cross-fiber friction. The stroke runs perpendicular to the muscle fibers (from **A** to **C**).

be very intense and uncomfortable, take great care to stay within the client's tolerance. Figure 11-3 shows XFF.

Circular friction (OF) is applied in small, circular motions to the affected tissue. It can be a very useful technique for addressing deep adhesions and scars (Fig. 11-4).

Longitudinal friction (LF) can help separate the randomly arranged fibers, freeing them up to allow more muscle movement. It differs from the other friction techniques because it is applied in the direction of the muscle fibers with a quicker and more superficial stroke. Figure 11-5 shows the application of LF.

Several principles guide the use of any type of friction. The principles are listed in Box 11-2.

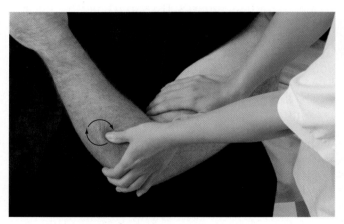

FIGURE 11-4   Circular friction.

Box 11-2

Principles for Applying Friction

- Educate the client about the technique. The therapist should explain that friction is a deep treatment designed to provide a controlled reinjury of the tissue and may induce pain. The therapist can explain that reinjury will allow the body to heal the tissue in a more functional manner.
- Obtain the client's consent to receive friction treatment.
- Fingernails must be short to apply this technique.
- The tissue must be warm prior to application.
- No lubricant is used, to allow the therapist to maintain the contact point.
- The client must be in a comfortable position that gives the therapist access to the affected tissues.
- Pressure is applied in one or more directions based upon the objective of the treatment.
- The pressure should be deep enough to penetrate the tissue and be annoying to the client yet remain within the client's pain tolerance.
- The therapist must tell the client that ice is recommended following treatment, to reduce inflammation.

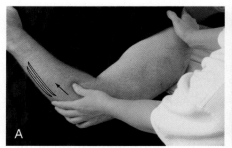
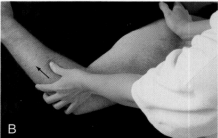
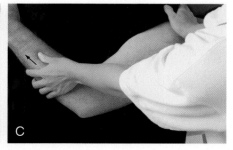

FIGURE 11-5   Longitudinal friction. The stroke runs parallel to the muscle fibers (from **A** to **C**).

Trigger Point Techniques

Usually activated by acute or repetitive overuse, a **trigger point** is a localized area of hypertonicity. Trigger points (TrPs) occur at the motor end unit, which is the neuromuscular junction, or meeting point between a nerve cell and the muscle cell it controls. TrP techniques are sometimes considered a subcategory of myofascial release and sometimes a form of neuromuscular (NOO-roh-MUSS-kyoo-lahr) therapy. In addition to treating fascial restrictions, TrP techniques address hypertonic areas of muscle tissue. Dr. Janet Travell, MD (1901–1997) developed trigger point therapy, and her research continues to be the most widely referenced in this type of treatment. Putting pressure directly on top of a TrP is usually painful for the client, and because of the nerve involvement, it refers vague, aching discomfort or an itchy sensation to the surrounding areas, in a specific pattern. It is usually painful for the client to actively move a muscle with a TrP, and the pain tends to limit the range of motion before reaching the end feel.

The difference between a tender point and a TrP is the involvement of a motor end unit. Tender points are areas of hypertonicity that do not refer pain. TrPs are so-named because the malfunctioning neuromuscular junction triggers pain patterns in specific patterns elsewhere on the body. Maps and charts of specific TrPs and their referred pain patterns are available for many muscles and can be very helpful. Figure 11-6 is a TrP map for the latissimus dorsi muscle.

Although they are not clinical pathology, TrPs do result from a hypertonic muscle. The decreased circulation in a hypertonic area reduces nutritional exchange to the area, causing it to be hypersensitive and hyper-

irritable. This is another example of the pain cycle in action. Several factors can create or perpetuate TrPs:

- Mechanical stresses, including skeletal misalignment
- Poor posture
- Long-term muscle constriction, such as compression by a purse or backpack
- Nutritional inadequacies
- Insufficient hydration
- Psychological factors, such as stress or the sympathetic nervous system response
- Inadequate sleep

TrPs that have existed longer than 3 weeks are considered chronic, and they can cause numbness and tingling along their specific referral patterns. They can also cause satellite TrPs in the synergists, created as a result of the original muscle being shortened and pulling the synergists into shortened positions.

The general benefits of wellness massage offer relief to clients suffering from TrPs, but specific TrP techniques can provide relief to the localized and referred pain, tingling, numbness, sensation of heat or cold, and itching. A TrP can feel like a nodule or localized area of hypertonicity amid a taut band of tissue running parallel to the muscle fibers. According to Dr. Travell, several methods can be used to release the hypertonicity at these troublesome neuromuscular junctions: PNF and friction techniques (discussed above), TrP pressure release, and strumming. A combination of techniques can also release a TrP.

TRIGGER POINT PRESSURE RELEASE

In the direct pressure release technique you first extend the target muscle to its comfort barrier and palpate the TrP. Increase your finger pressure on the TrP until you feel tissue resistance, and maintain that pressure until the tissues to release. This may take between 30 and 45 seconds. The release will feel like the nodule is melting as it lets go. Keep your contact finger on the original contact point on the client's skin and follow the release. The tissues may soften to allow your finger to sink deeper or the tissues may move in an irregular path at an irregular speed with fascial unwinding. There is a delicate balance between applying enough pressure to release it and applying so much pressure that the TrP worsens. The completion of the release is similar to the feeling you get at the bottom of a slide; initially there is a force that pulls you, and then the pull slowly fades away.

The release is effectively a neurological lengthening of the muscle fibers. To maintain the new length, the muscle and fascia must then be stretched for 5–10 seconds while you wait for a tendon reflex to relax the muscle further. Lengthening without stretching may

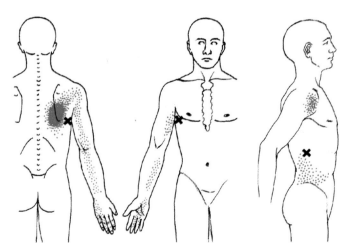

FIGURE 11-6 Trigger point map for the latissimus dorsi. (MediClip image copyright © 2003 Lippincott Williams & Wilkins. All rights reserved.)

cause the muscle to revert to its shortened position. Think of the longer loaf of bread in the shorter bag.

The more severe the TrP, the more it refers pain, so apply only minimal pressure to release the TrP. When spasm and muscle guarding are accompanied by satellite TrPs, release the satellite TrPs first. Your initial pressure on the TrP may be uncomfortable for the client but should not register as pain. As you continue to hold the point, the discomfort will diminish as the TrP releases. After circulation and nutrition are restored to the area, you may feel the area heat up. This TrP technique requires very little physical work and is a good approach to use when PNF is unsuccessful.

STRUMMING

If PNF and the pressure release technique do not release TrPs, you may need to try a more aggressive approach. Dr. Travell's strumming technique is very much like cross-fiber frictioning. It is most effective when the TrP is located near the center of the muscle belly. When you find a TrP, strum your finger perpendicular to the muscle fibers, at the level of the TrP until you come in contact with the TrP. Maintain light pressure on the TrP until it releases and melts under your finger. Following the release, continue the strum across the rest of the muscle's fibers. Finally, the tissues need to be elongated and stretched.

TRIGGER POINT RELEASE USING COMBINED TECHNIQUES

Sometimes a TrP is particularly persistent, and you will have to try several different approaches to facilitate its release. Using a combination of techniques in a single application can sometimes be the gentlest, quickest, most effective choice:

- TrP pressure and PR
- TrP pressure and reciprocal inhibition
- TrP pressure and PIR
- TrP pressure and connective tissue strokes
- Connective tissue strokes and CST

To combine TrP pressure with a PNF technique, apply pressure to the TrP with a monitoring finger (or knuckle or thumb) and use the pressure release technique while concurrently using the PNF technique. The combinations that use PNF along with the pressure release are very effective and typically last longer.

Combining TrP pressure release and connective tissue strokes often comes naturally. The primary difference between the 45° stroke and TrP pressure release is simply the monitoring finger. In both techniques, you apply pressure and wait for the client's tissues to deform, become more liquid, and release.

The combination of these techniques requires maintaining contact with the TrP with a monitoring finger while the connective tissue is being rearranged.

The combination of connective tissue strokes and CST is not used as much as the other combinations, because there is no monitoring finger on the TrP. Either technique can release a TrP using slow, steady pressure to facilitate a myofascial change. Basically, connective tissue strokes, craniosacral techniques, and TrP pressure release are variations of each other, the difference being the monitoring finger.

As with all PNF techniques and TrP releases techniques, the target muscle and its connective tissues should be elongated and stretched following treatment.

Treatment Plan

After you have taken a thorough history, completed the assessment process, and determined short- and long-term treatment goals, you develop a plan for the client's future treatment. This plan is based on all the information gathered in the initial session and should include the frequency and duration of future sessions and an estimated length of treatment. For example: 1 hour massage, once a week for 4 weeks. The plan can refer to treatment modalities that were successful on the client as well as modalities that could help achieve the treatment goals. Consult your plan at each session and adjust it as needed, depending upon how the client is responding to treatments. Each client is unique and may respond faster or slower than initially planned.

Also included in your treatment plan are recommendations for the client's self-care. These are exercises, stretches, and other homework activities that will help maintain the benefits of the massage between sessions. Recommendations should be relevant to the client's goals, simple, specific, and easy to follow. Clients are more likely to participate in their healthcare if you take time to educate them, and a demonstration of any stretches or exercises is especially helpful. These recommendations are not the same as goals, but they do help clients achieve their goals. Some suggested self-care activities include

- Exercises to strengthen the soft tissues and reduce the symptoms
- Stretches to retain elongated muscles and reset proprioceptors
- Proper hydration by drinking enough water
- Awareness exercises to help the client switch from focusing on the pain to focusing on periods of relief
- Any other activities that support the achievement of the client's goals

The treatment plan is important to the therapeutic massage arena because it demonstrates your understanding of the client's complete health condition, your comprehension of the benefits and limitations of massage therapy, and your ability to use massage most efficiently to attain the client's treatment goals. Most clients who suffer from some kind of dysfunction feel better knowing that there is a possibility of their health returning to a functional level. The massage treatment plan can provide that reassurance, showing that massage may be a means to the end. Understanding the massage techniques that may be used, the frequency of treatments, and the projected timeline for treatment, as well as activities clients can use between massage sessions will help clients see the light at the end of the tunnel and know that they may not have to suffer from their condition forever. Clients who want to restore function and return to a healthier condition will be more likely to participate in their own healthcare and will appreciate the components of the treatment plan.

As unusual as it may seem, not all clients look forward to eliminating their dysfunctions. Many persons who suffer from chronic symptoms become so accustomed to their symptoms that the symptoms actually become part of their identities. They complain about their symptoms and look for ways of eliminating them, but they resist improvement on a subconscious level.

Diagnosing or managing this psychological factor of health is not within the scope of practice of a massage therapist.

However, a massage therapist should recognize this phenomenon when it exists, because a client's resistance to improvement can be a source of frustration. You cannot force a client to accomplish a goal. In reality, you yourself do not make any changes to a client's tissues—you help the client's own body make the changes, or facilitate the changes, but you cannot force them. These are subtly different concepts, but they vastly affect your intent and play a large part in the effectiveness of the massage.

Treatment Documentation

After the massage session, document the techniques you used and their resultant changes in the Objective portion of the **SOAP** note. Record details of the treatment plan in the Plan section.

Chapter Summary

The therapeutic applications in this chapter are used for therapeutic massage rather than wellness massage. Massage students and massage therapists who understand the mechanisms of injury and repair and the pain cycle can use one or a combination of these techniques when a client is looking for more than a wellness massage. Techniques based on the concepts of lengthening muscles, stretching connective tissue, and going in the direction of ease minimize the amount of effort needed to change the musculature while increasing the effectiveness and permanence of changes. Clearly, it is important to address fascia when treating the muscles.

Your knowledge of medical terminology, anatomy, physiology, ethics, professionalism, documentation, and business practices as provided throughout this text are especially important for practicing therapeutic massage, because you are more likely to be communicating with persons in the medical, legal, and insurance fields.

The responses to therapeutic massage vary widely, but these more advanced techniques give you the opportunity to treat specific soft tissue conditions efficiently and effectively. Most clients respond well to these techniques, and some will be interested in knowing how the techniques work. Any time clients are interested in your work, you have the opportunity to educate them about massage. The more people know about the benefits of massage, the better.

 CHAPTER EXERCISES

1. Describe the events that occur in each of the three phases of healing.

2. Provide a real-life example of the pain cycle, including specific muscles or injuries for each stage of the cycle.

3. List at least five of the principles of therapeutic massage.

4. Define the following:
   a. Muscle guarding
   b. Target muscle
   c. Stretching
   d. Direction of restriction
   e. Tender point
   f. Unwinding
   g. Trigger point
   h. Lengthening

5. Practice the PNF procedures on a partner. First assess the joint range of motion moved by your target muscle, then perform each of the following techniques, and finish with a posttreatment assessment to determine whether any changes in muscle length occurred:
   a. Direct manipulation
   b. Positional release
   c. Postisometric relaxation
   d. Reciprocal inhibition

6. Describe the difference between the stretch reflex and the tendon reflex.

7. Practice each of the following connective tissue techniques on a partner, and ask your partner for feedback regarding discomfort, sensations, and responses:
   a. 45° stroke
   b. Skin rolling
   c. C-stroke
   d. S-stroke

8. Practice your palpation skills by trying to feel the craniosacral rhythm on several different people. With your "client" in a supine position, use a very light touch (the weight of a nickel) on the cranium, anterior superior iliac spines, the knees, and the toes.

9. List at least five of the principles for applying friction.

10. Practice the two different TrP release techniques on a partner. If your partner does not have a TrP, pretend that you found one and proceed with the techniques.

SUGGESTED READINGS

Chaitow L. Modern Neuromuscular Techniques. London: Churchill Livingstone, 1996.

Chaitow L, DeLany JW. Clinical Application of Neuromuscular Techniques, vol 1, The Upper Body. London: Churchill Livingstone, 2000.

Persad RS. Massage Therapy & Medications General Treatment Principles. Toronto: Curties-Overzet, 2001.

Scheumann DW. The Balanced Body A Guide to Deep Tissue and Neuromuscular Therapy. 2nd ed. Philadelphia: Lippincott Williams & Wilkins, 2002.

Thompson D. Hands Heal. Baltimore: Lippincott Williams & Wilkins, 2002.

Travell J, Simons DG, Simons LS. Myofascial Pain and Dysfunction: The Trigger Point Manual, 2nd ed. Baltimore: Lippincott Williams & Wilkins, 1999.

http://aaomed.org/awards/index.php, accessed 10/3/03.

http://archive.uwcm.ac.uk/uwcm/sr/whru/Phasebiology.html, accessed 9/17/02.

http://education.yahoo.com/reference/dictionary/entries/44/n0074400.html, accessed 9/16/02.

http://www.esomc.com/orthopaedic_medicine.htm, accessed 10/3/03.

http://medweb.bham.ac.uk/http/depts/path/teaching/foundat/repair/healing.html, accessed 9/15/02

http://w3.tvi.cc.nm.us/~katflies/patho1/patho1-wound-healing.htm, accessed 9/17/02.

http://www.bodyzone.com/custom/pain_cycle.html, accessed 9/15/02.

http://www.chiroweb.com/archives/19/08/21.html, accessed 11/5/02.

http://www.cityhealthcentre.nildram.co.uk/cranial.htm, accessed 9/18/02.

http://www.cofc.edu/~futrellm/healing.html, accessed 9/15/02.

http://www.cyriax.com/En-DrCyriax.htm, accessed 9/15/02.

http://www.e-antiinflammatory.com/, accessed 9/15/02.

http://www.efunda.com/materials/piezo/general_info/gen_info_index.cfm, accessed 11/5/02.

http://www.exrx.net/lists/Articulations.html, accessed 9/30.03.

http://www.focusonarthritis.com/script/main/art.asp?li=MNI&ArticleKey=11615, accessed 9/20/02.

http://www.frcc.cccoes.edu/~fsulliva/Lecture_The_Acute_Inflammatory_Response.htm, accessed 9/15/02.

http://www.hendrickhealth.org/rehab/strain.htm, accessed 11/04/02.

http://www.hsutx.edu/academics/eman/immun-ch5/tsld006.htm, accessed 9/15/02.

http://www.iol.ie/~alank/CROHNS/PRIMER/inflresp.htm, accessed 9/15/02.

http://www.jdaross.cwc.net/inflammatory_response.htm, accessed 9/15/02.

http://www.laredo.edu/jgoetze/General_Biology/3rd/TISSUES%20H.htm, accessed 9/15/02.

http://www.ma.psu.edu/~pt/renee160/pnf_files/frame.htm, accessed 9/15/02.

http://www.medhelp.org/glossary2/new/gls_2675.htm, accessed 9/15/02.

http://www.m-w.com/cgi-bin/dictionary?thixotropic, accessed 11/10/02.

http://www.myotherapy1.com/_myotherapy1/myotherapy_faq.htm, accessed 9/15/02.

http://www.naturalhealthnotebook.com/Anatomy_Physiology/Inflammatory_Response.htm, accessed 9/15/02.

http://www.nova.edu/~kimreed/inflammation.htm, accessed 9/15/02.

http://www.ortho-u.net/05/337.htm, accessed 9/30/03.

http://www.pathwaysmag.com/cranios.html, accessed 11/6/02.

http://www.ptcentral.com/muscles/, accessed 9/30/03.

http://www.qub.ac.uk/cm/pat/education/Inflamm/tsld004.htm, accessed 9/15/02.

http://www.repetitivemotion.com/cause.html, accessed 9/15/02.

http://www.simplesoap.net/phasesofhealing.htm, accessed 9/16/02.

http://www.thedrs.net/orthopaedic.htm, accessed 9/16/02.

http://www.time.com/time/innovators_v2/alt_medicine/profile_upledger2.html, accessed 11/6/02.

http://www.upledger.com/therapies/cst_faq.htm , accessed 11/6/02.

http://www.upledger.com/therapies/default.htm , accessed 11/6/02.

http://www.usabaseball.com/iceandheat.html, accessed 9/18/02.

http://www.vetmed.ufl.edu/path/pbteach/wlc/vem5161/inflect1.htm, accessed 9/15/02.

http://www.vetmed.ufl.edu/path/pbteach/wlc/vem5161/inflect3.htm, accessed 9/15/02.

http://www.woundcare.org/newsvol4n1/ar2.htm, accessed 9/16/02.

Special Populations

UPON COMPLETION OF THIS CHAPTER, THE STUDENT WILL BE ABLE TO:

- Explain the massage term "special population"
- Identify at least three research-proven benefits of massage in the workplace
- Identify at least three benefits of massage for athletes
- Demonstrate how to safely and comfortably position and bolster a pregnant client for massage
- List at least three special considerations for massaging a paralyzed client

KEY TERMS

Chronic illness: illness that lasts a year or longer, usually limits a patient's physical activity, and may require ongoing medical care and treatment

Corporate massage: a chair massage for persons in the middle of their workday, also called seated massage, on-site massage, and chair massage

Countertransference: your tendency to react emotionally when clients do not behave or respond to you or your treatment as you had expected

Hospice: a healthcare approach that caters to the quality of remaining life rather than the quantity of life when a person's life expectancy is limited by a life-threatening illness with no known cure

Postevent massage: a massage performed within 6 hours of the athletic performance that focuses on circulatory enhancement

Preevent massage: a massage performed up to 2 days before the client participates in an athletic event that focuses on circulatory enhancement and warming up the tissues.

Restorative massage: a massage performed 6–72 hours after the athletic performance that is intended to increase circulation and restore the normal resting length of muscles, also called curative massage and postrecovery massage

Transference: the client's dependence on you for friendship or companionship in addition to therapeutic treatment

Many segments of the population have special needs with regards to massage, such as special positioning, physical assistance, or a therapist who understands and can manage specific physiological characteristics. Various massage routines have been developed for some of these special populations, but a standard routine can significantly limit the benefit to the client. Standard routines do not allow the therapist to read and address the individual client's tissues, but they can serve as a good basis for the massage. A routine may include an efficient flow for the massage or a set of basic strokes that are appropriate. A qualified therapist can specialize and alter the routine to better accommodate each client.

The special circumstances and special populations discussed in this chapter include

- Fully clothed clients
- Athletes
- Pregnant women
- Infants
- Geriatric clients
- Chronically ill clients
- Disabled clients

Fully Clothed Clients

Almost anyone can receive massage in almost any setting. Persons who are fully clothed can benefit from massage, in casual or public venues such as airports or shopping malls, as well as in workplaces. A massage chair is a great piece of equipment to use to market your skills and gain access to persons who may not otherwise experience massage. It is a good first exposure for persons who have reservations or misconceptions regarding massage therapy and a good vehicle for educating clients about the benefits of regular massage. You can set up a massage chair at a public venue on your own, offer massages for free or for a nominal fee. Give people your business card and offer informative brochures and coupons for new clients. You can also charge a fee for chair massage at a rate that is comparable to your fee for table massage. For example, if you charge $60 for an hour-long table massage session, you might charge $15 for a 10- to 15-minute chair massage. Either way, your gross income is about $60 per hour. This kind of fee schedule is generally used for massage in the workplace or in a business organization.

CORPORATE MASSAGE

Corporate massage, also called seated massage, on-site massage, and chair massage, gives people an opportunity to receive massage in the middle of the work-day. Although some are concerned that a massage received at work may slow them down and make them sleepy for the rest of the day, this is not the case. **Research has found that massage in the workplace increases productivity and employee job satisfaction.** One of the leading researchers in the field of massage is Tiffany M. Field, PhD, of the Touch Research Institutes at the University of Miami School of Medicine (Box 12-1). Dr. Field's work is well received by the medical and scientific communities because her studies incorporate critical scientific methods, using control groups and objectively measured responses. By measuring hormone levels, blood pressure, brain wave activity, and math test performance, she showed that after a massage, employees were more alert, felt less job stress and anxiety, could perform more efficiently, and were more accurate with math calculations. Most people feel more relaxed and less anxious after chair massage, feel that they can think more clearly, and have increased energy. (Box 12-2 identifies some highlights of corporate massage.)

Box 12-1

Dr. Tiffany Field and the Touch Research Institute

The first Touch Research Institute (TRI) was formally established in 1992 by Director Tiffany Field, PhD, at the University of Miami School of Medicine via a startup grant from Johnson & Johnson. The TRI was the first center in the world devoted solely to the study of touch and its application in science and medicine. There is now a TRI in the Philippines whose neonatologists focus on preterm infants' weight gain and one in Paris that studies the role of touch in psychopathology.

The TRI's distinguished team of researchers, representing Duke, Harvard, Maryland, and other universities, strives to better define touch as it promotes health and contributes to the treatment of disease. Research efforts that began in 1982 and continue today have shown that touch therapy has numerous beneficial effects on health and well-being.

The institutes have completed over 80 studies on the positive effects of massage therapy. Physiological functions, chemical and hormone levels, and medical conditions in persons of all ages have been targeted in these studies. Some of the more significant research findings have shown enhanced growth in preterm infants, increased pulmonary function in asthmatics, increased natural killer cells in persons with HIV and cancer, lowered glucose levels in diabetics, and lowered blood levels of stress hormones.

More information about the Touch Research Institutes can be found on their web site: www.miami.edu/touch-research

---

Box 12-2

Corporate Massage to Invigorate Clients and Reduce Their Stress and Tension

- Clients are fully clothed
- Clients receive massage in the seated position, usually in a massage chair
- 10- to 15-minute treatment
- Fast-paced, brisk compression, and tapotement are the major strokes
- Focus on the neck, shoulders, upper back, arms, and hands
- No lubricant
- No draping

When clients are at work, they can be comfortably and modestly supported in a seated position using a massage chair (Fig. 12-1). They remain fully clothed, which means the massage is applied through their clothing. You use no lubricant. You work primarily on the client's posterior neck and shoulder muscles, the back muscles, and the arms and hands. This massage usually lasts only 10–15 minutes, the general pace of the massage is faster and brisker, and the flow follows somewhat of a routine. Often performed in a well-lit, open area, with upbeat or no music, the strokes used are quick and brisk to keep the client awake and invigorated (Procedure Box 12-1).

CORPORATE ACCOUNTS

Acquiring an account to provide corporate chair massage may be as simple as contacting local companies, educating them on the benefits of massage, and setting up an initial session for their employees. Corporations can justify the financial cost of massage therapy in the workplace with increased productivity and the ability to attract and retain high-quality employees, and improve employees' health and thereby minimize health insurance premiums. Many hospitals,

PROCEDURE BOX 12-1
Corporate Massage Routine

1. Welcome the client:
   a. Greet the client.
   b. Inquire about spine or neck injuries or conditions, wrist and shoulder issues, or recent surgeries.
   c. Orient the client to the massage chair and demonstrate how to sit in it.
   d. Ask client to sit in the chair, and adjust the chair to the client's body.
2. Apply a resting stroke to both of the client's shoulders.
3. Stand behind the client in an asymmetric position and warm up the shoulder and back muscles by applying compression and petrissage:
   a. With loose fists on either side of the spine, from shoulder to sacrum, 2–3 times
   b. With the heel of the hand, compressing the erector spinae muscles laterally, from shoulder to iliac crest, on one side of the spine at a time
   c. With the thumb, down the erector spinae muscles, working into the intercostal spaces, one side of the spine at a time
   d. With the forearm, into the upper trapezius and levator scapulae, one side at a time
4. Apply 8 seconds of moderate hacking over the whole upper back.
5. Stand by the client's right side, and apply compression to the right arm, from the deltoids to the hand, 2–3 times.
6. Apply compression and petrissage to the right hand, paying extra attention to the thenar eminence, and passively extend and stretch the hand and finger flexors.
7. Move to the client's left side and repeat steps 4–7 on the left arm.
8. Move to face the client and apply compression and petrissage strokes with both hands, moving medially from the shoulders toward the neck.
9. Apply circular friction to the base of the occiput, moving laterally.
10. Apply brisk effleurage strokes:
    a. Starting at the neck and brushing off the shoulders
    b. Starting at the shoulders and brushing down, toward the sacrum
11. Stretch the client's pectoral muscles:
    a. Ask client to sit up and take a deep breath.
    b. Ask client to place both hands behind the head and inhale slowly.
    c. Ask client to exhale slowly as you slowly pull the elbows back, toward you, to the end feel.
    d. Repeat 2–3 times.
12. Apply a resting stroke to the client's shoulders.
(Courtesy of Kathy Latimer, RRT, NCTMB)

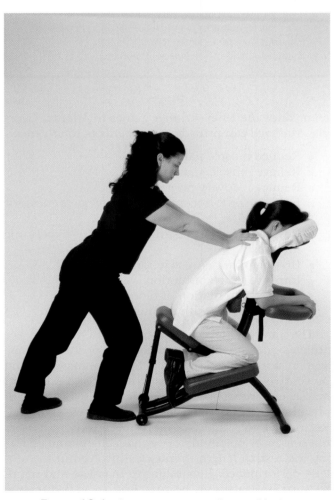
FIGURE 12-1 Corporate massage client positioning.

doctors' offices, pain clinics, regional conference gatherings, and schools provide chair massage.

Corporations and business organizations generally schedule your visits on a weekly or monthly basis with a contractual agreement, and they typically pay you directly, rather than requiring their employees to pay you individually. Make sure that you and the business both understand each other's expectations and accommodations:

- Your time commitment
- Specific location and space you will use
- Length of each appointment
- Appointment scheduling responsibility
- Payment arrangements
  - Fee schedule
  - Who is responsible for payment
  - When are payments made
- Sound system, or music
- Your parking arrangements
- Missed appointments
- Your tardiness or inability to meet the schedule

If you and the organization establish and clarify these responsibilities at the beginning, you can avoid potential complications and misunderstandings in the future.

Athletes

Athletes are especially prone to muscular strain and overuse. Sports massage is a general term that refers to massage for athletes, and it uses the basic massage strokes and therapeutic techniques. **The distinguishing factor of sports massage is that the therapist should know which muscles and motions athletes use most often in a particular sport** (Box 12-3). For example, the muscles actively used for running or jogging are the leg muscles. The massage therapist might focus on a runner's psoas major, hamstrings, quadriceps femoris group, tensor fascia latae, gastrocnemius, soleus, peroneus group, and anterior and posterior tibialis. Recognize also that the upper body counterbalances running with an arm swing. The postural muscles and the muscles responsible for shoulder flexion and extension are also involved in running. Particularly important to running is a normal gait pattern because if a runner deviates from an even, fluid gait pattern, compensations will result.

Massage is gaining popularity in all segments of the population, but athletes in particular often accept the importance of massage for flexibility, enhanced recovery from muscle fatigue and injury, and improved performance. Massage has been widely used in several amateur and professional sports for years and has been a part of the official Olympic medical

---

Box 12-3

Major Muscles Involved in Some Common Sports

- Basketball: gastrocnemius, anterior tibialis, quadriceps femoris, hamstrings, gluteal muscles
- Bicycling: neck extensors, trapezius, erector spinae, gastrocnemius, quadriceps femoris, hamstrings, gluteal muscles
- Bowling: finger flexors, wrist flexors, wrist extensors, anterior serratus, pectoralis major, anterior deltoids, triceps brachii
- Downhill skiing: quadriceps femoris, anterior tibialis, toe flexors, plantaris, peroneus group, adductor group, erector spinae, trapezius
- Golf: levator scapulae, triceps brachii, trapezius, infraspinatus, supraspinatus, rhomboids, quadratus lumborum
- Racquet sports: finger flexors, wrist flexors, triceps brachii, deltoids, subscapularis, trapezius, infraspinatus, pectoralis major, quadriceps femoris, gluteal muscles, hamstrings
- Rowing: most major muscle groups
- Running: anterior tibialis, psoas major, quadriceps femoris, hamstrings, gluteal muscles, gastrocnemius
- Swimming: infraspinatus, supraspinatus, subscapularis, teres minor, deltoids, pectoralis major, gluteal muscles, trapezius, latissimus dorsi, triceps brachii
- Volleyball: most major muscle groups

---

team since the 1996 summer games in Atlanta, Georgia. Massage can provide many benefits to athletes:

- Reduce muscle pain
- Relieve muscle spasms
- Reduce recovery period
- Enhance proprioception and body awareness for coordination
- Restore normal resting length to hypertonic muscles
- Break up fascial restrictions
- Improve range of motion
- Improve circulation of blood and lymph
- Enhance the health of muscle tissue

The many different applications of massage for athletes include preevent massage, postevent massage, restorative massage, rehabilitative massage, and preventive maintenance massage. Pre- and postevent massages involve special considerations, but the application involves a basic set of strokes and flow. Restorative massage is a more therapeutic massage, but it focuses on circulatory enhancement and restoring the resting length to muscles involved in the athletic performance. Rehabilitative massage and maintenance massage can be managed in a therapeutic massage session as long as the therapist understands the relevant anatomy, physiology, and mechanisms of injury repair and is experienced with range of motion and connective tissue manipulation. Sports massage is a growing field, and many workshops are available for learning more about this specialty.

If you plan to be at an event all day or for several hours, possibly doing both pre- and postevent massage, you must schedule breaks for yourself. You need to periodically rest and ground yourself. It can be overwhelming to touch so many bodies in a short time, and you need to stay grounded to maintain an emotional and energetic barrier. Sometimes food and drinks are provided for you, but not always. Come prepared with food and drink, and schedule breaks at least once an hour to take a walk or use the toilet.

PREEVENT MASSAGE

Preevent massage is performed before the client participates in an athletic event. Since the effects of preevent massage can last for a day or two, some athletes get their preevent massage up to 2 days before the event. The focus of the preevent massage is to increase circulation to the muscles, soften the connective tissue to prevent injury, increase the client's general kinesthetic awareness, and reduce general anxiety (Box 12-4). Also important are other benefits shown in Dr. Field's research, including reduced cortisol levels, lowered blood pressure, and changes in brain wave activity.

Box 12-4

Preevent Massage to Increase Circulation and Warm the Tissues

- Also applied to reduce muscular tension and increase flexibility and range of motion
- Can reduce anxiety and heighten the athlete's sense of well-being and ability to concentrate
- Usually on site
- Performed 2 days to 10 minutes before the event
- Clients are usually wearing athletic apparel or warm-up suits
- 15–20 minutes or less of brisk treatment
- Use light, nonspecific rhythmic compression, rhythmic compression, kneading, superficial friction, tapotement, vibration, and stretching and joint movements
- Focus on the primary muscles involved in the event
- Little or no draping
- No lubricant
- No changes are made to the length of muscles
- No comments are made regarding client's tissues unless you suspect an injury, at which point you refer them to the medical tent

---

Equipment

Preevent massage is usually performed on site, at the event, indoors or outdoors. For outdoor venues, you need to consider temperature and weather. Outdoor venues are not always warm and pleasant. Sometimes it is cold, windy, rainy, hot and humid, or especially dry. Dress appropriately with layers of clothing that you can add or remove to stay comfortable. Consider shelter to stay out of the bright sunlight or the rain. Highly coordinated events may provide a tent for you, but it is best to find out before you arrive. The larger the event, the more activity there is around you. Athletes and their supportive family members and friends, event organizers, vendors, music, loudspeakers, starting pistols, and roaring crowds are some of the aspects of a sports massage environment. You must stay grounded and centered throughout the day.

You typically bring your own table, but because clients often wear their athletic apparel or warm-up suits during the massage, you do not usually use linens. Instead, you need to bring supplies to properly disinfect your equipment between clients, as well as a trash container to dispose of your cleaning supplies. Some persons choose to bring towels and sheets to drape their equipment or clients, but because you must use new, clean linens for every client, it can add up to a lot of linens. Towels are always convenient to have on hand because they are so versatile. You can use towels for bolstering, to absorb sweat or spills, to cover clients for warmth, and to cover your equipment. Lubricants are not used for preevent massage because they can interfere with the skin's evaporative cooling mechanism, but it is always good to be prepared and have it with you.

Application

Preevent massage is often based on a routine similar to a corporate massage, but clients typically lie on a table, giving you access to the entire body. The routine usually lasts between 15 and 20 minutes or less, and its purpose is to warm the tissues, reduce muscular tension, enhance circulation, and increase flexibility and range of motion. Psychologically, the purpose is to reduce anxiety and heighten the athlete's sense of well-being and ability to concentrate. Because this massage is so brief, try to focus on the muscles that the athlete will use during the upcoming event and any muscles that might be held in passive contraction for extended periods.

The session should be light and nonspecific. The strokes used most often include rhythmic compression, kneading, superficial friction, tapotement, vibration, and stretching and joint movements to increase flexibility.

The techniques should not be deep or painful.

They are applied briskly, slightly faster than one compression stroke per second, and are intended to enhance circulation and energize the client (Procedure Box 12-2). Use joint movements to stimulate synovial fluid production for lubrication and shock absorption at the joints. Do not use joint movements to extend the ranges of motion or change the shape or position of soft tissues.

 No significant changes are made to the length of the muscles or fascia during preevent massage, because the client's kinesthetic awareness could be altered.

In other words, if a client has been training for a 10K run with a tight right psoas major muscle for 2 weeks, her body may have developed some compensation patterns that alter her posture and muscu-

lar coordination. The psoas major muscle is responsible for initiating a stride, slightly drawing the femur forward with hip flexion. If you were to lengthen the psoas and stretch the surrounding fascia immediately before the run, the athlete's body would be unfamiliar with the new length of the psoas muscle and the new body position. As a result, old patterns of coordination and kinesthetic awareness could cause the athlete to trip or otherwise negatively affect the performance.

Before an event, the athlete's mental state is often focused and possibly anxious. Athletes may be extrasensitive to comments regarding their physical condition. You can encourage the athlete to perform well but should not make any comments regarding an athlete's muscles or physical condition during a preevent massage. For instance, you might notice that your client's left hamstrings are a bit tighter than the right hamstrings or that the range of motion of the right shoulder is restricted. Instead of sharing that information before the event, keep that kind of information to yourself. Such thoughts can easily have a psychosomatic effect on a client. Be-

---

PROCEDURE BOX 12-2
Preevent Massage Routine for a Long-Distance Runner

Client in the prone position

1. Compression: 4 strokes that move distally along the client's left arm
2. Petrissage: 6 seconds to the left trapezius, levator scapula, and posterior deltoid
3. Tapotement: 6 seconds of hacking to the left upper back
4. Brisk effleurage: 2 strokes to brush down the left back
5. Compression:
   a. 6 strokes to the left gluteals
   b. 4 strokes that move inferiorly, to the left iliotibial band
   c. 4 strokes that move inferiorly, to the lateral side of the left hamstrings
   d. 4 strokes that move inferiorly, to the center of the left hamstrings
   e. 4 strokes that move inferiorly, to the medial side of the left hamstrings
6. Petrissage: 8 seconds to the left thigh
7. Tapotement: 8 seconds of hacking to the left gluteals and thigh
8. Compression:
   a. 3 strokes that move inferiorly, to the lateral side of the left calf
   b. 3 strokes that move inferiorly, to the lateral side of the left gastrocnemius
   c. 3 strokes that move inferiorly, to the medial side of the left gastrocnemius
9. Petrissage: 8 seconds to the left calf

10. Brisk effleurage: 2 strokes to brush down the left leg
11. Repeat steps 1–10 for the client's right side

Client turns over to the supine position

12. Compression:
    a. 3 strokes that move inferiorly, to the lateral side of the left quadriceps femoris
    b. 3 strokes that move inferiorly, to the center of the left quadriceps femoris
    c. 3 strokes that move inferiorly, to the medial side of the left quadriceps femoris
13. Petrissage: 8 seconds to the left thigh
14. Compression:
    a. 4 strokes that move inferiorly, to the left anterior tibialis
    b. 4 strokes that move inferiorly, to the left peroneus group
15. Joint movement:
    a. Passive left knee and hip flexion
    b. Passive left ankle rotation
16. Brisk effleurage: 2 strokes to brush down the left leg
17. Repeat steps 12–16 for the client's right leg
18. Brisk effleurage:
    a. 1 stroke, simultaneously with both hands, to brush down both of the client's arms
    b. 2 strokes, simultaneously with both hands, to brush down both of the client's legs

cause the athlete's mental state is so closely related to the physical state, negative thoughts can create a real physiological condition. As with a self-fulfilling prophecy, athletes who assume they cannot perform well may not try to perform well, believing that they are not capable. Then, when their performance is not successful, they have a "reasonable" explanation. If you notice a possible injury, however, you should suggest that the client visit the medical tent before the event.

POSTEVENT MASSAGE

Postevent massage is performed within 6 hours of the athletic performance. **Athletes should cool down and, if possible, put on dry clothes if they are receiving treatment immediately after their event.** The purpose of postevent massage is to encourage circulation in and around the muscles; reduce muscular tension, congestion, and potential muscle soreness; restore flexibility; and, if necessary, relieve muscle cramps. Immediately following performance, the athlete's musculature is often suffering oxygen debt. One of the greatest benefits of massage is increased circulation, which delivers oxygen to the tissues and greatly reduces the lactic acid buildup in the muscles. Lactic acid is the chemical that builds up in the muscle tissues and makes athletes feel sore and achy for the next few days. The stiffness and sore muscles, which often discourage people from exercise, can be prevented with massage. (Box 12-5 lists some of the highlights of postevent massage.)

Equipment

This massage is usually performed at the site of the event, on a massage table that you bring to the event, with the client still in athletic apparel or, if possible, in dry clothes. Ask the clients to remove their shoes, and massage them through their clothing. Be careful of broken and unbroken blisters.

> ⚠ *Open skin is an invitation for infection, and intact blisters can easily break open, so avoid massaging over broken and unbroken blisters.*

Be prepared for the environment with the proper clothing, shelter, food, and drink. Because clients are often sweaty, linens are not typically used for postevent massages. Instead, the athletes lie directly on the table and you properly disinfect your equipment with spray or disinfectant wipes between clients. Make sure you have a trash container, just in case one is not provided or nearby. As with preevent

---

Box 12-5

Postevent Massage to Increase Circulation

- Applied to reduce muscular tension, congestion, and potential muscle soreness and restore flexibility, and, if necessary, relieve muscle cramps
- Usually on site
- Performed within 6 hours after the event
- Clients are usually wearing athletic apparel or warm-up suits, or, if possible, dry clothes
- 15–20 minutes or less, moderately paced treatment
- Use effleurage, gentle compression, stretching, gentle joint movements, and fulling and lifting
- Focus on the major muscles involved in the athletic event
- Use lubricant
- Little or no draping
- No deep strokes

---

massage, you may be indoors or outdoors, on the deck of a swimming pool, in a locker room, in the grass at a rowing or track and field event, or next to a garage at a motorsports complex. Like the preevent environment, it is likely that there will be a lot of activity going on around you. Stay grounded, stay centered, and rest periodically.

Application

Postevent massage usually lasts 15 to 20 minutes or less. The session focuses on the muscles used during the athlete's event and is slower paced, providing relaxation and general relief from exhaustion. Effleurage is the primary stroke used in postevent massage, mostly applied toward the heart. Gentle compression and joint movements are commonly included in postevent massage routines. Avoid deep strokes because they can damage the fatigued tissues. Lubricant increases the comfort of effleurage strokes and enhances the slip, which can alleviate some of the pressure. Very gentle stretching and joint movement may also be applied to relax tense muscles and encourage circulation.

Some variations of the basic massage strokes that are commonly used in postevent massage include fulling and lifting. These two-handed strokes travel across the muscle fibers instead of along the length of the fibers. Fulling, also called broadening, spreads the muscle fibers out and away from each other. To perform fulling on the quadriceps femoris, bring your hands together and rest the heels or palms of your hands on the quadriceps femoris. Effleurage with both hands simultaneously so that one hand slides to the medial thigh and the other hand slides to the lateral thigh. Lifting is essentially the opposite of fulling, basically picking up the muscle and pulling it away from the underlying bone. Using the quadriceps femoris as an example, you start with one palm on the lateral side of the thigh and the other palm on the medial side of the thigh. Simultaneously slide both hands toward the front of the thigh, compressing and lifting the quadriceps femoris up and away from the femur. Together, fulling and lifting are similar to a petrissage stroke. As with all strokes, pay attention your body mechanics and make sure your wrist position does not put excessive pressure on the structures running through the carpal tunnel (Procedure Box 12-3).

 Sometimes athletes experience a muscle cramp after intense physical exertion in their event.

Because this might occur, you should be aware of what causes muscle cramping and how to alleviate it. Cramping is a forceful, painful, involuntary contraction of the muscle fibers that may be caused by trauma, overload, fluid loss, electrolyte imbalance, or excessive temperatures. You can alleviate cramping via ice massage, which decreases nerve impulses and muscle spindle cell activity, or you can use reciprocal inhibition, direct manipulation, or compression.

Athletes may also experience thermoregulatory conditions such as hypothermia (core body temperature that drops below the normal range), heat cramps, heat exhaustion, or heat stroke. Any time athletes complain of feeling excessively hot or cold, you notice that their tissues are abnormally hot or cold, or they feel faint, disoriented, or dizzy, you should refer them immediately to the emergency medical technicians (EMTs) or medical tent for treatment.

RESTORATIVE MASSAGE

Restorative massage, also called curative massage and postrecovery massage, takes place 6–72 hours after the athletic performance. The purpose of restorative massage is to increase circulation and restore the normal resting length of muscles. During an athletic event, some muscles contract repeatedly, usually with a lot of force. After the event, the muscles that have been contracting can easily develop a shorter resting length unless they are lengthened and their antagonistic muscles are activated. Restorative massage is the perfect opportunity to lengthen the muscles that were particularly active during the event and to stretch the fascia that surrounds those muscles. If an athlete is between events, *do not* do this. Between events, keep the client's muscles warm and flexible in preparation for another event (Box 12.6).

PROCEDURE BOX 12-3
Postevent Massage Routine for a Long-distance Runner

Client is in the supine position
Right leg:

1. Distal compression strokes to the quadriceps femoris
2. Proximal effleurage strokes to thigh
3. Fulling strokes to thigh
4. Lifting strokes to thigh
5. Distal compression strokes to the anterior tibialis
6. Proximal effleurage strokes to anterolateral lower leg
7. Passive joint movement to knee, hip, and ankle
8. Brisk effleurage strokes to brush down the leg

Left leg:
Repeat supine steps 1–8.

Client turns over to the prone position
Right leg:

9. Compression strokes to the gluteal muscles
10. Distal compression strokes to the hamstrings
11. Proximal effleurage strokes to thigh
12. Fulling strokes to thigh
13. Lifting strokes to thigh
14. Distal compression strokes to the gastrocnemius
15. Proximal effleurage strokes to calf
16. Brisk effleurage strokes to brush down the leg

Left leg:
Repeat prone steps 9–16.

Back:

17. Effleurage strokes across the low back
18. Effleurage strokes from the left iliac crest to the left shoulder
19. Effleurage strokes from the left shoulder to the occipital ridge (Walk to the client's right side)
20. Effleurage strokes from the right iliac crest to the right shoulder
21. Effleurage strokes from the right shoulder to the occipital ridge
22. Brisk effleurage strokes to brush down the back

Application

Restorative massage typically takes place in your standard treatment room because clients are not usually at the event 6–72 hours after their performance. You can use all of the basic massage strokes, ranges of motion, and therapeutic applications. Proprioceptive neuromuscular facilitation (PNF) techniques are especially effective during postevent massage to restore normal resting length to muscles. Remember to stretch the fascia in and around the muscles that are

Box 12-6

Restorative Massage to Increase Circulation and Restore Normal Resting Length to the Muscles

- Usually in your treatment room
- Performed 6–72 hours after the event
- Clients are usually undressed and modestly draped
- 30- to 60-minute treatment
- Use effleurage, petrissage, compression, range of motion, PNF techniques, and stretches
- Focus on the major muscles used in the athletic event
- Use lubricant

lengthened, and hold the stretch to allow a tendon reflex to further relax the muscle.

RECOVERY AND REHABILITATION

Part of your responsibility as a professional massage therapist is to be educated and to educate your clients. When clients come to you as a result of overexertion and muscle strain, ask about their physical activity patterns and goals, and try to understand their pain patterns. Different kinds of pain have different causes and thus require different treatment.

During and immediately following the physical activity, muscles may burn and feel fatigued as a result of oxygen debt. The pain subsides after exercise stops and the oxygen debt is repaid, which usually occurs within minutes. Lactic acid buildup and shortened muscles can cause the pain and discomfort that tends to worsen over 2–3 days before it gets better, but the soreness usually only lasts a few days. When muscle tissue is torn, the healing mechanism is initiated, and inflammation results.

 Localized areas of inflammation are contraindications for massage.

Depending on the client's health and the severity of the injury, healing can occur within several weeks or it can take up to a year or more. Clients who exercise regularly but are trying a new sport will heal differently and probably much quicker than someone who has been inactive for years and has started a strenuous exercise program. The pain cycle will aggravate the healing process, and clients who have been caught in a pain cycle for more than a month will benefit greatly from therapeutic massage. The more you understand your clients' physical activity, the better you can address their soft tissue complaints.

Discuss the healing mechanism and the effects of restricted fascia. Athletes frequently overuse and stress their muscles and suffer the resulting soreness, stiffness, range of motion limitations, muscle fatigue, and generalized body pain. Many people are familiar with the treatment of rest, ice, compression, and elevation (RICE), which speeds the healing process, but not everyone understands it. The rest prevents further injury, the ice provides pain relief and reduces circulation to the area, compression prevents lymph from accumulating, and elevation encourages lymph to drain away from the injured area. Once the ice is removed, the body floods the area with oxygenated blood to encourage healing, and the cellular and chemical wastes are removed. Remember that in phase III of healing, gentle movements of the injured area help create a functional scar. Persons who are seriously interested in healing will be grateful for information that helps them heal faster and more functionally.

During athletic activity, muscles contract repeatedly and can easily establish a shorter resting length once the activity stops. Lengthening and stretching muscles immediately after exercise is a very effective and beneficial technique clients can use for self-help. For example, to lengthen and stretch their gastrocnemius muscles, they can use a postisometric relaxation technique on their own:

1. Stand on the balls of the feet on the edge of a step or raised platform.
2. Let the heels slowly drop down to extend the gastrocnemius muscles to the end feel.
3. Rise up on the toes just a bit to contract the gastrocnemius muscles slightly.
4. Hold the position for 7–10 seconds.
5. Slowly relax the gastrocnemius muscles and let the heels drop down, extending the gastrocnemius to the end feel.
6. Hold the position for 7–10 seconds and wait for a tendon reflex to relax and lengthen the gastrocnemius muscles further.

Help clients help themselves. The combination of education, self-help activities, and massage treatment can be highly effective if your clients are willing to participate in their healthcare.

Pregnant Women

There is a lot of controversy regarding pregnancy and massage. Some suggest that women should not receive any massage at all during the first 3 months of pregnancy. However, others suggest that very light massage is appropriate and beneficial during the first

3 months. Many persons specifically avoid massaging women with a history or risk of miscarriage. Some recommend against the prone position at any point during the pregnancy, and others consider a bolstered prone position safe. Generally, healthy women with a low-risk pregnancy can receive the benefits of massage throughout their pregnancy, during labor, and through the postpartum period. Ask your pregnant clients to discuss the benefits of or contraindications to massage with their obstetricians before you agree to treat them.

The physical condition of pregnant women involves some important considerations and contraindications for massage. A pregnant body undergoes many changes that create stress, pain, and discomfort. Stress can complicate the pregnancy and delivery in numerous ways. Massage can provide relief from many of these symptoms, as long as it is applied carefully and knowledgeably.

FIRST TRIMESTER

The first trimester includes the first 3 months of pregnancy. Some women are unaware of their pregnancy for the first month or two. Once they are aware of their pregnancy, some women will openly inform you of it, but others keep their pregnancies private for some time. It is nearly impossible to be aware of every pregnancy during the first trimester, even if you ask every female client before every massage whether she is pregnant. At the same time, the embryo floats free in the uterus until it embeds itself in the uterine lining, which occurs within about 7 days. The embryo undergoes the important developmental stages of becoming a fetus during the first trimester. Considering the possibility that there is an undisclosed pregnancy, yet knowing that the first trimester is a critical time for the developing fetus, you can see why massage during the first trimester is so controversial.

Physically, the client may experience nausea, vomiting, taste and smell sensitivities, exhaustion, constipation, and mood swings, but her shape and size will be relatively unchanged. Assuming you are aware of your client's pregnancy, you must be sensitive to her emotions and her physical condition and especially attentive to her comfort.

Positioning

Although some persons recommend against the prone position during the first trimester, in reality, many women sleep in the prone position without being completely aware of it, and obstetricians do not typically recommend against the prone position during the first trimester. If you practice client-centered massage and pay attention to both verbal and nonverbal cues, you will know whether your client is comfortable or not and make appropriate adjustments to technique or client positioning.

SECOND TRIMESTER

The client may start "showing" during the second trimester, and she may feel the fetus moving. The mother's body has to make some physical changes to accommodate the size of the baby. Her ribs may start spreading apart, and her organs may get pushed aside. Connective tissues are stretched, sometimes past their limits. Stretch marks, shortness of breath, varicose veins, hemorrhoids, heartburn, frequent urination, and backaches are common symptoms that result from the physical changes of the second trimester. The lymph circulation is also affected. As the fetus gets larger, it puts pressure on the larger lymphatic vessels in the abdominal and pelvic cavities. The lymphatic vessels rely on gravity and skeletal movement to create lymphatic flow, and when the flow is restricted so close to the lymphatic ducts, lymph can accumulate in the tissues. This undrained lymph creates swelling, or edema (eh-DEE-mah), which is common during pregnancy, particularly in the areas that are least assisted by gravity, such as the ankles.

Unusual levels of hormones are produced during normal pregnancy, which affect a pregnant woman's emotions, body temperature, and ligaments. Because her body temperature may run a little higher than normal, fresh air or a breeze may help keep her comfortable. In the second trimester, the woman's body will start to manufacture relaxin, a hormone that changes the collagen composition, allowing the pubic symphysis to loosen and expand the pelvis for delivery of the baby. Unfortunately, relaxin affects ligaments as well. Be extra careful with joint movements because the ligaments will not stop the range of motion as normally occurs.

Positioning

The size of the client and the size of the fetus create a need for special positioning and bolstering. Because a pregnant woman's breasts often become sensitive and because her uterus may protrude during the second trimester, the prone position may not be favorable. Pregnant women who prefer the prone position for massage can be sufficiently bolstered to minimize pressure on the breasts and uterus, but the easiest and safest way to position clients during the second trimester is in a seated or side-lying position.

The supine position may be appropriate for the early part of the second trimester, but the fetus puts pressure on the aorta and lymph vessels, which restricts the delivery of oxygenated blood and lymph. Large or multiple fetuses put excessive pressure on the abdominal aorta when the mother is in the supine position, a condition sometimes called supine hypotension. With large and multiple fetuses and toward the later part of the second trimester, a woman's time spent in the supine position should be limited to 10–15 minutes. As a safer alternative, the client can be placed in a semireclined position.

Special massage tables have been designed for pregnant women that provide holes for an extended belly and for enlarged breasts. These tables allow pregnant women to lie prone, which otherwise can be uncomfortable and nearly impossible as the pregnancy progresses. As part of the controversy over the prone position, these pregnancy tables are considered ridiculous and worthless by some. Practically, these tables are more expensive than standard massage tables, and given the conflicting opinions, the side-lying position is a simpler alternative for clients in their second trimester of pregnancy.

THIRD TRIMESTER

During the final few months of pregnancy, the fetus grows considerably. The maternal conditions and symptoms of the second trimester continue and often are more pronounced. Edema can be a significant problem during the third trimester, particularly in the lower legs and feet, but also in the forearms and hands. Massage is especially effective at encouraging lymphatic flow. The size of the baby or unusual positioning of organs can also compress nerves and cause symptoms such as numbness, fatigue, tingling, a feeling of pins and needles, and sometimes pain. Compression on the brachial plexus can cause symptoms in the shoulders, arms, hands, or all three. Pressure on the tibial nerve can create similar symptoms in the feet or ankles.

Other common symptoms that can develop during the last trimester include muscular cramps, incontinence, sacroiliac joint pain, pelvic discomfort, indigestion, frequent urination, stress and worry, and sleeplessness. Massage can provide some relief to these symptoms, but it cannot eliminate them.

Positioning

Due to the size of the baby in the final trimester, the mother should be placed in the supine position for a maximum of 10–15 minutes. A slightly modified supine position, in which the woman's head, shoulders, and upper back are elevated with bolsters, can be used for a longer period, but the side-lying position is easiest and usually the most comfortable. Even in the side-lying position, the woman should be well bolstered for comfort.

CONSIDERATIONS FOR PRENATAL MASSAGE

Pregnant women can be massaged in a side-lying position with proper bolstering for most of their pregnancy. (See Fig. 9-3 for bolstering clients in the side-lying position.) During all stages of pregnancy, watch for the client feeling faint during the massage session. If this occurs, change the client's position; the therapist must pay close attention to the client's level of consciousness. Of course, this holds true for any client, pregnant or not, but there is a greater chance that woman whose baby is putting excessive pressure on her aorta will feel faint.

There are some contraindications for massaging pregnant women. Massage can interfere with the body's processes, aggravate conditions created by pregnancy, endanger anatomical structures, or encourage labor:

- Joints—because of the activity of relaxin, be cautious with any range of motion to prevent injury
- Abdomen—light abdominal massage is acceptable, but deep work can traumatize the uterus or fetus and should be avoided
- Connective tissue—the activity of relaxin can affect the fascia, so myofascial manipulation and connective tissue work should be avoided to prevent injury
- Varicose veins—caused by collapsed valves in the veins and resulting in blood collecting at the most distal functional valve, they are to be avoided at all times to prevent further injury to a faulty vein
- Acupressure points—a few are known to encourage uterine or cervical activity and should be avoided during pregnancy (See Chapter 13, Special Techniques, for maps of acupressure points.):
  □ Spleen 6—on the medial side of the tibia, approximately 3–5 inches from the medial malleolus
  □ Large intestine 4—in the web between the thumb and index finger, at the base of the crease created when adducting those two metacarpals
  □ Gall bladder 21—directly lateral of C7, midway between C7 and the acromion process
- Essential oils—a number of essential oils (not necessarily the raw ingredients from which they

originate) could be harmful to a pregnancy, including

- ☐ Angelica
- ☐ Basil
- ☐ Chamomile
- ☐ Clary sage
- ☐ Fennel
- ☐ Jasmine
- ☐ Juniper
- ☐ Peppermint
- ☐ Wintergreen

Massage is appropriate for most pregnant women and can be very beneficial. The same techniques used in a regular massage session can be used in a prenatal massage, but you must be aware of the client's special needs. Massage therapists should take additional training to specialize in prenatal massage.

POSTPARTUM

Having a baby is a physically, emotionally, and spiritually life-changing event. Labor and delivery can be both exciting and exhausting for new mothers who now must attend to their new baby or babies. There can also be changes in the dynamics of relationships with her partner, other children, family members, and friends. Postpartum mothers often experience exhaustion along with muscular tension and soreness in the neck, shoulders, arms, and upper back from delivering the baby and learning to breast-feed. Cesarean section (C-section) deliveries can result in a lot of back pain and discomfort because of the extended recovery from surgery and the prolonged inactivity. This tension may also increase when she starts moving around and hunches over to compensate for the abdominal pain associated with the surgery.

Use the basic massage strokes and lymphatic drainage techniques to facilitate relaxation, increase circulation to flush out chemical and cellular waste, and reduce edema. The side-lying position may be most comfortable for a new mother for up to 3 days postpartum, but the prone and supine positions are acceptable. Be sure to bolster your client so she is comfortable while receiving massage. Your focus should be on nurturing and supporting the mother during this time.

> ⚠️ *While postpartum massage is beneficial for many reasons, you should be aware that there are risks for deep venous thrombosis or blood clots for up to 6 weeks postpartum and no massage should be applied to the medial side of the legs.*

There is occasionally pain and soreness at and around the site where an epidural anesthetic was administered. Massage is indicated around, but not on the site, to relieve the pain and soreness. Consult with her physician if there have been complications with birth and prior to using any abdominal techniques on a mother who had a C-section delivery.

Infants

The benefits of massage are not limited to adults. **Increased circulation, more effective digestion, reduced stress, and deeper and more regular sleep patterns are some benefits that babies can appreciate just as much as adults.** Premature infants who receive massage have shown increased weight gain, reduced stress, and better developmental progress. Dr. Tiffany Field has scientifically studied the effects of massage on groups of infants in various stages of health or dysfunction. Babies born prematurely or with drug addictions, AIDS, breathing disorders, or diabetic conditions have all shown improved health after receiving regular massage while still hospitalized. Additionally, their improved health decreases the amount of medical intervention needed and reduces their hospital costs.

Massage can provide physical benefits to the baby as well as strengthen the bond between the baby and the person giving the massage (Fig. 12-2). Touch is a form of communication, and a new baby understands touch more than words. In fact, touch may be as important as food to babies, so the more they are touched with a caring, loving intent, the healthier they are. Ask the baby's parent or parents to be present while you massage their baby, for both professional courtesy and legal protection. While they observe, you

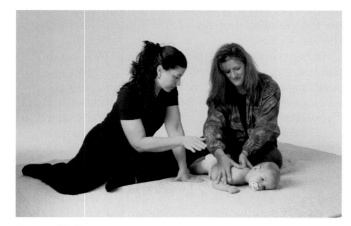

FIGURE 12-2 Massage therapist teaching a parent how to perform infant massage.

can describe some of the different strokes you use, explain the physiological benefits of the strokes, and encourage the parents to massage their baby on a regular basis, if not daily. Incorporating massage into the bedtime or bath routine is often easiest, but massage will provide quality time for the infant and parent whether it is used daily or weekly, regularly or not. There are infant massage videos, books, and classes available for parents who are interested.

INFANT MASSAGE

Therapists wishing to specialize in infant massage should receive additional training to learn techniques and flow. Keep in mind that to some degree, babies control the massage. The infant massage typically lasts only 15 minutes or so, but the duration is often determined by the baby's patience or willingness to accept the massage. An infant may dislike being touched in certain areas, may dislike particular strokes, or may dislike certain positions. Stay focused on the baby's comfort and change the massage as the baby expresses likes or dislikes.

During the massage, the baby may or may not wear a diaper. You may use a dry lubricant, such as cornstarch, or one of the many lotions and creams available for infant massage. Natural oils are better than synthetic or petroleum-based products, and vegetable or nut oils are preferable to mineral or animal-derived oils. Synthetic, mineral, and animal-based products are more likely to clog the baby's pores and irritate the skin.

Effleurage, petrissage, and tapotement can be used cautiously on infants. Some variations of these strokes have been specially developed for infant massage. One technique, called "milking," is commonly used. You hold the baby's hand or foot with one hand and form a sort of ring around the baby's limb with your other hand, gently squeezing the limb while sliding your hand toward the baby's body. It is like a long effleurage stroke of the entire limb. Another variation, wringing, is similar to milking, but has an added twisting action as the stroke moves proximally. Milking and wringing encourage both lymphatic and venous flow, they warm the tissues, and they are soothing strokes.

The baby can be positioned supine first, which allows you to see the baby's facial expressions and lets the baby fix his or her gaze on the person massaging. This positioning helps the baby trust the therapist and become familiar with the process. The strokes mentioned above may be used while the baby is supine. The baby's arms, legs, feet, face, and abdomen can all be massaged in this position. When massaging the abdomen, follow a clockwise pattern for abdominal massage as discussed in Chapter 13, Special Techniques. As the baby is supine with you at the baby's feet, looking at the baby's face, move your hands clockwise on the baby's abdomen. Clockwise effleurage strokes encourage peristaltic activity, which moves the contents of the intestines in the same direction.

You can attempt to put the baby in the prone position after the supine position for access to the baby's back, neck, scalp, legs, and arms. Wringing and milking might stress the baby's joints while prone, so limit your strokes to effleurage, petrissage, and tapotement of the baby's back and gluteal muscles in this position.

Return the baby to the supine position to complete the massage so that you can communicate to the baby that the massage is finished.

It should be common sense to use minimal pressure in infant massage. Being relaxed and patient will help the massage flow smoothly. Babies are very sensitive to emotions and will respond negatively if you are nervous or emotional. If the baby is not enjoying the experience or seems to be in pain, it may be best to stop the massage, comfort the baby, and try massage again at another time.

Geriatric Clients

The elderly population continues to grow as our life expectancy increases. Massage for senior clients is a specialty that provides them with both physical and mental benefits. Many health problems are associated with aging that range from mild discomfort to significant disease processes. Compounding existing problems, most elderly persons are not very physically active, which diminishes the circulation of blood and lymph. Without sufficient oxygen, cells suffer and eventually die.

GERIATRIC MASSAGE

Many seniors lead perfectly healthy, active lifestyles and can benefit from massage, but others have special needs. The condition of the client's tissues will determine the strokes and techniques used, but most of the work is accomplished with light, gentle effleurage strokes and passive range of motion (Box 12-7). For many elderly clients who are in very good health, are active in sports and other activities, and have healthy tissues, the massage can include faster, deeper, and more stimulating kinds of techniques.

All of the client's body systems are affected by increased circulation and the movements of the mas-

Geriatric Massage Highlights

- Clients may require physical assistance.
- Sessions usually last 30 minutes.
- Primarily gentle, more superficial strokes; use of deeper work depends on the client's health and condition of the soft tissues
- Almost always incorporates range of motion techniques, active or passive
- Hands and feet are gently massaged

sage. The body needs some time to readjust and recover, so the session should be shorter than usual to avoid overwhelming the client's body. Massage for seniors is typically 30 minutes instead of 60 minutes. Given by a therapist with proper training, geriatric massage can provide the following benefits:

- Increased circulation of blood
- Increased circulation of lymph
- Pain relief
- Reduced stress and anxiety
- Improved joint range of motion
- Personal attention and feelings of reassurance, which lead to a healthier disposition
- Improved sleep patterns
- Possible reduction of symptoms of Alzheimer's disease

The increased circulation of blood and lymph helps deliver oxygen and other nutrients to the cells of the body and remove cellular debris. As a result, healing processes are more efficient. Bedsores and other circulatory problems can be prevented by maintaining sufficient circulation.

Some senior clients are less modest and may attempt to undress while you are still in the treatment room. You may need to explain that the client should undress after you step out of the room. Occasionally, a client is unable to undress independently and requires assistance. Some senior clients, like persons of any age, prefer to remain clothed for the entire massage. Keep a wide, firm step stool nearby to help clients get on and off the table and be prepared to help clients turn from the supine to the prone position, or vice versa. Some clients are reserved and may be shy about asking for help, so it is better to offer assistance and not wait for the client to ask for it.

Receiving human touch along with someone's undivided attention for 30 minutes or more is a luxury many elderly clients may not have experienced for some time. Many have lost their spouses and feel lonely or depressed, confused, or anxious. Your presence and the massage combine to leave the geriatric client usually in a more positive mental state that facilitates health and well-being. Either active or passive range of motion techniques for the synovial joints promote the production of synovial fluid. The lubricating function of the fluid then improves range of motion.

Geriatric Massage Environment

Your geriatric clients may come to your office, but it is more convenient for those with special needs if you go to them. You can take your table and all of your supplies to their home, a nursing home, or an assisted living arrangement, just like any other outcall. Before you transport your table, ask about the special needs of your geriatric clients to find out if they are bedridden or unable to use your table. Clients who cannot get on the massage table are still able to enjoy the benefits of massage, but you have to adapt your massage to their needs. You can massage bedridden clients in their beds, despite the awkward body mechanics, because they cannot withstand a lot of pressure or a lot of movement. If they can get out of bed and sit in a chair, you can also offer them a massage in a wheelchair or household chair.

CONSIDERATIONS

The aging process affects all parts of an organism. As we get older and less physically active, it becomes more difficult to reach our feet to take care of them. Elderly clients commonly have feet that are in poor condition. Despite the shape and condition of their feet, massage and joint movement is very beneficial for their feet. Another common effect of aging is memory loss. Call or contact your elderly clients that morning to remind them of their appointment. Depending on the extent of their memory loss, you might want to contact them even an hour before the appointment. At the same time, if an elderly client misses an appointment, do not get frustrated or offended. You can talk to the nursing home administrators or family members to find out if there is an activities director or someone else who can help your clients make it to their appointments.

There are special geriatric conditions that present massage contraindications:

- Bedsores
- Arthritic joints
- Varicose veins
- Recent surgery
- Blood clots or history of blood clots
- Blood thinners

As with each special population, specialized training is available for geriatric massage that provides more detail. Every massage therapy student should experience geriatric massage. In many cases, students who never expected that they would enjoy the work end up loving it.

Chronically Ill Patients

A **chronic illness** is one that lasts a year or longer, usually limits the patient's physical activity, and may require ongoing medical care and treatment. Some chronic illnesses you may recognize include

- Alzheimer's disease
- Arthritis
- Asthma
- Cancer
- Diabetes
- Epilepsy
- Glaucoma
- Heart disease
- Hepatitis
- Human immunodeficiency virus (HIV)
- Lupus
- Multiple sclerosis
- Parkinson disease

Each of the above chronic illnesses has its own symptoms, but many chronically ill patients are commonly burdened with high medical costs, difficulty holding a job, family stress, and depression. Massage can offer relief from some of the associated physical and emotional stress and tension, but you must understand the anatomy and physiology of the illness before you incorporate massage into the client's treatment. Communicate with the client's other healthcare professionals and try to establish a team approach that includes the client's input. Ruth Werner's book *A Massage Therapist's Guide to Pathology* is an excellent resource that includes a number of illnesses, their causes, treatments, and the indications and contraindications for massage.

HOSPICE MASSAGE

There are many diseases and illnesses that cannot be cured with current medical treatment. When a person's life expectancy is limited because of a life-threatening illness and there is no known cure, **hospice** (HAHSS-PIHSS) care caters to the quality of remaining life rather than the quantity of life. It addresses all of the symptoms of the disease and provides emotional, spiritual, and practical support to the patient as well as the friends and family members. Massage therapy is frequently included in hos-

pice care to make patients more comfortable and reduce stress. It can also be helpful for the caretakers to ensure that their loved one is receiving caring touch when no true cure is available. Typically, relaxing techniques such as light effleurage, connecting strokes, and simply laying hands on the client may be used in this type of massage. As with most special populations, you can discuss the person's condition with the healthcare professionals to incorporate massage into the treatment plan safely.

Disabled Clients

Many persons with disabilities receive massage, including those with visual and hearing impairments, paralysis, amputation, and psychological issues. The massage itself is not so different, but your approach to caring for these clients requires that you understand their conditions and make special accommodations to ensure their safety and comfort.

VISUAL AND HEARING IMPAIRMENT

Visually or hearing impaired clients need some special assistance, but the massage itself is minimally affected by these disabilities. These clients may need a visual or auditory signal to let them know it is time to turn over during the massage, but the strokes and flow are the same as in a typical session. If the client has a companion dog that must stay in the treatment room, the dog can either lie in a corner of the room, out of the way, or under the table. These companion dogs are at work, so do not expect it to be playful and do not distract the dog by trying to play with it.

PHYSICAL DISABILITIES

With proper training and experience, massage therapists can specialize in massage for the physically disabled. For some massage therapists, working with the physically disabled is uncomfortable at first, but massage students are encouraged to experience the challenges and rewards of working with this special population.

Using crutches requires excessive use of the triceps brachii muscles, puts the wrists in an unnatural position, and can compress the structures running through the carpal tunnel. Manual wheelchairs also require a lot work from the arm muscles, particularly the latissimus dorsi, triceps, pectoralis, and coracobrachialis. You may need to alter your body mechanics to accommodate a client in a wheelchair or bed, but the correct principles of body mechanics are basically the same. In fact, massage is especially beneficial for clients who are bedridden and wheelchair-bound.

If you think about the joint movements involved in your client's physical limitations or compensation patterns, you can use the special muscle chart to determine which muscles to evaluate and treat. Table 11-1, Antagonistic muscle actions, can also help you determine other muscles to assess or to use in PNF techniques.

The flow of massage need not change if the client can lie on the massage table. If, however, the client must remain in a wheelchair or bed, a massage can still be given. The flow must change, and it may take a longer time to address the entire body. Shorten the session for a new client since the body needs to reestablish a balance following the soft tissue manipulation and circulatory enhancement. This can be an exhausting experience for anyone, but even more so for a client whose nervous and muscular systems are not functioning normally.

Paralysis

Paralysis is accompanied by a loss of sensation, the effects of which are important for the massage therapist. Since the client cannot sense pain, be especially careful to avoid injuring the tissues. To ensure the safety of the tissues, use enough bolstering to support the client's body. Position the client's muscles in passive contraction before working on them, to provide the softest, most relaxed position of the muscles. Strokes used for a person with paralysis are the same as those in a "regular" massage but must be gentler and more sensitive. Strokes have more therapeutic benefit for a paralyzed client if they are directed toward the heart to increase venous and lymphatic flow. Range of motion techniques are very beneficial but must be done with extreme care for a paralyzed client. The person's tissues are probably stuck together and shortened, significantly limiting the range of motion. Because of this hypertonicity, you *must* understand that the movements may be barely perceptible, and therefore you must pay close attention to feel the limits of the tissues.

The circulation of a paralyzed client and anyone bedridden or confined to a wheelchair is usually greatly compromised. Without muscular activity, small blood vessels do not receive normal amounts of blood flow, and the extremities can easily become ischemic. Likewise, the lymph, which does not have a pumping force behind it, does not flow well. Massage acts as an external pump that increases blood and lymph flow. Be extremely careful with clients who are significantly inactive, paralyzed, or bedridden. Their muscles are probably atrophied, their fascia severely restricted and bound down, and their joints very stiff; movement of any kind can hurt. Discuss their condition with their caretakers and/or physician to understand as much as you can about the client's health. Moving these clients into a chair or onto a table might not be appropriate, even if the client or the caretakers think it is. Use your best judgment, with a client-centered focus, and give your disabled clients a massage in the safest and most beneficial place.

Amputation

In the process of amputation, the surgical removal of part of a limb, nerves are severed. Many amputees, or persons who have undergone amputation, suffer a phenomenon called phantom pain, which is the sensation of pain in the missing limb. The point where the limb was amputated, called the stump, is often very sensitive to pain. In addition to coping with the emotional hardship of losing the limb, amputees must deal with the physical pain caused by faulty nerve signals. Massaging the stump can help quiet the pain, but you must go slowly and carefully, paying close attention to the client's tolerance.

The posture of an amputee is significantly affected, because the entire balance of the body is permanently offset. Whether the amputation occurs at an arm or leg, necessary compensation patterns develop to establish a posture that allows the amputee to balance and function normally. Address the muscular aches and pains, but use a knowledgeable approach when applying therapeutic techniques to ensure that you are not disturbing the necessary postural compensation patterns.

PSYCHOLOGICAL ISSUES

Treating mental impairment and emotional and psychological disturbances is not within the scope of practice for wellness or therapeutic massage. However, it *is* within the scope of practice massage on clients who suffer from emotional and psychological issues. Transference and countertransference can easily develop in relationships with psychological issues, so you need to recognize and avoid these situations. **Transference** is the client's dependence on you for friendship or companionship in addition to therapeutic treatment, and **countertransference** is your tendency to react emotionally when clients do not behave or respond to you or your treatment as you had expected. Offer clients your massage, education, and recommendations for self-care. Expect prompt payment, professional respect, and cooperation with your policies and business practices. Establish and maintain a professional client–therapist relationship to avoid complications and potential problems.

If you suspect that a client has a psychological impairment, emotional instability, or mental disturbance, you can neither diagnose nor treat it. You can gently refer clients to an appropriate healthcare professional, but you cannot force them to make or attend an appointment. **If you suspect that a client is being abused or that a client's life is in danger for any reason, you may have a legal responsibility to report it to the local authorities.** Check with your local government's child welfare, family services, or social services department to determine your legal responsibilities as a massage therapist.

Clients with psychological issues may respond to massage with defense mechanisms such as extreme laughter, sadness, introversion, or extroversion. They may have an emotional release, which is similar to a flashback of an emotional experience. Do not encourage clients to have emotional releases, but do not suppress them when they occur. You are not allowed to treat the emotional disturbance, but you can offer support, understanding, and patience to clients who experience an emotional release. There are advanced courses that teach massage therapists how to best handle and facilitate these emotional releases, but with the intent to relieve the fascial restrictions that affect the soft tissues of the body.

You must respect the coping mechanisms and behaviors of persons who have suffered abuse, be it physical or psychological. For example, they may want to leave all of their clothes on, they may ask for additional draping despite the room temperature, and they may be uncomfortable in certain client positions. You may or may not be informed of a client's abusive history, but by paying attention to nonverbal communication and using a client-centered approach, you can offer a safe massage to all clients.

Chemical imbalances such as depression, anxiety, and bipolar disorder can usually be treated medically, but persons with chemical imbalances commonly avoid their medications. If you notice that a client who is supposed to be taking medication is behaving inconsistently, carefully and cautiously inquire about the medication. You could casually ask the client about medication during the assessment process or as you set the next appointment by saying something like, "How are things going, anyway? Medications ok? Sleeping ok? Is anything new or interesting going on?" If they admit that they are not taking the medication, you could gently suggest they talk to their doctor about the medication or dosage to see if there might be a better alternative. If they are not willing to tell you about their use of medication, you cannot force the issue unless you suspect that they are endangering their life or someone else's.

Chapter Summary

The benefits of massage are available to anyone, male or female, young or old, pregnant, athletic, sedentary, healthy, ill, or disabled either physically or psychologically. The special needs of each population may require that you modify the massage in one way or another, but those needs should not prevent anyone from receiving the benefits of massage. Learn about the physical and psychological needs of those in these special populations and the contraindications for massage, cooperate with the other members of the client's healthcare team, and be careful to stay within the clients' tolerances. Students are encouraged to work with as many special populations as possible to learn about differences and face the challenges. Massaging members of these populations can be a very rewarding experience.

 CHAPTER EXERCISES

1. Compare and contrast preevent massage, postevent massage, and restorative massage. Include details of timing, duration of the massage, strokes used or techniques to avoid, purpose, location, and equipment.

2. Find at least three different volunteers on whom to practice a preevent massage routine. Ask them to identify a sport that they participate in so you can tailor their preevent massage to the muscles involved in that sport. Remember to incorporate grounding and centering techniques.

3. Use the same three volunteers from exercise 2 and practice an appropriate postevent massage routine on each of them. Include grounding and centering for each massage.

4. List at least five contraindications of massage for pregnant women.

5. List at least three benefits of massage for infants.

6. Describe some of the highlights of geriatric massage, including at least four contraindications, four benefits, and special considerations for the physical condition or mental capacity of elderly persons.

7. Describe how you can communicate with visually impaired clients during a massage session to ensure their safety and comfort.

8. Describe a scenario in which transference occurs and describe one in which countertransference occurs.

9. Go to the Touch Research Institute web site and find the research articles. Summarize at least two studies that are interesting to you.

10. Research hospice organizations and list at least five different services they offer for patients whose life expectancy is limited and the services they offer the friends and families of persons whose life expectancy is limited.

SUGGESTED READINGS

American Massage Therapy Association Sports Massage Tool Kit, American Massage Therapy Association, Evanston, IL 2003.

Cady SH, Jones GE. Massage therapy as a workplace intervention for reduction of stress. Percept Mot Skills 1997;84(1):157–158.

Field T, Ironson G, Safari F, et al. Massage therapy reduces anxiety and enhances EEG pattern of alertness and math computations. Int J Neurosci 1996;86:197–205.

Field T, Quintino O, Henteleff T, et al. Job stress reduction therapies. Alter Ther Health Med 1997;3(4):54–56.

Johnson J. The Healing Art of Sports Massage. Emmaus, PA: Rodale Press, 1995.

Osborne-Sheets C. Pre- and Perinatal Massage Therapy: A Comprehensive Practitioners' Guide to Pregnancy, Labor and Postpartum. San Diego, CA: Body Therapy Associates, 1998.

http://www.americanhospice.org, accessed 10/5/03.

http://www.amtamassage.org/about/terms.htm, accessed 10/12/02.

http://www.amtil.com/, accessed 10/15/02.

http://www.applesforhealth.com/AlternativeMedicine/agrowkn3.html, accessed 10/14/02.

http://www.childbirthsolutions.com/articles/birth/acupressure/index.php, accessed 10/12/02.

http://www.daybreak-massage.com/db02/aboutdaybreak.asp, accessed 10/15/02.

http://www.disabilitymuseum.org/lib/docs/954.htm, accessed 10/15/02.

http://www.essentialoils.co.za/pregnancy.htm, accessed 10/14/02.

http://www.findarticles.com/cf_dls/g2603/0003/2603000386/p1/article.jhtml, accessed 10/14/02.

http://www.findarticles.com/cf_dls/g2603/0004/2603000452/p1/article.jhtml?term=infant+massage, accessed 10/14/02.

http://www.findarticles.com/cf_dls/g2603/0006/2603000603/p3/article.jhtml?term=infant+massage, accessed 10/16/02.

http://www.hospicefoundation.org, accessed 10/5/03.

http://www.hospicenet.org, accessed 10/5/03.

http://www.injuryrehab.org.uk/preeventmassage.htm, accessed 10/12/02.

http://www.jorbins.com/baby_nursery_magazine/infantmassage.html, accessed 10/14/02.

http://www.montaine.com.au/corporate.htm, accessed 10/12/02.

http://www.ncbi.nlm.nih.gov/entrez/query.fcgi?cmd=Retrieve&db=PubMed&list_uids=8884390&dopt=Abstract, accessed 10/10/02.

http://www.pslgroup.com/dg/42772.htm, accessed 10/14/02.

http://www.synergy-studios.com/sys-tmpl/sportsmassage/, accessed 10/12/02.

Special Techniques

UPON COMPLETION OF THIS CHAPTER, THE STUDENT WILL BE ABLE TO:

- Name the three types of circulatory enhancement massage
- Describe at least three ways to enhance the flow of lymph
- Name and locate the major lymphatic ducts on an illustration of the skeleton
- Demonstrate an abdominal massage
- Name at least four benefits of reflexology
- Demonstrate a basic reflexology treatment
- Describe the Oriental concept of energy meridians
- Describe the concept of polarity therapy

KEY TERMS

Acupressure (AK-yoo-preh-sher)**:** a bodywork modality in which firm fingertip pressure is applied to points along the energy meridians to regulate the flow of Qi

Acupressure points: specific points along all of the meridians where the Qi can be most easily affected by pressure

Contrast therapy: heat application followed by cold application, also called alternating therapy

Lymph: interstitial fluid leaked into the tissues via capillaries carrying arterial blood

Meridians: precise and orderly channels or pathways through which Qi flows

Polarity (poh-LAIR-ih-tee) **therapy:** a modality in which very light massage strokes are applied on and off the client's body to balance electromagnetic fields

Reflexology (REE-fleks-AH-loh-jee)**:** a modality in which fingertip compression is applied to reflex points on the hand, foot, or ear that affect other parts of the body

Right lymphatic duct: a major drain that collects all of the lymph from the upper right quadrant of the body, including everything on the right side of the body above the diaphragm, and empties it into the right subclavian vein

Shiatsu (shee-AHT-soo)**:** a form of bodywork that uses a combination of acupressure with stretching, range of motion, and massage strokes

Thoracic duct: a major drain that collects the lymph from everywhere in the body except the right side of the head and thorax and empties it into the left subclavian vein

Yang (YAHNG)**:** energy that flows down from the sun and is associated with the active, bright, warm, consumptive, and outward activities of the body

Yin (YIHN)**:** energy that flows upward from the earth and is associated with the passive, dark, cool, supportive, and inward activities of the body

Many special techniques are often incorporated into massage sessions. These bodywork modalities have a specific intent and are applied for a specific purpose. Special techniques may use massage strokes, but others, such as hydrotherapy, may or may not. Hydrotherapy uses water of different temperatures and in various forms to aid in the treatment of soft tissue, and it can easily be used by massage therapists. On the other hand, some are special combinations of massage strokes that a therapist uses with a specific intent to serve a specific purpose. The activity of some organ systems can be enhanced by unique patterns of massage strokes. For example, the digestive system moves waste through the intestines via peristalsis, and a specific pattern of massage strokes can encourage that movement. Massage can also enhance the activity of the circulatory system by increasing the flow of arterial blood, venous blood, and lymph.

Reflexology (REE-fleks-AH-loh-jee) is a modality in which you apply fingertip compression to specific reflex points on the hand, foot, or ear to affect other parts of the body. Other bodywork modalities manipulate energy in and around the body. The concepts of Oriental medicine, including the philosophy of life force energy that flows through orderly patterns, can be incorporated into massage therapy via acupressure (AK-yoo-preh-sher) and shiatsu (shee-AHT-soo). **Polarity** (poh-LAIR-ih-tee) **therapy** uses very light massage strokes, both on and off the client's body, to balance those electromagnetic fields. There are too many specialized forms of energy therapy to introduce them all in this text, but they are certainly worth discovering.

Many special techniques require advanced study, and this chapter only serves as an introduction to some that are commonly used in massage practices. Additionally, before applying any new or special technique to a client, make sure the client has no pathological conditions for which the technique may be contraindicated.

Hydrotherapy

Hydrotherapy (HAHY-droh-THAIR-ah-pee) involves the external or internal use of water therapeutically. This text focuses on hydrotherapy applications you can use during massage sessions and those you can recommend as self-care activities, including applications of cold or heat, chemical substitutes that provide cold or heat, contrast therapy, or neutral baths. Box 13-1 describes the general categories of water temperatures. You must understand how the different temperatures affect a person's physiology so you can use hydrotherapy properly to enhance your massage treatments. Box 13-2 identifies the physiological effects of cold and heat.

COLD HYDROTHERAPY

Temperatures between 55 and 65°F are generally considered cold, and temperatures between 32 and 55°F are considered very cold. Cold and very cold temperatures applied for a short duration, a minute or less, cause vasoconstriction, or a narrowing of the blood vessels. When the cold is removed, vasodilation occurs, opening up the blood vessels and allowing arterial blood to rush into the blood vessels and supply the tissues with oxygen. Short applications of cold ultimately increase circulation.

The same mechanism occurs when cold temperatures are applied longer than a minute, but during the extended application, swelling (edema) decreases because of the reduced circulation, muscle spasms relax because of the reduced chemical activity of muscle contraction, and pain decreases because of the reduced chemical activity of nerve transmission.

Very cold temperatures, or ice packs, are particularly beneficial following an injury. Applications of very cold temperatures reduce capillary permeability and the amount of inflammatory substances produced, relieve muscle spasms, and decrease pain. As a result, very cold temperatures prevent swelling and encourage movement of the injured area to enhance circulation to the area. To successfully anesthetize or numb the tissues, ice or very cold temperatures must be applied for 20–30 minutes. Because of all these effects, ice is one of the most beneficial treatments during the acute phase of an injury (24–72 hours following the injury).

A couple of well-known postinjury treatments are RICE (rest, ice, compression, and elevation) and

Box 13-1		
General Categories of Water Temperatures		
Very cold	32–55°F	Painfully cold
Cold	55–65°F	Uncomfortable
Cool	65–92°F	Slightly below skin temperature, goose flesh
Neutral	92–98°F	Skin temperature, comfortable
Warm to hot	98–104°F	Tolerable, reddens skin
Very hot	104–110°F	Tolerable for very short periods
Painfully hot	Over 110°F	Possibly injurious, CONTRAINDICATED

Box 13-2

The Physiological Effects of Cold and Heat

Cold
Reduces
- Circulation (with prolonged use)
- Acute inflammation
- Swelling (edema)
- Muscle spasm via reduction of muscle spindle activity
- Nerve sensation and pain
- Metabolism
- Tissue damage
- Local oxygen supply (temporarily)

Increases
- Circulation and vasodilation (with short use)
- Urine production

Heat
Reduces
- Pain
- Stiffness and soreness
- Superficial fascia tightness

Increases
- Vasodilation
- Local blood flow/circulation (facilitates healing)
- Oxygen absorption
- Metabolism
- Relaxation
- Joint range of motion
- Sweating, creating a cooling effect on the body

Heat applications between 102 and 104°F
Increase
- Immune function via inhibition of bacterial and viral growth
- White blood cell count via creating an "artificial" fever

MICE (mobilization, ice, compression, and elevation). For the most part, RICE and MICE are the same treatment applied during the acute phase of an injury to facilitate healing. The "R" in RICE refers to the restricted activity that prevents further injury, and the "M" in MICE refers to the gentle, non-weight-bearing range of motion exercises that are recommended to prevent connective tissue adhesion.

- **Rest** allows the healing process to begin and prevents further injury.
- **Ice** causes vasoconstriction, reduces blood flow, prevents further inflammation, and creates an analgesic (pain-relieving) effect.
- **Compression** prevents lymph from accumulating, thus minimizing edema.
- **Elevation** of the injured area encourages lymph to return to the heart, which decreases inflammation.

Cold Applications

Cold and very cold temperatures can be applied with ice, cold packs, cold gel packs, baths, or stones. You can use them during the massage session or recommend them to clients as self-care activities. Ice can be applied directly to the skin, it can be contained and applied in a plastic bag, or it can be wrapped and applied in a cloth. Some people create their own ice applicators by freezing water in a small paper cup, peeling off some of the paper to expose the ice, and applying the ice by holding onto the ice with the paper cup that remains. With this method, it is good to have a small cloth or towel to collect the water from the melting ice.

Crushed ice or frozen vegetables in sealed plastic bags minimize the dripping, conform to the body part being treated, and can be refrozen. Frozen chemical gel packs are also easy to use, conform to the body part, and can be refrozen, but they are colder than ice and must be used cautiously.

> *When using a chemical gel pack, you* must *use a layer of fabric between the pack and the skin to avoid damage to the skin and nerves!*

Some other variations of cold or very cold temperatures include a cold bath, immersion of the body part in ice-cold water, or cold stones. Smooth, rounded stones can be chilled in a freezer or icy water for 15–20 minutes and placed directly on the body or over a thin cloth.

People may shy away from ice because it is initially uncomfortable, and the discomfort often becomes worse before numbness sets in. If the body part to be iced can be submersed in a bucket or bowl of water, you can reduce the shock of the cold by starting the water at room temperature and slowly adding ice cubes to drop the temperature. Another way to minimize the shock and discomfort of very cold temperatures is to take a warm bath or shower while applying the ice pack, or to apply a hot pack on another area of the body for distraction. While there are many benefits and indications for the use of cold applications, there are some contraindications as well. Box 13-3 lists indications and contraindications of cold and very cold applications.

HEAT HYDROTHERAPY

Temperatures between 98 and 104°F are considered warm to hot, they are usually tolerable, and they redden the skin. Very hot temperatures are generally between 104 and 110°F, and are tolerable only for

Box 13-3

Indications and Contraindications for Cold and Very Cold Applications

Indications
- Acute or chronic muscle spasm
- Acute or chronic pain
- Acute inflammation or injury
- Muscle strain
- Ligament sprains
- Tissue that has received any kind of myofascial work
- Bursitis, rheumatoid arthritis, osteoarthritis (unless cold aggravates the pain)
- Minor burns
- Fever

Contraindications
- Decreased cold sensitivity or hypersensitivity
- Compromised local circulation
- Circulatory or sensory impairment
- Spasm of the blood vessels (vasospastic disease)
- Cardiac disorders
- Respiratory disorders
- Use over chest during acute asthma
- Raynaud's syndrome
- Hypertension
- Uncovered open wounds, infections, or rash

very short periods. Temperatures above 110°F are dangerous and should be avoided for hydrotherapy purposes.

Heat applied for 5 minutes or less stimulates circulation by promoting vasodilation, which brings more oxygen and nutrients to the tissue and carries away lymphatic fluid and cellular waste. The increased oxygen can reduce muscle spasms, relieve muscle tension, and provide pain relief by breaking the pain cycle. Collagen fibers soften with heat, which increases tissue flexibility and range of motion. Heat applications used in the subacute phase of an injury (72 hours to 6 weeks following the injury) increase blood flow and promote healing in the injured area. In the chronic phase, which occurs between 6 weeks and 1 year after the injury, heat can be applied to tissues as long as the tissues are not swollen, because heat can increase edema. As the heat increases the temperature of the underlying tissues, cellular activity increases, and immune functions can be enhanced.

Interestingly, when heat is applied longer than 5 minutes, circulation decreases. The tissues get congested with prolonged exposure to heat because although vasodilation delivers more blood to an area, the venous and lymphatic flows are not equally en-

hanced. Unless there is enough muscular activity to encourage these flows toward the heart, you must use a cold application after long applications of heat. The cold temperatures help the blood and lymphatic vessels constrict to their normal size and return circulation to normal. Application of heat followed by cold is referred to as contrast therapy and is covered later in this section.

Heat Applications

Heat can be applied by using microwaveable or electrical hot packs or hot pads, hot water bottles, hot compresses, hot baths, whirlpool tubs, or hot stones. Hot packs, heating pads, and hot water bottles can be used for 5–20 minutes during a massage treatment to increase blood flow and soften fascia. As with frozen chemical gel packs, use a fabric barrier between chemical hot packs and the skin for safety. You can also recommend hot packs for self-care, again for 5–20 minutes at a time. A variation of a hot pack is a hot compress, which is a cloth immersed in warm-to-hot water, wrung out, and placed on the affected area until the heat dissipates and the compress is cool.

Mineral salts, Epsom salts, baking soda, and aromatherapy oils can be added to a hot bath (98°F) to enhance its effects or provide additional benefits. A common recipe to reduce muscle soreness uses 1 cup of Epsom salts and 1 cup of baking soda in a full tub of 98°F water. Many prepackaged mineral salts, often containing aromatherapy essences, are available at health food stores and spas and may be added to a hot bath to produce the effect listed on the package. Whirlpool tubs combine the benefits of warm-to-hot water with jets of water that mechanically massage the body.

 Keep the pressure of the jets off of an injured area to avoid further injury.

Smooth, rounded stones, usually made of basalt, can be heated in water or a special heating unit and used as a massage tool, but only after they are cooled to a safe temperature. They can be placed directly on the skin or over a thin cloth.

Any client who is being treated with temperatures above 99°F should be watched for nausea, splotchy discoloration on the skin, lightheadedness, dizziness, and headache. If any of those symptoms develop during heat application, stop the treatment immediately and monitor the client for improvement.

Despite the many benefits and indications for heat therapy, there are some important contraindications (Box 13-4).

CONTRAST THERAPY

Contrast therapy, sometimes called alternating therapy, involves the application of heat followed by the application of cold or very cold temperatures. By alternating vasodilation and vasoconstriction, and the associated benefits of each, contrast therapy is beneficial for reducing pain, promoting healing, and enhancing immune function. As long as you take into account the client's sensitivity and frailty and make sure there are no contraindications for applications of either heat or cold, you can safely apply and recommend contrast therapy.

NEUTRAL BATHS

Neutral baths are baths that use water at 92–98°F (body temperature) to increase relaxation and sedate the nervous system. Neutral baths are beneficial for reducing stress and anxiety and relieving chronic pain and insomnia. They are contraindicated for a client who has cardiac disease or skin conditions, which react badly to water.

INTERNAL HYDROTHERAPY

Another form of hydrotherapy is the simple act of drinking sufficient water. You have an opportunity to educate your clients on the importance of adequate hydration. Drinking water after a massage session can help the body rid itself of cellular and chemical wastes that are mechanically forced into the circulatory system, it can make scar tissue more functional, and it can help prevent fascial adhesion development. Proper hydration of the tissues enhances fluidity of movement and flexibility, whereas dehydration can lead to more tension, restricted movement, muscle soreness, headaches, and fatigue. Dehydration is the primary cause of a "hangover" headache. **(Drinking more water may be one of the most important self-care recommendations a therapist makes for the client's treatment plan.)**

Another form of internal hydrotherapy is drinking hot water or herbal tea. Hot beverages will warm the core of the body and stimulate blood flow and healing.

MEDICATION AND HYDROTHERAPY

Some pharmaceutical and hydrotherapy interactions should be avoided. Heat therapy should not be applied to any client who is taking medication that promotes vasodilation, including decongestants, migraine headache medications, blood-pressure-lowering medications, and attention-deficit/hyperactivity-disorder medications. The increased vasodilation could be dangerous for the client.

Similarly, any client taking medication that causes vasoconstriction such as migraine headache medications with caffeine should not be treated with cold applications that cause further vasoconstriction. Additionally, any nausea, splotchy discoloration on the skin, lightheadedness, dizziness, or headache may suggest that the client's body is having difficulty managing the temperature differential. If any of those signs or symptoms occur, stop the hydrotherapy treatment and wait for the client to return to normal.

Medications that provide pain relief, whether taken internally or applied topically alter the sensitivity of a person's skin. Hydrotherapy is not contraindicated, but the effects of treatment must be monitored carefully to prevent possible injury.

Some psychiatric medications that affect brain chemistry can compromise the body's ability to regulate a normal temperature. Hydrotherapy is contraindicated if the client's thermal regulation is not functioning normally.

Box 13-4

Indications and Contraindications for Heat Applications

Indications
- Muscle spasm
- Pain relief
- Increase range of motion
- Facilitate tissue healing in subacute and chronic injuries (3 days to 3 weeks after injury)
- Enhance immune function
- Increase mobility of tissues—benefits osteoarthritis and rheumatoid arthritis

Contraindications
- Acute inflammation or injuries (24–72 hours after injury), including open wounds, blisters, burns, and abrasions
- Area of a newly developed bruise
- Skin infections or rash
- Fever
- Impaired or poor circulation, including cardiac impairment and phlebitis
- Stroke, also called cerebrovascular accident (CVA)
- Impaired or poor sensation
- Impaired thermal regulation
- Area over implants, joint prosthetics, or pacemakers
- Tumor, cyst, or malignancy
- Autoimmune conditions

Circulatory Enhancement

Within the circulatory system, oxygenated blood, deoxygenated blood, and lymph circulate throughout the body in a network of vessels. Oxygenated blood is pumped from the heart, through the arteries, to the rest of the body. As the arteries get farther from the heart, they decrease in diameter and branch out until they become tiny capillaries. Oxygen molecules pass through the walls of the capillaries and diffuse from the blood to the body cells. From the capillaries, the deoxygenated blood is transported back to the heart through the veins. Lymph from around the cells and within the tissues travels toward the heart through the lymphatic vessels, eventually entering the heart through the subclavian vein and being added back to the blood. The veins and lymphatic vessels are supplied with valves to prevent backflow of the fluids, and the flow through the veins and lym-

---

Box 13-5

Cupping

Of all the important techniques used in TCM, only acupuncture and herbs have gained widespread popularity in the United States. However, cupping, a skin-surface therapy, also has been used effectively for many centuries in both the Orient and Europe. During the past three decades, improved instrumentation has made cupping even more useful for treating specific ailments. Cupping offers a chance for complete recovery to patients who cannot find relief through medication, surgery, and other traditional medical practices. For the healthy individual, cupping not only provides greater vitality and strength, but also prevents illness.

Cupping, or "body vacuuming," involves placing a few to several cups on the patient's skin. A vacuum is created by igniting a small amount of methanol alcohol in the cups and then quickly applying them to the skin. This vacuum causes the skin under the cups to rise, which causes skin pores to expand and discharge accumulated toxins and waste products from under the skin. The cups remain in place up to 20 minutes, forcing blood into the terminal ends of the capillaries.

The most essential and interesting benefit of cupping lies in its ability to improve blood circulation, thereby increasing the flow of oxygen to all the tissues of the body. Red blood cells, which transport oxygen through the arteries, must pass through a network of small capillaries of the cardiovascular system. While passing through the capillaries, the cells are dented, bruised, and cracked. This reduces their ability to carry oxygen and remove wastes. The spleen's job is to absorb these damaged blood cells. It is the bloodstream's filter, destroying old red blood cells and removing small particles from the blood. However, the blood cells must be badly broken for the spleen to absorb them. If the spleen doesn't absorb old red blood cells, the bone marrow doesn't produce new ones. During a cupping treatment, partially damaged blood cells are further broken down. This increased fragmentation stimulates the spleen to clear the old blood cells much faster, which in turn stimulates new red blood cell production by the bone marrow. New red blood cells carry more oxygen to every tissue and organ and boost a person's vitality.

Eastern physicians familiar with the practice of cupping have discovered a variety of additional benefits. Application of the cups usually creates short-term bruises, particularly if the patient is ill. To the practiced eye, this discoloration can be a valuable diagnostic clue. A skilled practitioner applying cups along the acupuncture meridians can recognize certain internal organ problems that may reside a considerable distance from the bruise.

The two cupping techniques are wet cupping and dry cupping. Wet cupping involves superficially puncturing an area of skin with a lancet before applying the cups. It is outside the scope of practice for massage therapists. A burning wick is placed over the punctured area and a glass cup is quickly applied over the wick to create a vacuum. Wet cupping is used mainly for localized musculoskeletal problems (athletic injuries, tendinitis, bursitis, low back pain, neck pain, arthritis, fibromyalgia, etc.). The treatment reduces inflammation and removes congested or stagnated blood (the underlying cause of the pain). The treated area then fills with fresh new blood, improving the flow of oxygen and relieving the pain.

Dry cupping, on the other hand, does not involve puncturing the skin before applying the cups and is within the massage therapy scope of practice. In dry cupping, a small amount of alcohol is ignited in each suction cup, which is then applied quickly to the skin. The vacuum extinguishes the flame and causes the skin under the cup to rise. The skin pores then expand and discharge wastes and toxins. Dry cupping is one of the best ways to improve general blood circulation and stimulate the immune system. It is also very effective in treating many internal chronic organ problems when the cups are applied along acupuncture meridians, which requires that massage therapists work in cooperation with a physician's medical diagnosis.

Today, many variations of cupping therapy are used. About 30 years ago, Joon Sung Ki patented a kind of cup that contains a porous material (gypsum) to absorb the alcohol. His fire-cupping method increases the speed and efficiency of the therapy, and those cups provide a much better vacuum than wine glasses. Another kind of cup used in modern treatment is a plastic cup with a check valve that can be attached to either an electric vacuum pump or a manual hand vacuum pump.

The healing principle of cupping is the cleansing of the blood. Cleansing improves circulation, and good circulation is essential to good health.

—Young Ki Park, D.O.

phatic vessels occurs via gravity and the skeletal muscle pump.

One of the primary benefits of massage is the increased circulation of blood and lymph. **Compression applied distally on the arteries, and effleurage strokes applied proximally over the veins and lymphatic vessels mechanically encourage the movement of fluids through the circulatory vessels.** By taking advantage of this mechanical concept, a therapist can intentionally increase circulation to a specific area of the body. Remember, however, that the massage therapist's scope of practice encompasses the soft tissues of the body, not the circulatory system. If the therapist is trying to encourage circulation in an effort to facilitate a change in the muscles and connective tissue, it is acceptable to incorporate circulatory enhancement into a session. The difference is in the therapist's intent and knowledge base. With increased circulation, there is an increased oxygenated blood supply, along with cellular and chemical waste removal. The health of the tissues, including the musculature, is promoted with enhanced circulation.

Another method of enhancing circulation is called cupping. (See Box 13-5 for more information about cupping.)

VENOUS ENHANCEMENT

Deoxygenated blood returns, against gravity, to the heart through the veins at the so-called end of the circulatory path. Many of the veins have a series of valves in them to prevent blood from flowing away from the heart. They are more prevalent where blood has a longer distance to travel back to the heart and are especially numerous in the veins of the lower extremities, where blood must be pumped against gravity. Remember, the heart does not pump blood through the veins. Instead, contraction of nearby muscles compresses the veins and squeezes the blood in the only direction the valves allow—toward the heart.

A massage therapist can enhance a client's venous return during a session by active or passive contraction of the client's muscles. Effleurage can also encourage blood movement through the veins. Since veins are more superficial than arteries, massage that addresses venous flow does not require deep pressure. Light effleurage strokes directed toward the heart encourage the blood to move through the veins. You can also use gravity to assist venous flow toward the heart. As long as the client is positioned with the heart inferior to the body part, gravity helps return blood to the heart. Elevating the arm or leg of a supine or prone client enhances venous return. Box 13-6 describes techniques for venous circulation enhancement.

Box 13-6

Venous Circulation Enhancement

- The individual effleurage strokes sweep proximally, toward the heart, but the series of strokes start progressively farther from the heart.
- Closer to the heart, use long effleurage strokes to encourage the blood to move through a series of valves.
- In the distal portions of the arms and legs, where there are more valves, use short, 1- to 2-inch effleurage strokes.
- Periodically use one long effleurage stroke that covers the area treated by the two or three previous effleurage strokes, ensuring that the blood still flows freely along the path.

ARTERIAL ENHANCEMENT

Fresh, oxygenated blood is pushed through the arteries by the forceful muscular contractions of the heart and continues with the help of gravity to flow to the cells and tissues throughout the body. The heart, as long as it is contracting, will continue to push blood into the arteries. Using the mechanical concept of pressure building behind a dam, a massage therapist can intentionally encourage arterial blood flow. In a massage session, the therapist can apply rhythmic, manual compression strokes that progressively move away from the heart along an artery. These compression strokes need moderate pressure to pinch off the blood supply without damaging the blood vessels. Procedure Box 13-1 describes the steps for arterial circulation enhancement.

LYMPH DRAINAGE

The lymphatic system, first identified in 1622, is a component of the circulatory system that transports nutrients and immune cells and cleans and filters

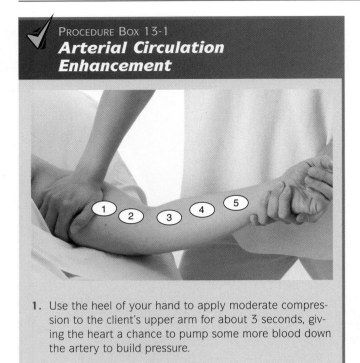

Arterial Circulation Enhancement

1. Use the heel of your hand to apply moderate compression to the client's upper arm for about 3 seconds, giving the heart a chance to pump some more blood down the artery to build pressure.

> **!** *Pay attention to your wrist position because it is easy to overextend the wrist while applying compression.*

2. Release the compression to allow the arterial blood to rush forward.
3. Move the heel of your hand a couple of inches distally and apply another 3-second compression stroke.
4. Repeat steps 1–3 until you reach the client's wrist, using less pressure as you move toward the wrist.

cellular waste, debris, and pathogens from the interstitial fluid, or fluid between the cells. The flow of interstitial fluid and lymph is vital to the health of the body; without it, blood would become thicker, blood volume would decrease, and blood pressure would fall.

The pressure of blood as it moves through the arterial capillaries is high enough that fluid, proteins, nutrients, and gases diffuse through the capillary walls into the interstitial spaces. There, the fluid and all of its components, including the waste products from the cells, is called interstitial fluid. Some of the proteins, cellular waste, and other ingredients cannot diffuse back into the capillaries and must be removed from the interstitial space. The very delicate ends of the lymphatic vessels pick up interstitial fluid and the larger constituents, at which point it is considered **lymph.** The lymphatic vessels form a drainage system that leads to the main veins that empty into the heart. Along the way, the lymph passes through lymph nodes, which house immune cells that engulf and neutralize the pathogens. Eventually the system of lymphatic vessels ends at ducts that drain the cleaned and filtered lymph directly into the bloodstream and into the heart. (Fig. 4-64 illustrates the lymphatic system.)

There are two separate "drains" for the lymph. The **right lymphatic duct** drains all of the lymph from the upper right quadrant of the body, including everything on the right side of the body above the diaphragm, into the right subclavian vein. The **thoracic duct** drains lymph collected from everywhere else on the body into the left subclavian vein (Fig. 13-1). Since lymph collection is divided into two separate paths, you must understand the direction of the lymph flow before attempting to enhance it.

Lymphatic vessels are like veins in several ways. They have valves that prevent lymph from flowing away from the heart, and the lymphatic system lacks a true mechanical pump to push lymph through the vessels. Instead, it uses the skeletal muscle pump mechanism, in which muscles and surrounding tissues put pressure on the lymphatic vessels and squeeze the lymph in the only direction the valves allow—toward the heart.

Emil Vodder, PhD, developed a system of lymphatic drainage in 1936, commonly called manual lymphatic drainage (MLD). The Vodder method uses light, rhythmic, spirallike movements to encourage the flow of lymph. More recently, Dr. Bruno Chikly developed and currently teaches Lymph Drainage Therapy (LDT), a technique based upon the work of Dr. Vodder, Alexander de Winiwarter (1891), and osteopath F. P. Millard (1922). LDT teaches therapists an anatomical approach that allows them to map the vessels, assess the quality and depth of overall circulation, and determine the best alternative pathways for draining stagnant body fluids. Therapists use all of the finger pads to simulate gentle, specific wavelike movements that activate lymph and interstitial fluid circulation and stimulate immune function and parasympathetic nervous system activity. Enhanced lymph drainage offers many benefits:

- Reduces edema
- Minimizes scarring
- Speeds up tissue healing, including burns, wounds, and wrinkles
- Relieves pain by relieving fluid pressure on nerve endings
- Relieves sinus congestion
- Reduces symptoms of chronic fatigue syndrome and fibromyalgia syndrome
- Relieves muscle hypertonicity
- Relieves some forms of constipation
- Increases relaxation to aid insomnia, stress, and loss of vitality

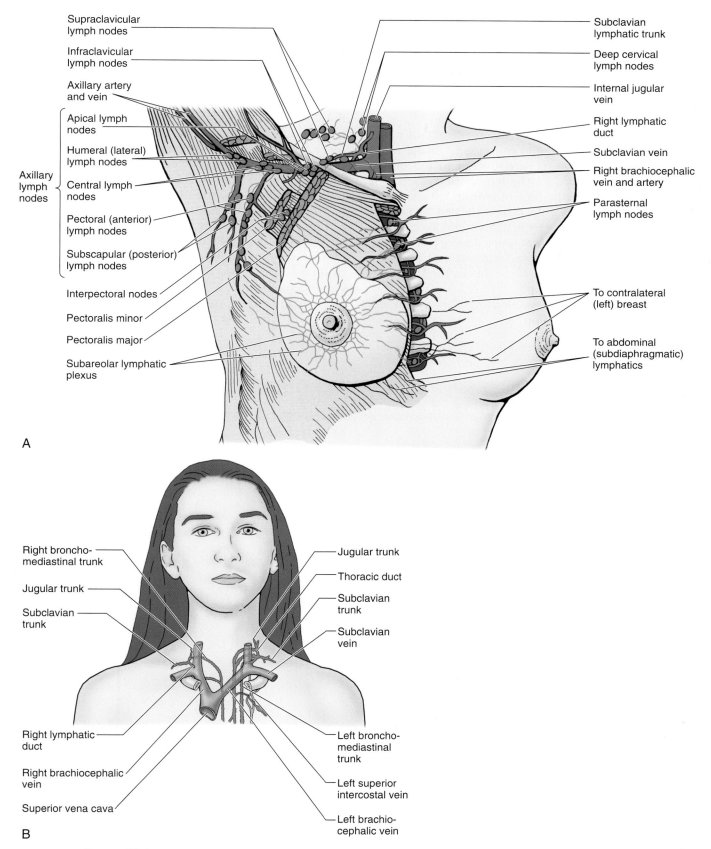

Supraclavicular
lymph nodes

Infraclavicular
lymph nodes

Axillary artery
and vein

Apical lymph
nodes

Humeral (lateral)
lymph nodes

Central lymph
nodes

Pectoral (anterior)
lymph nodes

Subscapular (posterior)
lymph nodes

Axillary
lymph
nodes

Interpectoral nodes

Pectoralis minor

Pectoralis major

Subareolar lymphatic
plexus

Subclavian
lymphatic trunk

Deep cervical
lymph nodes

Internal jugular
vein

Right lymphatic
duct

Subclavian vein

Right brachiocephalic
vein and artery

Parasternal
lymph nodes

To contralateral
(left) breast

To abdominal
(subdiaphragmatic)
lymphatics

A

Right broncho-
mediastinal trunk

Jugular trunk

Subclavian
trunk

Right lymphatic
duct

Right brachiocephalic
vein

Superior vena cava

Jugular trunk

Thoracic duct

Subclavian
trunk

Subclavian
vein

Left broncho-
mediastinal
trunk

Left superior
intercostal vein

Left brachio-
cephalic vein

B

FIGURE 13-1 Lymphatic drainage. (Reprinted from Moore KL, Dalley AF II. Clinical Oriented Anatomy. 4th ed. Baltimore: Lippincott Williams & Wilkins, 1999.

Enhancing Lymph Drainage

While the methods described earlier require advanced training, the beginning massage therapist can enhance lymph drainage with techniques similar to venous enhancement. The movement of lymph is encouraged by deep breathing, gravity, joint movement, muscular contraction, and general massage.

Full, deep breaths are beneficial for encouraging lymphatic flow. Not only do full breaths bring more oxygen into the lungs to be delivered to the blood, they also put pressure on the lymphatic vessels and organs to encourage the flow of lymph. **Lymphatic vessels are concentrated near the diaphragm, and the full contraction and relaxation of the diaphragm during deep breathing significantly enhances lymph drainage.** When the diaphragm contracts for inspiration, it puts pressure on the lymphatic vessels and organs in the thorax to encourage the flow of lymph.

Gravity can be used by elevating the client's extremities during the session.

 Maintain proper body mechanics while holding and lifting the client's extremities.

Because lymph nodes are more concentrated near joints, movement of the joints also encourages lymph flow. When the nodes are squeezed, as occurs with active and passive muscle movement, their valves force lymph toward the heart even more effectively than when the lymphatic vessels are squeezed. Joint movement goes hand in hand with muscle contraction, and isotonic contractions that create movement are more effective than isometric contractions.

Compression strokes applied in sets of three and very light effleurage strokes that sweep toward the closest lymph node or lymphatic duct enhance lymph drainage. There are different approaches to lymph enhancement, but ½- to 1-inch effleurage strokes or circular effleurage strokes are generally considered acceptable. Because of the location of the lymphatic

---

PROCEDURE BOX 13-2
Basic Lymph Drainage Enhancement

- Pumping—3 rhythmic compression strokes
- Sweeping—a series of short, superficial effleurage strokes that sweep proximally

Supine Position—Neck and Head Drainage

1. Place your relaxed, flat hands on the client's chest, just inferior to the client's clavicles, and apply 3 light compression strokes with a pumping rhythm.
2. Rotate the client's neck to the left, support the head with your left hand, and use your right hand to apply several sets of very light pumping and sweeping to the neck, starting at the client's right clavicle and gradually moving up to the occiput.
3. Rotate the client's neck to the right, supporting the head with your right hand, and use your left hand to apply several sets of very light pumping and sweeping to the neck, starting at the client's left clavicle and gradually moving up to the occiput.
4. Apply several sets of pumping and sweeping to the client's face, starting near the chin and gradually moving out and up to the client's forehead.

Supine Position—Arm Drainage

1. Use flat fingers to sweep the chest, starting near the client's sternum and gradually moving to the right axilla (armpit area).
2. Gently but firmly grasp your client's right hand, interlocking your thumb with theirs, support the client's elbow, and rhythmically flex and extend the client's right shoulder and elbow several times.

3. Use flat fingers to sweep the right arm, starting at the axilla and gradually moving to the hand.
4. Use flat fingers to sweep the thorax, starting at the right axilla and moving down the right side of the rib cage.
5. Repeat steps 1–5 on the left side.

Supine Position—Leg Drainage

1. Elevate the client's left leg with bolsters or, if possible, gently hold and support the client's left foot and lower leg to rhythmically flex the hip and knee several times.
2. Use your palms or flat fingers to pump and sweep the client's left leg, starting at the medial thigh and gradually moving to the ankle.
3. Repeat for the client's right leg.

Prone Position—Leg Drainage

 Do not put pressure on the popliteal fossa at the back of knee because it is an endangerment site.

1. Elevate the client's ankles with a small bolster.
2. Gently and firmly grasp the client's right ankle and rhythmically flex the knee several times.
3. Use your palms or flat fingers to pump and sweep the client's right leg, starting at the right iliac crest and gradually moving to the ankle.
4. Repeat for the client's left leg.

ducts and the high concentration of lymphatic vessels in the neck, begin treatment at the client's chest and neck. If you are not familiar with the lymphatic system, you will not know which node is closest, or which duct serves as the drain, and you could be working against the body. Since lymphatic vessels are more fragile than veins, use very little pressure so you do not compress the vessels and stop the flow altogether. Procedure Box 13-2 describes a basic lymph drainage enhancement procedure. Before applying any of these techniques, make sure there are no contraindications for lymph drainage enhancement. Some of the more common contraindications include

- Edema not related to soft tissue injury, which could indicate an overtaxed heart
- Liver or kidney congestion
- Blood clot
- Local infection or signs of local infection (pain, redness, heat and swelling)
- Red streaks from an infection site to the nearest lymph nodes

Deep pressure can damage lymphatic vessels, and damaged lymphatic vessels cannot drain lymph properly, which is why massage is contraindicated over areas of inflammation. Do not push fluids toward a developing scar, because the proteins in the interstitial fluid can agglomerate at the scar and form keloids. Instead, enhance lymph drainage proximal to the developing scar. If you are uncertain whether you should apply lymphatic techniques, do not proceed, and refer clients to their primary healthcare provider.

Abdominal Massage

The abdomen is often left untreated during a massage session. Properly draping the abdomen is slightly more complicated than draping the rest of the body, and a general unfamiliarity with abdominal massage can make it an uncomfortable experience for you and your clients. Not much scientific research has been conducted to confirm the benefits of abdominal massage, but many persons believe that it can provide relief from intestinal discomfort and nausea in adults, children, and infants.

Much scientific research shows that massage balances hormone levels, reduces stress, induces parasympathetic nervous system activity, leads to clarity of thought, and enhances concentration. The parasympathetic nervous response, induced by relaxation massage, stimulates digestive activity. When pressure is exerted on the abdomen, underlying structures are compressed and pushed out of the way.

An effleurage stroke can mechanically push intestinal contents through the intestines. Massage may also stimulate peristaltic contractions of the intestines, which is the body's natural mechanism for pushing contents through the digestive tract toward the rectum. The individual effleurage strokes must be applied in the same direction as peristalsis to enhance digestive progress.

Because clients are often unfamiliar with abdominal work, always ask them if they want the work done. With their permission, you can proceed. Draping requires at least one extra blanket or large towel, if not two, in addition to the standard sheets. (See Procedure Box 9-1 for the abdominal draping sequence.)

Abdominal massage for digestive enhancement uses an approach similar to that for venous enhancement and lymphatic drainage, in which you start closest to the outlet or drain, and progressively move farther away from it. The sequence of strokes is a counterclockwise pattern, but the individual strokes move clockwise along the large intestine (Fig. 13-2). These directions are determined as if the client is holding a clock on his or her abdomen so that you can read the face of the clock. Strokes should be slow and firm rather than quick and light. The abdominal massage backtracks through the large intestine, starting with the rectal area and moving counterclockwise toward the cecum. Clearing the exit end first is more effective than pushing from the other end, which could compact the contents in the passage.

Having the abdomen exposed often makes a person feel vulnerable and unsure. Be careful to help maintain the client's physical and mental safety, and be especially sensitive to the client's acceptance or discomfort with the work. Stay attuned to the client's verbal or nonverbal communication to be aware of the client's comfort level throughout the abdominal massage. Procedure Box 13-3 lists the steps for an abdominal massage.

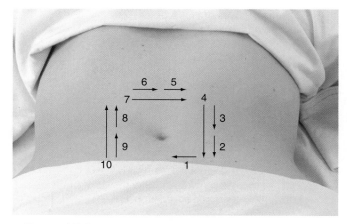

FIGURE 13-2 Sequence of strokes for digestive enhancement.

INDICATIONS AND CONTRAINDICATIONS FOR ABDOMINAL MASSAGE

Abdominal massage is beneficial for enhancing digestion and relief from constipation, diarrhea, colic, gas, and nausea. It also helps the uterus return to its normal size during the postpartum period.

For clients who are generally healthy, it is unnecessary to obtain a physician's consult before doing abdominal massage. If, on the other hand, the client is pregnant, has a history of diverticular disease, pelvic disorders such as endometriosis or pelvic in-

flammatory disease (PID), or fits the profile for aneurysm (history of heart disease, atherosclerosis, and high blood pressure), you should encourage that client to get clearance from his or her physician.

Reflexology

Reflexology is the bodywork modality in which defined points on the feet, hands, or ears are stimulated, resulting in specific reflexive activity of the nervous system. It is also thought that this pressure relieves blocked energy and allows the body to work more efficiently. Evidence suggests that people were applying manual therapy to the feet 5000 years ago in ancient India. A wall carving in the ancient Egyptian tomb of Ankhmahor, dated about 2350 BCE, shows a person manipulating a patient's foot, and although many claim that reflexology is being depicted, there is some dispute over the actual subject (See Fig. 1-5). History indicates the use of foot massage in China around 300 BCE and also in Japan, where it was called sokushinjutsu.

Dr. William Fitzgerald was an ear, nose, and throat surgeon who developed a system of reflexive work called Zone Therapy in 1917. Based on his discovery that pressure on a specific area on the body resulted in a referred anesthetic effect somewhere else, he mapped a pattern of longitudinal zones on the body that had related referral effects. He used pressure points on the tongue, palate, and the back of the pharynx wall to relieve pain, and he discovered that application of pressure on the zones also relieved the underlying cause in most cases. Shelby Riley, MD, worked closely with Dr. Fitzgerald and identified additional horizontal zones across the hands and feet.

In the 1930s, Eunice Ingham, a physical therapist who worked closely with Dr. Riley, refined the familiar modern-day system of foot reflexology. She noticed that congestion and tension in specific points on the foot, called reflex points, corresponded to congestion and tension in specific areas elsewhere on the body. By applying focused pressure to the reflex points, she could create stimulating effects on the body. She integrated all of her findings into the Ingham Method of Reflexology, which improves nerve function and blood supply to normalize body processes and relieve tension.

Reflexology maps and charts are widely available that identify specific reflex points and areas on the hands and feet. They also indicate the body parts that are affected when pressure is applied to those specific reflex points (Fig. 13-3). With sensitive, trained hands, your fingertip pressure on reflex points can

---

> ### PROCEDURE BOX 13-3
> ## *Abdominal Massage Procedure*

1. Position your fully draped client supine, with both knees bent to relax the abdomen, and place a towel across the chest, on top of the draping.
2. Ask your client to rest the hands on the chest. Explain that the hands act as a physical barrier to stop you from touching the abdomen any higher than the hands. (Some clients will rest their hands close to their navel while others may not need a barrier. Whatever your client's modesty, keep your work inferior to the xyphoid process.)
3. Establish the inferior limit for your work by tucking the sheet tightly under the client's hips, just inferior to the ASIS. You can place a second towel over the client's pelvis to cover the area inferior to the ASIS for additional modesty or warmth.
4. With the superior and inferior borders determined, ask the client to firmly hold onto the towel on the chest.
5. Gently pull the draping sheet out from under the towel to expose the abdomen down to the pelvis, stopping at the inferior barrier.
6. Stand at your client's side and apply superficial effleurage strokes to spread the lubricant and help the client get used to abdominal contact.
7. Place the palms of both hands against the close side of your client's abdomen and firmly effleurage across the abdomen, your hands moving away from you.
8. Before your fingertips reach the client's midline, relieve some of the pressure by lifting your hands slightly, and reach across the gathered tissue to the far side of the client's abdomen.
9. Use both of your flat hands to slowly and firmly effleurage the abdomen toward you. Slowly and rhythmically repeat steps 8 and 9 several times with wave-like strokes across the abdomen.
10. Apply effleurage strokes to enhance peristaltic activity, as in Figure 13-2.
11. Apply a resting stroke to the abdomen with both hands.
12. Pull the draping sheet up, leaving the chest drape in place underneath the sheet.

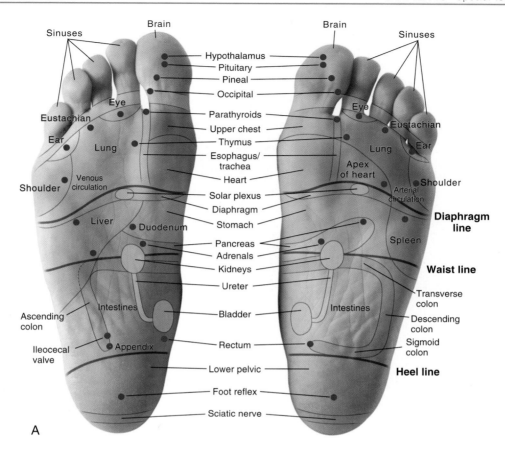

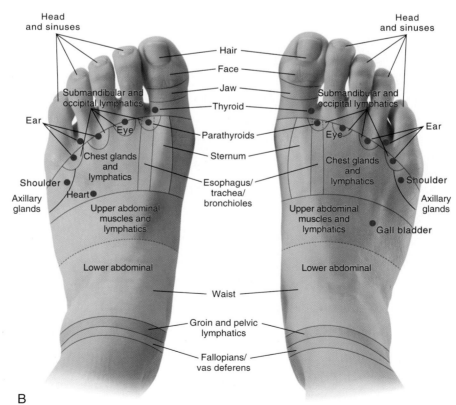

FIGURE 13-3 Reflexology foot charts. **A.** Bottoms of feet. **B.** Tops of feet.

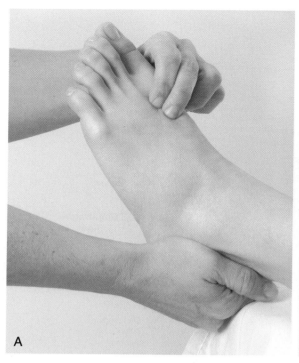

A. Finger walking—apply pressure with your thumb or index finger and slide it forward in an "inchworm" movement across the client's foot.

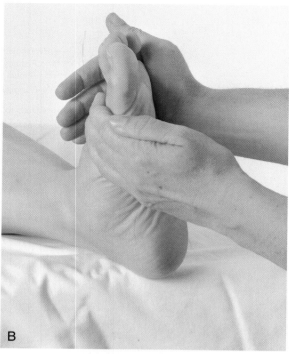

B. Back-and-forth technique—use one hand to grasp the medial edge of the client's foot and the other hand to grasp the lateral edge. Flex the metatarsals by moving your right hand up and your left hand down, and then switch.

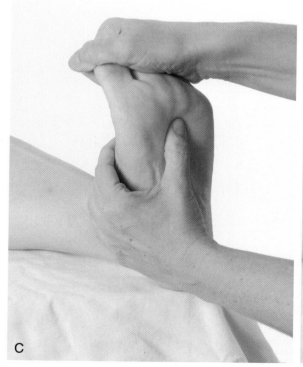

C. Diaphragm and solar plexus flexing—apply thumb pressure to the diaphragm and solar plexus reflex point and flex the toes toward you. Then, maintain thumb pressure and extend the toes away from you.

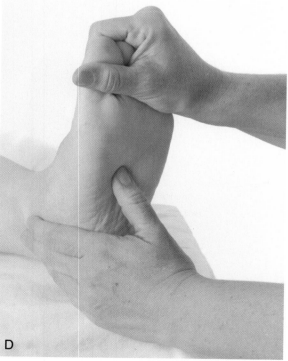

D. Holding—place your thumb along the base of the toes and wrap your hand around the toes, resting your fingers on the top of the foot. With your other hand, apply pressure to the desired reflex point.

FIGURE 13-4 Basic reflexology techniques.

relieve stress, pain, and muscular tension; it can restore and maintain homeostasis; and it can encourage healing. While reflexology techniques can be applied to the hands, ears, or feet, working on the feet is the most common. Learn some of the major reflex points. It is simple to incorporate reflexology into a standard massage session, and many clients are familiar with the technique and request it. Reflexology workshops and certification courses are available worldwide that provide more thorough information and training.

INCORPORATING REFLEXOLOGY INTO A MASSAGE SESSION

There are three lines you can use as landmarks on the foot to orient you to a person's feet and guide your reflexology work: the diaphragm line, the waist line, and the heel line. Just below the ball of the foot is the diaphragm line. The waist line is an imaginary line from the 5th metatarsal (protrusion on lateral edge of the foot) to the arch. The point above the heel where the lighter and softer skin becomes the darker, thicker skin of the heel is the heel line (Fig. 13-3A).

The basic foot reflexology techniques include holding, thumb walking, finger walking, and joint movement. Specific passive joint movements of the ankle, metatarsals, and toes are incorporated into reflexology, as are specific deep effleurage strokes (Fig. 13-4). Start and end your reflexology sessions with the back-and-forth technique, ankle rotation, and diaphragm and solar plexus flexing. The back-and-forth technique is a joint movement that does not occur with normal use of the feet, making it particularly beneficial for loosening up the foot at the beginning of a reflexology session. Clockwise and then counterclockwise ankle rotation increases the production of synovial fluid in the ankle joint and also loosens up the fascia in the client's foot. Diaphragm and solar plexus flexing is a tension reliever that should be used at the beginning and end of a reflexology session.

When you apply pressure to a reflex point, use your free hand to apply the holding technique to stabilize the client's foot. You can apply pressure to a reflex point with your thumb or finger, or you can modify the basic pressure technique to cover a larger reflex area by "inchworming" your thumb or finger across the desired area.

More-advanced techniques can be learned and used with advanced training and practice. No oil, cream, or lotion is used for reflexology, but you can use powder if the client's feet are damp. Combine techniques into a basic reflexology flow. Procedure Box 13-4 describes a basic reflexology procedure.

PROCEDURE BOX 13-4
Basic Reflexology Flow

1. Sit at the client's feet, undrape one foot, and find the diaphragm line, waist line, and heel line.
2. Apply back-and-forth movements, ankle rotation, and diaphragm and solar plexus flexing to warm up the client's foot.
3. Grasp the client's foot with both hands so that the flats of your fingers are on the top of the foot and your thumbs on the soles.
4. Effleurage several times with both hands from the toes to the ankles and from the ankles back to the toes.
5. Using thumb or finger walking in different areas while holding with your other hand:
   a. The base of all the toes, from the big toe to the little toe
   b. Each toe, from the tip to the base, and from the base to tip, from the big toe to the little toe, and back to the big toe
   c. The ball of the foot to the base of each toe
   d. The top of the foot, from the base of each toe and along each metatarsal, from the big toe to the little toe
   e. From the arch to the lateral portion of the foot, between the waist line and the diaphragm line
   f. On the left foot, from the heel line to the waist line, moving from the arch to the lateral portion of the foot, then up the lateral portion of the foot
      On the right foot, from just below the heel line to the arch of the foot at a 45° angle, then up the lateral portion of the foot
   g. The arch of the foot, from the heel line to the big toe
   h. From the base of the 5th metatarsal, just below the little toe, down to the heel line
   i. Across the heel, just below the heel line
   j. Around the lateral malleolus and medial malleolus (ankle protrusions)
6. Apply back-and-forth movements.
7. Grasp the foot so that the flats of your fingers are on the top of the foot and your thumbs are on the sole, and effleurage several times with both hands from the toes to the ankles, and from the ankles back to the toes.
8. Redrape the foot.
9. Expose the other foot and repeat steps 1–8.
(Adapted from Lidell L, Thomas S, Cook CB, Porter A. The Book of Massage. New York: Gaia Books Limited/Simon and Schuster, 1984.)

INDICATIONS AND CONTRAINDICATIONS FOR REFLEXOLOGY

Reflexology relieves tension, and it stimulates the lymphatic and nervous systems by reflexively affecting different points or zones in the body. Plantar warts, bunions, and musculoskeletal injuries on the feet are local contraindications for reflexology, as are any areas of numbness and neuromas. If the client has a foot condition that contraindicates reflexology, you can alternatively use hand or ear reflexology techniques.

East Meets West

The concept of energy is important in the Eastern philosophy of health. It is challenging to understand the Eastern terminology because there is no direct translation in the English language for many words. To make matters worse, a single Chinese term can have different meanings when used in different contexts. Because of the language discrepancy, many of the explanations and descriptions of Eastern healthcare seem vague or abstract. Keeping this in mind, this section is a very simplified introduction to the Eastern healthcare philosophy and some of the associated bodywork approaches.

Traditional Chinese medicine (TCM) approaches healthcare quite differently from the Western medical approach. Both Eastern and Western medicine have their unique advantages, and sometimes one system may be more effective than another. TCM practitioners evaluate the whole person as an entire universe or a masterpiece painting. It is difficult to isolate a single factor that keeps a painting from being a work of art, and it is just as complicated to determine exactly what has created dysfunction within the body. In the Western medical approach to evaluation, a painting's lack of success might be analyzed with high-technology testing and attributed to a single ingredient of the paint being wrong or to the wrong kind of bristles on the paintbrush. Oriental assessment, in contrast, might look at how the lighting and shapes and textures interact, and the practitioner might look for an imbalance somewhere.

YIN AND YANG

There are moving, dynamic, and opposing energetic forces that exist within us. Consider the difference between dark and light, fast and slow, hot and cold, moving and stationary, or large and small. They are relative terms, one helping define the other, and TCM refers to these opposites as **yin** (YIHN) and **yang** (YAHNG). Yin energy is associated with passive, dark, cool, supportive, female, and inward activities of the body. Conceptually flowing from the earth, this energy runs up the front of the body, and continues flowing down the posterior aspect of the body. The contrasting yang energy conceptually emanates from the sun, flowing down the front of the body and up the back of

the body, and it is associated with the active, bright, warm, consumptive, male, and outward activities of the body. Again, these descriptions of yin and yang are conceptual rather than literal translations.

The symbol of yin and yang is a two-dimensional representation of the concept of dynamic balance of opposites within an organism. The smaller dots within opposites represent the influence and presence of the opposition, however small (Box 13-7). When opposites exist in relatively equal amounts, they are considered balanced. TCM theory suggests that when yin and yang are balanced, the body enjoys good health.

ENERGY

One view of energy, more common in Western cultures, is that it is a scientific, physical property that can be measured and qualified. Another view, more

---

BOX 13-7

Yin and Yang Symbol

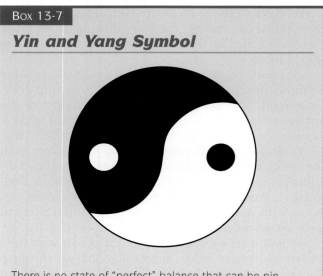

There is no state of "perfect" balance that can be pinpointed in the TCM approach to healthcare. Instead, a person's health and well-being is a constantly moving and changing interaction of opposing forces. The only time there is no relative movement is when there is no life.

Understanding the Eastern and Oriental concepts as dynamic, moving processes instead of fixed and isolated objects can be represented by one of those rectangular wave machines that contain a layer of clear oil above a layer of blue water. As the container rocks back and forth, the oil and water constantly move in relation to each other. The molecular structures of the oil and water have opposite polarities, which keep them separated. Despite their opposition, the shape and movement of the oil is defined and influenced by that of the water, and vice versa. There is no condition of isolated, balanced stillness unless the container has been at rest for some time.

common in Eastern and Oriental cultures, understands energy as a dynamic, changing force commonly called Qi (CHEE) that supports and is supported by the other processes of the body. TCM practitioners skillfully palpate Qi to evaluate the processes and structures of the body to develop an understanding of how they work together in a balanced or imbalanced sense. **Balance is the essence of TCM and many energetic therapies.**

In Chinese medicine, organs are conceptually different from anatomical structures because they have energetic as well as physical presence. In fact, some of the TCM organs do not exist as anatomical organs in the human body. To maintain the yin and yang balance, there are six yin organs paired with six yang organs.

Generally, Qi flows through the body in precise and orderly channels most often referred to as **meridians.** There are 12 bilateral, paired primary meridians that flow in a specific pattern and are associated with body organs (Table 13-1). In addition to the 12 organ meridians, there are 2 extraordinary meridians called the Governing vessel, which flows along the spine, and the Conception vessel, which flows along the anterior midline. These meridians can be loosely mapped on a model of the human figure, but like anatomical structures, their exact locations vary among individuals (Fig. 13-5).

As Qi travels through the meridians, it passes through and affects organs and structures along the way. The lung meridian is the most superficial and opens to the pores and body hair. Understand that

TABLE 13-1

Descriptions of the Energy Meridian Pathways

MERIDIAN	STARTING POINT	PATH	ENDING POINT
Stomach (ST)	Eye	Down the front of the body	Second toe
Spleen (SP)	Big toe	Up the medial leg and up the front of the body	Axilla
Heart (HT)	Axilla	Up the inside of the arm	Little finger
Small intestine (SI)	Little finger	Up the arm, over to C7, up the neck, and zigzags inferior and then superior to the zygomatic process	Just anterior to the ear
Bladder (BL)	Eye	Over the top of the cranium and down the back and leg	Little toe
Kidney (K or KI)	Bottom of the foot	Up the medial side of the leg and thorax	Middle of the clavicle
Pericardium (P or PC), also called heart governor (HG) and circulation sex	On the chest, medial to the axilla	Up the inside of the arm	At the middle finger
Triple heater (TH), also called triple warmer (TW)	Ring finger	Up the back of the arm and the lateral neck	At the lateral edge of the eyebrow ridge
Gall bladder (GB)	Lateral corner of the eye	Zigzags around the ear, up and down the back of the head, and zigzags down the side of the body	Fourth toe
Liver (LV or LR)	Big toe	Up the medial leg	Front of the thorax at the eighth rib
Lung (LU)	Middle of the clavicle	Up the front of the arm	Thumb
Large intestine (LI)	Index finger	Up the arm, up the neck, around the edge of the mouth	Base of the nose
Conception vessel (CV), also called central vessel	Perineum, anterior to the anus	Up the anterior midline of the body	Center of the lower lip
Governing vessel (GV)	Coccyx	Up the posterior midline of the body, and over the head	Center of the upper lip

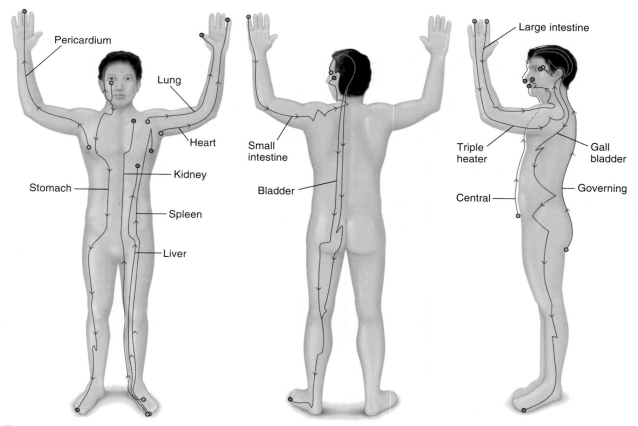

FIGURE 13-5 Energy meridians.

pain or tension along the lung meridian indicates an imbalance in the lung energy and that the anatomical lungs may not be affected. In contrast, the kidney meridian is where the vital and genetic energy runs. Tsubos (SOO-bohz), also called **acupressure points,** acupuncture points, and potent points, are defined points along all of the meridians where the interior energy can easily be affected by an external source. They are identified as a numbered point along the organ meridian. For example, stomach 36 is the 36th acupressure point along the stomach meridian and can be abbreviated ST36 or St36. Originally there were 365 of these points, but some claim that 2000 points have since been determined. The names of the original points referred to their usage or their location. For example, LI4 is called the Great Eliminator because it is a powerful point that can relieve constipation, headache, toothaches, and colds. Some of the most powerful acupressure points are located on the hands and feet. Scientific studies have shown that there is, indeed, a lower electrical resistance at these points. Some theorize that acupressure points and trigger points are one and the same and cannot be distinguished from each other. According to Dr. Janet Travell, 70% of acupressure points coincide with trigger points.

ACUPRESSURE

The practice of acupuncture uses needles inserted into the acupuncture points to stimulate and balance the flow of Qi through the meridians. It is not within the scope of practice of massage therapy to use needles, but similar results can be obtained with acupressure and shiatsu, which both use pressure to influence the flow of Qi through the meridians.

Acupressure is a bodywork modality in which firm fingertip pressure is applied to points along the energy meridians to regulate the flow of Qi. When you feel an area or acupressure point that is deficient in Qi, the tissue may yield to your touch, and feel somewhat hollow. As you apply pressure to an energy-deficient area, you supply and activate energy flow to the area, and it typically feels good to the client. Conversely, areas that have excessive Qi may feel hard or resistant when you touch them, and they are usually painful or hypersensitive.

In another example of yin and yang, the body compensates for a Qi deficiency by redirecting an excess of Qi to another area. The pain and hypersensitivity in the area of excess Qi is considered a symptom of the deficiency. One approach to acupressure recommends that you treat the painful points until they are no longer painful, but some clients cannot or do not want to tolerate pressure on the areas with excess energy. Another approach to TCM focuses on treating the deficient areas, since the deficiency is considered the cause for the symptoms. By treating the cause, you can eliminate the symptoms of pain and hypersensitivity without aggravating the painful area.

To perform acupressure, you apply firm pressure to a specific acupressure point, and hold it for about 30 seconds, once a day, until the flow of Qi is restored. It is best to apply pressure to both bilateral acupressure points at the same time, but some find it effective to treat one side at a time. Occasionally the pressure is delivered with a knob or other device or supplemented with circular motions or vibration to activate stagnant Qi or regulate excessive Qi. There are several acupressure points that can be used for self-treatment and clients can use these between massage sessions (Table 13-2).

TABLE 13-2

Acupressure Points for Self-Care (This is a very small sample—many more exist)

ACUPRESSURE POINT	LOCATION		SELF-CARE APPLICATIONS
LI4 (large intestine 4)	Base of webbing between thumb and index finger		Sinus problems Headaches Constipation ⚠ *Contraindicated during pregnancy*
P6 (pericardium 6)	On forearm, about three finger widths from the crease at the base of the hand, between two tendons		Nausea Anxiety
ST36 (stomach 36)	Front of leg, about four fingers below the kneecap, just lateral to the tibia		Fatigue Depression Lack of grounding Instability
SP6 (spleen 6)	Medial side of tibia, about four fingers above medial malleolus		Irritability Worry Cold and flu Fear ⚠ *Contraindicated during pregnancy*
GB20 (gall bladder 20)	Base of skull, in the hollow on either side of the neck, about 2–3 inches apart		Shoulder pain Depression Neck tension Irritability

SHIATSU

Shiatsu (shee-AHT-soo) is literally translated "finger pressure" and is a variation of acupressure. The purpose of shiatsu is to increase Qi and circulation of blood throughout the body, but it can also increase endorphin levels and stimulate nerve function. Whereas acupressure uses focused pressure directly on an acupressure point, **shiatsu** is a form of bodywork that uses a combination of acupressure with stretching, range of motion, and massage strokes. You can use your finger or thumb to deliver pressure in shiatsu, or you can use a broader surface, such as the heel or palm of your hand, your elbow, your knee, or your foot, to cover a more general area on the client's body. If you do use your knee or your foot, apply pressure carefully and gradually to avoid hurting your client. Since the breath encourages the flow of Qi, you can synchronize your application of pressure with the client's exhalation to pay more attention to the breathing pattern.

When you apply a series of compression strokes to a client's limb, one of your hands maintains contact with the client's body while the other hand moves down the limb. The stationary hand, called the mother hand, does not move and it does not apply pressure. You use your mother hand as an assessment tool, to sense any changes or reactions occurring in the client's body.

The body mechanics differ from those in traditional massage because the work requires significant compression applied perpendicularly (90°), and no oil or gliding pressure is used. The pressure for all of your strokes and techniques originates in your hara (HAHR-uh), which is the center of your energy, located in the abdomen, below the navel, and is directed through your relaxed but stable body. It is the same practice as using proper body alignment for body mechanics, but with a different philosophy. Because you use so many compression strokes in shiatsu, you must maintain proper body mechanics:

- Pay special attention to your wrist position.
- Make sure that your shoulders stay relaxed.
- Avoid putting excessive pressure on your cubital tunnel.
- Keep your joints stacked.
- Support your fingers and thumbs when using them to apply pressure.

You and your client should wear clothes that allow you to move easily. You do not need a massage table for shiatsu, and you do not need lubricant. Clients can remain fully clothed during a shiatsu session and they can lie on the floor, a shiatsu mat, a shiatsu table, or a lowered massage table, allowing you to use good body mechanics. A basic shiatsu routine is shown in Procedure Box 13-5.

Both acupressure and shiatsu claim to relieve stress, tension, muscular aches and pains, nausea, depression, and headaches. Both techniques can be integrated into a standard massage session and can help you accomplish your client's treatment goals with techniques that are more effective for them or that they prefer. A wealth of information is available on the topics of TCM, acupuncture, acupressure, and shiatsu. Classes, courses, and programs of various lengths are offered worldwide to provide more information and training on these topics.

FIVE PHASES

The five elements, fire, earth, metal, water, and wood, are an integral part of the Oriental philosophy of health. As with the Qi and the organs, these elements are dynamic, energetic, relative processes that are better described as phases. There are qualities to each of these phases that can be loosely described in English:

- Wood—active growth
- Fire—peak activity just before diminishing
- Metal—diminishing activity
- Water—period of rest between different activities
- Earth—balanced state of activity and rest

The five phases can be considered parts of a cycle, all interacting to create a complete universe, an organism, or a masterpiece painting. There is a cycle of production, in which the different phases feed each other, and a cycle of control, in which the phases limit each other. Figure 13-6 illustrates the cycles of the five phases. The association of the yin and yang organs with the phases involves a theoretical connection between the phases and health. When either cycle is imbalanced or disrupted, Qi will not flow properly, and the person's health will be affected. Manipulating the Qi from an external source using points on the meridians can restore flow and balance.

Polarity

Polarity therapy was developed in the early 1900s by Randolph Stone, DO, DC, ND. He found that electromagnetic fields of the human body are affected by touch, diet, movement, sound, attitudes, experiences, trauma, and environmental factors and suggested that balanced, regular electromagnetic fields allow the body to function properly in a healthy state. When these energy fields are imbalanced or blocked, pain and disease can result. The objective of polarity therapy is to adjust the energy flow to create a bal-

Start with your client in the prone position, on a clean blanket, shiatsu mat, or shiatsu table.

1. Kneel at the client's left side and perform a diagonal stretch to the client's back.
   a. Place your left hand on the client's left scapula and your right hand just below the client's right iliac crest.
   b. Lean forward and apply pressure to move your hands away from each other, and hold for 5–10 seconds.
   c. Lean back to relieve the pressure.
   d. Move your left hand to the client's right scapula and your right hand to just below the client's left iliac crest.

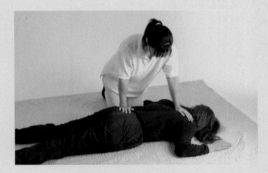

   e. Lean forward and apply pressure to move your hands away from each other, and hold for 5–10 seconds.
   f. Lean back to relieve the pressure.
2. Perform a lumbar stretch to the client's back.
   a. Cross your arms, placing your right hand on the upper thoracic spine and your left hand on the sacrum.
   b. Lean forward and apply pressure to separate your hands, and hold for 5–10 seconds.

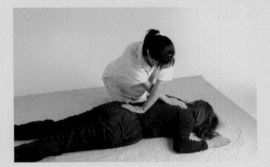

   c. Lean back to relieve the pressure.
3. Apply rhythmic compression strokes to the client's back.
   a. Starting at the top of the back, place the heels of your hands on either side of the spine and let your fingers rest along the client's ribs.
   b. Lean forward to apply pressure and hold for 5 seconds.
   c. Lean back to relieve pressure and move your hands 1–2 inches down the spine.
   d. Repeat steps b and c until you reach the low curve of the client's back.

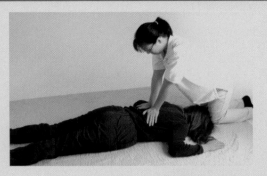

4. Still on your knees, straddle or sit beside the client's thighs and squeeze the gluteal muscles.
   a. With your fingers pointing inward, place the palms of your hands on the client's gluteal muscles.
   b. Lean forward to apply compression with the heels of both hands, squeezing the gluteal muscles between your hands for 5 seconds.

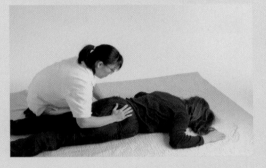

   c. Lean back to relieve pressure, and repeat the squeeze two more times.
5. Kneel at the client's left side to apply compression to the back of the client's left leg.
   a. Place your left hand on the client's sacrum and leave it there as the mother hand while you proceed with steps b through e.
   b. Place the palm of your right hand just beneath the ischial tuberosity.
   c. Lean forward and apply pressure for 5 seconds.
   d. Lean back to relieve the pressure, and move your right hand 1–2 inches down the leg.

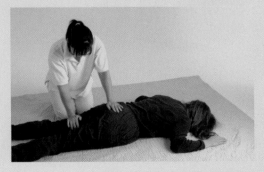

   e. Repeat steps c and d until you reach the Achilles tendon.

 Do not apply pressure to the popliteal fossa.

(continued)

6. Perform a 3-step stretch to the client's left leg.
   a. Your left hand remains on the client's sacrum as the mother hand.
   b. Grasp the client's left ankle with your right hand and carefully flex the client's knee to the end feel.
   c. Extend the client's left knee and pull the client's ankle toward you, medially rotating the client's left femur.
   d. Carefully flex the knee with the client's foot lateral to the thigh, stopping at the end feel.

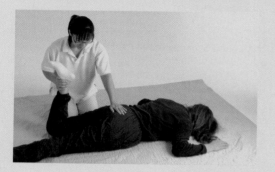

   e. Extend the client's knee and push the ankle away from you, laterally rotating the client's left femur.
   f. Carefully flex the knee with the client's left foot directed toward his or her right gluteals.
   g. Extend the client's knee and place the left foot next to the right foot.

7. Repeat steps 5 and 6 for the client's right leg.

Ask your client to turn over, into a supine position.

8. Kneel at the client's head and apply thumb compression strokes to the client's face.
   a. Place your thumbs together at the hairline at the center of the client's forehead, apply pressure, and hold for 5 seconds.

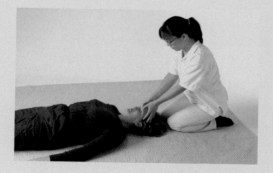

   b. Move both of your thumbs laterally about an inch, apply pressure, and hold.
   c. Continue to move your thumbs laterally, applying pressure at 1-inch intervals until you reach the brow line.
   d. Move both of your thumbs to the center of the forehead, apply pressure, and hold.
   e. Move your thumbs laterally about an inch, apply pressure, and hold.
   f. Continue to move your thumbs laterally, applying pressure at 1-inch intervals until you reach the brow line.

   g. Move your thumbs to the inside edges of the eyebrows, apply pressure, and hold.
   h. Repeat the thumb pressure at the center of the eyebrows and the outside ends of the eyebrows.
   i. Place your thumbs just to the side of the nostrils, apply pressure, and hold for 5 seconds.
   j. Move your thumbs laterally, applying pressure to the underside of the cheekbones at 1-inch intervals.

9. Kneel at your client's right side and apply rhythmic compression strokes to the client's right arm.
   a. Position your client's right arm out to the side, perpendicular to the body, palm up.
   b. Place your right hand around the client's right shoulder as the mother hand, and leave it there while you proceed with steps c through f.
   c. Place your left palm on the client's arm, just distal to the axilla.
   d. Lean forward to apply pressure for 5 seconds.
   e. Lean back to relieve the pressure, and move 1–2 inches down the arm.
   f. Repeat steps d and e until you reach the client's wrist.
   g. Move to the client's left side and repeat step 9 for the client's left arm.

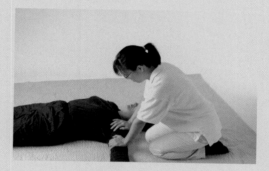

10. Kneel at your client's right side and rock the hara.
    a. With both of your palms down, overlap your hands and place them on the right side of the client's abdomen.

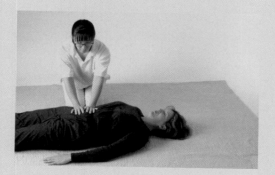

    b. Lean forward and push the abdomen away from you with the heels of your hands.
    c. Lean back and pull the abdomen toward you with your flat fingers.
    d. Repeat steps b and c several times in a fluid, wavelike movement.

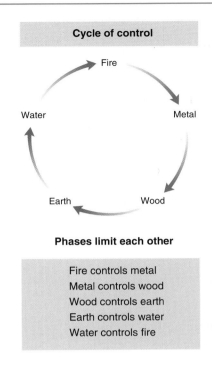

Cycle of production

Fire

Wood

Earth

Water   Metal

Phases feed each other

Fire produces earth
Earth produces metal
Metal produces water
Water produces wood
Wood produces fire

Cycle of control

Fire

Water   Metal

Earth   Wood

Phases limit each other

Fire controls metal
Metal controls wood
Wood controls earth
Earth controls water
Water controls fire

FIGURE 13-6 Production and control cycles involving the five phases. The five phases can be considered parts of a cycle, all interacting to sustain an organism.

anced field in an effort to facilitate healthy, normal function to all parts of the body. Some clients experience profound relaxation and relief from problematic situations following polarity therapy. Following the work, clients may feel more clear-headed, exhausted, extremely relaxed, or dizzy.

There is a lot of electrical activity in the body. For example, nerves and muscles depend on the flow of negatively and positively charged molecules to function. All of this electrical activity creates general patterns of energy flow through the body called energy fields. The fields around one person can alter the fields of another person, which is why polarity therapy does not necessarily require touch.

With practice, you can learn to sense the fields surrounding a person's body. Some persons compare the feeling to the repulsion of two magnets, some sense more of a tingling or electrical shock sensation, and others feel vibrations as they approach the fields. Once you can sense energy fields, you can try to manipulate them. Apply your hands directly to the client's body or to the energy fields surrounding the client's body, and focus your energy on your intent to balance the fields. This is a subtle technique that uses your own energy fields and your conscious intention to redirect the client's energy flow to balance the fields. Because the work is so subtle, you may want to explain the theory and technique to your client before using polarity therapy in a massage session.

Specific polarity therapy techniques are based on principles of energy flow in and around the body, and they can be applied to specific areas of pain. In one

technique, you gently place your left hand or left index finger on a client's area of pain, and place your right hand or right middle finger on the area directly across the body from the area of pain, and maintain contact for several seconds until the energy is released. As the energy releases, you may feel heat, tingling, or a pulse that is faster than the cardiac pulse, often called a therapeutic pulse.

This is only an introduction to the basic applications of polarity therapy. With advanced training and experience, you can learn how to perform a true polarity therapy session that lasts between 60 and 90 minutes and allows clients to remain fully clothed. Certified polarity therapists learn how to evaluate a person's energetic attributes with palpation, observation, and interviewing skills and to use various forms of touch and intent to manipulate the energy flow with the intent to enhance their clients' self-healing mechanisms. You can seek more-advanced training to apply the principles more specifically.

Chapter Summary

The special techniques discussed in this chapter are only some of the techniques you can incorporate into a standard massage session. Most of these techniques can and should be studied in depth, and many therapists continue their education and training to specialize in a particular technique. For a massage therapist, they are good techniques to be familiar with and to have available. Most of them can be incorporated into a massage session easily, and clients often request some of these special techniques. Client education and client participation is a big part of healthcare, and these special techniques can serve as good teaching tools to help clients take responsibility for their own health.

CHAPTER EXERCISES

1. Name three indications and three contraindications for
   a. Cold hydrotherapy applications
   b. Heat hydrotherapy applications

2. Name three physiological effects of
   a. Cold hydrotherapy
   b. Heat hydrotherapy

3. Explain the importance of recommending that clients increase their water intake after a massage.

4. Explain why it is beneficial to enhance circulation.

5. Explain why the flow of lymph is vital to health.

6. List at least three benefits of abdominal massage.

7. Explain the concept of reflexology.

8. Explain the concepts of yin and yang.

9. Describe the starting and ending points for the following energy meridians:
   a. Heart
   b. Lung
   c. Spleen
   d. Liver
   e. Kidney
   f. Small intestine
   g. Large intestine
   h. Conception vessel
   i. Governing vessel

10. Describe how to apply the specific polarity technique described in this chapter.

SUGGESTED READINGS

Anderson MK. Fundamentals of Sports Injury Management. 2nd ed. Baltimore: Lippincott Williams & Wilkins, 2003.

Ashton J, Cassel D. Review for Therapeutic Massage and Bodywork Certification. Baltimore: Lippincott Williams & Wilkins, 2002.

Chaitow L, DeLany JW. Clinical Application of Neuromuscular Techniques, vol 1. The Upper Body. London: 2000.

Chikly B, Welfley S. Lymphedema and lymph-drainage techniques. AMTA Massage Ther J 2001;Fall: pp.80–88.

Cohen BJ, Wood DL. Memmler's Structure and Function of the Human Body. 7th ed. Philadelphia: Lippincott Williams & Wilkins, 2000.

Eisenberg D. Encounters with Qi: Exploring Chinese Medicine. New York: WW Norton, 1985.

Fritz S. Fundamentals of Therapeutic Massage. 2nd ed. St. Louis: Mosby, 2000.

Gray H, Lewis WH. Anatomy of the Human Body. 23rd ed. Philadelphia: Lea & Febiger, 1936.

Kaptchuk TJ. The Web That Has No Weaver: Understanding Chinese Medicine. Chicago: Congdon & Weed, 1983.

Knaster M. Energy Eastern Style. AMTA Massage Ther J 1998;36, 40–46

Lidell L, Thomas S, Cook CB, Porter A. The Book of Massage. New York: Gaia Books Limited/Simon and Schuster, 1984.

Maxwell-Hudson C. K.I.S.S. Guide to Massage. New York: DK Publishing, 2001.

Salvo SG. Massage Therapy: Principles and Practice. 2nd ed. St. Louis: Saunders/Elsevier Science, 2003.

Scheumann DW. The Balanced Body: A Guide to Deep Tissue and Neuromuscular Therapy. 2nd ed. Philadelphia: Lippincott Williams & Wilkins, 2002.

Simons DG, Travell JG, Simons LS. Travell and Simons' Myofascial Pain and Dysfunction: The Trigger Point Manual, vol 1. Upper Half of Body. 2nd ed. Baltimore: Lippincott Williams & Wilkins, 1999.

Werner R. A Massage Therapist's Guide to Pathology. Philadelphia: Lippincott Williams & Wilkins, 1998.

Wright J. Reflexology and Acupressure: Pressure Points for Healing, Summertown, TN: CRCS Wellness Books/Book Publishing, 2000.

http://healthplusweb.com/alt_directory/polaritytherapy.html, Health Plus Web Directory of Alternative Medicine Your Unbiased Health Information Source on the Web, "Polarity Therapy," accessed 11/20/02.

http://qi-journal.com/TCM.asp?-token.SearchID=TuinaFAQ, accessed 12.18.02.

http://reflexologycollege.tripod.com/whatis2.htm. Ontario College of Reflexology web site, accessed 11/20/02.

http://www.aaaom.org/HPIRREGULAR%20PERIOD.htm, The American Academy of Acupuncture and Oriental Medicine web site, "Treating Irregular Periods with Traditional Chinese Medicine," accessed 12/19/02.

http://www.acupressure.com/, Acupressure.com web site, accessed 12/3/02.

http://www.acuxo.com/index.asp, accessed 10/17/03.

http://www.aor.org.uk/ The Association of Reflexologists web site, accessed 11/20/02.

http://www.aworldofacupuncture.com/acupuncture-frequently-asked-questions.htm, A World of Acupuncture web site, "Acupuncture" and "Acupressure," accessed 12/3/02.

http://www.bbc.co.uk/science/scienceshack/backcat/multimedia/fllymph.shtml, BBCi web site, accessed 11/27/02.

http://www.chiroweb.com/archives/17/09/34.html, Chiroweb.com web site, "Spectacular Acupuncture Points in Diffuse Musculoskeletal Pain—with or without Needles" accessed 12/19/02.

http://www.chiroweb.com/archives/17/12/14.html, Chiroweb.com web site, "What Points Do You Use For _____?" by John Amaro, DC, FIAMA, Dipl.Ac. (NCCAOM), accessed 12/19/02.

http://www.findarticles.com/cf_dls/g2603/0006/2603000658/p1/article.jhtml, Gale Encyclopedia of Alternative Medicine web site, "Shiatsu" by Greg Annussek, accessed 12/3/02.

http://www.healerwithin.com/articles/rc-lymph.htm, Feel the Qi.com web site, "Lymph" by Roger Jahnke, O.M.D., accessed 11/27/02.

http://www.holisticonline.com/Remedies/Depression/dep_acupressure.htm, Holistic-online.com web site, "Acupressure," accessed 12/19/02.

http://www.howstuffworks.com/question138.htm, accessed 11/26/02.

http://www.jdaross.mcmail.com/lymphatics2.htm, accessed 11/27/02.

http://www.lymphatics.net/, accessed 11/27/02.

http://www.mythos.com/webmd/Content.aspx?P=LYMPHA&E=4, Mythos Anatomy web site, Lymphatic system, accessed 11/28/02.

http://www.orientalmedicine.com, accessed 12.18.02.

http://www.orientalmedicine.com/acu_points.htm, Orientalmedicine.com web site, "Acupuncture Points," accessed 12/19/02.

http://www.orientalmedicine.com/bt_five_elems.htm, Orientalmedicine.com web site, "The Five Elements," accessed 12/19/02.

http://www.polaritytherapy.org/polarity/, accessed 10.11.03.

http://www.polaritytherapy.org/polarity/index.html, American Polarity Therapy Association web site, accessed 11/21/02.

http://www.reflexology-research.com/, The Reflexology Research Project web site, accessed 11/20/02.

http://www.reflexology-usa.net/facts.htm, accessed 10.10.03.

www.iahe.com/html/therapies/ldt.jsp, accessed 10.10.03.

GLOSSARY

Accountability: the quality of accepting the consequences of your actions and claiming responsibility for your decisions

Active range of motion (AROM): joint movement that requires clients to actively use their own energy to demonstrate how much of the full range can be completed comfortably and without restriction

Acupressure (AK-yoo-preh-sher)**:** a bodywork modality in which firm fingertip pressure is applied to points along the energy meridians to regulate the flow of Qi

Acupressure points: specific points along all of the meridians where the Qi can be most easily affected by pressure

Acute: refers to a condition that has existed for up to 3 days or has developed very quickly and severely

Anatomical position: describes a person standing up, feet shoulder-width apart, arms at the sides, and palms facing forward

Anatomy: the study of the structures of plants and animals

Antagonist: muscle whose contraction moves the body in the opposite direction from that of the prime mover

Anterior (ventral)**:** refers to something on or toward someone's front side, or on the navel side

Artery: a tube that carries blood away from the heart

Assessment: the process of evaluating a client's condition

Asymmetric stance (also called archer, bow, and lunge stance): standing position in which both feet are on the ground, shoulder-width apart, one foot is in front of the other, and the back foot is laterally rotated

Atrophy (AT-roh-fee)**:** a condition that results when a muscle is not used either by choice or by lack of nerve stimulation (e.g., with nerve damage)

Body mechanics: the careful, efficient use of your body by incorporating the principles of leverage and structural alignment to prevent injury and reduce fatigue

Bodywork: treatment that involves manipulation of the client's body as a way to maintain or improve health

Bony landmark: site for muscle attachment or safe passageway for nerves and blood vessels

Centering: a technique that helps you focus your attention on your clients

Chronic illness: illness that lasts a year or longer, usually limits a patient's physical activity, and may require ongoing medical care and treatment

Chronic: refers to a condition that develops slowly, recurs, or persists longer than 3 weeks

Client-centered: when attitudes, decisions, and activities of a practice are in the best interest of the client's health and well-being

Code of ethics: commonly accepted guidelines or principles of conduct that govern professional conduct.

Compensation pattern: a postural offset that is the body's attempt to correct an imbalance or protect a primary dysfunction or injury

Compression: a stroke that applies pressure to soft tissues to squeeze them together without any slip

Concentric contraction: muscle shortens and the attachment sites of the muscle move closer together

Confidentiality: the principle that client information revealed to a health professional during an appointment is to be kept private and has limits on how and when it can be disclosed to a third party

Contraindication: a situation or condition in which massage is inappropriate

Contrast therapy: heat application followed by cold application, also called alternating therapy

Corporate massage: a chair massage for persons in the middle of their workday, also called seated massage, on-site massage, and chair massage

Corporation: a business arrangement that has one or more owners who are legally separate from the business

Countertransference: your tendency to react emotionally when clients do not behave or respond to you or your treatment as you had expected

Deep fiber friction: a stroke that is applied with deep, localized pressure without any slip on the skin to break up fascial adhesions and separate the muscle fibers

Deep: refers to something farther from the surface of the skin, or more toward the inside of the body

Direct manipulation (DM): a proprioceptive neuromuscular facilitation (PNF) technique in which you use the muscle spindles and Golgi tendon organs to relax a hypertonic muscle

Direction of ease: the direction in which tissues move with least resistance

Direction of restriction: the direction in which tissues resist movement the most

Distal: refers to something that is farther away from the torso, toward the fingers or toes

Draping: the use of sheets and towels to cover clients during the massage for warmth and modesty

Eccentric contraction: muscle contraction in which the distance between the muscle attachments increases and the muscle effectively gets longer

Effleurage (EF-lur-ahzh)**:** a slow, gliding stroke along the client's skin

Endangerment sites: particular areas of the body that contain superficial or unprotected organs, nerves, and blood vessels and require caution to prevent injury

End feel: a unique feel when a joint reaches the end of its passive range of motion (PROM) determined by specific structures that stop the movement

Ergonomics: the science that designs and coordinates people's activities with the equipment they use and the working conditions of their environment

Ethics: conduct rules based on integrity and differentiating right from wrong

Excursion: the physical length of one stroke along the client's skin

Fascia (FASH-uh)**:** a fibrous band or sheetlike tissue membrane that provides support and protection for the body organs

Fascial adhesion (fascial restriction): an area where the fascia has adhered to nearby tissues or has been crumpled or kinked

Fixator: special synergist (also called stabilizer) that holds a part of the body steady while the prime mover contracts to move that part

Flow: a routine-like sequence of steps that leads the massage from one body part to the next in a systematic, fluid pattern that often specifies stroke sequences

Friction: the physical resistance between two surfaces as they rub against each other and create heat

Functional limitation: a normal activity of daily life that is limited by muscular or connective tissue conditions

Gait: a walking pattern, including qualities of the footstep, armswing, and, postural alignment

Grounding: a technique you can use to establish an emotional and energetic boundary between you and your clients

Gymnastics: activity at ancient gymnasiums that included exercise, massage, and baths

Homeostasis: The body's constant monitoring and adjustment of metabolic processes in an effort to maintain an internally balanced state of equilibrium

Hospice: a healthcare approach that caters to the quality of remaining life rather than the quantity of life when a person's life expectancy is limited by a life-threatening illness with no known cure

Hydrotherapy: the use of water as a treatment

Hypertonic (HAHY-per-TAHN-ik)**:** excessively tense or tight

Indication: when a particular technique could improve the health and healing process

Inferior (caudad): refers to something being more toward the feet, or below

Informed consent: a client's agreement to participate in an activity after the purpose, methods, benefits, risks, and rights to withdraw at any time have been explained

Insertion of a muscle: the point of attachment that moves most during contraction, often at the distal end

Intake form: a form that documents a client's contact information, health history, or informed consent for care

Laterally recumbent (also called side-lying)**:** lying on one's side

Leading question: a question that focuses the client's attention to clarify or specify information and to recall missing or forgotten details

Lengthening: the neurological process that lengthens myofibrils and results in a longer muscle

Leverage: the mechanical use of your body as a rigid structure that can apply a lot of pressure without doing a lot of muscular work

Licensure: legal authority or permission to practice massage when the state laws or regulations require it

Local contraindication: a condition in which massage is appropriate except in the affected area

Lubricants: wet and dry products that reduce friction between your skin and the client's skin and increase the comfort of the massage strokes

Lymph: interstitial fluid leaked into the tissues via capillaries carrying arterial blood

Massage treatment record: the document containing input from clients, your objective assessments of the clients' condition, the massage techniques you use, results of the treatment session, and plans for future massage treatment

Massage: manual therapy involving pressure applied with the hands (term started by the French explorers in the 1700s)

Mechanical effects: therapist applies pressure or manipulation to physically change the shape or condition of the client's tissues

Metabolic effects: combined result of mechanical and reflex effects on the whole body

Meridians: precise and orderly channels or pathways through which Qi flows

Metabolism: the overall cellular activity that breaks down nutrients to generate energy for building essential molecules

Modality: a collection of manual therapies that tends to use similar applications of movement or massage strokes to reach a similar goal

Motor neuron: neuron that carries messages away from the central nervous system (CNS) to the muscle or organs that must react (also called an efferent neuron)

Motor unit: one motor neuron and all of the muscle cells it stimulates

Movement Cure: American version of Ling's movement system

Muscle energy techniques (MET): massage applications that use the nervous system to change a muscle's resting length, also called proprioceptive neuromuscular facilitation

Muscle guarding: hypertonic muscles stabilizing or splinting an injured area

Muscle: A specially organized and packaged group of muscle cells, connective tissue wrappings, and blood vessels

Nerve plexuses: large networks of intertwined nerves

Nerve: A specially organized and packaged bundle of neurons (individual nerve cells), connective tissue wrappings, and blood vessels

Networking: the practice of establishing mutually beneficial professional relationships with other persons in a business or networking group

Neuron: the basic unit of the nervous system, also called a nerve cell

Open-ended question: a question that requires a descriptive answer instead of a one-word answer

Origin of a muscle: the attachment on the bone or connective tissue structure that is more stationary during muscle contraction

Outcall: a massage appointment in which you take your massage table to a client's home, hotel, or office

Palpation: the skillful art of client evaluation that uses touch to locate and assess the quality of different structures

Parasympathetic response: autonomic nervous system response that stimulates organs to work in a "rest and digest" mode

Partnership: a company in which two or more persons share ownership and personal liability for all business transactions

Passive contraction: a stationary muscle position created when you move the origin and insertion of a client's muscle closer together while the client relaxes

Passive range of motion (PROM): joint movement that requires the therapist to move the relaxed client through a range of motion to determine how much of the full range can be completed comfortably and without restriction

Pathogen (or pathogenic microorganism)**:** a microscopic organism that can cause disease in other organisms, commonly called a germ

Pathology: the study of disease processes or of any deviation from a normal, healthy condition

Petrissage (PET-rih-sahzh)**:** a stroke that kneads soft tissues with a grasping and lifting action

Pharmacology: the science of the preparation, usage, and effects of medications

Physiology: the study of the normal functions of the organism or any part of the organism

Polarity (poh-LAIR-ih-tee) **therapy:** a modality in which very light massage strokes are applied on and off the client's body to balance electromagnetic fields

Positional release (PR): a PNF technique that relieves hypertonicity by holding the body in a painless position and waiting for the nervous system to trigger relaxation, also called strain/counterstrain

Posterior (dorsal): refers to something on or toward someone's back

Postevent massage: a massage performed within 6 hours of the athletic performance that focuses on circulatory enhancement

Postisometric relaxation (PIR): a PNF technique that uses active contraction and relaxation of the target muscle to lengthen the muscle

Preevent massage: a massage performed up to 2 days before the client participates in an athletic event that focuses on circulatory enhancement and warming up the tissues

Prime mover: muscle that performs most of the intended movement, also known as an agonist

Professionalism: ethical conduct, goals, and qualities characterized by a profession

Prone: lying on one's stomach, or face down

Proprioceptive neuromuscular facilitation (PROH-pree-oh-SEP-tive NOO-roh-MUSS-kyoo-lar fah-SIHL-ih-TAY-shun) (PNF): bodywork applications that use the nervous system to change a muscle's resting length, also called muscle energy techniques

Proprioceptor (PROH-pree-oh-SEP-tor): sensory neuron responsible for detecting body position, muscle tone, and equilibrium

Proximal: describes something toward the attachment point of the limb to the body

Qi (CHEE): a dynamic, changing energy force that runs through the whole body, supplying and being supplied by body processes and activities

Range of motion (ROM): the end-to-end distance of a specific joint movement that is structurally possible

Rapport: mutual trust in a relationship

Reciprocal inhibition (RI): a PNF technique in which the client contracts a target muscle's antagonists to reflexively relax the target muscle

Reflective listening: a method with which you reiterate the client's words to convey your comprehension or to clarify a misunderstanding

Reflex effects: therapist stimulates the client's sensory neurons, which triggers the client's nervous system to change the shape or condition of the tissues in areas that were addressed as well as other, related areas

Reflexology (REE-fleks-AH-loh-jee): a modality in which fingertip compression is applied to reflex points on the hand, foot, or ear that affect other parts of the body

Repetitive stress injury (RSI): an injury that occurs when a particular body movement is repeated often enough to damage the structures involved in the movement

Resting length: the length to which a relaxed, inactive muscle can be safely extended

Resting stroke: a stroke that requires you to stop moving and lightly rest your relaxed hands, fingers, or arms on your client for several seconds

Restorative massage: a massage performed 6–72 hours after the athletic performance that is intended to increase circulation and restore the normal resting length of muscles, also called curative massage and postrecovery massage

Right lymphatic duct: a major drain that collects all of the lymph from the upper right quadrant of the body, including everything on the right side of the body above the diaphragm

Scope of practice: a practitioner's service limits and boundaries as determined by legal, educational, competency, and accountability factors

Self-care (self-help): activities that clients can use between massage sessions to participate in their healing process and help them achieve their treatment goals

Sensory neuron: neuron that receives sensory input and transmits that information to the CNS, also called an afferent neuron

Shiatsu (shee-AHT-soo): a form of bodywork that uses a combination of acupressure with stretching, range of motion, and massage strokes

Side-lying (laterally recumbent): refers to a person lying on his or her side

Slip: the sliding of your skin over the surface of the client's skin

SOAP: an acronym for Subjective, Objective, Activity and Analysis, and Plan that refers to a format for documentation

Sole proprietorship: a business arrangement in which one person owns the business and is personally liable for all business transactions

Standard precautions: specific procedures that maintain a hygienic and sanitary practice and reduce the risk for germ transmission

Standards of practice: specific rules and procedures for professional conduct and quality of care that are to be followed by all members of a profession

Strain/counterstrain (SCS): a PNF technique that relieves hypertonicity by holding the body in a painless position and waiting for the nervous system to trigger relaxation, also called positional release

Stretching: an elastic deformation of the fascia that extends its length

Stretch reflex: a protective muscle contraction that occurs when the tissues are stretched too far and/or too fast

Subacute: the period from about 3 days to 3 weeks after a health condition started

Superficial: refers to something closer to the surface of the skin

Superficial friction: a brisk variation of light effleurage that increases circulation in the superficial tissues and dissipates body heat

Superior (cephalad): refers to something being more toward the head, or above

Supine: lying on one's back or spine, face up

Swedish Gymnastics: a therapeutic movement system developed by Per Henrik Ling

Swedish Movements: Europe's version of Ling's movement system

Symmetric stance (also called the horse stance and warrior stance): standing position in which both feet are placed as if the toes are on a line, pointing forward, shoulder-width apart

Synergist: a muscle that assists the prime mover by contracting at the same time to facilitate more effective movement, also called an accessory muscle

Systemic contraindication: a condition or situation in which massage should be avoided altogether

Tapotement (tuh-POHT-ment): a fast rhythmic stroke that uses both hands, like rapid drumming

Target muscle: the muscle being treated in a therapeutic technique

Tender point: a small, painful area of hypertonicity, also called a tender spot

Tendon reflex: a reflex that relaxes a muscle when a muscle and its tendon are subjected to slow and gentle tension

Thoracic duct: a major drain that collects the lymph from everywhere in the body except the right side of the head and thorax

Tissue: a group of cells with similar structure and function

Transference: the client's dependence on you for friendship or companionship in addition to therapeutic treatment

Treatment goal: a specific goal that is determined after therapeutic massage treatment to clarify progress toward restoring functional limitations

Treatment plan: your recommendations for future treatment, self-care activities, and referrals to other healthcare professionals

Trigger point: a localized area of hypertonicity at the motor end unit, or neuromuscular junction, that refers symptoms to other areas of the body

Unwinding: the process in which soft tissues move in different directions, circles, or wavy lines as the collagen fibers change shape and the fascia softens

Vein: a tube that transports blood from the capillaries of the body back to the heart

Vibration: a stroke that involves high-frequency shaky hand movements and is capable of deep effects

Yang (YAHNG): energy that conceptually flows down from the sun and is associated with the active, bright, warm, consumptive, and outward activities of the body

Yin (YIHN): energy that conceptually flows upward from the earth and is associated with the passive, dark, cool, supportive, and inward activities of the body

INDEX

In this index, *italic* page numbers designate figures; *italic* page numbers followed by the letter *P* designate plates; page numbers followed by the letter "b" designate text boxes; page numbers followed by the letter "t" designate tables.